DIAGNOSTIC ATLAS OF

the heart

DIAGNOSTIC ATLAS OF

the
heart

EDITORS

J. WILLIS HURST, M.D.

Consultant to the Division of Cardiology
Professor and Chairman of the Department of Medicine (1957–1986)
Emory University School of Medicine
Atlanta, Georgia

JOSEPH S. ALPERT, M.D.

Robert S. and Irene P. Flinn Professor of Medicine
Head, Department of Medicine
University of Arizona Health Science Center
Tucson, Arizona

ASSOCIATE EDITORS

ROBERT H. ANDERSON, M.D.

Director and Joseph Levy Professor of Paediatric Cardiac Morphology
The National Heart and Lung Institute
Royal Brompton Hospital
London, United Kingdom

ANTON E. BECKER, M.D.

Professor of Pathology
Department of Cardiovascular Pathology
Academic Medical Center
Amsterdam, The Netherlands

BENSON R. WILCOX, M.D.

Professor of Surgery
Chief
Division of Cardiothoracic Surgery
University of North Carolina School of Medicine
Chapel Hill, North Carolina

RAVEN PRESS

New York

Raven Press, Ltd., 1185 Avenue of the Americas, New York, New York 10036

Printed and bound in Hong Kong

Library of Congress Cataloging-in-Publication Data

Diagnostic atlas of the heart / editors, J. Willis Hurst, Joseph S. Alpert; associate editors,
Robert H. Anderson, Anton E. Becker, Benson R. Wilcox.
        p. cm.
 Includes bibliographical references and index.
 ISBN 0-7817-0058-2
 1. Heart Diseases—Diagnosis. 2. Cardiological manifestations of general diseases
Diagnosis-Atlases. I. Hurst, J. Willis (John Willis), 1920-. II. Alpert Joseph S.
 [DNLM: 1. Heart Diseases—diagnosis—atlases. WG 17 D536 1992]
RC683.D46 1994
616.1'2075—dc20
DNLM/DLC
for Library of Congress   92-48357
CIP

Some of the material contained in this volume has been revised and updated from *Atlas of the
Heart*, Hurst JW, Anderson RH, Becker AE, and Wilcox BR, eds. Gower Medical Publishing,
New York, 1988.

9 8 7 6 5 4 3 2 1

To all students of medicine, young and old, who appreciate the value of visual images as they try and try to learn medicine

CONTENTS

CONTRIBUTING AUTHORS

WALTER H. ABELMANN, M.D.
Professor of Medicine
Department of Medicine
Harvard Medical School
Physician
Beth Israel Hospital
330 Brookline Avenue
Boston, Massachusetts 02215

JAMES K. ALEXANDER, M.D.
Professor of Medicine
Department of Medicine
Baylor College of Medicine
Chief of Cardiology
Veterans Administration Hospital
6550 Fanin, Suite 447
Houston, Texas 77030

JOSEPH S. ALPERT, M.D.
Robert S. and Irene P. Flinn Professor of
    Medicine
Department of Medicine
University of Arizona
    Health Science Center
1501 N. Campbell Avenue
Tucson, Arizona 85724

ROBERT H. ANDERSON, M.D.
Director and Joseph Levy Professor of
    Paediatric Cardiac Morphology
The National Heart and Lung Institute
Royal Brompton Hospital
Dovehouse Street
London SW3 6LY
United Kingdom

ANTON E. BECKER, M.D.
Professor of Pathology
Department of Cardiovascular Pathology
Academic Medical Center
1105 AZ Amsterdam-Zuidoost
The Netherlands

HARISIOS BOUDOULAS, M.D.
Professor of Medicine
Division of Cardiology
Department of Internal Medicine
The Ohio State University
    College of Medicine
1654 Upham Drive
Columbus, Ohio 43210

A. JAMES BRADLEY, M.D.
Doctors Clinic
2300 5th Avenue
Vero Beach, Florida 32960

BRAD S. BURLEW, M.D.
Associate Professor of Medicine
Department of Medicine
Director of Catheterization Laboratory
The University of Tennessee
    College of Medicine
951 Court Avenue, Room 353D
Memphis, Tennessee 38163

CAROLYN A. BURNS, M.D.
Instructor of Clinical Medicine
Medical College of Virginia
Box 150
Richmond, Virginia 23298

STUART R. CHIPKIN, M.D.
Associate Professor of Medicine
Director
Clinical Endocrinology, Diabetes, and
    Metabolism
Thorndike #1
Boston University School of Medicine
Boston City Hospital
818 Harrison Avenue
Boston, Massachusetts 02118

DAVID M. CLIVE, M.D.
Associate Professor of Medicine
Division of Renal Medicine
Department of Medicine
University of Massachusetts Medical Center
55 Lake Avenue North
Worcester, Massachusetts 01655

ANDREW J. COHEN, M.D.
Professor of Medicine
Division of Renal Medicine
Department of Medicine
University of Massachusetts Medical Center
55 Lake Avenue North
Worcester, Massachusetts 01655

JAMES E. DALEN, M.D.
Professor of Medicine
Vice Provost, Health Sciences
Dean, College of Medicine
University of Arizona College of Medicine
1501 North Campbell Avenue
Tucson, Arizona 85724-0001

DAVID T. DURACK, M.B., D.PHIL
Professor of Medicine
Department of Medicine, Microbiology and
    Immunology
Chief, Division of Infectious Diseases
Duke University Medical Center
Box 3867
Durham, North Carolina 27710

MARC FISHER, M.D.
Professor of Neurology
Department of Neurology
The Medical Center of Central
    Massachusetts
119 Belmont Street
Worcester, Massachusetts 01605

JOHN F. GOODWIN, M.D.
Emeritus Professor of Clinical Cardiology
Honorary Consulting Physician
Royal Postgraduate Medical School
Hammersmith Hospital
London, United Kingdom

THOMAS W. GRIFFIN, M.D.
Director of Clinical Research
Associate Professor of Medicine
University of Massachusetts Medical Center
55 Lake Avenue North
Worcester, Massachusetts 01655

ROBERT J. HALL, M.D.
Clinical Professor
Department of Medicine
Baylor College of Medicine and the
    University of Texas Medical Center at
    Houston
Medical Director
Texas Heart Institute
Chief of Cardiology
St. Luke's Episcopal Hospital
6720 Bertner Avenue (MC 1-102)
Houston, Texas 77030

BERNADINE P. HEALY, M.D.
Director
Cardiovascular Research
The Cleveland Clinic Foundation
Cleveland, Ohio 44195

HOWARD R. HORN, M.D.
L.W. Diggs Professor of Medicine
Vice Chairman and Program Director
Department of Medicine
Chief of Medicine
The University of Tennessee College of
    Medicine
951 Court Avenue
Memphis, Tennessee 38163

S.K. STEPHEN HUANG, M.D.
Professor of Medicine
Director, Section of Cardiac
    Electrophysiology and Pacing
Division of Cardiovascular Medicine
Department of Medicine
University of Massachusetts Medical Center
55 Lake Avenue North
Worcester, MA 01655

J. O'NEAL HUMPHRIES, M.D.
O.B. Mayer Sr. and Jr. Professor of Medicine
Dean, School of Medicine
University of South Carolina
Garners Ferry Road
Columbia, South Carolina 29208

J. WILLIS HURST, M.D.
Consultant to the Division of Cardiology
Professor and Chairman of the Department
    of Medicine (1957–1986)
Emory University School of Medicine
1462 Clifton Road, NE
Suite 301
Atlanta, Georgia 30322

JEFFREY M. ISNER, M.D.
Professor of Medicine
Chief, Cardiovascular Research
Tufts University School of Medicine
St. Elizabeth's Hospital
736 Cambridge Street
Boston, Massachusetts 02135

STEPHEN L. KEITH, M.D.
Fellow, Vascular Surgery
Department of Surgery
University of Massachusetts Medical Center
55 Lake Avenue North
Worcester, Massachusetts 01655

HIROSHI KUIDA, M.D.
Professor of Medicine
Associate Dean, Student Programs
University of Utah School of Medicine
50 N. Medical Drive
Salt Lake City, Utah 84132

CARL V. LEIER, M.D.
James W. Overstreet Professor of Medicine
    and Pharmacology
Director
Division of Cardiology
Department of Internal Medicine
The Ohio State University Hospitals
1654 Upham Drive, 6th Floor, Means Hall
Columbus, Ohio 43210

KAZUO MINEMATSU, M.D.
Chief
Cerebrovascular Laboratory
Department of Pathogenesis
National Cardiovascular Center
    Research Instutute
5-7-1 Fujishirodai
Suita, Osaka 565
Japan

ROBERT S. MITTLEMAN, M.D.
Assistant Professor of Medicine
Division of Cardiovascular Medicine
Department of Medicine
Associate Director
Section of Cardiac Electrophysiology and
    Pacing
University of Massachusetts Medical Center
55 Lake Avenue North
Worcester, Massachusetts 01655

JOHN H. NEWMAN, M.D.
Associate Professor of Medicine
Elsa S. Hanigan Chair in Pulmonary
    Medicine
Vanderbilt University School of Medicine
Vanderbilt University Medical Center North
Nashville, Tennessee 37232

JOHN V. NIXON, M.D.
Professor of Medicine
Division of Cardiology
Department of Medicine
Director
Echocardiography Laboratory
Medical College of Virginia
Virginia Commonwealth University
MCV Station, Box 128
Richmond, Virginia 23298

ELIZABETH W. NUGENT, M.D.
Associate Professor of Pediatrics
Department of Pediatrics
The Children's Heart Center
Emory University School of Medicine
Division of Cardiology
2040 Ridgewood Drive, NE
Atlanta, Georgia 30322

CHARLES E. RACKLEY, M.D.
Anton and Margaret Fuisz Professor of
   Medicine
Department of Medicine
Georgetown University Medical Center
3800 Reservoir Road, NW
Washington, D.C. 20007

TIMOTHY REGAN, M.D.
Professor of Medicine
Department of Medicine
Director
Division of Cardiovascular Diseases
University of Medicine and Dentistry of
   New Jersey
New Jersey Medical School
185 South Orange Avenue
Newark, New Jersey 07103-2757

JAMES M. RIPPE, M.D.
Associate Professor of Medicine
Division of Cardiovascular Medicine
Department of Medicine
Director
Exercise Physiology and Nutrition
   Laboratory
University of Massachusetts Medical Center
55 Lake Avenue North
Worcester, Massachusetts 01655

MICHAEL J. ROHRER, M.D.
Assistant Professor of Surgery
Division of Vascular Surgery
Department of Surgery
55 Lake Avenue North
Worcester, Massachusetts 01655

JOSEPH C. ROSS, M.D.
Professor of Medicine
Associate Vice-Chancellor for Health Affairs
Vanderbilt University Medical Center
D-3300 Medical Center North
Nashville, Tennessee 37232

MARY ELLEN M. RYBAK, M.D.
Director, Clinical Research
Schering-Plough Research Institute
Building K-61, Mailstop G-14
2000 Galloping Hill
Kennilworth, New Jersey 07033

RALPH SHABETAI, M.D.
Professor of Medicine
Department of Medicine
Cardiology Section (111-A)
VA Medical Center
3350 La Jolla Village Drive
San Diego, CA 92161

JAY M. SULLIVAN, M.D.
Professor of Medicine
Department of Medicine
Chief
Division of Cardiovascular Diseases
The University of Tennessee College of
   Medicine
951 Court Avenue
Memphis, Tennessee 38163

PANAGIOTIS N. SYMBAS, M.D.
Professor of Surgery
Chief of Cardio-Thoracic Surgery
Emory University School of Medicine
Grady Memorial Hospital
69 Butler Street, S.E.
Atlanta, Georgia 30303

ANN WARD, Ph.D.
Associate Professor
Department of Kinesiology
University of Wisconsin
2000 Observatory Drive
Madison, Wisconsin 53706

NANETTE KASS WENGER, M.D.
Professor of Medicine (Cardiology)
Emory University School of Medicine
Director
Cardiac Clinics
Grady Memorial Hospital
69 Butler Street, S.E.
Atlanta, Georgia 30303

BENSON R. WILCOX, M.D.
Professor of Surgery
Chief
Division of Cardiothoracic Surgery
University of North Carolina School of
   Medicine
108 Burnett-Womack Building
CB# 7065
Chapel Hill, North Carolina 27599-7065

PREFACE

One picture is worth more than a thousand words

Chinese Proverb

The cliché above is true; communication is enhanced enormously when it is possible to fill a book with carefully chosen color illustrations that teach the reader. In the practical world we live in it is not easy to accomplish this feat. Accordingly, many excellent textbooks on cardiology have an abundance of excellent text, but in order to create a book that can be lifted by the reader, it is often necessary to limit the number of illustrations.

This book, *Diagnostic Atlas of the Heart*, is mainly a picture book. The illustrations, many of which are in color, have been chosen carefully to teach the readers, while the text serves to guide them.

Diagnostic Atlas of the Heart evolved from a previous book, *Atlas of the Heart*, a joint venture of Gower Medical Publishing and McGraw-Hill, which in turn was based on the sixth edition of *The Heart*. Robert Anderson and Anton Becker, superb pathologists and teachers, supplied some of the text and the illustrations related to cardiac pathology. Benson Wilcox, a creative cardiac surgeon, provided some of the text and illustrations that teach the nuances of cardiac surgery. This new book is larger than *Atlas of the Heart* and the focus is slightly different. New chapters have been added that cover many subjects that were not discussed in the original *Atlas of the Heart*. This book concentrates on a discussion of the anatomy, physiology, clinical manifestations, and diagnostic testing needed to understand cardiac diagnosis. Treatment, which was abbreviated in *Atlas of the Heart*, has been eliminated entirely in order to emphasize the more basic aspects of the physician's diagnostic efforts.

Diagnostic Atlas of the Heart should be useful to students, house officers, and cardiology fellows because it enables them to create "mental images" of cardiovascular diseases and disorders. The book, for the same reason, should be useful to the seasoned physician who wishes to "keep up" with the rapid changes in concepts that are occurring in cardiovascular medicine. Finally, the book would be of considerable value to the teacher of cardiovascular medicine because it really is true—a picture is worth more than a thousand words.

J. Willis Hurst, M.D.

Joseph S. Alpert, M.D.

ACKNOWLEDGMENTS

We thank our colleagues at Emory University, the University of Massachusetts, and the University of Arizona for their assistance and advice. We also thank the many individuals who contributed to the original *Atlas of the Heart* as well as McGraw-Hill and Gower Medical Publishers for their permission to utilize material from *Atlas of the Heart* and other publications. A book of this type also draws from many sources. We have, in an obsessive manner, meticulously cited the sources and obtained permission from publishers and authors to use material from other sources. The sources of such figures are cited in a special section at the end of each chapter.

We thank Mary Rogers, President of Raven Press, for having faith in the project. She has vision and, with hard work, produces excellent books. We thank Bernadine Richey, Cassie Moore, and Mattie Bialer of Raven Press for doing their jobs in the most professional manner.

Finally, and most importantly, we thank our wives Nelie Wiley Hurst and Helle Mathiasen. Without them there would be no book.

J. Willis Hurst, M.D.

Joseph S. Alpert, M.D.

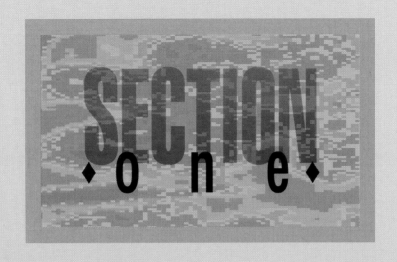

SECTION ·one·

THE NORMAL HEART AND CARDIAC RESPONSE TO DISEASE

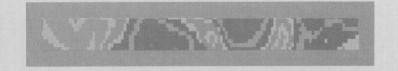

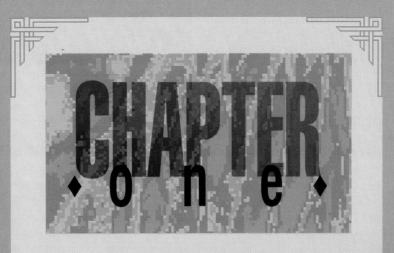

CHAPTER
·one·

ANATOMY OF
THE HEART

ROBERT H. ANDERSON, MD

BENSON R. WILCOX, MD

ANTON E. BECKER, MD

To understand the normal action of the heart and to diagnose its abnormalities, it is necessary to have a complete and full knowledge of the usual arrangement of cardiac structure.

This knowledge starts with a consideration of the *position of the heart* within the chest. A mediastinal structure, the heart lies within its pericardial sac with one third of its bulk to the right of the midline (Fig. 1.1). The long axis of the heart is oblique, with the base in right-sided superior location and the apex extending well to the left. The right atrial appendage is a key landmark on the right border of the silhouette, while the pulmonary trunk occupies the left superior border, lying anteriorly and to the left of the aorta.

The arrangement of the covering pericardial sac ensures smooth action of cardiac contraction. The *pericardium* has a firm fibrous layer, which encloses and fuses with the outer membrane of a double serous layer. The inner layer of the serous sac fuses with the surface of the heart itself to form the epicardium. The pericardial cavity therefore is between the epicardium and the outer layer of serous pericardium, itself fused with the tough fibrous pericardium. Within the overall cavity thus formed are two distinct recesses, namely the oblique and transverse sinuses of the pericardium (Fig. 1.2).

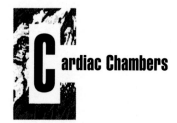

ardiac Chambers

The *arrangement of the cardiac chambers* themselves can be understood on the basis of the structure of the short axis. Figure 1.3 shows the structure of the atrio-ventricular valves relative to the aortic root. The latter structure is wedged deeply between the mitral and tricuspic orifices; the atrioventricular junctions are then encircled by major branches of the coronary arteries.

FIGURE 1.1   The heart within its pericardial cavity, with the anterior thoracic wall removed and the fibrous pericardium incised. Note that the pericardial cavity is between the fibrous layer and the epicardium (see Fig 1.2), and that the pulmonary trunk is anterior and to the left of the aorta. (Reproduced with permission; see Figure Credits)

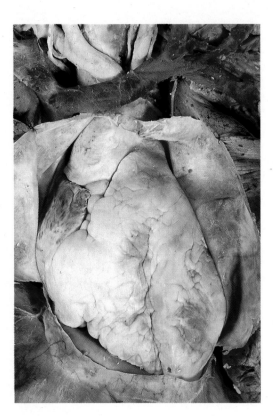

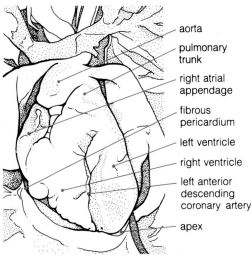

aorta

pulmonary trunk

right atrial appendage

fibrous pericardium

left ventricle

right ventricle

left anterior descending coronary artery

apex

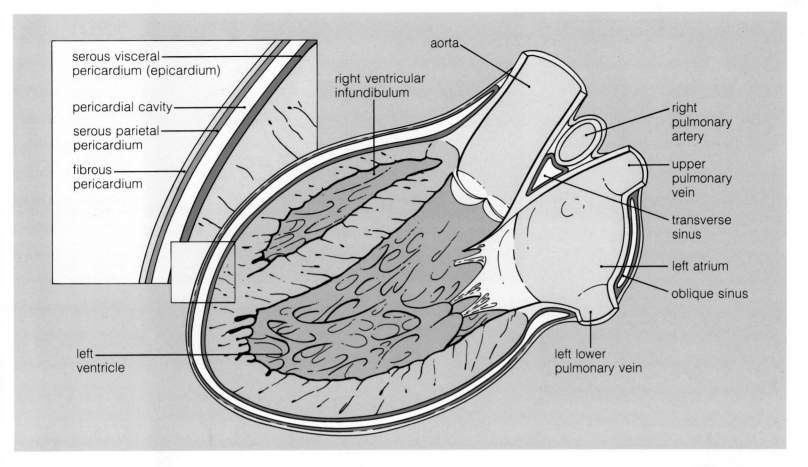

serous visceral
pericardium (epicardium)

pericardial cavity

serous parietal
pericardium

fibrous
pericardium

aorta

right ventricular
infundibulum

right
pulmonary
artery

upper
pulmonary
vein

transverse
sinus

left atrium

oblique sinus

left lower
pulmonary vein

left
ventricle

FIGURE 1.2 The long axis of the heart at right angles to the outlets, showing the arrangement of the pericardium. The outer fibrous sac is firmly attached to the great arteries and veins at the base. The heart itself invaginates a second sac, the serous pericardium. The two layers of this serous membrane, however, are densely adherent to other structures. The inner layer (visceral) is attached to the surface of the myocardium as the epicardium. The outer layer (parietal) is attached to the fibrous pericardium. Effectively, the pericardial cavity is located between the tough fibrous layer and the surface of the heart. Within this cavity are two recesses: the transverse and oblique sinuses. As shown in the diagram, the transverse sinus is in the inner heart curvature while the oblique sinus is behind the diaphragmatic aspect of the left atrium, limited by the attachments of the pulmonary veins (see Fig. 1.19). (Reproduced with permission; see Figure Credits)

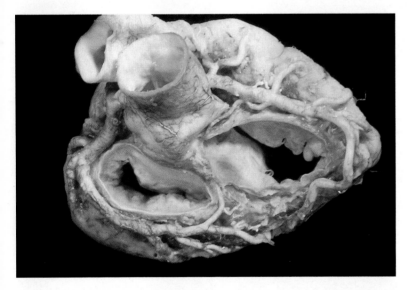

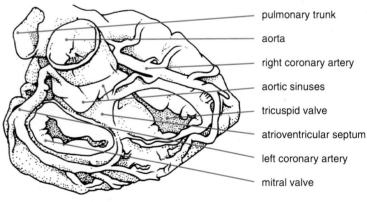

pulmonary trunk

aorta

right coronary artery

aortic sinuses

tricuspid valve

atrioventricular septum

left coronary artery

mitral valve

FIGURE 1.3 The superior aspect of the base of the heart after removal of the atrial chambers. This view reveals the interrelationships of the aortic, tricuspid, and mitral valves, which underscores the arrangement of the fibrous skeleton (see Figs. 1.4–1.6). The aorta is deeply wedged between the two atrioventricular orifices. The coronary arteries emerge from the two aortic sinuses closest to the pulmonary trunk and proceed in the atrioventricular grooves. The leaflet arrangements of the atrioventricular valves are well seen, with mural and aortic (anterior) leaflets guarding the mitral orifice, and septal, anterosuperior, and inferior (mural) leaflets in the tricuspid orifice. (Reproduced with permission; see Figure Credits)

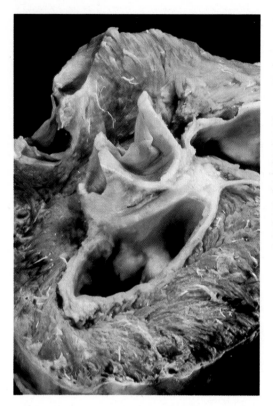

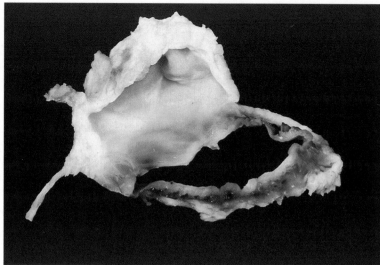

FIGURE 1.5
The fibrous skeleton (shown in Fig. 1.4) removed from the heart and photographed from below. Note the firm annulus of the mitral valve, the limited extensions around the tricuspid valve, and the subvalvar fibrous skirt of the aortic valve (see Fig. 1.6). The central fibrous body is made up of the fusion of the right fibrous trigone and the membranous part of the septum. Examination of this figure together with Figure 1.4 shows that the fibrous skeleton has no relationship to the pulmonary valve. As demonstrated in Figure 1.13, the leaflets of the pulmonary valve arise directly from the musculature of the right ventricular outlet component and have no fibrous support. (Reproduced with permission; see Figure Credits)

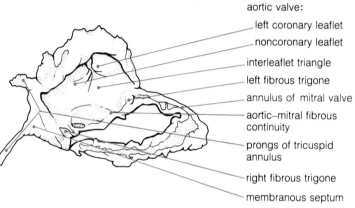

aortic valve:
- left coronary leaflet
- noncoronary leaflet

interleaflet triangle

left fibrous trigone

annulus of mitral valve

aortic–mitral fibrous continuity

prongs of tricuspid annulus

right fibrous trigone

membranous septum

FIGURE 1.4   Dissection of the fibrous skeleton. The heart is in the same orientation as the specimen in Figure 1.3. The atrioventricular junction is bared down to the annulus of the mitral valve, while the aortic valve leaflets are removed to the level of their semilunar attachments. (Figure 1.5 shows these attachments from the ventricular aspect.) The fibrous skeleton is made up of the aortic–mitral unit together with much weaker extensions around the tricuspid orifice. The keystone of the skeleton is the central fibrous body, formed from fusion of the aortic, mitral, and tricuspid orifices. The dissection also shows the extensive area of fibrous continuity between the aortic and mitral valves. This is thickened at each end to form the right and left fibrous trigones. The right trigone is then incorporated into the central fibrous body. The atrioventricular conduction axis penetrates through this body to reach the subaortic outflow tract (see Fig. 1.30). (Reproduced with permission; see Figure Credits)

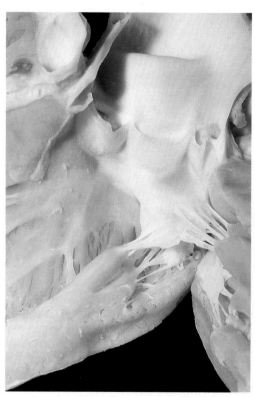

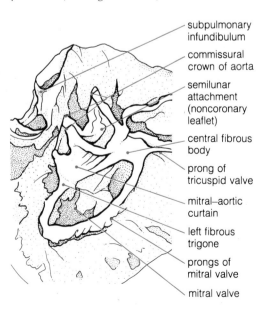

subpulmonary infundibulum

commissural crown of aorta

semilunar attachment (noncoronary leaflet)

central fibrous body

prong of tricuspid valve

mitral–aortic curtain

left fibrous trigone

prongs of mitral valve

mitral valve

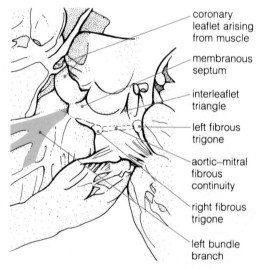

coronary leaflet arising from muscle

membranous septum

interleaflet triangle

left fibrous trigone

aortic–mitral fibrous continuity

right fibrous trigone

left bundle branch

FIGURE 1.6   The subaortic outflow tract. The dissection shows that the aortic root is a partly fibrous, partly muscular structure sculpted by the semilunar attachments of the leaflets of the aortic valve. There is no annulus as such supporting these leaflets. Anteriorly they arise directly from the musculature of the ventricular septum. Posteriorly they arise from the membranous septum, the fibrous trigones, and the area of aortic–mitral fibrous continuity. Fibrous sheets fill the interleaflet triangles in these areas and contribute to the fibrous skeleton. It is a mistake to conceptualize the skeleton itself as ascending in the form of tricorn cords to support the attachments of the valve leaflets. (Reproduced with permission; see Figure Credits)

Further dissection (Fig. 1.4) shows the firm fibrous continuity existing between the sinuses of the aortic valve and the annulus of the mitral valve; this is the *cardiac skeleton*, which is much less well formed around the leaflets of the tricuspid valve. There is a very well-formed block of fibrous and collagenous tissue where the support structures of the mitral, tricuspid, and aortic valves are all continuous. This is the central fibrous body, shown from its atrial aspect in Figure 1.4 and from the ventricular aspect after removal of the skeleton from the ventricular mass in Figure 1.5. The leaflets of the aortic and mitral valves are then continuous, forming the roof of the subaortic outlet; they also form a block of fibrocollagenous tissue within the left margin of the outflow tract. This thickening strengthens the left margin of fibrous continuity and is called the *left fibrous trigone*. It complements the right trigone, which is incorporated into the central fibrous body. The remainder of the fibrous body is the membranous septum, which separates the subaortic outlet from the right atrium and ventricle, respectively (see below).

The function of the fibrous skeleton is to support the leaflets of the various valves and bind them to the myocardial masses. As can be seen in Figure 1.5, the skeleton is less well formed around the tricuspid valve orifice. In this position, the leaflets spring from the fibro-fatty atrioventricular groove and are directly apposed to the right ventricular muscle mass. By and large, it is the substance of the atrioventricular grooves that serves to isolate the atrial from ventricular musculature at all points, save the site of the atrioventricular conduction axis (bundle of His). This insulates the atrial and ventricular segments of myocardium, except at the point of normal conduction (see below). The fibrous elements of the skeleton are well represented in the aortic root, where they form its roof and border with the right-sided heart chambers (Fig. 1.6).

The overall arrangement of the *cardiac valves* in short axis is shown in Figure 1.7, while the ventricular short-axis equivalent is seen in Figure 1.8. The key feature is the deeply wedged position of the aortic valve between the tricuspid and mitral valves.

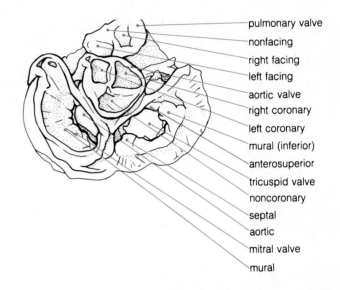

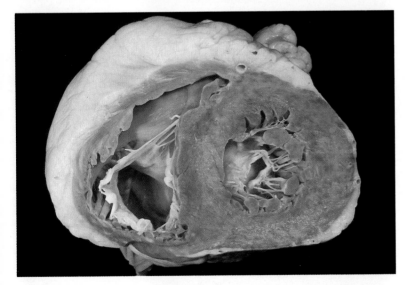

FIGURE 1.7   Dissection of the heart revealing the atrial aspect of the short axis, with both atrial chambers and both arterial trunks removed (see Fig. 1.3). The deeply wedged position of the aortic valve between the atrioventricular valves is apparent, as is its central position within the outline of the heart. Note the different appearance of the mural and aortic leaflets of the mitral valve, the mural leaflet occupying two thirds of the annular circumference. Note also that two of the com-

missures of the arterial valves face each other, permitting two of the leaflets of each valve accurately to be described as the facing leaflets while the third leaflet in each case is the nonfacing leaflet. The coronary arteries arise from the sinuses supporting the facing leaflets of the aortic valve. Because of this, it is customary in the aortic valve to identify the leaflets and sinuses as right coronary, left coronary, and noncoronary, respectively. (Reproduced with permission; see Figure Credits)

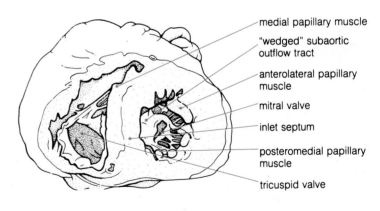

FIGURE 1.8   A short–axis section of the heart viewed from below, replicating the view obtained by the echocardiographer. The section is through the ventricular mass, just above the junction of inlet and apical trabecular components (see Figs. 1.12, 1.20). The section shows how the mural (inferior) leaflet of the tricuspid valve hugs the diaphragmatic wall of the right ventricle. The septal leaflet, in contrast, firmly adheres to the ventricular septum. The third anterosuperior leaflet hangs as a curtain between the inlet and outlet components of the ventricle. In the left ventricle the section shows how the wedged position of the subaortic outflow tract lifts the mitral valve away from the

septum, giving it an oblique orientation. Its leaflets are described most accurately as being aortic and mural in location. The valve commissures are attached to the paired anterolateral and posteromedial papillary muscles. The mitral valve does not have cordal attachments to the ventricular septum. Note the extensive swing of the septum itself; the inlet part is virtually in the sagittal plane while the outlet component is in the coronal plane. Note also the characteristic medial papillary muscle (of Lancisi) in the right ventricle and the extensive supraventricular crest separating the tricuspid and pulmonary valves (see Fig. 1.14). (Reproduced with permission; see Figure Credits)

The expression of this within the ventricles is that the subaortic outlet lifts the leaflets of the mitral valve away from the septum so that a crevice of the outlet reaches to the diaphragmatic surface of the heart. In contrast, the inlets and outlets of the right ventricle are widely separated by the muscular roof of the right ventricle (the supraventricular crest); the outlet extends out to the left border of the heart; and the septum—seen in short axis—has a considerable curvature.

Taken in isolation, each of the *cardiac chambers* possesses intrinsic features that permit its unequivocal recognition. In the case of the atrial chambers, each possesses a venous component, an appendage, and an atrioventricular vestibule. It is the appendage that most constantly retains its structure in congenitally malformed hearts and therefore is most reliable for identification.

The morphologic right appendage (Fig. 1.9) is a triangular structure having a broad base, with the venous component marked externally by the terminal groove and internally by the terminal crest. The crest is the junction of the trabeculated appendage with the smooth-walled venous component, which receives the superior and inferior caval veins together with the coronary sinus (Fig. 1.10).

The venous orifices surround the septal surface of the right atrium, this being the oval fossa characterized by its broad rim and smooth floor. The oval fossa is of vital significance during fetal life, when it is patent. Then its proximity to the inferior caval vein permits the richly oxygenated blood coming from the placenta (reaching the inferior caval vein through the venous duct) to pass directly into the left atrium and then to the left ventricle, aorta, and brain. In contrast,

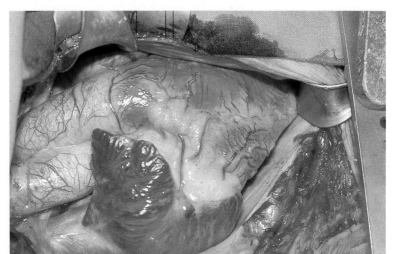

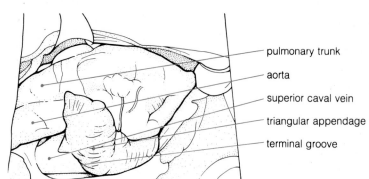

FIGURE 1.9 Surgical view taken through a median sternotomy of the right atrial appendage, illustrating its triangular shape and the extent of its junction with the venous component of the right atrium. Note the upper end of the terminal groove marking this junction. (Reproduced with permission; see Figure Credits)

- pulmonary trunk
- aorta
- superior caval vein
- triangular appendage
- terminal groove

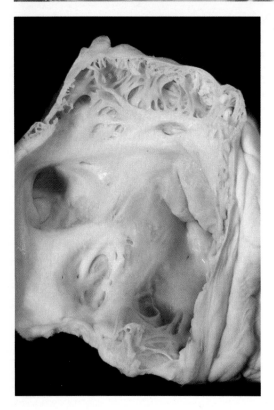

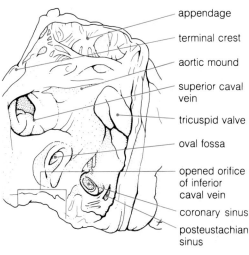

- appendage
- terminal crest
- aortic mound
- superior caval vein
- tricuspid valve
- oval fossa
- opened orifice of inferior caval vein
- coronary sinus
- posteustachian sinus

FIGURE 1.10 The internal appearance of the morphologic right atrium. The photograph was taken obliquely from behind the heart after opening the atrium through the orifice of the inferior caval vein. The broad opening of the superior caval vein is sandwiched between the terminal crest (the muscle bundle marking internally the site of the terminal groove; see Fig. 1.9) and the superior infolding of the atrial roof, which makes up the upper rim of the oval fossa. The oval fossa itself is the site of the atrial septum. The oval fossa is far less extensive than often thought, the septum itself being confined to the floor of the fossa and its immediate surrounds. The fossa is separated from the orifice of the coronary sinus by the sinus septum. More anterosuperiorly, both these structures abut on the atrioventricular septum (see Figs. 1.12, 1.13), which separates both from the vestibule of the tricuspid valve. The internal aspect of the triangular appendage is distinguished by its prominent trabeculations in contrast to the smooth lining of the venous sinus and the vestibule. In the morphologic right atrium, these pectinate muscles extend around the atrioventricular junction to its posterior aspect (compare with Fig 1.17). (Reproduced with permission; see Figure Credits)

the deoxygenated blood returning from the brain through the superior caval vein is deflected away from the fossa by its extensive rim, being directed instead toward the right ventricle, pulmonary trunk, and arterial duct. The vestibule of the right atrium contains and supports the tricuspid valve with leaflets in septal, anterosuperior, and inferior (or mural) location; the valve orifice is encircled by the right coronary artery (see Fig. 1.3).

The major distinguishing feature of the right ventricle is the coarse nature of its apical trabeculations, together with the fact that the septal leaflet of the tricuspid valve has extensive attachments distally to the ventricular septum, a feature lacking in the mitral valve (Fig. 1.11). This is well seen in the simulated four-chamber cut of the heart, which, when taken posteriorly (Fig. 1.12), demonstrates also the offsetting of the proximal attachments of the atrioventri-

cular valves. Because of this offsetting, there is overlapping of the atrial and ventricular septal structures, producing a muscular atrioventricular septum between the right atrium and left ventricle. However, the extent of this muscular septum is limited because of the posterior extension of the subaortic outlet. For their larger part, therefore, four-chamber sections reveal the subaortic outflow tract interposed between the mitral valve and the septum. These sections also demonstrate well the part of the central fibrous body that is interposed between the subaortic outlet and the right-sided heart chamber. As described above, this component of the cardiac skeleton is called the *membranous septum*. It is crossed on its right ventricular aspect by the attachment of the septal leaflet of the tricuspid valve, thus dividing it into interventricular and atrioventricular components (Fig. 1.13).

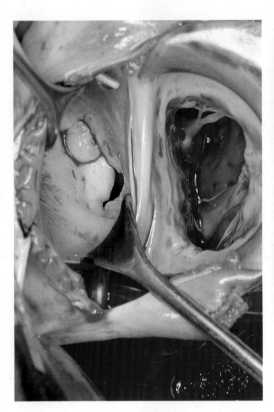

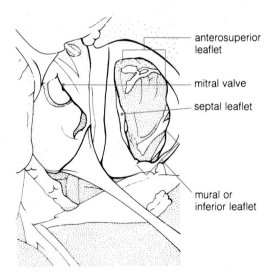

FIGURE 1.11   Surgical view of the arrangement of the leaflets of the atrioventricular valves. The tricuspid valve has septal, anterosuperior, and mural (or inferior) leaflets while the mitral valve has aortic and mural leaflets. (Reproduced with permission; see Figure Credits)

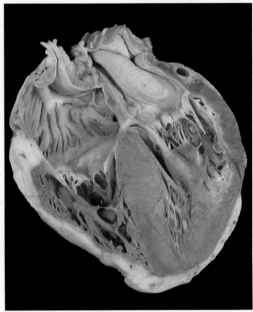

FIGURE 1.12   Long-axis section of the heart taken at right angles to the inlet part of the ventricular septum. This section produces the so-called four-chamber view of the echocardiographer since it displays the four cardiac chambers. The significant point in this posterior cut is the offsetting of the attachments of the mitral and tricuspid valve leaflets at the atrioventricular junction. The leaflet of the tricuspid valve is attached more toward the ventricular apex. Because of this, part of the atrial septum overlaps the muscular ventricular septum, with a sloping junction between them. This part of the septum therefore is neither atrial nor ventricular but is the muscular atrioventricular septum. (Reproduced with permission; see Figure Credits)

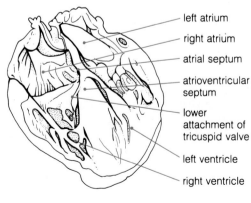

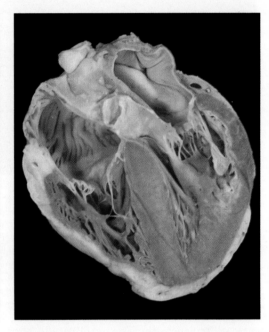

FIGURE 1.13   Section taken immediately anterior to section shown in Figure 1.12. It shows the limited extent of the muscular atrioventricular septum since, in this cut, the subaortic outflow tract has intervened between the mitral valve and the septum, lifting the leaflet of the mitral valve away from the septum. The space of the muscular atrioventricular septum is now occupied by another atrioventricular septal structure, since the septum immediately below the aortic valve continues to separate the left ventricle from the right atrium. This part of the septum, however, is made up of fibrous tissue and is part of the central fibrous body (see Figs. 1.4–1.6). Specifically, it is the atrioventricular component of the membranous septum. (Reproduced with permission; see Figure Credits)

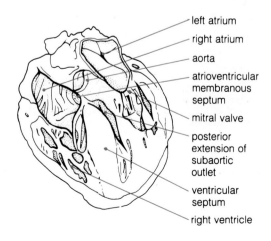

Although a ventricle is traditionally thought to have only inlet (or sinus) and outlet (or conus) components, it is advantageous to recognize the extensive apical trabecular component (Fig. 1.14), thus describing the ventricle in tripartite fashion. There are no discrete boundaries between the components, but the overall arrangement of inlet, apical trabecular, and outlet por-

tions is readily appreciated. The outlet component is extensive in the right ventricle, the leaflets of the pulmonary valve being exclusively attached to the ventricular musculature and having no connection with the cardiac skeleton. Because of this, the larger part of the subpulmonary infundibulum can be completely removed from the heart without disturbing any left ven-

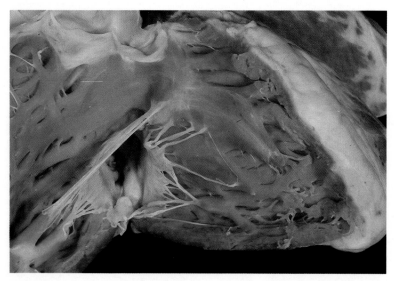

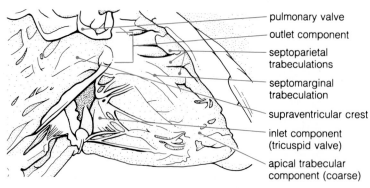

pulmonary valve
outlet component
septoparietal trabeculations
septomarginal trabeculation
supraventricular crest
inlet component (tricuspid valve)
apical trabecular component (coarse)

FIGURE 1.14   The vestibule of the tricuspid valve in the normal heart connecting with the morphologic right ventricle. As shown in this photograph, the right ventricle can readily be analyzed in terms of three components: the inlet, apical trabecular, and outlet portions. The inlet part contains the tricuspid valve and extends from the atrioventricular junction to the attachments of the valvular tension apparatus. The outlet component is the smooth sleeve of muscle supporting the semilunar attachments of the pulmonary valve leaflets. The apical trabecular component merges with these other components and has more obvious boundaries at the inlet than the outlet. Nonetheless, it is recognized because of its heavy and coarse trabeculations. The nature of these trabeculations also serves to distinguish it from the morphologic left ventricle (see Fig. 1.20). One muscular trabeculation is much more obvious in the morphologic right ventricle: it is a strap-like structure that extends down from the area of the membranous septum, having two limbs at this site that extend into the inlet and outlet components, respectively. The body of this strap then runs down toward the ventricular apex where it gives rise to

the prominent anterior papillary muscle of the tricuspid valve. This structure is the septomarginal trabeculation (or septal band). From its anterior surface, a further series of trabeculations originates and runs to the parietal wall of the ventricle; these are the septoparietal trabeculations. One of these is usually prominent and is described as the moderator band. This section also shows the characteristic arrangement of the tricuspid valve and its papillary muscles. The septal leaflet has extensive cordal attachments directly to the inlet part of the muscular septum. It is limited by the medial papillary muscle (of Lancisi) anteriorly and by the prominent inferior papillary muscle posteriorly. The anterosuperior valve leaflet extends across like a curtain between ventricular inlet and outlet to the more prominent anterior papillary muscle. The inferior leaflet is then seen also to be mural, running along the diaphragmatic surface of the inlet. Note the extensive muscle shelf that separates the tricuspid and pulmonary valves. This is made up of the inner curve of the heart wall and is called the *supraventricular crest*. (Reproduced with permission; see Figure Credits)

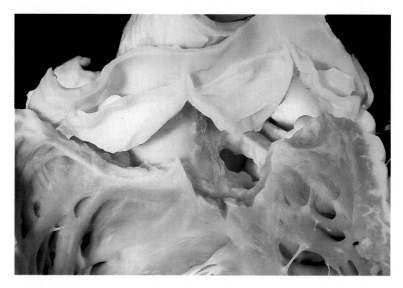

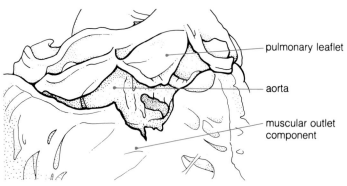

pulmonary leaflet
aorta
muscular outlet component

FIGURE 1.15   Dissection of the heart illustrating the anatomy of the outlet component of the morphologic right ventricle. It shows the three semilunar attachments of the leaflets of the pulmonary valve. These are exclusively connected to the sleeve of outlet musculature. There is no annulus supporting these leaflets in the sense that the fibrous skeleton forms a ring around the mitral valve (see Fig. 1.5). The dissection also shows that the area often considered to be septum in the region below the two facing leaflets of the valve is in reality the inner wall of the heart. There is a space in this position between the right ventricular infundibulum and the aorta. The origin of the coronary arteries from the aorta can be seen through the incision which liberated the leaflets from the ventricular outlet (see Fig. 1.32). (Reproduced with permission; see Figure Credits)

tricular structures (Fig. 1.15). It follows also that the pulmonary valve has no annulus in terms of a discrete fibrous ring. Instead, the leaflets are simply supported in semilunar fashion by the infundibular musculature.

The left atrium, like the right, has an appendage, a venous component, and a vestibule. The appendage is long, tubular, and usually crenellated and has a narrow junction with the venous component (Fig. 1.16). The junction is not marked, either internally or externally, by a terminal crest or groove such as seen on the right side (Fig. 1.17). The venous component receives the four pulmonary veins at its corners (Fig. 1.18). The septal surface of the atrium is roughened and has no rim, as in the right atrium (Fig. 1.17).

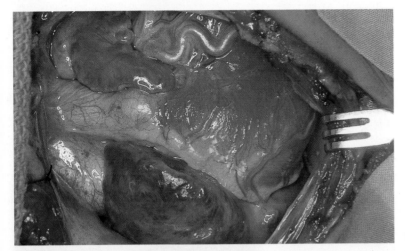

FIGURE 1.16 Surgical view through a median sternotomy, contrasting the long, tubular shape of the left atrial appendage with the broad, triangular right appendage. (Reproduced with permission; see Figure Credits)

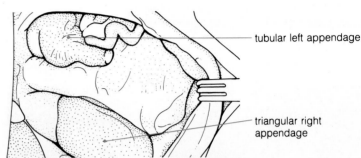

— tubular left appendage

— triangular right appendage

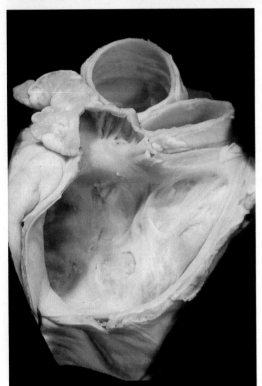

FIGURE 1.17
Dissection of the heart depicting the narrow junction of the appendage with the vestibule of the mitral valve. Note how the pectinate muscles are confined within the appendage. There is no prominent terminal crest in the left atrium (compare with Fig. 1.10). The four pulmonary veins enter the corners of the smooth walled venous component (see Fig. 1.18). Note that the left atrial aspect of the septum is roughened and has no rim to the oval fossa, such as that found in the right atrium (see Fig. 1.10). (Reproduced with permission; see Figure Credits)

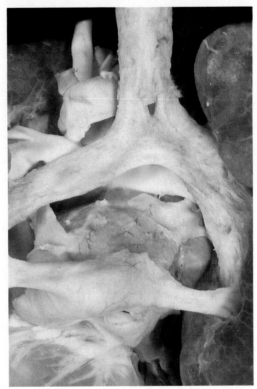

FIGURE 1.18
Dissection of the posterior aspect of the heart showing the pulmonary veins entering the four corners of the diaphragmatic surface of the left atrium. The four venous connections limit the oblique sinus of the pericardium (see Fig. 1.2). This dissection also shows the site of the descending aorta (left aortic arch) and the typical pattern of the normal tracheal bifurcation. The left bronchus is twice as long as the right bronchus and is crossed by the lower lobe pulmonary artery before bifurcation. (Reproduced with permission; see Figure Credits)

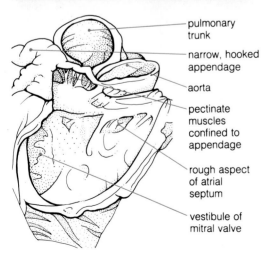

— pulmonary trunk

— narrow, hooked appendage

— aorta

— pectinate muscles confined to appendage

— rough aspect of atrial septum

— vestibule of mitral valve

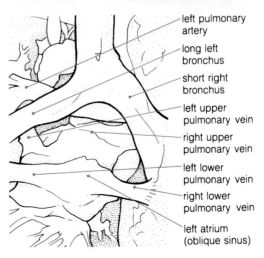

— left pulmonary artery

— long left bronchus

— short right bronchus

— left upper pulmonary vein

— right upper pulmonary vein

— left lower pulmonary vein

— right lower pulmonary vein

— left atrium (oblique sinus)

Dissection shows that the greater part of the rim of the oval fossa is simply a deep groove between the venous components of the two atria (Fig. 1.19). This crevice, termed *Waterston's groove*, is important since it can be dissected during surgery to provide one means of access into the left atrium.

Although not as obviously differentiated as the right ventricle, the left ventricle can also conveniently be described in terms of inlet, apical trabecular, and outlet components (Fig. 1.20). This tripartite approach highlights the fine apical trabeculations that are the most characteristic and constant feature of the left ventricle in congenitally malformed hearts (see Chapter 3). In the normal heart, however, both the inlet and outlet components of the left ventricle have their own distinctive characteristics. The major distinguishing feature of the inlet is that the leaflets of the mitral valve have no distal attachment to the septum. The two leaflets themselves are supported by paired papillary muscles and are located such that one is in direct fibrous continuity with the aortic valve while the other springs from the parietal part of the left atrioventricular junction (see Fig. 1.13). For this reason, the leaflets are best described as being aortic and mural. They have grossly dissimilar circumferential extent, the aortic leaflet guarding one third and the mural leaflet two thirds of the junction (see Fig. 1.3). Because the aortic leaflet is much deeper, they have similar areas (Fig. 1.21). Usually the mural leaflet is divided into three components called *scallops*, but this arrangement is variable.

An important feature of the left ventricular outlet is its abbreviated nature due to the aortic wedge position and its interposition between the inlet and the septum (Fig. 1.22). Unlike the pulmonary valve, the leaflets of the aortic valve are intimately related to the fibrous skeleton such that the overall circumference of the valve orifice is half fibrous support. Despite this, the leaflets of the aortic valve do not have an annulus in the sense of a complete ring, such as exists in the mitral valve. The leaflet support is again conditioned by the semilunar attachments, the zenith of the commissures being appreciably higher than the nadir of the leaflet troughs. The leaflets of both arterial valves are unsupported by tension apparatus so that they close simply due to the hydrostatic pressure of the column of blood they support during ventricular diastole (Fig. 1.23).

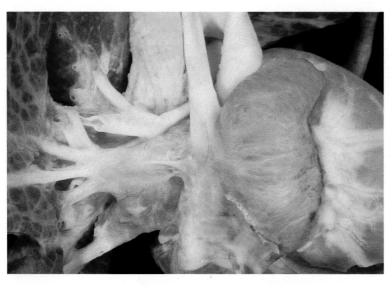

FIGURE 1.19   Dissection of the heart illustrating the important relationships between the right pulmonary veins and the venous sinus of the right atrium. There is a deep furrow (Waterston's groove) between the pulmonary veins and the caval veins, which forms the upper margin of the oval fossa. In this position it is often taken to be a septal structure instead of the infolding of the atrial roof. Note also that the site of the terminal groove is lateral to the venous sinus of the right atrium, separating it from the appendage. This groove marks the site of the terminal crest and contains the sinus node (see Fig. 1.27). (Reproduced with permission; see Figure Credits)

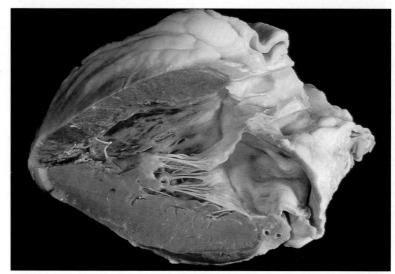

FIGURE 1.20   The morphologic left ventricle opened through an incision in its parietal wall. Like the right ventricle, it can readily be described in terms of inlet, apical trabecular, and outlet components (see Fig. 1.14). The inlet component contains the mitral valve with its two leaflets supported by prominent paired papillary muscles. As shown in this dissection, the anterior or aortic leaflet is separated by the subaortic outflow tract from the ventricular septum. The mitral valve, unlike the tricuspid valve, never has direct attachments to the ventricular septum. The apical trabecular component in the left ventricle is characteristically fine and has no septomarginal trabeculation reinforcing its smooth septal surface. The outlet component is abbreviated in comparison with that of the right ventricle, since there is fibrous continuity between the mitral and aortic valves. Thus there is no muscular supraventricular crest within the left ventricle. There is, however, a marked posterior extension of the outflow tract that separates the mitral valve from the septum. (Reproduced with permission; see Figure Credits)

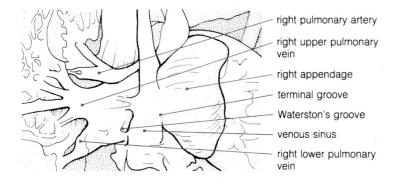

- right pulmonary artery
- right upper pulmonary vein
- right appendage
- terminal groove
- Waterston's groove
- venous sinus
- right lower pulmonary vein

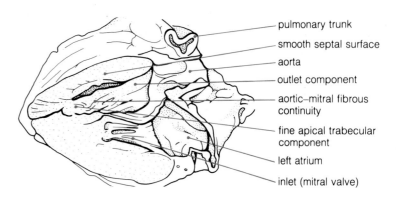

- pulmonary trunk
- smooth septal surface
- aorta
- outlet component
- aortic–mitral fibrous continuity
- fine apical trabecular component
- left atrium
- inlet (mitral valve)

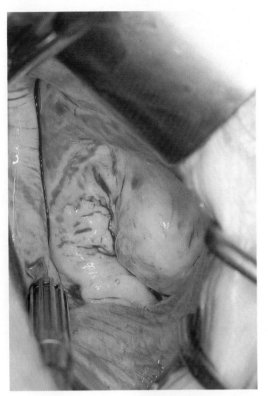

FIGURE 1.21
Surgical view of the leaflets of the mitral valve, oriented in anatomic fashion. Note the annular attachment of the two leaflets is markedly different, the aortic leaflet taking up only one third of the overall circumference. This leaflet, however, is much deeper than the mural leaflet so that the overall area of the two is comparable. (Reproduced with permission; see Figure Credits)

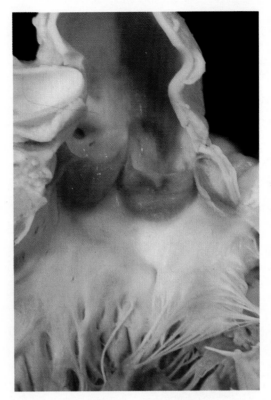

FIGURE 1.22
Dissection showing the outlet component of the left ventricle. The anatomy is determined by the semilunar attachments of the leaflets of the aortic valve. Unlike the pulmonary valve, which has exclusively muscular attachments, the leaflets of the aortic valve are attached in part to the muscular walls of the ventricle and in part to the fibrous skeleton (see Figs. 1.4–1.6). Note also the extensive posterior extension of the subaortic outflow tract, which is bordered on one side by the mitral valve and on the other by the atrioventricular septal structures (see Figs. 1.12, 1.13). (Reproduced with permission; see Figure Credits)

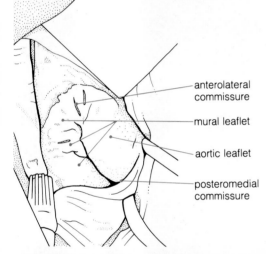

- anterolateral commissure
- mural leaflet
- aortic leaflet
- posteromedial commissure

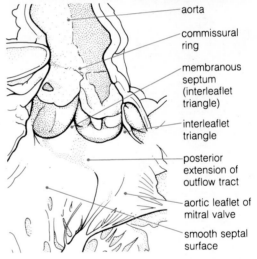

- aorta
- commissural ring
- membranous septum (interleaflet triangle)
- interleaflet triangle
- posterior extension of outflow tract
- aortic leaflet of mitral valve
- smooth septal surface

FIGURE 1.23   The aortic valve viewed from above, illustrating the simple closing mechanism of an arterial valve. The three leaflets are forced together by the hydrostatic pressure of the column of blood they support during ventricular diastole. The function of the valves, however, depends on the normal formation of the subvalvular supporting tissues, the integrity of the leaflets, the normal arrangement of the commissural ring, and the normal configuration of the sinuses of Valsalva. (Reproduced with permission; see Figure Credits)

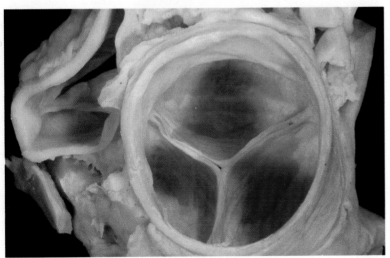

Arterial Trunks

The arterial trunks in the normal heart ascend into the mediastinum in a particular fashion called *normal relations*. Because of the wedge location of its root (see Fig. 1.3), the aorta springs from the cardiac base posteriorly and to the right of the pulmonary trunk (Fig. 1.24). The trunks then spiral around one another as they pass to supply the systemic and pulmonary circulations, respectively. The arch of the aorta gives off brachiocephalic (innominate), left common carotid, and left subclavian arteries from its superior aspect while the pulmonary trunk divides into right and left branches (Fig. 1.25). During fetal life an important channel connects the arterial trunks so that deoxygenated blood returning through the right side of the heart from the head can be shunted into the descending aorta, to be returned to the placenta for reoxygenation. This chan-

nel is the arterial duct, which runs from the left pulmonary artery to the aorta, marking the origin of the descending component of the aorta. The segment of the aortic arch between the left subclavian artery and the junction of the duct with the descending aorta is called the *isthmus* (see Fig. 1.25). The arterial duct stays patent only during fetal life, normally becoming constricted and closed in the first days after birth. Within the next six weeks it becomes converted into the arterial ligament and, by adult life, is simply a fibrous cord.

Conduction System

Normal action of the heart demands the synchronous activity of the *cardiac subsystems*, namely the conduction system, the arteries and veins, and the nervous and lymphatic systems. The conduction system generates

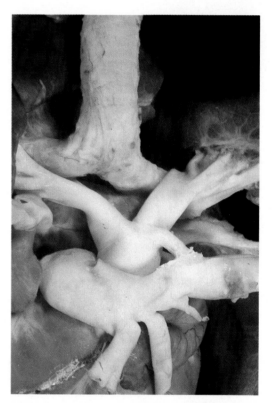

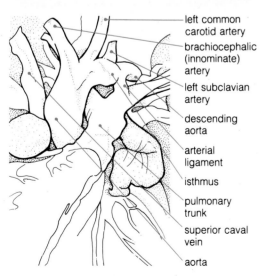

FIGURE 1.24
An infant heart illustrating the normal relationships of the great arteries as they leave the base of the heart. The pulmonary trunk is to the left and anterior relative to the centrally positioned aorta. The trunk having bifurcated, the right pulmonary artery swings beneath the aortic arch. The arch gives rise superiorly to the brachiocephalic (innominate), left common carotid, and left subclavian arteries. It then continues as the isthmus until it becomes the descending aorta at the site of the arterial ligament. This structure, arising from the left pulmonary artery, is the remnant of the arterial duct, which in fetal life conveys the right ventricular output to the placenta. In this specimen the duct has already closed and is in the process of conversion to a fibrous cord. (Reproduced with permission; see Figure Credits)

- left common carotid artery
- brachiocephalic (innominate) artery
- left subclavian artery
- descending aorta
- arterial ligament
- isthmus
- pulmonary trunk
- superior caval vein
- aorta

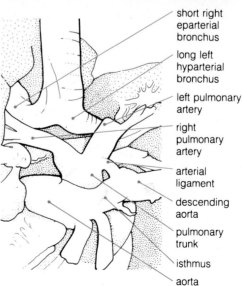

FIGURE 1.25
Superior view of the arterial trunks shown in Figure 1.24, with the aorta deflected forward. The smooth bifurcation of the pulmonary trunk is seen along with the site of the arterial duct. It demonstrates further the anatomy of the tracheal bifurcation shown from behind in Figure 1.18. This view shows how the lower lobe artery of the left lung crosses over the long left bronchus before it has given rise to any branches. The short right bronchus gives rise to its eparterial branch prior to being crossed by the pulmonary artery of the lower lobe. (Reproduced with permission; see Figure Credits)

- short right eparterial bronchus
- long left hyparterial bronchus
- left pulmonary artery
- right pulmonary artery
- arterial ligament
- descending aorta
- pulmonary trunk
- isthmus
- aorta

and dissipates the cardiac impulse (Fig. 1.26). A vital part of this system is the fibro-fatty atrioventricular tissue plane which insulates the atrial from the ventricular muscle masses at all points except the penetration of the specialized conduction axis. When speaking of the conduction tissues, however, we usually refer only to the nodes and their ramifications. The impulse is generated by the sinus node, a small, cigar-shaped structure lying within the terminal groove, usually lateral relative to that part of the lateral sino-atrial junction marked by the crest of the right atrial appendage (Fig. 1.27).

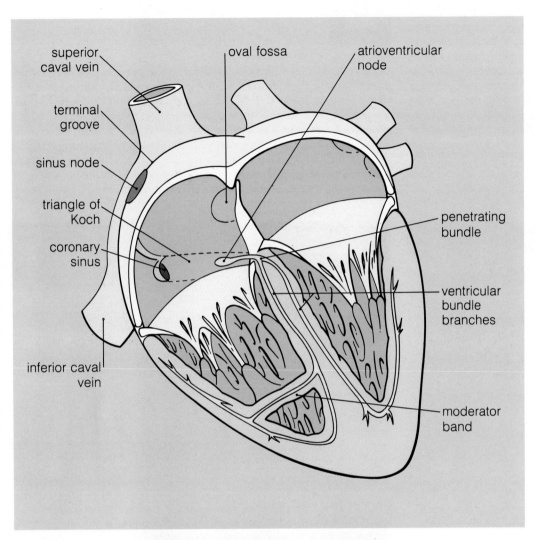

FIGURE 1.26   Arrangement of the conduction system in the normal heart. The sinus node sits laterally in the terminal groove (see Fig 1.27). It gives rise to the cardiac impulse, which is then carried through the atrial myocardium toward the ventricles, at the same time activating the myocardium. Conduction through the atrial chambers occurs through the working atrial myocardium, the geometric arrangement of the muscle bundles in the septum, and the terminal crest, being responsible for any preferential spread that exists. There is no evidence to support the concept of histologically discrete tracts of specialized conduction tissue extending between the sinus and atrioventricular nodes. The atrioventricular node, which produces the greater part of atrioventricular delay, is located within the triangle of Koch (see Fig. 1.29). The atrioventricular conduction axis continues from the node into the ventricles with penetrating and branching components before becoming the ventricular bundle branches. These branches are insulated from the septum in their proximal portions, activating the myocardium of the trabecular components through the so-called Purkinje cell network. The Purkinje cells in the human heart have small dimensions and do not resemble the large and clear cells found in the hearts of cattle and related mammals. (Reproduced with permission; see Figure Credits)

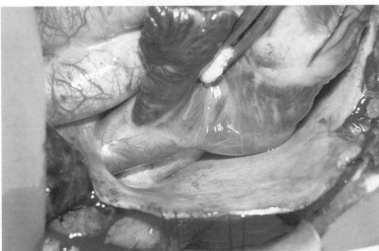

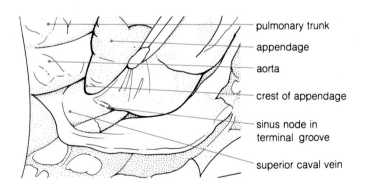

FIGURE 1.27   Surgical view showing the location of the normal cigar-shaped sinus node within the lateral extent of the terminal groove at the superior cavoatrial junction. (Reproduced with permission; see Figure Credits)

The node is discrete histologically, is immediately subepicardial, and is generally arranged around a prominent nodal artery (Fig. 1.28). Although several textbooks now illustrate "specialized tracts" emanating from the sinus node in triradiate fashion, there is no convincing evidence, either anatomic or electrophysiologic, to support the existence of these purported structures.

Instead, preferential conduction through the atrial musculature is governed by the geometric arrangement of the ordinary atrial muscle cells. The atrial impulse is gathered together, delayed, and distributed to the ventricular myocardium by the specialized atrioventricular conduction axis. The atrial component is the atrioventricular node, which produces the greater part of atrioventricular delay. It is located within the triangle of Koch, a most useful surgical landmark (Fig. 1.29). The node penetrates through the central fibrous body at the apex of the triangle, being no more than the size of a strand of cotton as it penetrates (the bundle of His) (Fig. 1.30). Having penetrated, it reaches the subaortic outflow tract and extends into right and left bundle branches. The left branch spreads out in fan-like fashion (Fig. 1.31), while the right branch is a thin cord-like structure. Both branches, however, pass out to the ventricular apices before arborizing into the myocardial masses as the so-called Purkinje networks.

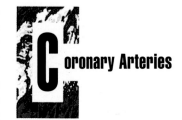

Coronary Arteries

Equally important as the conduction system is the arrangement of the *coronary arteries* supplying the heart. The two major arteries, right and left, arise from the sinuses of the aortic root (Fig. 1.32). Since there are usually three sinuses but only two arteries, and since each artery usually arises from a separate aortic sinus, one sinus does not give rise to an artery. Always, irrespective of the relationship of the arterial trunks in congenitally malformed hearts, the sinus lacking an artery is the one most distant from the pulmonary trunk (see Fig. 1.3). This sinus is therefore conveniently designated as the nonfacing sinus while in the normal heart the other sinuses are designated right coronary and left coronary, respectively.

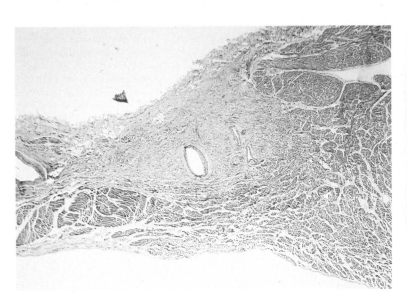

FIGURE 1.28   Histologic section, stained by the trichrome technique so that muscle appears red and fibrous tissue blue, taken at right angles to the cigar-shaped sinus node. It shows how, in short axis, the node is a wedge-shaped structure set in the angle between the wall of the superior caval vein and the terminal crest. Note the discrete boundaries between node and muscle and the arrangement of the node around a prominent artery. (Reproduced with permission; see Figure Credits)

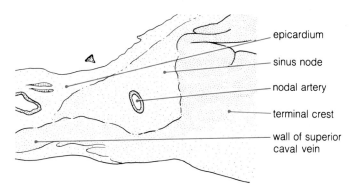

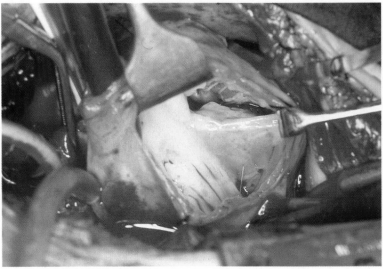

FIGURE 1.29   Surgical view showing the landmarks of the triangle of Koch. The triangle itself is clearly visible, limited distally by the septal attachment of the tricuspid valve and proximally by the sinus septum. If the surgeon scrupulously avoids this area, the atrioventricular conduction axis will not be damaged. (Reproduced with permission; see Figure Credits)

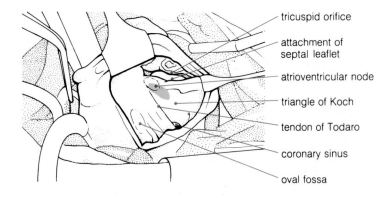

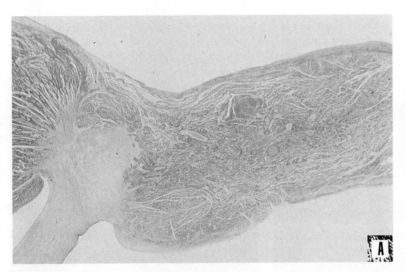

FIGURE 1.30   Sections stained by the trichrome technique demonstrating the position of the atrioventricular node within the triangle of Koch **(A)** and the penetrating atrioventricular bundle (of His) within the central fibrous body **(B)**. (Reproduced with permission; see Figure Credits)

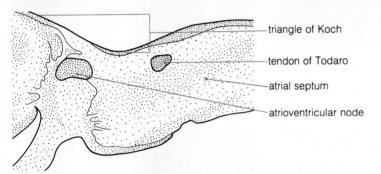

- triangle of Koch
- tendon of Todaro
- atrial septum
- atrioventricular node

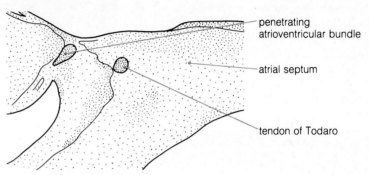

- penetrating atrioventricular bundle
- atrial septum
- tendon of Todaro

FIGURE 1.31   Diagram taken from the monograph of Tawara (1906), which established and elucidated the significance of the atrioventricular conduction axis. It shows the fan-like arrangement of the left bundle branch. The clinical value of the so-called concept of hemiblocks should not be extended to presume that the left bundle branch is arranged anatomically in bifascicular fashion. As shown here, it is arranged as a fan and, if it divides at all, it forms three rather than two divisions. (Source, see Figure Credits)

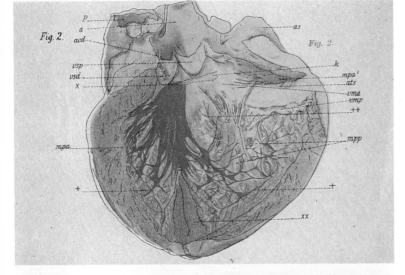

FIGURE 1.32   Dissection showing the origin of the coronary arteries from the aortic root. As shown in Figure 1.3, these arteries emerge from the two aortic sinuses that face the pulmonary trunk. The left coronary artery immediately divides into anterior interventricular and circumflex branches. The interventricular artery is well seen in this dissection along with its septal perforating branches. The circumflex and right coronary arteries encircle the orifices of the atrioventricular valves as shown in Figure 1.3. (Reproduced with permission; see Figure Credits)

The two mainstem coronary arteries then extend and branch to irrigate the atrioventricular and interventricular grooves (Fig. 1.33). In most hearts this is accomplished by the right coronary artery continuing as a solitary channel encircling the right atrioventricular junction (Fig. 1.34; see also Fig. 1.3) and descending within the posterior interventricular groove. In contrast, the left artery runs a very short course prior to its bifurcation into anterior interventricular and circumflex branches (Fig. 1.35). The interventricular branch then occupies the anterior interventricular groove while the circumflex branch extends to

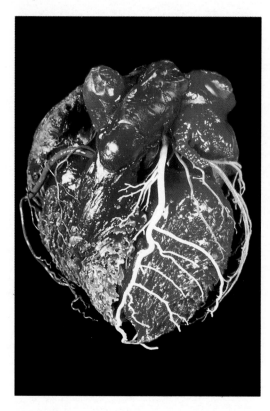

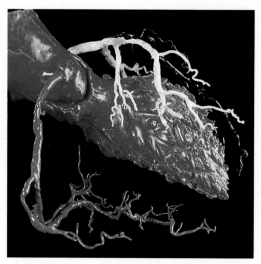

FIGURE 1.34 Anatomy of the coronary arterial tree in the right anterior oblique angiographic projection. The extent of the right coronary artery is well seen, along with its posterior interventricular artery. As in this cast, the posterior artery is a branch of the right artery in nine tenths of individuals, an arrangement termed *right dominance*. In one-tenth of cases, as shown in Figure 1.3, the circumflex artery gives rise to the posterior descending artery—left dominance. (Reproduced with permission; see Figure Credits)

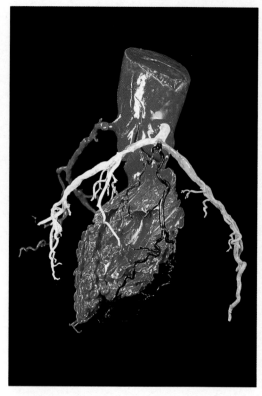

FIGURE 1.33 Anterior view of a cast showing the position of the coronary arteries and ventricles. The anterior interventricular branch of the left coronary artery is in white, together with its infundibular and diagonal branches. The circumflex branch of the left coronary artery together with its obtuse marginal branches are shown in yellow. The right coronary artery and its acute marginal branch are depicted in green. (Reproduced with permission; see Figure Credits)

FIGURE 1.35 Left lateral projection of the same heart shown in Figure 1.34 depicting the left mainstem artery and its anterior interventricular and circumflex branches. Also present in this heart is a so-called intermediate artery, shown in black. It is usual now to consider such arteries as diagonal branches of the anterior interventricular artery. (Reproduced with permission; see Figure Credits)

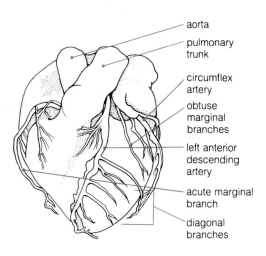

aorta

pulmonary trunk

circumflex artery

obtuse marginal branches

left anterior descending artery

acute marginal branch

diagonal branches

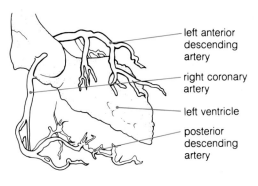

left anterior descending artery

right coronary artery

left ventricle

posterior descending artery

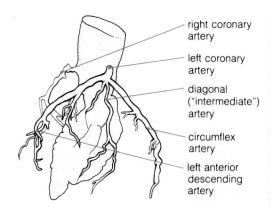

right coronary artery

left coronary artery

diagonal ("intermediate") artery

circumflex artery

left anterior descending artery

varying points around the left atrioventricular junction. In a minority of individuals (perhaps one tenth), it is the circumflex artery that reaches the crux and runs down into the posterior interventricular groove (see Fig. 1.3). The *coronary* *veins* also occupy the atrioventricular and interventricular grooves, returning blood into the coronary sinus, which itself runs along the left atrioventricular groove and opens into the right atrium (Fig. 1.36).

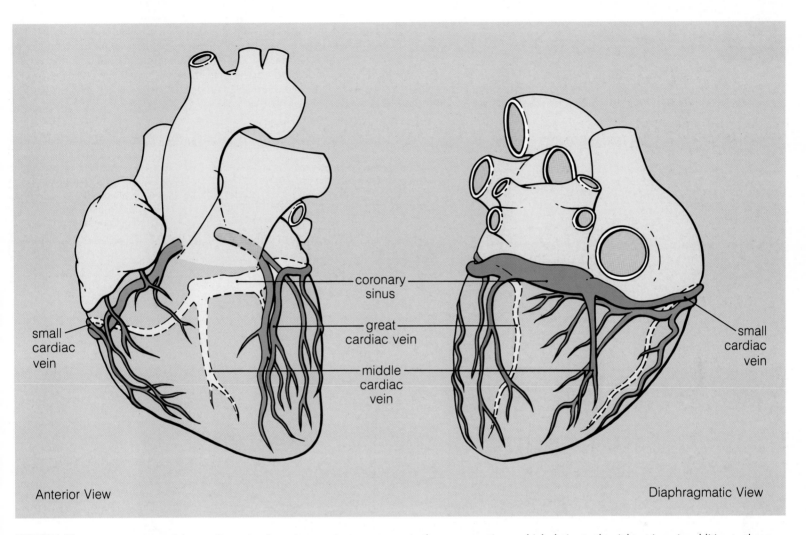

Anterior View

Diaphragmatic View

small cardiac vein

coronary sinus

great cardiac vein

middle cardiac vein

small cardiac vein

FIGURE 1.36 Arrangement of the cardiac veins from the anterior aspect (left) and the diaphragmatic aspect (right). The veins follow the great arteries, running in the interventricular and atrioventricular grooves. They terminate in the coronary sinus, which drains to the right atrium. In addition to these larger veins, smaller veins, called *thebesian veins*, drain directly to the right atrium. (Reproduced with permission; see Figure Credits)

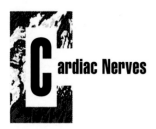

Cardiac Nerves

In terms of *nerves*, the heart is supplied from both sympathetic and parasympathetic sources. Although it was at first thought that the nerves may conduct the cardiac impulse, this impression had been shown to be spurious by the start of the twentieth century. The nerves monitor the function of the heart, being intimately related to the conduction system, and are also widely distributed along the coronary arteries. The supply to the musculature of the heart itself is relatively limited compared with these richly supplied areas. The parasympathetic nerves come from the vagus and are relayed via ganglion cells confined to the atrial tissues. Indeed there are few, if any, vagal fibers within the ventricles of the human heart. In contrast, the sympathetic fibers, derived from the cervical and upper thoracic ganglia of the sympathetic chains, are distributed more widely within the atria and ventricles. running primarily in concert with the branches of the coronary arteries (Fig. 1.37).

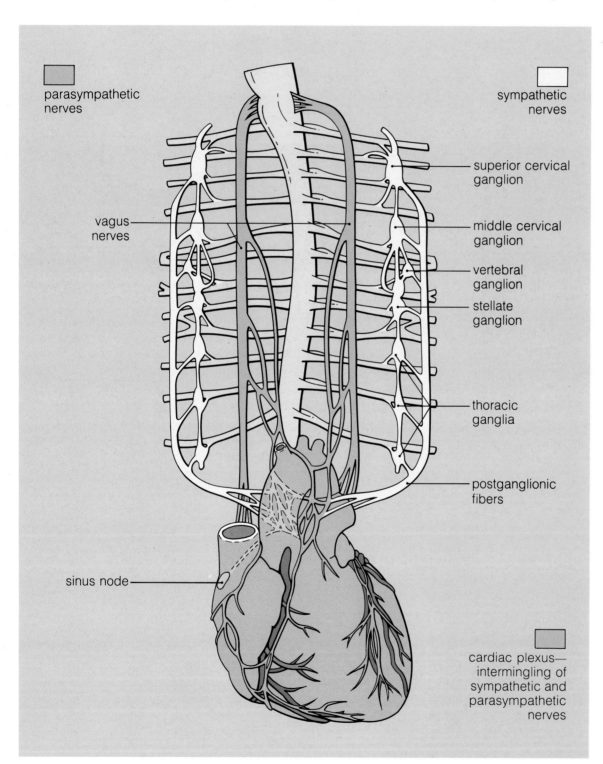

parasympathetic
nerves

sympathetic
nerves

vagus
nerves

superior cervical
ganglion

middle cervical
ganglion

vertebral
ganglion

stellate
ganglion

thoracic
ganglia

postganglionic
fibers

sinus node

cardiac plexus—
intermingling of
sympathetic and
parasympathetic
nerves

FIGURE 1.37 Diagram of the extent and origin of the cardiac nerves. The sympathetic nerves supply both ventricles and atria, while the parasympathetic supply is largely confined to the atrial chambers. (Reproduced with permission; see Figure Credits)

Histology of the Heart

Histologically, the heart is made up of masses of *myocardial fibers*, which are intermediate in their structure between voluntary (striated) and involuntary (smooth) muscle. Although the cardiac muscle is involuntary, it has marked cross striations, which are readily visible using the light microscope. Examination with the electron microscope shows that, as with skeletal muscle, the striations are due to the interdigitation of actin and myosin fibrils (Fig. 1.38). Thought at one time to be syncytial in nature, the cardiac cells are now known to be multiple individual units joined by intercalated disks (Fig. 1.39). Each cell therefore originates from and inserts into its neighbors. The cardiac skeleton is in no way analogous to the appendicular skeleton in terms of giving origin and insertion to the muscles. Instead, the cardiac skeleton supports most of the leaflets of the atrioventricular valves and helps in the insulation of the atrial and ventricular muscle masses (Fig. 1.40). The specialized conduction system of the heart is less obviously cross-striated than the ordinary "working" myocardium, although the precise arrangement differs within the different components of the system.

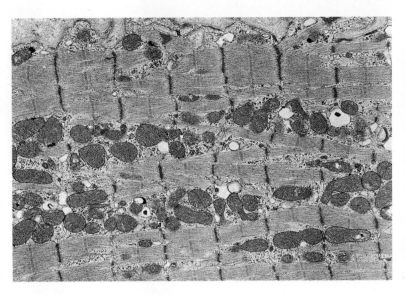

FIGURE 1.38   Electron micrograph showing the typical striated arrangement of normal cardiac muscle. The cross striations are due to the interdigitation of actin and myosin fibrils. (Reproduced with permission; see Figure Credits)

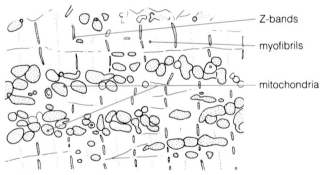

- Z-bands
- myofibrils
- mitochondria

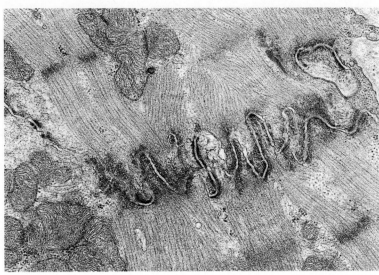

FIGURE 1.39   Electron micrograph showing the structure of an intercalated disk. (Reproduced with permission; see Figure Credits)

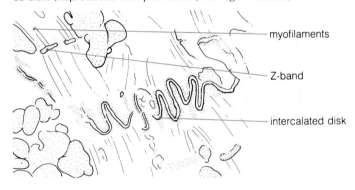

- myofilaments
- Z-band
- intercalated disk

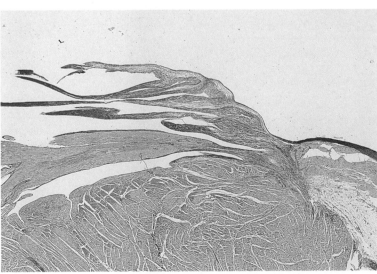

FIGURE 1.40   Histologic section showing the structure of the left atrioventricular junction. Note that the fibrous skeleton supports the leaflet of the mitral valve and insulates the atrial from the ventricular muscle masses. (Reproduced with permission; see Figure Credits)

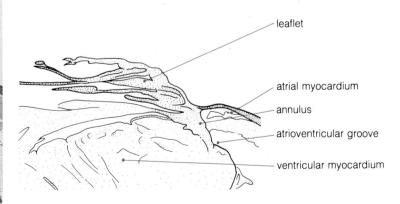

- leaflet
- atrial myocardium
- annulus
- atrioventricular groove
- ventricular myocardium

The coronary arteries are arranged as typical arteries with intima, muscular media, and adventitia (Fig. 1.41). The arterial trunks are characterized by the presence within their walls of multiple elastic lamellae while the arterial duct, during fetal life, is a muscular artery (Fig. 1.42).

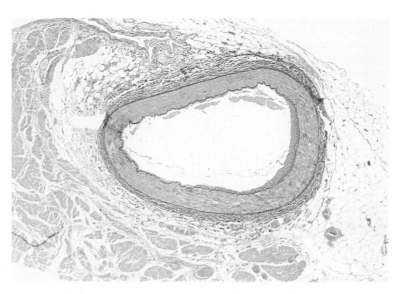

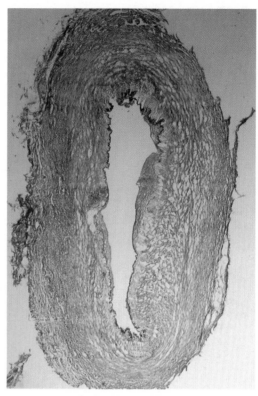

FIGURE 1.42
Cross section of the arterial duct. This duct has the typical muscular arterial arrangement. (Reproduced with permission; see Figure Credits)

FIGURE 1.41 Cross section of a coronary artery showing the typical arterial arrangement with intima, muscular media, and adventitia. (Reproduced with permission; see Figure Credits)

FIGURE CREDITS

Figs. 1.1–1.3, 1.5–1.19, 1.21–1.28, 1.30, 1.36, 1.38–1.42 from Hurst JW: Atlas of the Heart. Gower, New York, 1988.

Figs. 1.4, 1.20, 1.32–1.35, from Anderson RH, Becker AE: Cardiac Anatomy. Churchill Livingstone, Edinburgh, 1980.

Fig. 1.29 from Wilcox BR, Anderson RH: Surgical Anatomy of the Heart. Raven Press, New York, 1985.

Fig. 1.31 from Tawara S: Das Reizleitungssystem des Saugetierherzens. Gustav Fisher, Jena, Germany, 1906.

Figs. 1.33, 1.34, 1.35: Cast prepared by and photograph courtesy of Sally Allwork, PhD,. London, England.

Fig. 1.37 adapted from Anderson RH, Becker AE. Cardiac Anatomy. Churchill Livingstone, Edinburgh, 1980; Schlant RC, Silverman ME: Anatomy of the Heart. In Hurst JW (ed): The Heart, 6th ed. McGraw-Hill, New York, 1986.

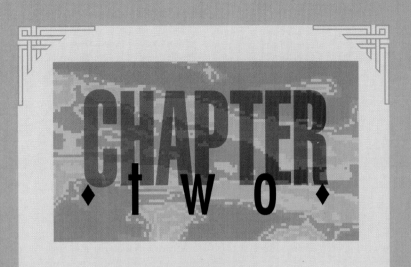

CHAPTER ·two·

MYOCARDIAL REMODELING AND ITS COMPLICATIONS

ANTON E. BECKER, MD

The morphologic mechanisms that underlie remodeling of the heart as an adaptive phenomenon are limited. The cardiac chambers may dilate, often due to an increased volume load, or the myocardial wall may hypertrophy as an expression of increased work load.

Several factors are important when considering the pathophysiologic effects of remodeling. The time available for adaptation plays an important role. For example, adaptation in response to a sudden change in left ventricular volume load, as in a patient with ruptured cords of the mitral valve, differs from adaptation in a patient who develops a gradually progressive mitral insufficiency on the basis of rheumatic heart disease. Heavy chain isozymes of myosin may differ among various forms of remodeling. The adjustment of the capillary network may not necessarily keep pace with myocardial hypertrophy. Moreover, little is known about the role of the fine fibrillar connective tissue meshwork that wraps around individual heart muscle cells, forming a tensile element that resists stretch and provides a restoring force that may cause individual muscle cells to return to their original length after contraction.

Myocardial remodeling therefore is a process that involves many of the elements that normally constitute the heart as a whole, both at the cellular and subcellular levels. Although basically reversible in nature, the adaptive changes may in themselves introduce secondary alterations that render the heart prone to injury.

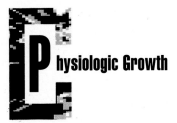

Physiologic Growth

During intrauterine life the heart supports fetal circulation. The myocardium initially develops mainly by cellular multiplication. Functional organization of the myocytes occurs very early during development. At this early stage, cellular enlargement, e.g., increased myocyte diameter and length, becomes an important mechanism contributing to the augmentation of the myocardial mass. Myocardial cellular enlargement is accompanied by growth of capillaries.

In this context two important aspects merit further consideration. During intrauterine development the growing myocardium adapts to the presence of cardiac malformations to guarantee the optimal functional capacity of the heart. Secondly, fetal myocytes also have the capacity to adapt to abnormal circumstances by hypertrophy. This implies not only that myocytes increase their

dimension but also that they expand their cellular organelles, which are responsible for oxygen consumption and adenosine triphosphate synthesis and utilization. Subsystems, such as the vascular network and the fine fibrillar connective tissue support, should also adapt to these changes.

Little is known at present about intrauterine remodeling and its functional implications. Nevertheless, the considerations discussed above imply that the myocardium in a case of congenital malformation may function at a different level from that of a normal heart. This aspect may be important when considering myocardial vulnerability in the postnatal state, such as myocardial susceptibility to hypoxia.

The transition in postnatal myocardial growth from the fetal to the adult circulatory system is accompanied by a progressive increase in volume load affecting both sides of the heart. There is marked increase in pressure load on the left ventricle. The main morphologic counterpart of these functional changes is further enlargement of myocytes, producing a left ventricle that rapidly outgrows the right (Fig. 2.1). At the cellular level the myocyte organelle composition changes rapidly after birth. There is a significant increase in the volume fractions of mitochondria and myofibrils, which reach adult levels shortly after birth, together with a proportional increase in the capacity of the vascular bed.

The normal maturation of myocardium is a well-balanced compensatory response in which the myocytes, including their cellular organelles, and the capillary microvasculature grow in proportion to the work load. As a side effect the compensatory response may render vulnerable the myocardium of hearts with congenital heart malformations.

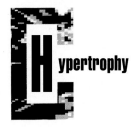

Hypertrophy

Hypertrophy is defined as increased myocardial muscle mass due to enlargement of myocytes (Fig. 2.2). Ultrastructurally the hypertrophied myocyte is characterized mainly by an increase in mitochondria (Fig. 2.3), which are responsible for oxygen consumption and adenosine triphosphate synthesis. Myocardial cell hypertrophy is accompanied by dilation of the main coronary arteries (Fig. 2.4) and expansion of the capillary network in order to maintain adequate oxygen supply. This produces a rise in the total myocardial oxygen consumption demand, which may become highly significant in the clinical setting (see later discussion).

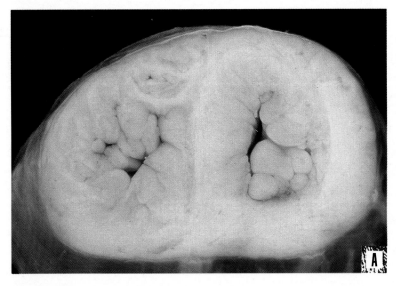

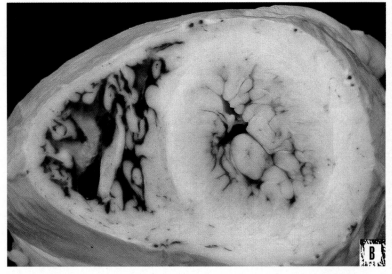

FIGURE 2.1   Cross sections made perpendicular to the long axis of the heart. Specimens from a newborn baby **(A)** and a one-year-old child **(B)**. In the newborn, the thickness of the right and left ventricular wall is about equal, and the interventricular septum is almost straight. In the older infant, the thickness of the left ventricular wall has increased over that of the right ventricle, and the septum is now convex toward the right ventricular cavity. (Reproduced with permission; see Figure Credits)

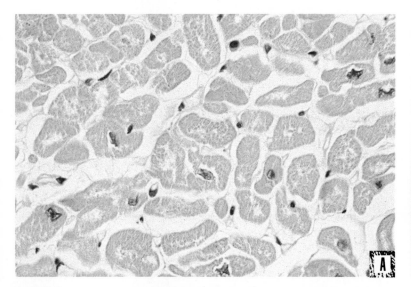

FIGURE 2.2   Histologic sections of normal **(A)** and hypertrophic **(B)** myocardium. The myocardial cells are shown in cross section at the same

magnification. Hypertrophied myocytes are considerably larger than their normal counterparts. (Reproduced with permission; see Figure Credits)

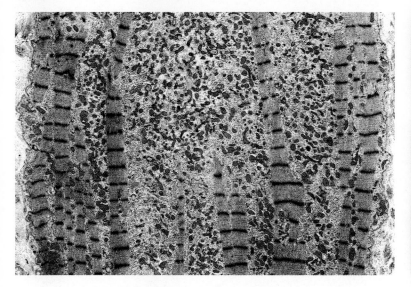

FIGURE 2.3   Electron micrograph of a hypertrophied myocyte with a marked increase in mitochondria. This accommodates for increased demands in oxygen consumption and adenosine triphosphate synthesis. (Reproduced with permission; see Figure Credits)

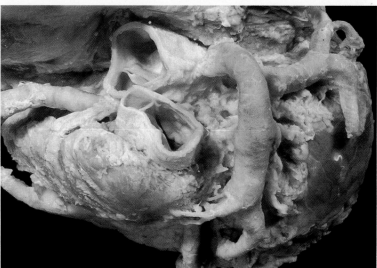

FIGURE 2.4   Superior view of the heart showing the aorta and main coronary arteries. The latter are markedly dilated as an adaptive phenomenon related to myocardial cell hypertrophy. (RCA = right coronary artery; Ao = aorta; PA = pulmonary artery; LCA = left main coronary artery; LCF = left circumflex coronary artery; LAD = left anterior descending coronary artery) (Reproduced with permission; see Figure Credits)

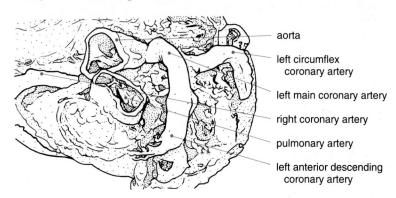

aorta

left circumflex
    coronary artery

left main coronary artery

right coronary artery

pulmonary artery

left anterior descending
    coronary artery

Myocardial hypertrophy often is categorized morphologically as concentric or eccentric. In concentric ventricular hypertrophy the wall thickness is increased without chamber enlargement. Such a response is encountered in patients with compensated pressure load hypertrophy of the left ventricle (Fig. 2.5). Eccentric ventricular hypertrophy is marked by a hypertrophic wall associated with an enlarged chamber volume, although the ratio between ventricular volume and wall thickness remains unaltered (Fig. 2.6). This arrangement is often encountered in compensated volume load hypertrophy of the left ventricle, e.g., aortic regurgitation.

PRESSURE LOAD HYPERTROPHY

The classic conditions producing pressure load hypertrophy of the left ventricle include systemic hypertension, aortic coarctation, and aortic valve stenosis (see Fig. 2.5B). Right ventricular pressure load may be due to pulmonary valve stenosis, disease of the left side of the heart (with heart failure), or primary pulmonary disease. Pulmonary vascular resistance is increased in the latter two examples.

An increase in pressure load induces concentric ventricular hypertrophy as previously defined. The degree of myocyte hypertrophy differs in the various layers of the myocardium, although the overall effect is an increase in wall thickness. The thicker wall counteracts the elevated systolic pressures and the potentially high peak systolic wall stress according to Laplace's law (Fig. 2.7).

Growth adaptation is accompanied by hyperplasia of myofibrillar units and initially exceeds myofibrillar growth. Eventually there is a reduction of the mitochondrial-to-myofibrillar volume ratio. A critical perimitochondrial radius, which is necessary to supply adenosine triphosphate to the contractile proteins, may become a limiting factor in myocardial adaptation. This ultimately may impair the energy supply and compromise myocardial function. The capillary bed then increases concomitantly with the increase in dimension of myocytes. In these instances the perfusion of heart muscle increases in proportion to the mass of muscle and the work it must perform. Lack of microvascular adaptation may severely impair myocardial function.

VOLUME LOAD HYPERTROPHY

Adaptation to exercise, particularly in dynamic forms of conditioning as seen in endurance athletics (running or swimming), may be accompanied by an elevated preload and eccentric hypertrophy as a compensatory mechanism. Examples of pathologic conditions that cause volume load hypertrophy of the left ventricle are aortic and mitral valve regurgitation (see Fig. 2.6B).

Structurally, volume load hypertrophy consists of chamber enlargement and accompanying myocardial hypertrophy, expressed mainly as increased myocyte length. The latter counteracts the increased end-diastolic wall stress by accommodating the enlarged chamber volume that otherwise may lead to spatial

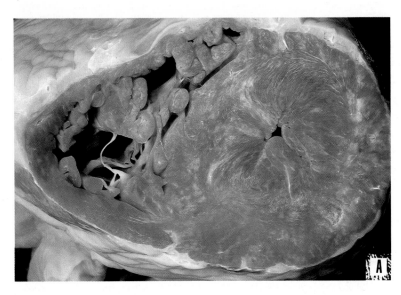

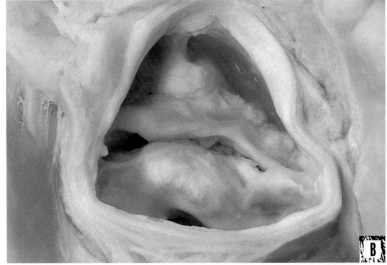

FIGURE 2.5 Cross sections through a heart with isolated aortic stenosis. **(A)** Concentric ventricular hypertrophy is characterized by an increase in wall thickness without chamber enlargement. **(B)** A calcified and stenotic congenitally bicuspid aortic valve. (Reproduced with permission; see Figure Credits)

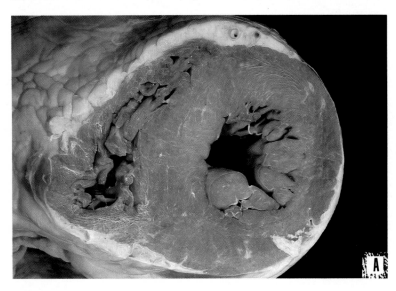

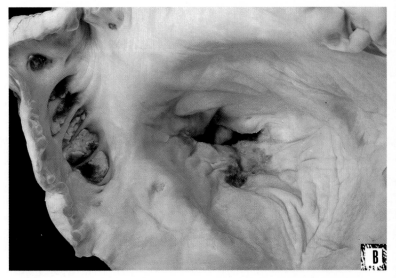

FIGURE 2.6 **(A)** Cross section through a heart with eccentric ventricular hypertrophy. Note increased wall thickness in the presence of an enlarged chamber volume. The ratio between ventricular volume and wall thickness remains unaltered. **(B)** Left atrial view of the regurgitant mitral valve. (Reproduced with permission; see Figure Credits)

rearrangement and lateral slippage of the myocytes (see Fig. 2.7). The volume fractions of mitochondria and myofibrils remain almost constant. This may constitute the morphologic counterpart for the normal or improved contractile and relaxation properties of the myocardium.

Moderate exercise hypertrophy is associated with expansion of the capillary network in proportion to the increased muscle mass. In contrast, there is evidence that strenuous exercise may be accompanied by inadequate capillary compensation, thus jeopardizing oxygen supply to the myocardium.

Hence, excessive volume load hypertrophy may lead to a state in which the myocardium is more susceptible to ischemia than expected from hypertrophy alone.

▓▓▓ REACTIVE HYPERTROPHY

The classic examples of this form of myocardial remodeling are ischemic cardiomyopathy and myocardial infarction (Fig. 2.8). Under these circumstances muscle cells are lost, either diffusely or focally, and replaced by scar tissue.

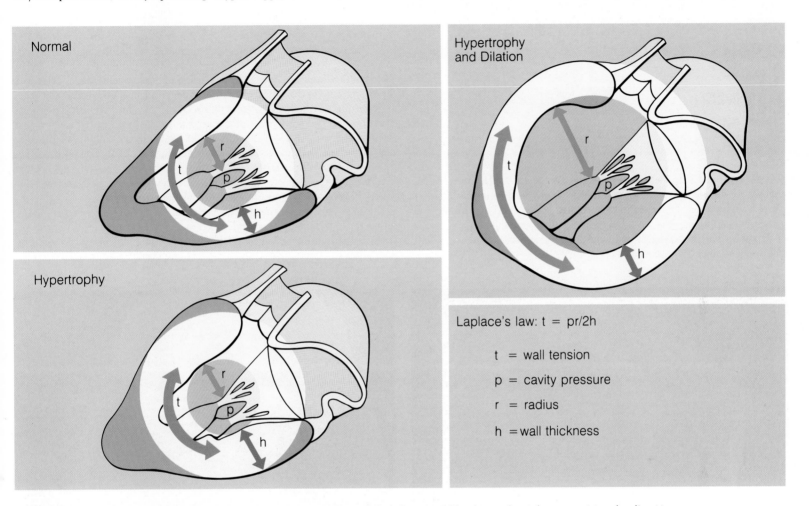

FIGURE 2.7   Laplace's law: the load on the myocytes (wall tension = t) is determined by the product of pressure (p) and radius (r), divided by twice the wall thickness (h). (Reproduced with permission; see Figure Credits)

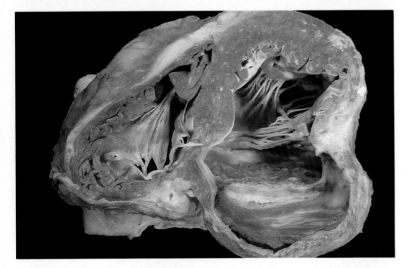

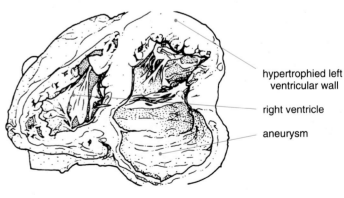

FIGURE 2.8   Cross section of heart with a left ventricular inferior wall aneurysm filled with thrombus due to previous myocardial infarction. There is marked reactive hypertrophy of the remaining viable left ventricular myocardium. (Reproduced with permission; see Figure Credits)

Compensatory hypertrophy of viable myocytes occurs, probably proportionally to the amount of myocardial cell loss. Under the given circumstances the ability of the myocardium to become hypertrophic is largely determined by the underlying vascular obstructive disease. In general myocytes will increase in mean diameter while the mitochondrial-to-myofibrillar volume ratio remains constant in proportion to cell growth. Depending on the extent of myocardial cell loss, however, the ventricle may suffer chronic volume overload and subsequent lengthening of myocytes may occur. Moreover, the capillary vascular response to infarction lags behind the adaptive growth of the myocytes. Hence, the hypertrophied infarcted ventricle is more vulnerable to subsequent ischemic episodes.

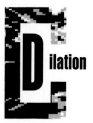

Dilation

Dilation is defined as an increase in the volume of the cardiac chamber. Sudden changes in volume load affecting a chamber usually lead to instant dilation. Chronic dilation may be related to compensated volume load hypertrophy (see above) or heart failure (Fig. 2.9). Depending on the cause dilation may resolve or persist, either as a compensated adjustment or as part of chronic volume overload with impaired hemodynamics.

Complications of Myocardial Remodeling

Hypertrophy of myocardium and dilation of cardiac chambers induced as compensatory mechanisms may ultimately set the scene for secondary complications.

Dilation of a ventricular chamber, whether acute or chronic, may initiate papillary muscle dysfunction and, hence, mitral regurgitation (see Fig. 2.9). The latter condition itself causes further remodeling of the left ventricle, as evidenced by enlargement of the ventricular chamber due to augmented volume load.

Hypertrophy, whether concentric or eccentric, may affect ventricular geometry. This becomes particularly pronounced in cases of marked right ventricular hypertrophy with chamber dilation. In this circumstance, the interventricular septum assumes an almost straight configuration (Fig. 2.10). The reverse situation, an extreme hypertrophy of the left ventricular wall with a bulging septum transforming the geometry of the right ventricle, is known as Bernstein's disease, which may be a cause of right ventricular impairment.

The most important consequences of the aforementioned compensatory mechanisms relate to impaired myocardial perfusion. Marked volume load of the left ventricle with distinct chamber dilation in the setting of eccentric hypertrophy may affect the transmural perfusion pressure and may lead to impaired oxygena-

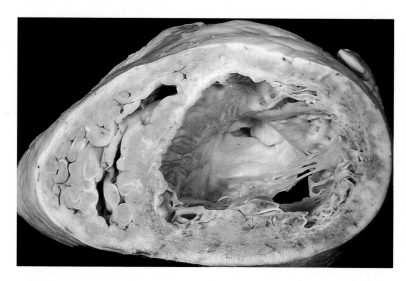

FIGURE 2.9   Cross section of a heart with marked increase in left ventricular chamber volume as an expression of chronic ischemia leading to a failing heart. Chronic dilation under these circumstances may lead to papillary muscle dysfunction and mitral regurgitation. The latter in itself may further jeopardize myocardial perfusion, which may aggravate left heart failure already present. (Reproduced with permission; see Figure Credits)

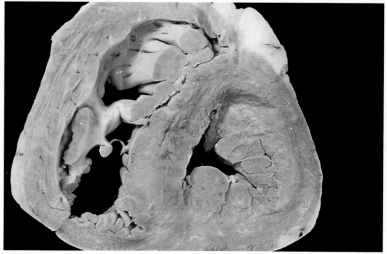

FIGURE 2.10   Cross section through a heart with marked right ventricular hypertrophy and right ventricular chamber dilation. Note an almost straight configuration of the interventricular septum, thereby affecting left ventricular geometry. (Reproduced with permission; see Figure Credits)

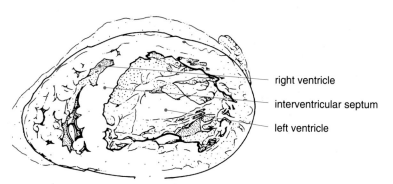

right ventricle

interventricular septum

left ventricle

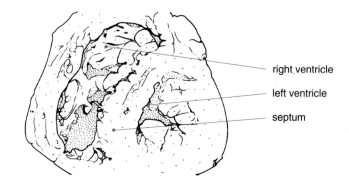

right ventricle

left ventricle

septum

tion of the subendocardial myocardial layers. This phenomenon is particularly prone to occur when volume load and dilation coexist with obstructive coronary artery disease (Fig. 2.11). Hence, compensated chronic volume load hypertrophy may ultimately transform into a diseased state consequent to myocardial ischemia. Once induced, this process will further aggravate the impairment of myocardial perfusion by further dilation of the ventricular chamber; this allows increased end-diastolic left ventricular volume and concomitant increased pressure (Fig. 2.12). The consideration that volume load hypertrophy due to strenuous exercise may not necessarily be compensated by adequate adaptation of the microvasculature makes this sequence of events more likely.

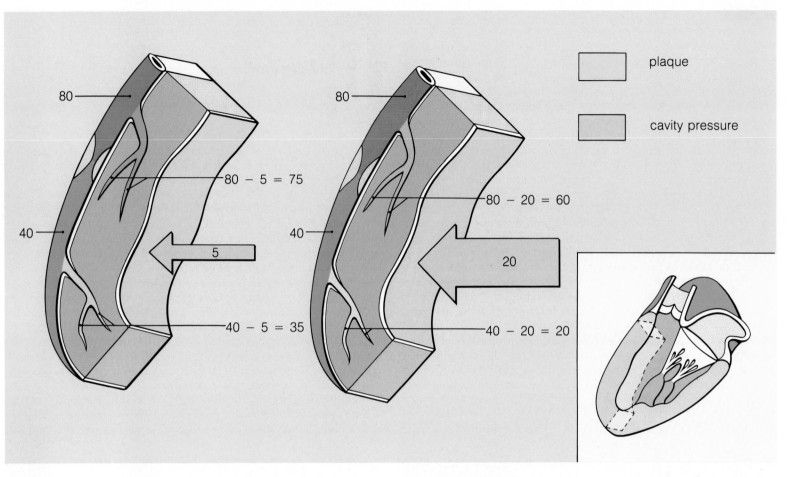

FIGURE 2.11 Interaction between myocardial perfusion and intracavitary and diastolic pressures in the presence of an obstructive coronary artery lesion. Elevated end-diastolic pressure may lead to impaired subendocardial perfusion of the left ventricular myocardium; ischemia and infarction may result. (Reproduced with permission; see Figure Credits)

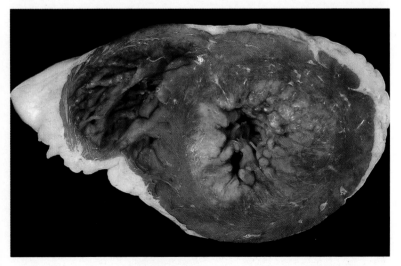

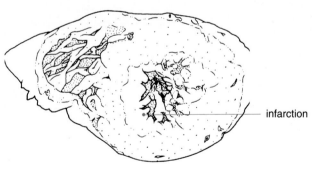

FIGURE 2.12 Cross section through a heart with impairment of left ventricular subendocardial perfusion and circumferential infarction. The infarction was caused by increased end-diastolic left ventricular pressure with chamber dilation in the setting of critical obstructive coronary artery lesions. (Reproduced with permission; see Figure Credits)

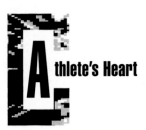

Athlete's Heart

The term *athlete's heart* is used to describe the cardiac effects of long-term conditioning as it occurs in highly trained competitive athletes. Enlargement of the heart is the most important feature from a morphologic viewpoint. The enlargement is due to hypertrophy of the myocardial wall, particularly in the left ventricle, and enlargement of the ventricular cavities. These features are easily demonstrated with cross-sectional echocardiography. Particularly in endurance athletes, such as marathon runners, cavity dimension is increased almost constantly. The hypertrophy of the left ventricular wall under such conditions is symmetric and the compensatory conditioning may well be summarized as eccentric hypertrophy. Occasionally an asymmetric pattern of left ventricular hypertrophy may ensue. The absolute thickening of the septum is usually minimal and the echocardiographic septal/free wall ratio remains below one to three. This suggests disproportionate septal thickening rather than asymmetric septal hypertrophy as part of hypertrophic cardiomyopathy (see Chapter 8). Nevertheless, once noticed, this particular aspect should always be carefully evaluated.

It remains speculative whether the type of exercise is important with respect to the changes in cardiac structure. It has been demonstrated that athletes participating in dynamic endurance sports are exposed primarily to conditions producing a volume load and thus develop eccentric hypertrophy. On the other hand, athletes involved in sports that are primarily static, such as weight lifting, are conditioned to produce primarily a pressure load hypertrophy. In view of these considerations, one may expect that endurance athletes will be more prone to secondary myocardial complications, at least when additional pathologic circumstances, such as obstructive coronary artery disease, are present. Indeed, sudden death in competitive athletes is almost always caused by additional cardiovascular abnormalities which may have passed unnoticed clinically. Nevertheless, one may occasionally encounter instances of sudden death in athletes where no addi-

tional abnormalities can be detected other than chamber enlargement and myocardial hypertrophy without obstructive coronary disease. In some of these instances the heart shows extensive fibrosis and, occasionally, definite scars, indicating previous infarction clinically unrecognized (Fig. 2.13). In other cases, however, there is no detectable abnormality and the mechanisms underlying sudden death remain unclear.

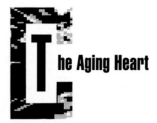

The Aging Heart

The increased longevity of humans in the western world has led to interest in geriatric cardiology. The myocardium of the elderly may be expected to atrophy unless other circumstances prevail to induce compensatory changes. As such, systemic hypertension is a frequent disorder, and a substantial number of elderly patients have myocardial hypertrophy on that basis. With increasing age, moreover, major abnormalities can occur in the fibrous tissues that constitute the cardiac skeleton, including the cardiac valves. In elderly patients, therefore, morphologic abnormalities of the valves, particularly of the aortic and mitral valves, are the rule rather than the exception.

In a significant proportion of patients these alterations are functionally important although not necessarily clinically manifest. Not infrequently, severe isolated calcific aortic stenosis with colossal myocardial hypertrophy is detected at autopsy. This can underscore sudden death in an elderly patient in whom the valve abnormality was never apparent clinically. Likewise, a calcified mitral ring may induce mitral valve regurgitation and volume load hypertrophy of the left ventricle that, in the presence of obstructive coronary artery disease, may easily lead to myocardial ischemia, infarction, and death.

At a cellular level, it is still uncertain whether the adaptive phenomena are equal in children and adults. Such features may nonetheless prove to be important in the future for better understanding of the pathophysiology in this category of patients.

![Cross section of heart specimen]

FIGURE 2.13　　Cross section through the heart of an endurance athlete with left ventricular chamber dilation and hypertrophy of the left ventricular wall. There is extensive almost circular and band-like scarring of the left ventricular myocardium without evidence of obstructive coronary artery disease. (Reproduced with permission; see Figure Credits)

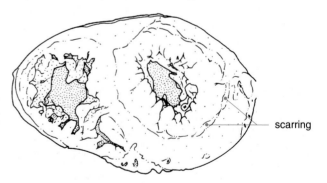

scarring

ACKNOWLEDGMENTS

This chapter is based in part on Becker AE, Anderson RH: Cardiac adaptation and its sequelae. In Cardiac Pathology. Edinburgh, Churchill Livingstone, 1983; Anversa P, et al: Quantitative structural analysis of the myocardium during physiologic growth and induced cardiac hypertrophy: A review. J Am Coll Cardiol 7:1140, 1986; Maron BJ, Epstein SE (eds): Symposium on the athlete heart. J Am Coll Cardiol 7:189, 1986.

FIGURE CREDITS

Figs. 2.1, 2.4–2.6, 2.8, 2.10, 2.12, 2.13 from Hurst JW (ed): Atlas of the Heart. Gower, New York, 1988.

Figs. 2.2, 2.3, 2.7, 2.9, and 2.11 from Becker AE, Anderson RH: Cardiac adaptation and its sequelae. In Cardiac Pathology. Edinburgh, Raven Press, 1983. Figs. 2.7 and 2.11 have been redrawn. Fig. 2.3 courtesy of Dr. KP Dingemans.

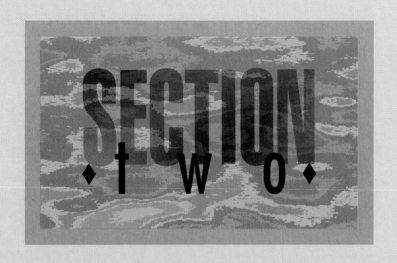

SECTION
·two·

DISORDERS OF THE CARDIOVASCULAR SYSTEM

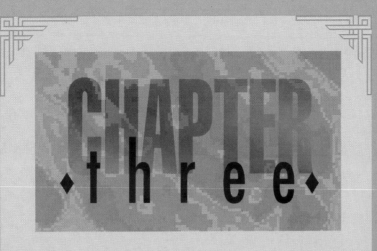

CHAPTER three

PART ONE:
HEART FAILURE

A. JAMES BRADLEY, MD
JOSEPH S. ALPERT, MD

PART TWO:
HIGH OUTPUT
HEART FAILURE

CARL V. LEIER, MD
HARISIOS BOUDOULAS, MD

Congestive heart failure is a complex clinical entity in which an abnormality in cardiac function is responsible for failure of the heart to deliver blood at a rate sufficient to meet the demands of metabolizing tissues or to function at normal filling pressures. Heart failure may result from many types of cardiac disease and, as such, does not lend itself to simple definitions. Congestive heart failure should be regarded as a constellation of signs and symptoms with a diversity of etiologies. Cardiac output may be low, normal (as in diastolic dysfunction), or elevated (as in high output cardiac failure). Most patients, however, demonstrate reduced left ventricular systolic function.

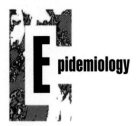

Epidemiology

In the United States, heart failure is responsible for approximately 497,000 hospital admissions and 4.8 million hospital days annually. Despite research advances and insights into the pathophysiology of heart failure in the past decade, congestive heart failure portends an overall poor prognosis, with less than 50% of patients surviving 5 years after diagnosis. In addition, there is a strong correlation of heart failure with advancing age; up to 80% of patients are over 60 years of age. The Framingham study suggests a prevalence of heart failure of 1% in persons between 50 and 59 years of age and 10% in persons 80 to 89 years of age. Based on physician surveys, the U.S. census, and projections from the Framingham study, over 2 million persons in the United States currently carry the diagnosis of heart failure. The incidence of cardiac failure in men exceeds that in women at all ages, presumably because of the higher incidence of coronary atherosclerotic heart disease in men. Heart failure remains the primary diagnosis-related group for in-patients over the age of 65 and contributes to the almost $100 billion cost of treating heart disease each year in the United States.

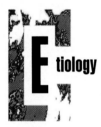

Etiology

Heart failure should be differentiated from circulatory failure: the former is due to an intrinsic abnormality of the heart whereas the latter may be due to an abnormality of any component of the circulation, including the heart, vascular bed, or blood volume. These syndromes are often interrelated, such as in hypertensive crisis with an excessively high peripheral resistance leading to left ventricular dysfunction, in hypovolemia secondary to blood loss leading to inadequate cardiac output, or even in hypovolemic shock in the presence of an otherwise normal heart.

Heart failure encompasses a wide range of conditions that have varying etiologies, prognoses, and therapeutic implications. Differentiation between predominant systolic and diastolic dysfunction and low and high cardiac output states is critical to selection of the appropriate management. The majority of patients with symptoms of heart failure have impaired left ventricular systolic function, a dysfunction discussed in detail later in this chapter.

The causes of heart failure are diverse, with many possible etiologies (Fig. 3.1). Over 75% of patients with the diagnosis of congestive heart failure in the Framingham study, however, were noted to have either hypertension or coronary atherosclerotic heart disease. Heart failure in patients with coronary atherosclerotic heart disease without hypertension occurred in only 10% of patients. Risk for development of heart failure has been shown in patients with diastolic or isolated systolic hypertension.

DIABETES

Diabetes was present in 16% of patients with heart failure in the Framingham study, with greater incidence in women than in men. Diabetes remained a significant independent risk factor in the multivariate analysis for the development of heart failure, apart from the increased risk of developing coronary atherosclerosis. Pathologic studies reveal small coronary artery involvement in up to 70% of diabetic hearts with endothelial proliferation, subendothelial fibrosis, hyaline deposition, and atheromatous involvement similar to the microangiopathy seen elsewhere in the body. Involvement of the intramural myocardial circulation may impair both systolic and diastolic myocardial function leading to the "small stiff heart" syndrome seen in diabetic patients, and eventually to pulmonary edema.

VALVULAR HEART DISEASE

Following the decline and control of rheumatic fever over the past several decades, valvular heart disease has decreased dramatically as a cause of chronic heart failure. Valvular heart disease currently accounts for 10% or fewer of patients referred to medical centers for heart failure management. The development of congestive heart failure is dependent upon the severity and duration of the valvular abnormality. Heart failure may occur when compensatory mechanisms are overwhelmed (e.g., in chronic aortic insufficiency with progressive left ventricular dilatation), or when compensatory mechanisms have not had sufficient time to develop (e.g., in acute aortic insufficiency with infective endocarditis). The recognition of valvular disease in patients with congestive heart failure is important, as correction of valvular abnormalities occurring before irreversible myocardial decompensation may alleviate the heart failure—one of the few potentially correctable instances of congestive heart failure.

Mitral regurgitation alone seldom produces a left ventricular ejection fraction <0.40. Mitral regurgitation is present in as many as two thirds of patients with dilated cardiomyopathy and is usually of mild or moderate severity. A dilated cardiomyopathy, as opposed to primary mitral valvular disease, should be considered when mitral regurgitation is present with a markedly depressed left ventricular ejection fraction.

DILATED CARDIOMYOPATHY

Dilated cardiomyopathy refers to a group of disorders in which the myocardium is diseased in a diffuse or multifocal fashion. Dilated cardiomyopathy is characterized by a reduction of the left ventricular ejection fraction, as well as reductions in ventricular and often atrial dilatation. This group of disorders causes symptoms of heart failure primarily through a reduction in systolic performance. Symptoms are not generally seen until the left ventricular ejection fraction falls below 0.40. The most common cause of dilated cardiomyopathy in the United States and Europe is coronary atherosclerotic heart disease with multiple areas of infarction. Wall motion abnormalities develop together with left ventricular dilatation and reduced left ventricular ejection fraction. Some authorities object to the inclusion of ischemic cardiomyopathy within the category of dilated cardiomyopathy. However, the prognosis for ischemic cardiomyopathy is thought to be similar to that for idiopathic dilated cardiomyopathy, with only 40% to 50% of patients surviving 5 years after diagnosis. Treatment tends to be similar as well; selected patients should be considered for cardiac transplantation.

Idiopathic dilated cardiomyopathy may have a variety of causes, since it is the common expression of diverse myocardial afflictions. Endocrinologic, nutritional, chemical, and immunologic causes have been suggested as possible etiologic factors. The progression of viral myocarditis to dilated cardiomyopathy has gained wide acceptance as a pathogenic source of this entity. An inflammatory infiltrate is frequently, but variably, reported in the early course of the illness, and immunologic abnormalities have been detected in some patients with dilated cardiomyopathy (e.g., abnormalities of T-cell subsets and circulating antibodies to myocardium). Pathologic examination of myocardial biopsy specimens reveals interstitial fibrosis, cellular enlargement, myocardial cell degeneration, and occasionally an inflammatory infiltrate with lymphocyte predominance. An aberrant or on-going immune response may occur after viral myocarditis with eventual progression to cardiomyopathy. Most patients with dilated cardiomyopathy have no clear history of viral myocarditis, however, and no single virus has been identified with any frequency. Common cardiomyopathic viruses include Coxsackie viruses A and B, echovirus, and polio virus.

Nonviral infections of the myocardium may lead to heart failure and cardiomyopathy as well. *Toxoplasma gondi* produces sporadic cases of dilated cardiomyopathy. *Trypanosoma cruzi* is responsible for Chagas disease and is found almost exclusively in Central and South America. The parasite is transmitted via triatoma insects and leads to an acute illness in only 1% of those infected. Thirty percent of those infected have signs of cardiac disease after a latent period of 20 to 30 years. Patients with Chagas disease commonly have electrocardiographic changes, such as right bundle branch block, bilateral bundle branch block (or atrioventricular first-, second-, and/or third-degree block), various arrhythmias, or heart failure secondary to a dilated cardiomyopathy. Immunologic factors have been implicated in the chronic form of the disease. It is estimated that over 3 million people in Central and South America have electrocardiographic or clinical evidence of chronic myocardial involvement.

Two forms of dilated cardiomyopathy deserve specific attention: alcoholic cardiomyopathy and peripartum cardiomyopathy. Both of these entities have a favorable prognosis in contrast to idiopathic dilated cardiomyopathy. Alcohol is a direct myocardial toxin and is known to depress contractility through a variety of metabolic derangements. Abstinence from alcohol can result in an improvement in left ventricular function, and some studies have reported a 4-year survival rate of up to 80% of patients. The propensity for improvement with abstinence is in contradistinction to idiopathic dilated cardiomyopathy. Failure to abstain from alcohol results in a grim prognosis, with survival curves similar to those for patients with idiopathic dilated cardiomyopathy. Nutritional defects secondary to alcoholism, particularly thiamine deficiency, may lead to myocardial damage as well. Cobalt was at one time added by brewers to beer to stabilize the foam, leading to a toxic cardiomyopathy termed *beer-drinker's cardiomyopathy*. No cases have been reported since brewers ceased using cobalt as an additive.

Peripartum cardiomyopathy typically presents in the last month of pregnancy or within 6 months of delivery. Histologic features are indistinguishable from those of other causes of cardiomyopathy; a mononuclear cell infiltrate is often seen. Although an immunologic basis for the cardiomyopathy is presumed, 50% of patients have a history of hypertension. Two outcomes are common: (1) in approximately 50% of individuals, the heart size and function may return to normal within 6 months, with a high likelihood of long-term survival, or (2) patients may follow a course similar to that of idiopathic dilated cardiomyopathy.

A number of other etiologies may lead to dilated cardiomyopathy, including toxins; medications such as the anthracyclin derivatives (including doxorubicin); metabolic disorders such as uremia, hypophosphatemia, hypocalcemia and pheochromocytoma; infiltrative diseases such as sarcoidosis, hemochromatosis, and amyloidosis; and endocrine disorders such as thyroid disease.

DIASTOLIC LEFT VENTRICULAR DYSFUNCTION

Thirty to forty percent of patients who present with classic symptoms of heart failure are subsequently found to have normal left ventricular systolic function (left ventricular ejection fraction >0.45). Diastolic dysfunction is the predominant abnormality in this subset of patients. Diastolic filling is an energy-dependent process requiring adenosine triphosphate. Abnormal diastolic filling may result from myocardial cell energy depletion and incomplete relaxation, as in coronary atherosclerotic heart disease. A number of variables affect diastolic filling, including preload, heart rate, size of the left ventricular chamber, wall thickness, compliance properties of the myocardium, and presence of pericardial disease. Many symptoms of heart failure are due to abnormal myocardial diastolic properties with a resultant abnormally steep diastolic ventricular pressure–volume curve, resulting in high left ventricular filling pressures. This may produce pulmonary congestion similar to that observed with abnormalities of systolic function.

Many of the clinical manifestations of heart failure are more closely related to diastolic than to systolic properties of the myocardium. Several studies have shown that a resting left ventricular ejection fraction does not necessarily predict treadmill exercise duration in patients with symptoms of heart failure. In addition, diastolic dysfunction often precedes the development of systolic dysfunction and may be an important clinical marker for early coronary atherosclerotic heart disease and/or hypertensive heart disease.

The major causes of heart failure without demonstrable systolic dysfunction are ischemic heart disease and disorders that result in myocardial hypertrophy, particularly hypertension and hypertrophic cardiomyopathy. Other causes of abnormal diastolic function include restrictive cardiomyopathy and infiltrative diseases, uremia, valvular disease, and pericardial disease such as constrictive pericarditis. A distinction should be made between patients with predominant systolic failure and those with abnormal diastolic function. Despite similar symptoms and degrees of exercise intolerance in such patients, therapeutic and prognostic implications differ markedly.

HIGH OUTPUT HEART FAILURE

The final group of disorders that may lead to heart failure are those associated with an abnormally high cardiac output. These disorders are discussed in detail in the second part of this chapter.

FIGURE 3.1 PRINCIPLE CAUSES OF HEART FAILURE

CORONARY ATHEROSCLEROTIC HEART DISEASE

MYOCARDITIS

VALVULAR HEART DISEASE

PERICARDIAL DISEASE

CARDIOMYOPATHY
Idiopathic dilated
Infiltrative
Toxic
Endocrine   **HYPERTENSION**
Nutritional
Infectious
Hypersensitivity
Postpartum
Alcohol-induced
Hypertrophic
Neuromuscular
Radiation-induced
Metabolic
Restrictive

HYPERTENSION

ALTERED CARDIAC RHYTHM OR CONDUCTION

PRESBYCARDIA

HIGH OUTPUT CARDIAC STATES

Pathophysiology of Heart Failure Secondary to Left Ventricular Dysfunction

In considering the patient with heart failure, a distinction is commonly made between forward heart failure (i.e., a reduced forward flow of blood from the left ventricle) and backward heart failure (i.e., an increase in left atrial pressure that results from impaired left ventricular function). The former leads to fatigue and symptoms related to poor tissue perfusion, whereas the latter causes symptoms of pulmonary congestion, which include dyspnea, orthopnea, and pulmonary edema. Forward and backward failure generally coexist to some degree in the patient with heart failure, although one component may predominate. These hemodynamic alterations are helpful in conceptualizing heart failure but ultimately the pathogenesis of heart failure occurs at the cellular level, where complex derangements are present in the structure and function of myocardial cells.[2]

The myocyte is incapable of cell division following neonatal life; myocytes enlarge by hypertrophy as a compensatory mechanism in early heart failure. New sarcomeres are added within the myocyte, thereby decreasing the amount of energy expenditure required by an individual sarcomere. However, myocyte enlargement is associated with increased cytoplasmic volume and increased dis-

tance between capillaries, which may impair the supply of oxygen and nutrients required for energy expenditure by the hypertrophied heart. Moreover, an increased number of myofibrils are supplied by a decreased number of mitochondria. An imbalance of energy production and energy expenditure may subject the heart to chronic work overload. Eventually, cellular exhaustion, or "the cardiomyopathy of overload," occurs. Later, myocyte necrosis may result with fibroblast infiltration and production of collagen, leading to cardiosclerosis and ultimately left ventricular dilatation.

A number of alterations in the function and cellular energetics of the myocyte develop in response to chronic hemodynamic overload. The myocardial contractile state is closely coupled to cellular energetics. Myocyte contraction is stimulated by cellular membrane depolarization, resulting in the release of calcium from the sarcolemma into the myoplasm. This triggers an interaction between actin and myosin that, in the presence of adenosine triphosphate, leads to a contractile state with shortening and the development of force. Relaxation occurs with reaccumulation of calcium ions by the sarcolemma and repolarization of the cellular membrane by calcium and sodium ion pumps, respectively, both of which are ATP dependent. Therefore, myocyte contraction and relaxation are both energy-dependent processes.[1]

Abnormalities in these processes result in the abnormal contractile and diastolic function which can be seen in chronic heart failure. Although our knowledge of altered myocyte energetics in heart failure is still incomplete, a number of cellular alterations have been reported: (1) myosin ATPase is decreased along with altered myocyte protein isoforms (including myosin, actin, and tropomyosin); (2) reduced concentrations of calcium pump ATPase in the sarcoplasmic reticulum membrane may lead to impaired relaxation; (3) levels of myocar-

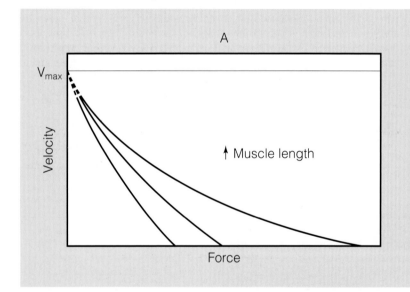

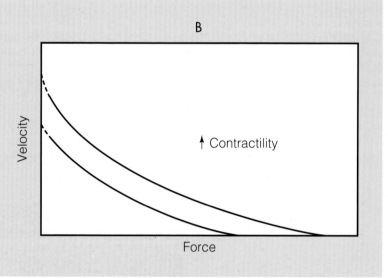

FIGURE 3.2 **(A)** Representative force–velocity relations in isolated heart muscle at three different muscle lengths. **(B)** Representative changes in the force–velocity relation following an increase in contractile state. (Reproduced with permission; see Figure Credits)

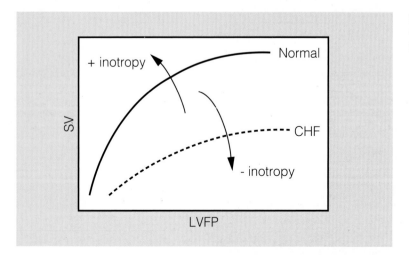

FIGURE 3.3 Frank Starling left ventricular function curve relating left ventricular filling pressure (LVFP) to stroke volume (SV) in both normal and failing hearts.

dial norepinephrine stores are reduced; and (4) an imbalance occurs of inhibitory and stimulatory G proteins, which couple receptor stimulation by a variety of hormones and neurotransmitters to the intracellular production of second messenger systems such as cyclic AMP. These cellular and molecular abnormalities are at present incompletely understood but appear to underlie the myocardial dysfunction that ultimately produces many of the symptoms and signs of chronic heart failure.

Both chronic pressure overload and chronic volume overload lead to depressed myocardial contractility. Depression of the velocity of isotonic shortening of heart muscle, an increase in the duration of time to peak muscle tension, a slowed rate of force development (dP/dt), and a decrease in isometric contraction have been observed in the in vivo heart and in vitro heart muscle preparations. These changes can be demonstrated by means of the length–tension curve (Fig. 3.2), in which muscle length is plotted against developed muscle tension. In cardiac muscle, as in all forms of striated muscle, actively developed tension (force of contraction) is a function of initial muscle length. The force placed on the muscle to stretch it to its initial length is termed *preload*. A preload can be determined for a muscle at which a maximal force of contraction is produced. The ascending limb of the curve is defined as the length–tension relation below the optimal preload; the descending limb is the length, or preload, above the optimally determined length. Studies reveal that the failing heart functions on the ascending limb of a depressed length–tension curve rather than on the descending limb of a normal curve.[2]

The tension at a given myocardial fiber length, or end-diastolic volume, is reduced in failing hearts compared with normal hearts. An elevated left ventricular end diastolic volume is therefore necessary to develop a force of contraction equivalent to that of a normal heart with a normal end-diastolic volume. This principle underscores the benefit of compensatory left ventricular dilatation in patients with heart failure as homeostatic mechanisms seek to preserve the force of myocardial contraction. This dilatation occurs at the expense of increased left ventricular end-diastolic volume and pressure. However, sarcomere length, as measured by electron microscopy, is not increased in muscle from failing hearts. Ventricular dilatation results from the addition of sarcomeres in series to myocytes.

Depression of contractility appears to be an intrinsic property of the failing heart muscle itself. Force of contraction, at the expense of elevated end-diastolic volume, is maintained through ventricular dilatation in early heart failure. Starling's Law states, "the mechanical energy set free on passage from the resting to the contracted state is a function of the length of the muscle fiber." This applies to beat-to-beat variation in contractility seen at various preloads rather than to the chronic compensatory left ventricular dilatation that occurs with chronic heart failure.

A Starling curve relates preload to left ventricular performance. Preload, as noted earlier, is analogous to left ventricular end-diastolic wall tension and is a principal determinant of resting sarcomere length. End-diastolic volume and pressure, however, may not bear a predictable relation to wall tension, particularly in chronic heart failure. Figure 3.3 demonstrates a Starling curve relating stroke volume to left ventricular filling pressure. Stroke volume rises as left ventricular filling pressure increases on the ascending limb of the curve. The depressed curve observed in heart failure is associated with a reduced stroke volume for any particular left ventricular filling pressure. These curves may be shifted up or down by positive and negative inotropic stimuli. The existence of a descending limb of the Starling curve is controversial.

Contractility, heart rate, and afterload, in addition to preload, are important determinants of cardiac performance. Afterload is the tension or wall stress within the ventricular wall that is present during systolic shortening of muscle. Stroke volume generally declines with increasing afterload, though stroke volume is also dependent on the preload and contractile state of the ventricle.

Pressure–volume loops provide another way of examining cardiac dynamics in heart failure (Fig. 3.4). In the normal heart (Fig. 3.4A), contraction begins at point A and ends at point C. Point A to point B represents a change in pressure without a change in volume, or isovolumic contraction. Point B to point C represents the ejection phase, and point C represents end-systolic pressure–volume. Diastole commences with isovolumic relaxation (point C to point D) and ends with diastolic filling (point D to point A). The upper curve represents the isovolumic pressure–volume relation for the ventricle; it may be shifted up or down by positive or negative inotropic influences. The lower curve represents the diastolic pressure–volume curve.

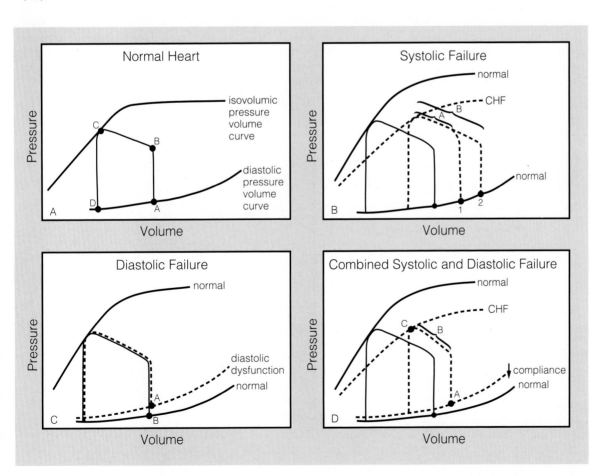

FIGURE 3.4 Pressure–volume diagrams. **(A)** Normal heart. **(B)** Systolic failure. **(C)** Diastolic failure. **(D)** Combined systolic and diastolic failure. (See text for explanation.)

The pressure–volume relation in a ventricle with depressed contractility is shown in Figure 3.4B. Despite an elevated end-diastolic volume at point 1, stroke volume A is reduced compared with the normal heart. Stroke volume may be restored to normal (B), but only at the expense of a further increase in end-diastolic volume (point 2). The pressure–volume relation associated with pure diastolic dysfunction (Fig. 3.4C) shows a shift upward of the diastolic pressure–volume curve, reflecting a decrease in diastolic compliance. Left ventricular end-diastolic pressure is elevated (point A) at any given end-diastolic volume compared with a normal heart (point B).

As noted previously, both systolic and diastolic dysfunction commonly coexist in the patient with heart failure (Fig. 3.4D). In the heart with systolic and diastolic dysfunction, left ventricular end-diastolic pressure and volume (point A) are elevated compared with the normal heart. Stroke volume (line B) is reduced, end-systolic volume (point C) is elevated, and diastolic filling is accomplished at a higher pressure and volume, reflecting reduced ventricular compliance.

The development of a ventricular aneurysm following an occlusion of a coronary artery and subsequent myocardial infarction may contribute to heart failure. Initially, the aneurysm may undergo paradoxical expansion during ventricular systole with a subsequent reduction in forward stroke volume (Fig. 3.5). With healing and formation of a fibrous scar, the length–tension properties of the aneurysmal wall are altered, with a reduction in compliance and a subsequent decrease in paradoxical systolic aneurysmal expansion.

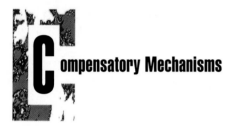

Compensatory Mechanisms

The heart depends upon a number of compensatory mechanisms in order to meet increased demands or periods of depressed contractility. These compensatory mechanisms have a limited ability to sustain cardiac performance in the face of continuing hemodynamic function. The clinical syndrome of heart failure develops when these compensatory mechanisms are overwhelmed. Meerson[9] has described three stages of cardiac response to a sudden hemodynamic overload. The first stage, termed *transient breakdown*, occurs when acute heart failure develops with low cardiac output, pulmonary congestion, and acute left ventricu-

ular dilatation. A period of *stable hyperfunction* follows, brought about by myocardial hypertrophy. During this stage, cardiac output is improved, with subsequent relief of pulmonary congestion. Over time, however, *cardiac exhaustion* occurs, accompanied by myocardial cell death. This leads to progressive fibrosis and decompensated heart failure.

The heart responds to a pressure or volume load through the development of hypertrophy, i.e., an increase in the size of individual myocytes rather than an increase in the number of myocytes. Mitochondrial numbers increase as the myofibrillar mass increases. The stimuli that induce the nuclear DNA to initiate this hypertrophic response are still poorly understood.

In response to a volume load, sarcomere length initially increases by an amount that leads to maximal force of contraction in accordance with Starling's Law. An increase in the number of sarcomeres arranged in series results in an increase in left ventricular mass with consequent ventricular dilatation. The left ventricular wall may show little increase in thickness. An elevated left ventricular end-diastolic volume results, often associated with a normal left ventricular end-diastolic pressure and normalization of end-systolic wall tension. This compensatory process is known as *eccentric hypertrophy*.

In response to a pressure overload, myofibrils are laid down parallel to one another and myocardial wall thickness increases with little change in the size and shape of the left ventricular cavity. This process is termed *concentric hypertrophy*. Left ventricular systolic wall tension is reduced and a temporary period of compensation and stabilization results. Following myocardial infarction, the surviving myocytes undergo hypertrophy with an increase in myocyte diameter and length, as would be seen in pressure and volume overload combined.

As clinical decompensation occurs in a heart subjected to chronic volume overload, left ventricular end-diastolic volume shows little further increase; stroke volume declines with an increase in end-systolic volume secondary to an impairment of myocardial contractility. In the heart exposed to a chronic pressure overload, ejection fraction and end-diastolic volume remain nearly normal until late in the course, when left ventricular dilatation occurs.

A rightward shift in the oxygen–hemoglobin dissociation curve occurs in patients with heart failure, resulting in improved oxygen delivery to peripheral tissues. The sympathetic nervous system is activated, redistributing peripheral blood flow away from the skin, extremities, and splanchnic organs toward vital organs such as the heart and brain. Venoconstriction occurs in the extremities, increasing blood flow to the central circulation. These changes are apparently mediated through humoral vasoconstriction and increased stimulation of the sympathetic nervous system. An elevation in systemic vascular resistance results. In addition, renal retention of sodium and water also occurs.

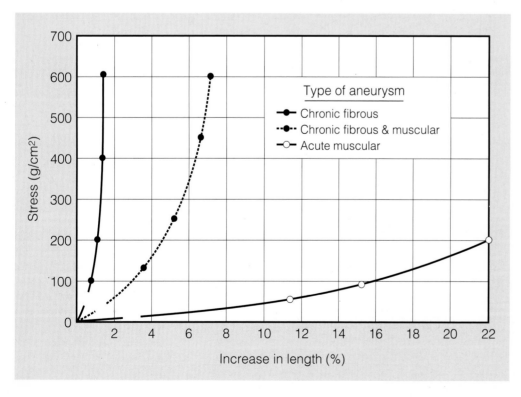

FIGURE 3.5   Representative length–tension relations of three different types of left ventricular aneurysms removed from patients. The chronic fibrous aneurysm is the stiffest, while the acute infarction zone aneurysm is extremely compliant. The chronic aneurysm composed of fibrous and muscle tissue is intermediate. (Modified with permission; see Figure Credits)

Fluid volume in the body is strictly regulated and is important in the maintenance of homeostasis. Normally, an expansion of body fluid volume in the extracellular, intracellular, and/or intravascular compartments, results in compensatory increases in renal sodium and water excretion, thereby normalizing body fluid volume. In certain conditions, including congestive heart failure, renal sodium and water retention persist despite increases in total body fluid volume. The kidneys are influenced by extrarenal stimuli that enhance sodium and water retention. Teleologically, this may have developed from primitive reflexes acting to maintain perfusion pressure in the face of loss of blood volume. In congestive heart failure, perfusion pressure and effective blood volume are decreased; neurohumoral compensatory changes result in an avid renal resorption of sodium and water. In fact, these reflexes may override the usual signals of body fluid overload, resulting in a vicious cycle of fluid retention, cardiac decompensation, and resultant intensification of congestive heart failure (Fig. 3.6).

Elevated systemic vascular resistance induced by neuroendocrine mechanisms results in an increased impedance to ejection in an already failing left ventricle. This, in turn, causes a decline in stroke volume and further increases in systemic vascular resistance. The syndrome of congestive heart failure when viewed in this manner is a gradual progression of cardiac decompensation, with dilatation and impaired performance based more on overshooting physiologic compensatory mechanisms than on a continuation of the originally inflicted damage to the myocardium. Neuroendocrine activation occurs early in the course of patients with left ventricular dysfunction even in asymptomatic or mildly symptomatic patients.

Circulating catecholamines are elevated in heart failure, and plasma norepinephrine levels have been shown to correlate with survival (Fig. 3.7).[1] Norepinephrine is synthesized in postganglionic sympathetic neurons from l-tyrosine and is released following stimulation of the sympathetic nerve. Release of norepinephrine into the synaptic cleft occurs with binding of norepinephrine to postsynaptic receptors. Neuronal re-uptake of norepinephrine occurs by active transport. A small amount of norepinephrine diffuses from the synaptic cleft into the circulation and is taken up by muscle tissue. Plasma norepinephrine is, therefore, thought to be an index of activation of the sympathetic nervous system.

In contrast to elevated plasma levels of norepinephrine, myocardial stores of norepinephrine are found to be depleted in heart failure. Epinephrine is also released from the adrenal medulla when there is an increased demand. Epinephrine levels are otherwise usually normal in heart failure. Variations in norepinephrine levels are only weakly correlated with the severity of left ventricular dysfunction. Acute periods of cardiac decompensation prior to stabilization may precipitate high circulating levels of norepinephrine, and thus, individual measurements may not necessarily predict long-term prognosis. Moreover, elevated norepinephrine levels are more than just a marker of increased sympathetic drive; they may contribute to arrhythmias. In addition, elevated catecholamine levels have been noted to be directly toxic to the myocardium in humans and in animal models. Plasma catecholamines appear to be better predictors of overall survival than hemodynamic variables.

A decrease in myocardial beta-adrenergic receptor density, referred to as *down regulation*, has been observed in chronic heart failure. There is a concomitant decrease in myocardial responsiveness to beta-adrenergic stimulation. Elevated plasma catecholamines and increased sympathetic drive are not necessarily adaptive responses. Acute withdrawal of sympathetic stimulation in patients with heart failure through low-dose beta blockade (or bromocriptine, which inhibits norepinephrine release) is not necessarily associated with hemodynamic deterioration. Indeed, clinical improvement occurs in some patients. An increase in myocardial beta-adrenergic receptor density (up regulation) has been noted in these patients.

Activation of the renin–angiotensin–aldosterone axis occurs in heart failure and contributes to arterial vasoconstriction and sodium retention. Angiotensinogen is an inactive serum alpha-2 globulin produced in the liver. Renin is a proteolytic enzyme produced by the juxtaglomerular apparatus of the kidney, whose release is stimulated by activation of the sympathetic nervous system, decreased sodium delivery to the distal tubule, and/or afferent renal arteriolar tone. Renin cleaves amino acids from angiotensinogen, thus forming angiotensin I, which is weakly vasoactive. Angiotensin-converting enzyme, present throughout the body (with high levels in the lung, vessels, and myocardial tissue), cleaves two more amino acids to form the potent vasoconstrictor angiotensin II. Angiotensin II has a number of pivotal effects on the peripheral circulation besides its vasoconstrictive effects on vascular smooth muscle. One such effect includes the stimulation of aldosterone release from the adrenal cortex, which, in turn, causes sodium and water retention in the kidney. Angiotensin II increases norepinephrine release by sympathetic neurons, blocks neuronal norepinephrine re-uptake, increases catecholamine synthesis by the adrenal medulla, and is a stimulus for arginine vasopressin release. In addition, angiotensin II has been noted to stimulate cardiac myocyte growth and thereby may contribute to myocardial hypertrophy and remodeling. Levels of plasma renin activity, angiotensin, aldosterone, and arginine vasopressin (the posterior pituitary hormone and vasoconstrictor) are often elevated in patients with heart failure.

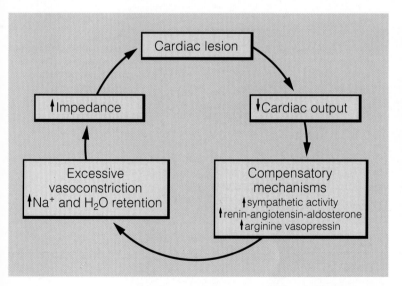

FIGURE 3.6   Cycle of decompensation in heart failure initiated by a cardiac lesion and decline in cardiac output, leading to activation of compensatory systems and further myocardial failure.

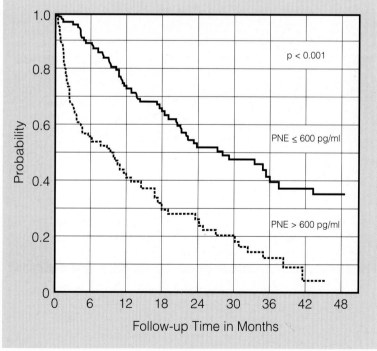

FIGURE 3.7   Survival curves relating plasma norepinephrine levels to probability of survival. A cutoff value of 600 pg/ml provided the most prognostic information. (Redrawn with permission; see Figure Credits)

Activation of the sympathetic nervous system—both central and peripheral—is increased in the presence of heart failure. A blunted response to orthostatic tilt and depressed activation of the baroreceptor reflex to hypotensive stimuli have been observed in patients with heart failure. The significance of these blunted autonomic responses in heart failure is incompletely understood, but it may relate to reduced responsiveness of baroreceptors and of the heart to sympathetic stimulation.

Atrial natriuretic factor (ANF) is a protein released from the atria in response to myocardial stretch. This hormone has a natriuretic effect on the collecting ducts of the kidneys and a vasodilatory effect on the peripheral vasculature. ANF levels are increased in patients with heart failure. The hormone also antagonizes the peripheral actions of angiotensin II. A blunted natriuretic effect of ANF has been reported in heart failure, possibly secondary to a decrease in sodium delivery to the renal collecting ducts. In general, the vasodilatory and diuretic effects of ANF are overwhelmed by the sum of other vasoconstrictive and sodium-retaining influences in patients with heart failure. ANF may serve as a marker of elevated cardiac preload; high ANF levels correlate with decreased survival in patients with heart failure. Conversely, a decrease in ANF levels may herald clinical improvement.

In summary, the compensatory responses of the neurohumoral and sympathetic nervous system support the failing heart. However, they are often excessive and contribute to the clinical picture of heart failure.

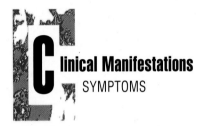

Clinical Manifestations
SYMPTOMS

Backward heart failure leads to an elevation in left atrial pressure with resultant pulmonary congestion. Dyspnea is common with exertion or at rest in patients with heart failure. Because dyspnea is common in normal individuals during strenuous exertion, it is important to elicit the degree of activity necessary to induce dyspnea in patients with heart failure. Orthopnea is a manifestation of elevated pulmonary venous pressure with consequent interstitial pulmonary edema. Cough without sputum production is a common concomitant of orthopnea. Paroxysmal nocturnal dyspnea is the sudden onset of shortness of breath occurring during sleep at night. Wheezing may accompany any of the symptoms mentioned above;

it is associated with bronchial mucosal edema. Pulmonary edema may result from sudden, severe, and/or prolonged elevation of pulmonary venous and capillary pressures with resultant alveolar edema: patients are severely short of breath and cyanotic, with cough producing pink frothy sputum.

Manifestations of forward heart failure include fatigue, weakness, and poor exercise tolerance associated with diminished cardiac output and poor skeletal muscle perfusion, and deconditioning. Confusion and memory impairment may be related to reduced cerebral perfusion. Nocturia is a common occurrence in patients with heart failure and relates in part to diminished renovascular vasoconstriction at rest and during sleep.

Symptoms of right heart failure include fatigue, weakness, and poor exercise tolerance secondary to low cardiac output. In addition, right upper quadrant tenderness and a sense of abdominal fullness is common secondary to congestive hepatomegaly. Nausea and anorexia are manifestations of liver and gastrointestinal tract edema.

The classification of functional capacity as designated by the New York Heart Association (Fig. 3.8) is a useful method for comparing the clinical status of patient groups with heart failure or the status of a single patient at differing points in time.

PHYSICAL FINDINGS

The patient with mild-to-moderate heart failure may appear comfortable at rest with a mildly elevated heart rate. The patient with more severe heart failure may appear acutely ill with resting tachycardia and evidence of peripheral vasoconstriction (i.e., cool, clammy skin, dusky discoloration, and cyanosis). Cachexia with loss of lean body mass may be present in patients with chronic heart failure. Pulses may be weak with diminished pulse pressure. *Pulsus alternans* may be present in severe heart failure and is distinguished by the alternation of regularly timed strong and weak pulses believed to be secondary to alternation in the magnitude of left ventricle stroke volume with each beat. Jugular venous distension is present in patients with elevated right heart filling pressures: 4 to 5 cm above the sternal angle at a 45° incline is the upper limit of normal. An S_3, or low frequency protodiastolic left ventricular filling sound, is frequently audible at the apex in patients with heart failure. An S_3 gallop may be normal in healthy children or young adults, but is generally abnormal in individuals over 40 years of age. The P_2 component of S_2 may be increased in intensity with elevated pulmonary artery pressure. A thorough cardiac examination is important to rule out the presence of valvular heart disease (as previously mentioned, a potentially curable cause of heart failure). Pulmonary rales are frequently present at the lung bases in chronic heart failure; dullness to percussion over the right lower lung field often signifies the presence of a right pleural

FIGURE 3.8 NEW YORK HEART ASSOCIATION FUNCTIONAL CLASSIFICATION

CLASS I: No limitation.
Ordinary physical activity does not cause symptoms.

CLASS II: Slight limitation of physical activity. Ordinary physical activity results in symptoms.

CLASS III: Marked limitation of physical activity. Less than ordinary activity leads to symptoms.

CLASS IV: Inability to carry on any activity without symptoms. Symptoms may be present at rest.
(Reproduced with permission; see Figure Credits)

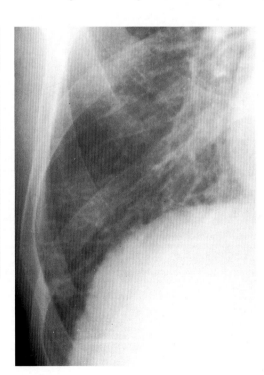

FIGURE 3.9
Chest x-ray demonstrating pulmonary interstitial edema with Kerley B lines. (Reproduced with permission; see Figure Credits)

effusion. Hepatomegaly may be palpable in the right upper abdominal quadrant secondary to hepatic congestion; abdominojugular reflux may be present with expansion of the jugular veins during compression over the liver. Dependent peripheral edema may be present symmetrically in the lower extremities or sacral area of bedridden patients.

LABORATORY STUDIES
CHEST RADIOGRAPHY

The chest x-ray in patients with heart failure often reveals cardiomegaly, defined as a cardiothoracic ratio (ratio of transverse diameter of heart to thorax) >0.6. Left ventricular dilatation may be recognized by the downward and leftward enlargement of the cardiac silhouette in the anteroposterior view. Atrial enlargement may be seen in patients with cardiomyopathy or valvular heart disease. Pulmonary interstitial edema results in edematous interlobular pulmonary septa. When viewed on end, these septa are seen as Kerley B and Kerley A lines (Fig. 3.9).

Peribronchial cuffing is caused by edema of the bronchial walls and surrounding connective tissue. Alveolar edema is manifest by inhomogeneous patchy pulmonary densities, resulting from interspersed air- and fluid-filled alveoli. A butterfly-wing appearance of pulmonary edema extending out from the mediastinum usually involves the inner two thirds of the lung fields.

ELECTROCARDIOGRAPHY

The electrocardiogram is frequently abnormal in patients with heart failure. Ventricular conduction blocks, including left bundle branch block, left anterior fascicular block, and/or bifascicular block, are often noted. Left ventricular hyper-

trophy is often present in patients with hypertension or aortic stenosis. Nonspecific ST-segment and T-wave changes are commonly present.

Infarction patterns are also common in patients with ischemic heart disease although pseudoinfarction patterns are present in 5% to 10% of patients with idiopathic dilated cardiomyopathy. Low voltage is seen with idiopathic cardiomyopathy, amyloidosis, pericardial effusions, and endomyocardial fibrosis.

In Chagas disease, the most common finding is right bundle branch block and left anterior fascicular block. Atrial enlargement is common in heart failure as is atrial fibrillation, which occurs in 15% to 20% of patients.

ECHOCARDIOGRAPHY

Echocardiography is useful in quantifying the degree of left ventricular dysfunction. The left ventricle is commonly dilated and uniformly hypokinetic. Regional variations in wall motion are common in ischemic heart disease, although this finding is not specific; wall motion may be heterogenous in patients with dilated cardiomyopathy. Several M-mode criteria are useful in quantifying the degree of ventricular dysfunction: fractional shortening, mean velocity of circumferential fiber shortening, posterior left ventricular wall velocity, ventricular wall thickening, and E-point septal separation. Ventricular chamber dimensions and wall thickness can be quantified. Reduced mitral valve and aortic valve leaflet excursions are seen with reduced cardiac output; abnormal early closure of the mitral valve may be noted with elevated left ventricular end-diastolic pressure. The two-dimensional apical, four-chamber view frequently reveals incomplete closure of the mitral valve leaflet in systole, leading to mild-to-moderate mitral regurgitation (Fig. 3.10). Mural thrombi may be detected in apical views.

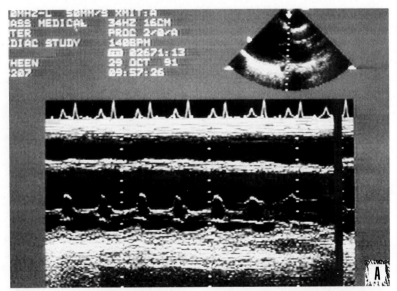

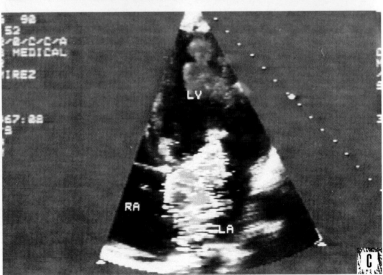

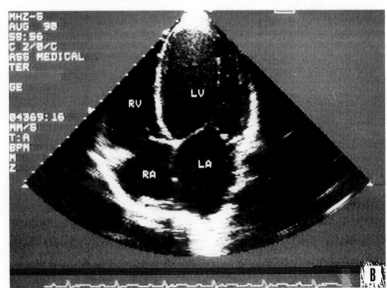

FIGURE 3.10 **(A)** M-mode echocardiogram demonstrating increased E-point septal separation. **(B)** Apical four-chamber echocardiogram demonstrating left ventricular dilatation in a patient with idiopathic cardiomyopathy. **(C)** Apical two-dimensional echocardiogram demonstrating left ventricular dilatation and mitral regurgitation.

Doppler examination of mitral valve inflow often reveals abnormal patterns in these patients, reflecting reduced myocardial compliance. However, diastolic filling can be affected by a number of other variables, including loading conditions, ischemia, hypertrophy, aging, inotropic state, and the force of left atrial contraction.

CARDIAC CATHETERIZATION

Cardiac catheterization and angiography undertaken in patients with heart failure often supplies important diagnostic information. Elevated left and/or right ventricular filling pressures and reduced cardiac output are usually documented. Valvular gradients and/or regurgitation, ventricular wall motion abnormalities, and coronary arterial obstruction may be observed.

OTHER RADIOLOGIC STUDIES

Magnetic resonance imaging is particularly well suited for the examination of the heart and cardiovascular system in heart failure. Natural inherent contrast is present between the soft tissues and chamber walls and the flowing blood (due to the minimal MRI signal of blood). Since the heart is in motion, the study must be gated to an electrocardiogram or peripheral pulse. Since MRI is a three-dimensional imaging technique, it provides accurate measures of ventricular mass, ventricular chamber size, wall thickness, systolic and diastolic volumes, stroke volume, and ejection fraction. Disadvantages to its use include high cost, requirement that patients be supine for 10 to 20 minutes, and inaccessibility for the critically ill or mechanically ventilated patient.

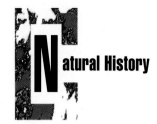

Natural History

Despite advances in the management of congestive heart failure, the prognosis is generally poor. Sudden death occurs in 40 to 50% of patients; progressive pump failure occurs in approximately 40%; and morbid clinical events such as myocardial infarction, stroke, or pulmonary embolism are common.

The New York Heart Association has provided a rough index of prognosis for patients with heart failure, giving 1-year mortalities to 34 to 58% of those in classes III and IV (Fig. 3.11).[3] The Framingham study followed a cohort of patients who were initially free of symptoms and subsequently developed heart failure. Overall 5-year mortality was 62% for men and 42% for women.[8]

Left ventricular function at rest only weakly correlates with exercise tolerance, and it appears to be a significant prognostic variable with regard to survival. The Seattle Heart Attack Registry revealed a sixfold increase in mortality rate in patients with increases in end-diastolic volume index >110 mL/m²; this finding has subsequently been confirmed by other studies.[4] Both the Veterans Administration V-HEFT trial[6] and the Duke Data Bank[3] observed that resting left ventricular ejection fraction was a significant predictor of survival in patients with heart failure.

FIGURE 3.11   Data from the Duke Data Bank relating survival to New York Heart Association functional class. Class IV patients have a particularly poor prognosis. (o = noCHF (1728 pts); [Δ] = class I (36 pts); [●] = class II (79 pts); [▲] = class III (62 pts); [■] = class IV (59 pts). (Redrawn with permission; see Figure Credits)

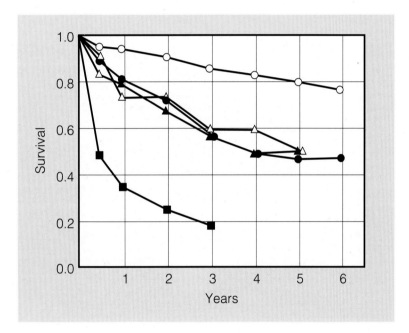

Hemodynamic variables have also been shown to predict survival in patients with heart failure: systemic vascular resistance, left ventricular filling pressure, cardiac output, and stroke-work index all carry prognostic implications.

Elevated levels of neurohumoral factors, including plasma norepinephrine, arginine vasopressin, atrial natriuretic factor, and various components of the renin–angiotensin–aldosterone system, correlate with decreased survival of patients with heart failure. Lee and Packer found that serum sodium levels mEq/L were associated with decreased survival.[7]

Ventricular arrhythmias are common in heart failure and their presence carries prognostic implications. Up to 95% of patients with heart failure have frequent complex ventricular premature beats during 24-hour Holter monitoring; up to 80% of patients will have nonsustained ventricular tachycardia. Most of this ectopy is asymptomatic. As many as 50% of deaths in patients with heart failure are sudden and are most likely due to ventricular tachycardia/ventricular fibrillation. The pathogenesis of arrhythmias in heart failure is complex and multifactorial and includes altered conduction, abnormal automaticity, increases in triggered activity secondary to left ventricular dilatation, ischemia, and scarring. Electrolyte abnormalities are common (e.g., hypokalemia and hypomagnesemia during diuretic therapy). Elevation of components of the neurohumoral system and high levels of circulating catecholamines can exert important arrhythmogenic influences. In addition, many of the drugs used to treat heart failure can exacerbate arrhythmias (i.e., digitalis, diuretics, and inotropic agents). Antiarrhythmic drugs may further depress left ventricular function. Indeed, the incidence of proarrhythmia is greater in patients with heart failure. This is particularly the case in patients with a history of sustained ventricular arrhythmia.

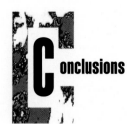

Conclusions

The clinical syndrome of heart failure is the result of a number of pathogenic entities and compensatory responses. Despite great gains in the understanding of the pathophysiology and treatment of heart failure in recent decades, chronic heart failure remains associated with high mortality, frequent physician visits and hospitalizations, and substantial economic burden to the patient and society in general. The final stage of heart failure appears to be one of cardiac exhaustion after compensatory mechanisms have been depleted or overwhelmed. It is largely irreversible. In spite of therapy, mortality rates are high (e.g., 35% over 3.5 years in the enalapril treatment arm of the SOLVD study).[10]

The optimal approach to heart failure appears to be prevention of predisposing risk factors (e.g., hypertension, left ventricular hypertrophy, coronary atherosclerotic heart disease, and adult-onset diabetes). Detection of impaired left ventricular function should be sought in high-risk individuals before cardiac decompensation occurs.

FIGURE CREDITS

Fig. 3.2 from Chatterjee K, et al: Cardiology: An Illustrated Text–Reference. Gower, New York, 1992.

Fig. 3.5 modified from Parmley WW, et al: In vitro length–tension relations of human ventricular neurysms: The relationship of stiffness to mechanical disadvantage. Am J Cardiol 32:887, 1973.

Fig. 3.7 redrawn from Rector TS, et al: Predicting survival for an individual with congestive heart failure using the plasma norepinephrine concentration. Am Heart J 114:148, 1987.

Fig. 3.8 from Criteria Committee of the New York Heart Association, Inc. Diseases of the heart and blood vessels (Nomenclature and Criteria for Diagnosis), 6th ed. Little, Brown and Company, Boston, 1964.

Fig. 3.9 from Kassner, EG: Atlas of Radiologic Imaging. Gower, New York, 1989.

Fig. 3.11 redrawn from Braunwald E, Mock MB, Watson J (eds): Congestive Heart Failure: Current Research and Clinical applications. Grune & Stratton, New York, 1982.

REFERENCES

1. Braunwald E, Mock MB, Watson J (eds): Congestive Heart Failure: Current Research and Clinical Applications. Grune & Stratton, New York, 1982.

2. Braunwald E, Ross J, Sonnerblick EH (eds): Mechanisms of Contraction of the Normal and Failing Heart. Little, Brown, Boston, 1976.

3. Califf RM, Bounous P, Hamell FE, et al: The prognosis in the presence of coronary artery disease. In Braunwald E, Mock MB, Watson J (eds): Congestive Heart Failure: Current Research and Clinical Applications. Grune & Stratton, New York, 1982.

4. Cohn JN, Archibald DS, Ziesche S, et al: Effect of vasodilation therapy on mortality in chronic congestive heart failure: Results of a Veterans Administration Cooperative Study. N Engl J Med 314:1547, 1986.

5. Cohn JN, Levine TB, Olivari RT, et al: Plasma norepinephrine as a guide to prognosis in patients with chronic congestive heart failure. N Engl J Med 311:819, 1984.

6. Hammermeister KE, DeRouen TA, Dodge HT: Variables predicting survival in patients with coronary artery disease. Circulation 59:421, 1979.

7. Lee WH, Packer M: Prognostic importance of serum sodium concentration and its modification by converting enzyme inhibition in patients with severe chronic heart failure. Circulation 73:257, 1986.

8. McKee PA, Castelli WP, McNamara PM, et al: The natural history of congestive heart failure: The Framingham study. N Engl J Med 285:1441, 1971.

9. Meerson FZ: On the mechanism of compensatory hypertension and insufficency of the heart. Cor Vasa 3:161, 1961.

10. SOLVD investigators: Effect of enalapril on survival in patients with reduced left ventricular ejection fractions and congestive heart failure. N Engl J Med 325:294, 1991.

Normal values for cardiac output in humans vary somewhat between laboratories, but generally range from 2.5 to 5.0 L/min/m² for ages 20 to 80 years. Cardiac output in excess of 6.0 L/min/m² is regarded as elevated beyond the usual variance of normal.

It is important to distinguish between the many factors and conditions that cause a simple elevation of cardiac output[7,15,16] (Fig. 3.12) from those, considerably fewer in number, that cause high-output heart failure if allowed to remain marked in degree and/or prolonged in duration[1-6,17-33] (Fig. 3.13). Of course, any of the factors that simply increase cardiac output (see Fig. 3.12) can precipitate heart failure in patients with underlying cardiovascular disease (e.g., valvular or occlusive coronary artery disease); these clinical conditions and situations are not addressed in this discussion.

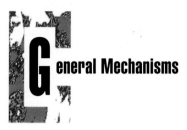

General Mechanisms

Since cardiac output equals the product of stroke volume and heart rate, a rise in cardiac output can be evoked by a fall in aortic impedance and peripheral vascular resistance (increasing stroke volume), an elevation in central blood volume or venous return (increasing stroke volume), stimulation of heart rate and contractility (increasing stroke volume), or a combination of these factors (Fig. 3.14). These hemodynamic modulators have been respectively designated *afterload reduction*, *preload elevation*, *positive chronotropy* and *inotropy* ("cardiostimulation"), or a combination of these (Figs. 3.15, 3.16). These modulators allow the cardiovascular system to rapidly and appropriately adjust to the demands and moment-to-moment energy and metabolic requirements of the entire organism, and they serve as the primary means whereby various physiologic and pathologic conditions (see Fig. 3.12) evoke an elevation of cardiac output.

The determinants of an elevated cardiac output are causally interrelated at various steps in the process of increasing output (see upper panel of Fig. 3.17). For example, the activation of sympathetic nervous system activity (and fall in parasympathetic activity) following a decrease in vascular resistance evokes positive inotropy and chronotropy and stimulates the renin–angiotensin–aldosterone axis; thus, a state of low vascular resistance augments cardiac output via ventricular afterload reduction, increased venous return (increasing preload), and, by activating the sympathetic nervous system, elevation of heart rate, contractility, and preload (via aldosterone-induced fluid retention and possibly venoconstriction).

The pathophysiologic mechanisms that cause a marked and/or chronic high cardiac output state to become high output heart failure have not been fully elucidated and likely differ somewhat for each provocation (i.e., the causal steps to high output heart failure from thyrotoxicosis differ from those of chronic anemia or large arteriovenous fistulas). A general overview of the major events and

---

FIGURE 3.12 STATES OF HIGH CARDIAC OUTPUT*

A. PHYSIOLOGIC CONDITIONS
1. *Stress, excitement, pain, discomfort*
2. *Meals*
3. *Physical activity*
4. *Warm/cold environment*
5. *Pregnancy*

B. PATHOLOGIC DISORDERS
1. *Cardiovascular*
   a. Arteriovenous shunting/fistulas
   b. Labile hypertension
   c. Hyperkinetic heart syndrome

2. *Endocrine*
   a. Hyperthyroidism
   b. Hyperadrenal conditions
   c. Carcinoid syndrome

3. *Hematologic/oncologic*
   a. Reduced oxygen-carrying capacity
   b. Anemia
   c. Hemoglobinopathies
   d. Polycythemia
   e. Various neoplastic conditions

4. *Gastrointestinal/visceral*
   a. Hepatitis
   b. Hepatic cirrhosis
   c. Pancreatitis

5. *Pulmonary*
   Conditions of impaired gas exchange

6. *Dermatologic*
   a. Psoriasis
   b. Exfoliative dermatitis
   c. Generalized erythroderma
   d. Kaposi's sarcoma

7. *Infectious*
   a. Infection
   b. Sepsis

8. *Miscellaneous*
   a. Fever
   b. Anaphylactic reactions
   c. Obesity
   d. Nutritional deficiencies, early stages
   e. Pharmacologic agents
   f. Smoking
   g. Caffeine-containing substances
   h. Renal failure
   i. Skeletal disorders (e.g., Paget's disease, fibrous dysplasia)

The conditions listed above do not in themselves cause high output heart failure but can evoke heart failure when present in patients with underlying cardiovascular disorders or diseases.

FIGURE 3.13 PATHOLOGIC CONDITIONS CAPABLE OF CAUSING HIGH OUTPUT HEART FAILURE

A. SYSTEMIC ARTERIOVENOUS FISTULAS, COMMUNICATIONS, OR MALFORMATIONS

1. *Congenital*
   a. AV fistulas of large vessels
   b. Hemangioma/hemangioendothelioma of liver, skin, and other structures
   c. Hereditary hemorrhagic telangiectasia (Osler–Weber–Rendu disease)

2. *Acquired*
   a. Post-traumatic
   b. Surgical placement (e.g., renal dialysis access)
   c. Spontaneous arterio-venous communication (e.g., erosion or rupture of arterial lesion into adjacent vein)
   d. Neoplastic disease (e.g., Wilm's tumor, hypernephroma)

B. CHRONIC ANEMIA
1. *Long-term hemoglobin <5 g %*
2. *Sickle cell anemia*
3. *Other hemoglobinopathies*

C. CHRONIC HYPERTHYROIDISM, THYROTOXICOSIS

D. OTHER CONDITIONS

1. *Severe skeletal disorders*
   a. Osteitis deformans (Paget's disease)
   b. Polyostotic fibrous dysplasia

2. *Beriberi (thiamine deficiency) heart disease*

3. *Neoplastic/paraneoplastic disease (mechanisms other than arteriovenous fistulas)*

4. *Marked obesity*

5. *Chronic tachycardia*

causal steps evoking high cardiac output conditions and high output heart failure as proposed by the authors is presented in Figures 3.16–3.20.

Most primary causes of high output heart failure (see Fig. 3.13) have several pathophysiologic features in common. Basically, all evoke an excessive increase in cardiac volume load over time with the progressive development of relative or absolute cardiac dysfunction (Figs. 3.19, 3.20). Most causes are associated with a low systemic vascular resistance and a greatly expanded intravascular volume, although the mechanisms leading to these hemodynamic adjustments vary among the different etiologies. Dilated cardiac chambers and progressive systolic and diastolic dysfunction are common to all high output heart failure conditions and are probably secondary to a marked, chronically elevated ventricular (and atrial) preload and wall stress and disturbed myocardial energetics (increasing myocardial oxygen consumption and decreasing coronary diastolic perfusion time). The cardiac chambers enlarge and assume a more spherical shape.

Myocardial remodeling consists of cellular hypertrophy and elongation, new sarcomeres placed in series, and accentuated interstitial fibrosis.

The critical pathophysiologic mechanisms, events, and conditions (other than underlying cardiac disease) that push a high cardiac output state into symptomatic, chronic heart failure are unknown, but, based on the usual clinical presentation, they probably include a varying combination of chronic activation of the sympathetic nervous system and the renin–angiotensin–aldosterone axis, chronically expanded intravascular volume, elevated preload, cardiac wall stress, and myocardial oxygen consumption, and cardiac/ventricular/myocardial remodeling (see lower panel of Fig. 3.17). Other factors (such as downregulation or uncoupling of myocardial adrenoceptors, alteration in myocardial G proteins, local endothelin release, and tissue/vascular renin-angiotensin activity) are likely to contribute to developing chronic heart failure, but data in humans are currently limited regarding the involvement of these and other local mechanisms.

FIGURE 3.14 PRIMARY PHYSIOLOGIC MODALITIES THAT AUGMENT CARDIAC OUTPUT

AFTERLOAD REDUCTION (↑ STROKE VOLUME)
1. Fall in aortic impedance.
2. Fall in systemic vascular resistance.

PRELOAD ELEVATION (↑ STROKE VOLUME)
1. Increased intravascular volume and venous return increase ventricular diastolic volume.

2. Ventricular systolic performance is augmented via Frank–Starling forces.

CARDIOSTIMULATION
1. Positive inotropy (↑ stroke volume).
2. Positive chronotropy (↑ heart rate).

COMBINATION OF ABOVE

Cardiac output = stroke volume x heart rate.

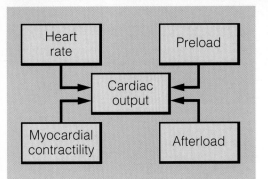

FIGURE 3.15
Cardiac output is most influenced and modulated by changes in preload, afterload, heart rate (chronotropy), and contractility (inotropy).

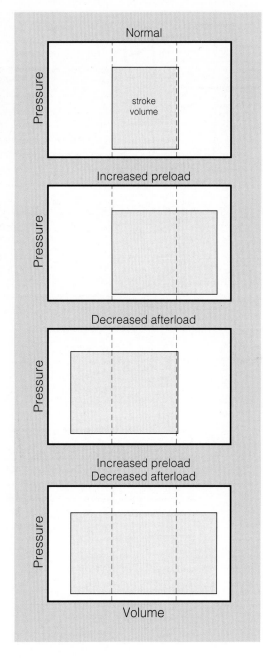

FIGURE 3.16
Effects of increased preload and reduced afterload, two common features of high output heart failure, on left ventricular stroke volume.

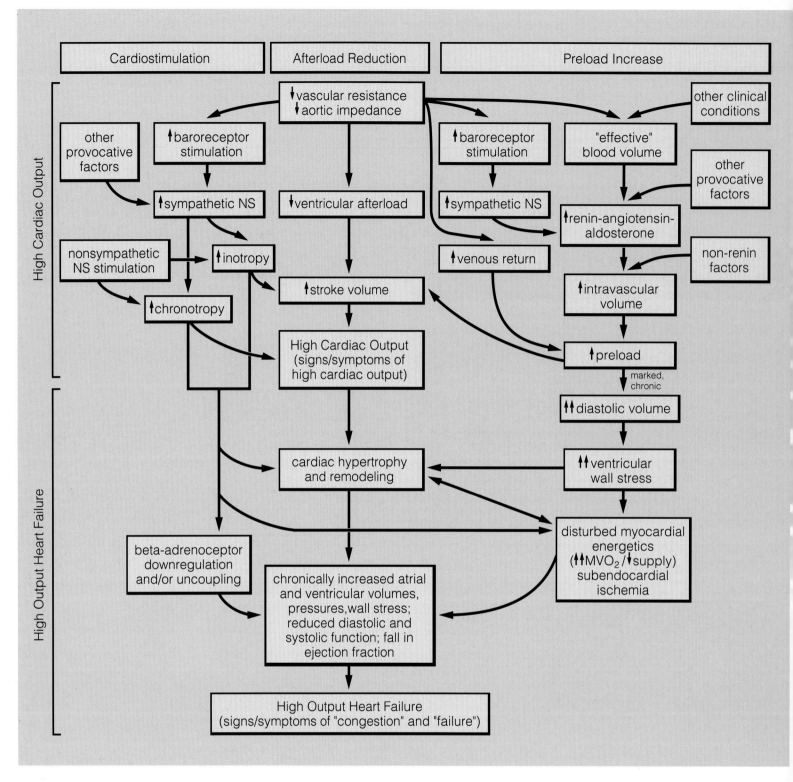

FIGURE 3.17   The authors' proposal for mechanisms, and their inter-relationship, involved in the development of states of high cardiac output (upper panel) and high output heart failure (lower panel). The fundamental starting point in most instances is excessive cardiostimulation (↑ heart rate and/or ↑ contractility), afterload reduction, preload elevation, or a combination of these.

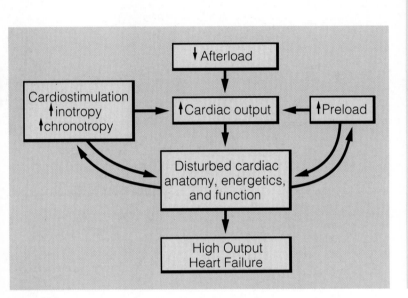

FIGURE 3.18 Overview of the mechanisms presented in Figure 3.17.

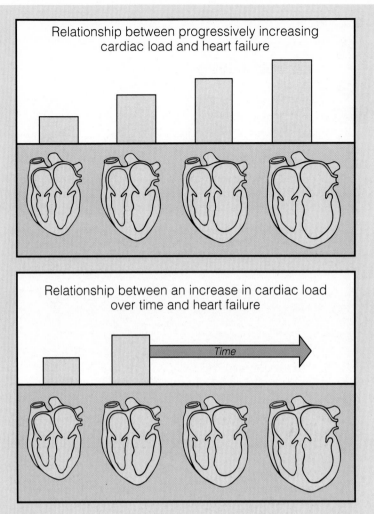

FIGURE 3.19 High output cardiac failure developing from a progressive rise in cardiac volume load (upper panel) or from a simple elevation of cardiac volume load over an extended period of time (lower panel).

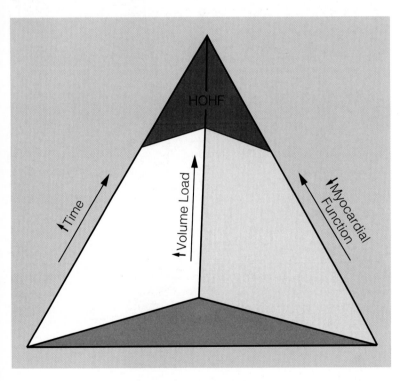

FIGURE 3.20 Development of high output heart failure (HOHF): the presence of an excessive volume load and the evolution of myocardial dysfunction over a period of time are generally required.

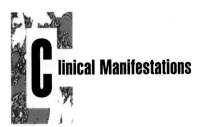

Clinical Manifestations

A number of clinical manifestations are common to most types of high output failure (Figs. 3.21, 3.22) and others are unique to certain etiologies. It is important to note that the clinical manifestations are not only dependent on the specific etiology, but also on the degree of severity, the duration of the problem, and the stage of heart failure. Presenting features generally include varying degrees of exercise intolerance due to easy fatigability or exertional dyspnea, "heart awareness" and palpitations early in the course and dyspnea at later stages, resting tachycardia and an exaggerated rise in heart rate with physical activity, bounding pulses with other peripheral signs of an elevated stroke volume and reduced vascular resistance (e.g., Quincke's pulses of capillary beds, "pistol shot" sounds, Duroziez's sign, venous hums), elevated systemic systolic pressure and reduced diastolic pressure, hyperkinetic precordium, cardiomegaly with four-chamber dilatation, high flow gallops (right and left heart S_3), and ejection murmurs (see Fig. 3.22).

As the disease process advances into stages of decompensation and the terminal phase of heart failure, symptoms and signs of high cardiac output evolve into those of inadequate cardiac output (relative or absolute) and congestion.

FIGURE 3.21 CLINICAL MANIFESTATIONS COMMON TO MOST FORMS OF HIGH OUTPUT HEART FAILURE

DURING GENERAL COURSE

Symptoms
1. Exercise intolerance, dyspnea or exertion, easy fatigability
2. "Heart awareness" and palpitations

Physical Findings
3. Resting tachycardia
4. Exaggerated rise in exertional heart rate
5. Bounding pulses, Duroziez's sign, Quincke's pulses, pistol shot sounds
6. Venous hums
7. Elevated systolic blood pressure, reduced diastolic pressure
8. Hyperkinetic precordium and apical impulse
9. Four-chamber cardiomegaly
10. Protodiastolic and presystolic gallop sounds
11. Loud first heart sound
12. Ejection flow murmurs
13. Occasional regurgitation of mitral and tricuspid valves

ADVANCED STAGES: DECOMPENSATED HEART FAILURE

Symptoms
1. Dyspnea and fatigue at rest or with mild exertion, malaise
2. Extremely poor exercise tolerance

Physical findings
3. Resting tachycardra
4. Reduction or loss of bounding pulses, Duroziez's sign, Quincke's pulses, venous hums, hyperkinetic precordium, ejection flow murmurs
5. Jugular venous distention
6. Systolic and diastolic blood pressures move toward "normal" levels (i.e., ↓ systolic blood pressure, ↑ diastolic blood pressure)
7. Accentuated cardiomegaly
8. Prominent protodiastolic gallops
9. Mitral and tricuspid regurgitation
10. Marked fluid retention with peripheral and pulmonary edema
11. End-organ dysfunction, azotemia

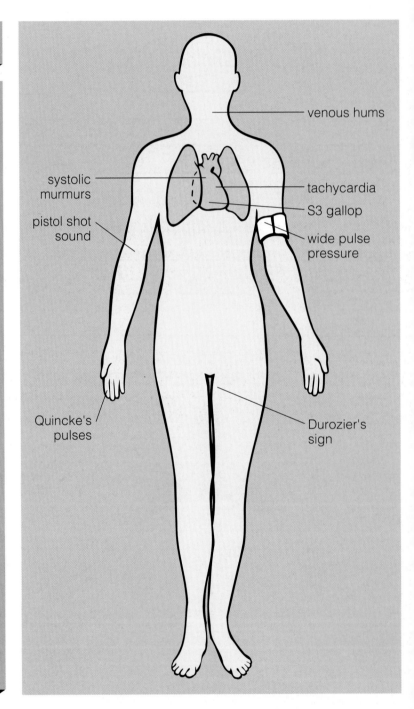

FIGURE 3.22   Common physical findings in patients with elevated cardiac output and high output heart failure.

The pivotal factor is loss of ventricular systolic and diastolic performance such that the heart cannot sustain the demands of the high output condition in terms of a high stroke volume, cardiac output, and ventricular diastolic capacity. At this stage, patients develop dyspnea, malaise, and fatigue at rest or with minimal activity; systolic blood pressure falls and diastolic pressure rises toward "normal values"; signs of congestive, "less-than-adequate output" heart failure appear (e.g., peripheral cutaneous vasoconstriction, jugular venous distention, peripheral and pulmonary edema, and prominent gallop sounds); mitral and tricuspid regurgitation often occur secondary to ventricular annular dilatation and anatomic distortion of the valvular apparatus; and end-organ dysfunction (e.g., prerenal azotemia) eventuates.

Roentgenographic, echocardiographic, hemodynamic, and angiographic studies are used to confirm the presence of a high cardiac output condition, to determine its cause, to exclude primary cardiac etiologies and underlying cardiac disease, and to assess the status of ventricular systolic and diastolic function[11,14,18,19] (Figs. 3.23–3.25; see also Fig. 3.28). In general, the cumulative laboratory findings are 4-chamber cardiomegaly, high velocity ventricular ejection, ejection fraction ≥ 0.60, resting cardiac outputs in excess of 8 L/min/m^2, normal biventricular diastolic filling pressures, and reduced systemic and pulmonic vascular resistances. Normal coronary anatomy and high coronary blood flow are noted during coronary angiography. As the condition evolves into a state of cardiac decompensation, ejection velocity and ejection fraction fall toward normal values or below, cardiac output falls toward (but generally remains above) the normal range, right and left heart diastolic filling pressures rise to ≥ 6 and ≥ 14 mmHg, respectively, and vascular resistances rise into the normal range and above.

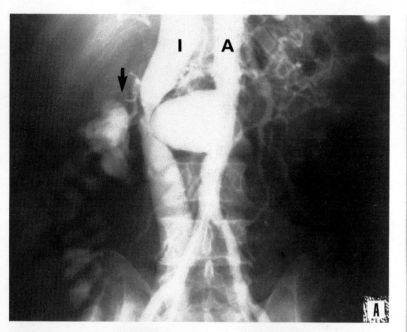

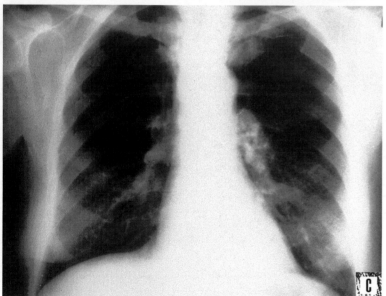

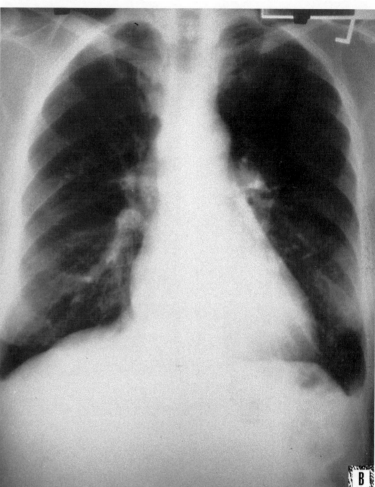

FIGURE 3.23 (A) Contrast injection of the aorta (A) demonstrated a large saccular aneurysm with prompt contrast opacification of the inferior vena cava (I) secondary to a fistula between the aortic aneurysm and the inferior vena cava. The 65-year-old male presented with recent-onset dyspnea with moderate exertion and resting tachycardia. The size of the cardiac silhouette on the chest roentgenogram at the time of presentation (B) decreased substantially over 4 weeks following aneurysmectomy and fistula repair (C). (Reproduced with permission; see Figure Credits)

SPECIFIC ETIOLOGIES

In addition to the clinical manifestations common to virtually all types of high output heart failure (see Fig. 3.21), each type or cause has its own unique clinical and laboratory features; the characteristics and features of the most common types of high output heart failure are presented below.

ARTERIOVENOUS FISTULAS

The clinical presentation of high output heart failure secondary to arteriovenous fistulas ranges from a gradual and prolonged course for medium-sized arteriovenous fistulas or multiple, small fistulas (e.g., hereditary hemorrhagic telangiectasia) to a more abrupt course for aortocaval fistulas caused by rupture of an ather-osclerotic aortic aneurysm into the inferior vena cava[1,3,5,6,8,11,13,14,18,19,25,28,32] (see Figs. 3.23–3.25). The most common arteriovenous communications leading to high output failure are large hemangiomas/hemangioendotheliomas (most common cause in infants and children), excessively large arteriovenous fistulas constructed surgically for vascular access (renal dialysis), iatrogenic fistulas (e.g., arteriovenous injury during vascular catheterization, surgical procedure, laminectomy, biopsies), spontaneous fistulas between atherosclerotic arterial lesions (e.g., aneurysm) and an adjacent vein, gunshot and knife wounds, and fistulas present within neoplastic structures.

Stroke volume and cardiac output increase in proportion to the size of the fistula; the increase is secondary to the fall in aortic impedance and overall systemic vascular resistance (both decreasing afterload), baroreceptor activation of

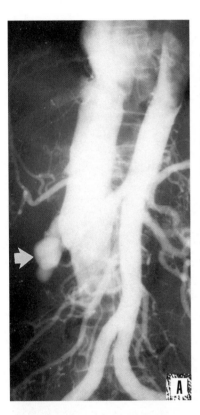
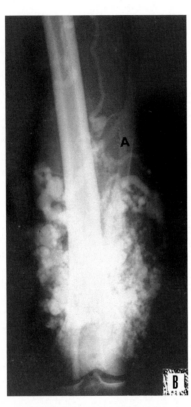

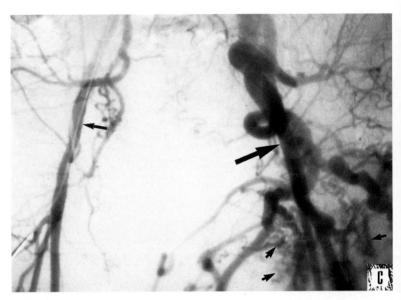

FIGURE 3.24 Arteriograms of patients who presented with high output heart failure secondary to arteriovenous fistulas and communications. **(A)** Postnephrectomy fistula of right renal artery-vein *(arrow).* **(B)** Extensive arteriovenous communications in the region of the distal right femoral artery **(A)**. **(C)** Left iliac and femoral arteriovenous communications *(arrowheads).* Note the disparate sizes of the left *(large arrow)* and right *(small arrow)* iliac vessels. (Reproduced with permission; see Figure Credits)

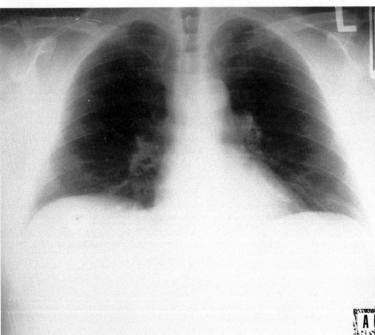
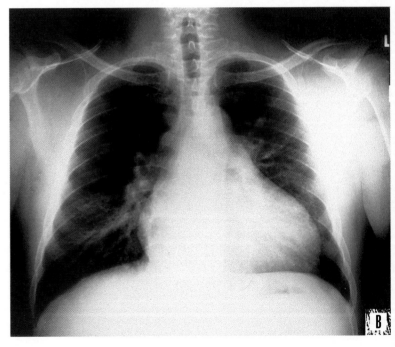

FIGURE 3.25 Chest roentgenograms of a 36-year-old male with hereditary hemorrhagic telangiectasia, multiple arteriovenous communications, and chronic anemia (hemoglobin values from 7 to 9 g %). X-rays were taken in 1978 **(A)** and again in 1990 **(B)**, when he presented with high output congestive heart failure. (Reproduced with permission; see Figure Credits)

sympathetic nervous tone, and augmented venous return (increasing preload) (see Fig. 3.17). The augmented sympathetic nervous system activity increases heart rate, ventricular contractility, stroke volume, and renin release with expansion of intravascular volume.

In addition to the general clinical presentation of high cardiac output states and failure (see Fig. 3.21), the arteriovenous fistula conditions have unique physical characteristics. Large arteriovenous fistulas and malformations of the liver, lungs, and brain in children are frequently accompanied by obvious cutaneous arteriovenous malformations. Large arteriovenous malformations and multiple diffuse telangiectasias in hereditary hemorrhagic telangiectasia are often suspected in patients with small telangiectasias of mucous membranes, skin, and nailbeds and an occasional history of chronic gastrointestinal bleeding. A scar or a history of trauma (e.g., gunshot, surgery, catheterization) are important clues to the presence of post-traumatic fistulas in a patient with high output heart failure.

Sizable arteriovenous fistulas involving the limbs (e.g., femoral artery–vein) often present with warm skin, palpable thrill, and audible systolic–diastolic bruit over the lesion. Venous varicosities, representing the high-flow and high-pressure veins receiving the shunted blood, may be seen around the lesion (see Fig. 3.31). The oxygen saturation of the blood contained in these venous structures is elevated above the usual venous oxygen saturation of that locale. In children, the involved limb is greater in size and length than its counterpart. Size differences (without changes in length) may also be noted in adults. Edema, venous engorgement, and status dermatitis commonly occur distal to the lesion. Occlusive pressure over the artery proximal to or at the shunt will generally slow the heart rate in patients with a hemodynamically significant arteriovenous communication; this maneuver and its response are referred to as *Branham's sign.*

Doppler flow studies are confirmatory of the etiology and may be useful in following the course of the arteriovenous malformation. Anatomic definition is provided by arteriography. Good angiographic delineation, exclusion of other fistulas, assessment of cardiac function, and evaluation of associated systemic conditions are advised prior to major intervention (e.g., corrective surgery or selective embolization).

FIGURE 3.26 PROPOSED MECHANISMS LINKING CHRONIC ANEMIA TO HIGH CARDIAC OUTPUT HEART FAILURE

Chronic Afterload Reduction
1. Peripheral vasodilatation (metabolic demand–supply mismatch)
2. Reduced blood viscosity

Chronic Preload Elevation
1. Enhanced venous return
2. Increased blood volume ($\uparrow$ sympathetic nervous tone, $\uparrow$ renin)

Chronic Cardiostimulation by Baroreceptor and Other Reflex-mediated Mechanisms
1. Tachycardia
2. Augmented contractility

Other Pathophysiologic Factors
1. Elevated wall stress
2. Disturbed myocardial energetics ($\uparrow$ oxygen consumption, $\downarrow\downarrow$ oxygen delivery)
3. Cardiac/ventricular/myocardial remodeling

FIGURE 3.27 MECHANISMS OF THYROID-INDUCED ELEVATION IN CARDIAC OUTPUT

Afterload Reduction
1. Systemic vasodilatation (secondary to increased metabolic demands of tissues and organs)
2. Cutaneous vasodilatation for heat dissipation

Preload Increase
1. Increased blood volume
2. Increased venous return

Cardiostimulation
1. Direct effect of thyroid hormone on cardiomyocytes
2. Augmentation of sympathetic nervous system tone and activity

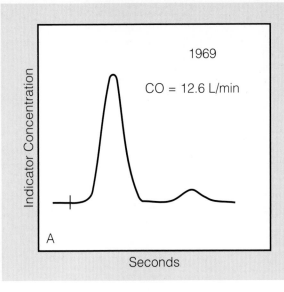

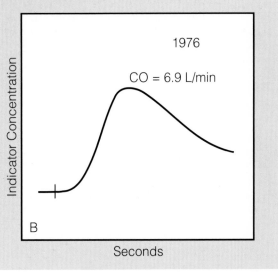

FIGURE 3.28 Cardiac output curves (indocyanine green) of a 32-year-old woman who presented with thyrotoxicosis and a Means–Lerman scratch murmur in 1969 (**A**). She refused therapeutic intervention until she reappeared in 1976 (**B**) with symptoms and signs of congestive heart failure, cardiomegaly, ventricular gallop sounds, mitral and tricuspid regurgitation, and peripheral edema. Echocardiography and cardiac catheterization demonstrated four-chamber enlargement, ventricular systolic and diastolic dysfunction, mild-to-moderate mitral and tricuspid regurgitation, and normal coronary arteries. The marked elevation of cardiac output in 1969 (**A**) decreased over the ensuing 7 years (**B**) as heart failure became superimposed on her high output state.

Blood hemoglobin levels <8 g % are associated with a rise in cardiac output. Unless a patient has underlying cardiovascular disease or sickle cell anemia, a chronic hemoglobin level ≤5.0 g % is usually required for the development of high output cardiac failure.[4,9,12,17,27] The rise in cardiac output in chronic anemia is related to a number of factors (Fig. 3.26), including reduced oxygen delivery (decreased DO_2) secondary to loss of oxygen-carrying capacity, afterload reduction secondary to reduced systemic vascular resistance (myogenic and local mechanisms) and reduced blood viscosity, increased preload secondary to increased venous return and elevated total blood volume, and activation of the sympathetic nervous system. Marked depression of oxygen delivery (via depressed hemoglobin levels) to myocardium in the setting of elevated oxygen consumption likely contributes to other mechanisms (see Fig. 3.17) in the eventual development of ventricular systolic and diastolic dysfunction. The degree of hematocrit depression required to cause heart failure is less in sickle cell anemia because this form of anemia is also accompanied by higher blood viscosity, micro-

vascular pathology, pulmonary ventilation–perfusion defects, and an earlier appearance of ventricular diastolic dysfunction. A number of other hemoglobinopathies (e.g., thalassemia major) are complicated by hemochromatosis.

In addition to the clinical features common to most types of high output heart failure (see Fig. 3.21), the severely anemic patient is noticeably pale and, oftentimes, "pasty" or "waxy" to touch. Mucous membranes, conjunctiva, and skin creases (in palms) are quite pale, an important finding in non-Caucasian patients in whom cutaneous pallor is more difficult to detect.

CHRONIC HYPERTHYROIDISM–THYROTOXICOSIS

Elevated thyroid hormones greatly augment cardiac output through an integration of several mechanisms (Fig. 3.27). Increased metabolic demands of virtually all tissues increase local blood flow requirements and lower regional (and thus, systemic) vascular resistance. The general increase in metabolic activity produces heat and, therefore, a need to augment cutaneous blood flow for heat dissipation. Venous return and, thus, preload are increased. The peripheral vasodilation and

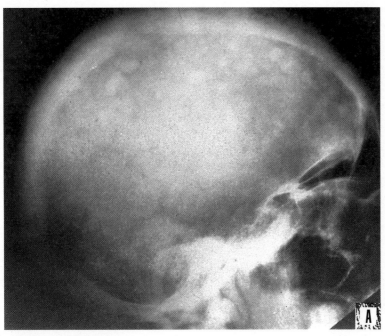

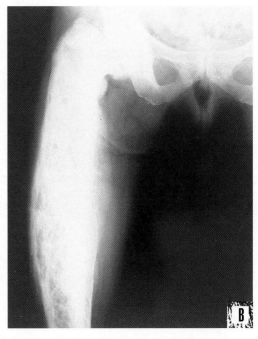

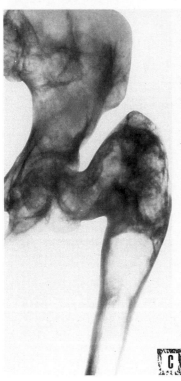

FIGURE 3.29 Skeletal lesions that can lead to the development of high output heart failure. **(A)** Skull roentgenogram of a patient with Paget's Disease. Note the thickened calvarium, dense basilar regions, indistinct bony margins, and irregular densities.
(B) Marked osteitis deformans (Paget's) of the right femur of a 56-year-old patient who presented with high output heart failure. Well over 25% of the skeleton was involved by the disease process, including skull, spine, pelvis, left humerus, radius and ulna, right radius, both femurs, and several ribs. **(C)** Left pelvis and femur of a 36-year-old woman with Albright's syndrome (polyostotic fibrous dysplasia, hyperpigmented irregularly edged macules, and sexual precocity). The roentgenogram demonstrates the typical radiolucent areas and a shepherd's crook deformity of the femur. (Figures A and C reproduced with permission; see Figure Credits)

thyroid hormone enhance activity and tone of the sympathetic nervous system at several levels. Thyroid hormone also has a direct positive inotropic effect and further disturbs already threatened myocardial energetics by greatly increasing myocardial oxygen consumption. Changes in cardiac output over time in a patient with untreated thyrotoxicosis are presented in Figure 3.28.

The diagnosis of high output heart failure secondary to chronic thyrotoxicosis is usually made by recognizing the clinical manifestations unique to hyperthyroidism;[24,26,29,31] these manifestations include nervousness, anxiety, personality changes, heat intolerance, weight loss in spite of enhanced appetite and caloric intake, tremor, hyper-reflexia, exophthalmos and lid lag, and other signs. The cardiovascular manifestations are similar to those presented earlier in Figure 3.21. A venous hum is often present over the jugular veins. The systolic ejection murmur along the left sternal border in some thyrotoxic patients has a characteristic sound referred to as a *Means–Lerman scratch*. Atrial fibrillation, commonly associated with hyperthyroidism, is usually accompanied by a rapid ventricular response relatively refractory to digitalis. The diagnosis is confirmed by detecting elevated serum T4 and T3 levels and depressed concentrations of thyroid-stimulating hormone.

The clinical diagnosis of hyperthyroidism can be difficult to make in some patients with high output heart failure, particularly in the elderly.[31] Elderly patients often present with malaise, lassitude, listlessness, and chronic fatigue rather than nervousness, anxiety, and an overall "hyper" state; the term *apathetic hyperthyroidism* has been applied to this patient group. Weight loss, malaise, listlessness, and atrial fibrillation in an elderly patient with heart failure should arouse suspicion of this clinical condition. Hyperthyroid heart failure in elderly patients can also be caused by the superimposition of hyperthyroidism on an underlying cardiovascular disease (e.g., atherosclerotic coronary artery disease, myocardial changes of aging) rather than by the effects of chronic thyrotoxicosis alone.

OTHER CONDITIONS

Certain skeletal disorders have been associated with high output heart failure; however, the mechanisms linking these disorders to high output failure have not been convincingly established.[2,21,22] Fifteen percent of the skeleton must be afflicted with osteitis deformans (Paget's disease) before high cardiac output and eventual cardiac failure become a part of this condition. The high cardiac output is probably related to the high metabolic rate (likely enhanced heat production) of the disease process, although arteriovenous communications in the diseased bone may also contribute to the development in some patients. Multiple arteriovenous sinusoids are a pathologic feature of polyostotic fibrous

dysplasia of bone, but whether this finding is the sole explanation for high output cardiac failure in this condition remains to be determined. Osteitis deformans and polyostotic fibrous dysplasia produce rather characteristic x-ray findings (Fig. 3.29).

Chronic thiamine deficiency (beriberi) remains one of the more classic causes of high output heart failure.[2,20] The causal link between thiamine deficiency and high output heart failure has not been established. Degeneration of sympathetic ganglia with consequent generalized vasodilatation is the leading hypothesis at the present time. The current prevalence of high output heart disease associated with beriberi in western societies is relatively low, although individuals with long-term, low-vitamin, high-carbohydrate diets ("junk" food, polished rice, sweet drinks, alcohol) may be most susceptible to its development. This form of high output cardiac failure is commonly accompanied by considerable fluid retention and edema, symptoms and signs of nutritional deficiencies, and, occasionally, disorders of the nervous system (e.g., peripheral neuropathy, Wernicke–Korsakoff's psychosis). Thiamine and supportive dietary measures reverse most of the manifestations of beriberi heart disease. A rare fulminant form referred to as *Shoshin beriberi* presents with severe refractory hypotension, lactic acidosis, circulatory shock, and pulmonary edema, and carries a high mortality rate.

Neoplastic and paraneoplastic diseases (e.g., carcinomas, sarcomas, lymphomas, hyperviscosity disorders) can evoke high output heart failure through mechanisms other than arteriovenous fistulas and shunting. Alternative explanations include elevated metabolic rate and high blood viscosity.

Marked obesity is associated with increased cardiac output and heart failure; however, the heart failure is only partially related to the chronically elevated cardiac output.[10,23] Other common contributory insults include systemic hypertension and elevated pulmonary artery pressures and pulmonary vascular resistances secondary to alveolar hypoventilation.

Chronic tachycardia has been shown to cause heart failure in humans and, interestingly, serves as a reliable means of inducing heart failure in canine models.

COMBINATION OF MECHANISMS

A number of clinical conditions are complicated by high output heart failure caused by several distinct etiologies. Chronic renal failure serves as a good example (Figs. 3.30, 3.31). High cardiac output in many of these patients is caused by chronic anemia (hemoglobin levels of 7 to 9 g %), expanded intravascular volume, tachycardia, and chronic high flow through the surgically constructed, dialysis-access arteriovenous shunt.

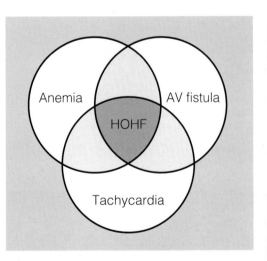

FIGURE 3.30   Conditions that often interact in chronic renal failure to cause high output heart failure. A combination of disorders are often responsible for evoking high output heart failure (HOHF).

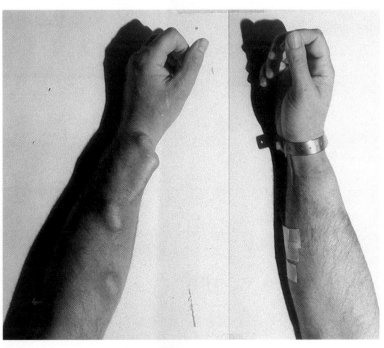

FIGURE 3.31
A 46-year-old patient with high output heart failure secondary to the triad present in Figure 3.30. Tachycardia, chronic anemia (hemoglobin 7.4 g %), and the dialysis-access shunt (left forearm) led to a resting cardiac output of 15 L/min. Occlusion of the arterial segment of the shunt evoked an 18% fall in cardiac output and a 10% drop in heart rate (Branham sign). Note the sizable venous segments of the surgical shunt and the darker pigmentation in the left forearm. The right arm is included as the control limb.

FIGURE CREDITS

Fig. 3.23 courtesy of William Smead, MD, Columbus, Ohio.

Fig. 3.24, 3.25 courtesy of Michael Van Aman, MD, Columbus, Ohio.

Fig. 3.29A,C from Shands AR, Raney RB (eds): Handbook of Orthopedic Surgery, 7th ed. St. Louis, CV Mosby, 1986

REFERENCES

1. Ahearn DJ, Maher JF: Heart failure as a complication of hemodialysis arteriovenous fistula. Ann Intern Med 77:201, 1972.

2. Akbarian M, Yankopoulos NA, Abelmann WH: Hemodynamic studies in beriberi heart disease. Am J Med 41:197, 1966.

3. Anderson CB, Codd JR, Graff RA, et al: Cardiac failure and upper extremity arteriovenous dialysis fistulas. Arch Intern Med 136:292, 1976.

4. Balfour IC, Covitz W, Davis H, et al: Cardiac size and function in children with sickle cell anemia. Am Heart J 108:345, 1984.

5. Baranda MM, Perez M, DeAndres J, et al: High-output congestive heart failure as first manifestation of Osler-Weber-Rendu disease. J Vasc Dis 35:568, 1984.

6. Branham HH: Aneurysmal varix of the femoral artery and vein following a gunshot wound. Int J Surg 3:250, 1890.

7. Burch GE, DePasquale N, Hyman A, et al: Influence of tropical weather on cardiac output, work, and power of right and left ventricles of man resting in hospital. Arch Intern Med 104:553, 1959.

8. Burckhardt D, Stalder GA, Ludin H, et al: Hyperdynamic circulatory state due to Osler-Weber-Rendu disease with intrahepatic arteriovenous fistulas. Am Heart J 85:797, 1973.

9. Denenberg BS, Criner G, Jones R, et al: Cardiac function in sickle cell anemia. Am J Cardiol 51:1674, 1983.

10. DeVitis O, Fazio S, Petito M, et al: Obesity and cardiac function. Circulation 64:477, 1981.

11. Dorney ER: Peripheral AV fistula of fifty-seven years' duration with refractory heart failure. Am Heart J 54:778, 1957.

12. Duke M, Abelmann WH: The hemodynamic response to chronic anemia. Circulation 39:503, 1969.

13. Epstein FH, Post RS, McDowell M: The effect of an arteriovenous fistula on renal hemodynamics and electrolyte excretion. J Clin Invest 32:233, 1953.

14. Fee HJ, Levisman J, Doud RB, et al: High output congestive heart failure from femoral arteriovenous shunts for vascular access. Ann Surg 183:321, 1976.

15. Gillum RF, Teicholz LE, Herman MV, et al: The idiopathic hyperkinetic heart syndrome: Clinical course and long-term prognosis. Am Heart J 102:728, 1981.

16. Gorlin R, Brachfeld N, Turner JO, et al: The idiopathic high cardiac output state. J Clin Invest 38:2144, 1959.

17. Graettinger JS, Parsons RL, Campbell JA: A correlation of clinical and hemodynamic studies in patients with mild and severe anemia with and without congestive failure. Ann Intern Med 58:617, 1963.

18. Gupta PD, Singh M: Neural mechanism underlying tachycardia induced by nonhypotensive A-V shunt. Am J Physiol 236:H35, 1979.

19. Hildreth DH, Turcke DA: Postlaminectomy arteriovenous fistula. Surgery 81:512, 1977.

20. Kawai C, Wakabayashi A, Matsumura T, et al: Reappearance of beriberi heart disease in Japan; a study of 23 cases. Am J Med 69:383, 1980.

21. Lequime J, Denolin H: Circulatory dynamics in osteitis deformans. Circulation 12:215, 1955.

22. McIntosh HD, Miller DE, Gleason WL, et al: The circulatory dynamics of polyostotic fibrous dysplasia. Am J Med 32:393, 1962.

23. Messerli FH, Ventura HO, Reisin E, et al: Borderline hypertension and obesity: Two prehypertensive states with elevated cardiac output. Circulation 66:55, 1982.

24. Miller GJ, Serjeant GR, Sivapraqasam S, et al: Cardioventricular function and hyperthyroidism. Br Heart J 46:137, 1982.

25. Peery WH: Clinical spectrum of hereditary hemorrhagic telangiectasia. Am J Med 82:989, 1987.

26. Pietras RJ, Real MA, Poticha GS, et al: Cardiovascular response to hyperthyroidism. Arch Intern Med 129:426, 1972.

27. Richardson TQ, Guyton AC: Effects of polycythemia and anemia on cardiac output and other circulatory factors. Am J Physiol 197:1167, 1959.

28. Sanyal SK, Saldivar V, Coburn TP, et al: Hyperdynamic heart failure due to A-V fistula associated with Wilms' tumor. Pediatrics 57:564, 1976.

29. Shapiro S, Steiner M, Dimich I: Congestive heart failure in neonatal thyrotoxicosis: A curable cause of heart failure in the newborn. Clin Pediatr 14:1155, 1975.

30. Shuster S: High output cardiac failure from skin disease. Lancet 1:1338, 1963.

31. Thomas FB, Mazzaferri EL, Skillman TG: Apathetic thyrotoxicosis: A distinctive clinical and laboratory entity. Ann Intern Med 72:679, 1970.

32. Vaksmann G, Rey C, Marache P, et al: Severe congestive heart failure in newborns due to giant cutaneous hemangiomas. Am J Cardiol 60:392, 1987.

33. Voight GC, Kronthal HL, Crounse RG: Cardiac output in erythroderma skin disease. Am Heart J 72:615, 1966.

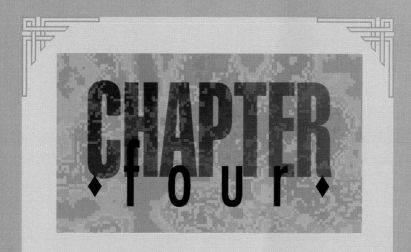

CHAPTER four

ARRHYTHMIAS

ROBERT S. MITTLEMAN, MD

S. K. STEPHEN HUANG, MD

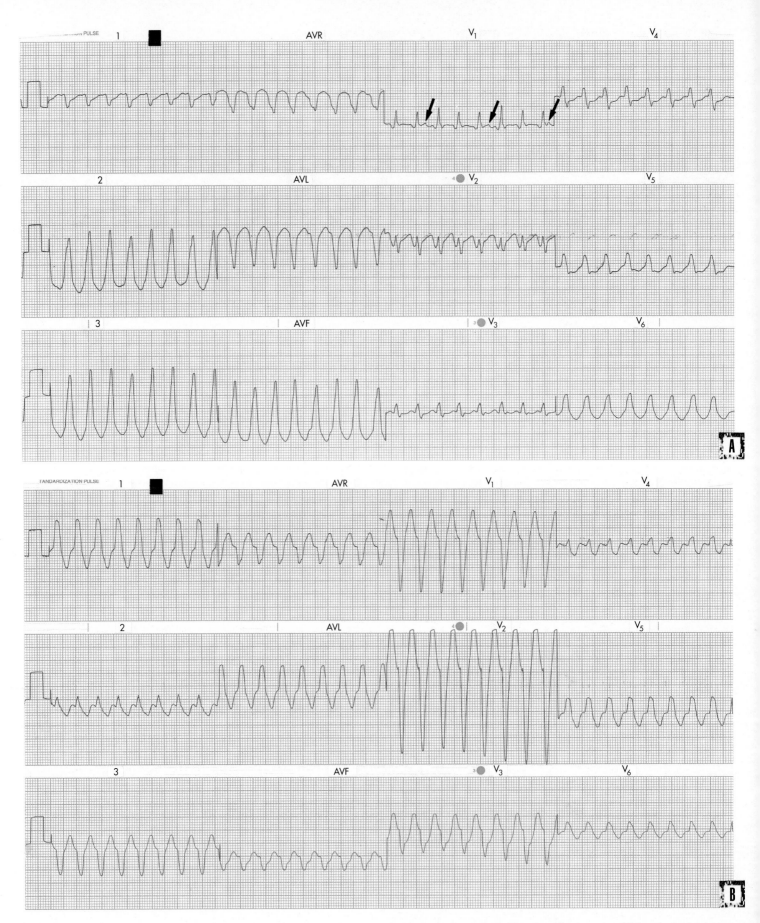

FIGURE 4.1 **(A)** Wide-complex tachycardia, that proved to be a sustained monomorphic ventricular tachycardia, in a 55-year-old male with a history of myocardial infarction. It is regular at a rate of 180 BPM, with a right axis deviation. Careful inspection of the ECG produced the definitive diagnosis—the P waves are dissociated from the tachycardia. This is clearly demonstrated in lead V_1 where P waves (*arrows*) are seen after the second, fifth, and eighth complexes. **(B)** A similar wide-com-

plex tachycardia recorded in a healthy 22-year-old female with a history of palpitations. The rate and the morphology of the precordial leads are similar to those seen in Figure 4.1(A), but the axis is leftward and there is a more apparent left bundle branch block pattern compared to the previous ECG. By invasive electrophysiologic evaluation, an AV-reciprocating tachycardia was diagnosed with aberrant conduction due to a concealed accessory pathway.

Our understanding of cardiac arrhythmias has evolved greatly in the past two decades, particularly with the availability of intracardiac recordings and programmed electrical stimulation to reproduce clinical arrhythmias. However, the basic skills such as the detailed collection of a medical history and physical examination remain a valuable part of the data base. For example, the onset of a wide-complex tachycardia in a 55-year-old man with a history of a large myocardial infarction is likely to be due to ventricular tachycardia, while a similar tachycardia in a 22-year-old female with a long-standing history of palpitations and no cardiac disease is likely to be a supraventricular tachycardia with aberrancy; consequently the two would be managed very differently (Fig. 4.1). In both cases programmed electrical stimulation might be necessary to confirm the diagnosis, to guide drug therapy, and even potentially to deliver treatment.

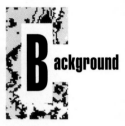

Background

In order to diagnose arrhythmias properly, it is important to be aware of the anatomy of the conduction system, as well as the pathophysiology of arrhythmia formation. Cardiac depolarization generally begins at the sinoatrial (sinus) node, an oblong structure that lies along the sulcus terminalis near the junction of the superior vena cava and the lateral portion of the right atrium (Fig. 4.2).[4] The rest of the conduction system is illustrated in Figure 4.3. The route of conduction to the atrioventricular (AV) node is still not clarified; specialized atrial conduction pathways have been hypothesized to exist, but have never been demonstrated anatomically. The AV node is an elongated structure found in the most anterior portion of the triangle of Koch, on the right side of the atrial septum just above the tricuspid ring (Fig. 4.4; see also Figs. 1.29–1.30). The superior limit of the triangle of Koch is the tendon of Todaro, which continues posteriorly as the eustachian valve of the inferior vena cava. The inferior limit is the tricuspid valve annulus. The os of the coronary sinus defines the posterior border. Conduction through the AV node is slow compared to the rest of the specialized conduction pathways, and this property generally controls the maximal rate of ventricular response, preventing the heart rate from being dangerously elevated in the event of supraventricular tachycardia.

Conduction from the AV node to the ventricular myocardium occurs by way of the His–Purkinje conduction system, a set of specialized fibers that are able to conduct very rapidly (3 cm/sec). Those fibers first leave the AV node to enter the bundle of His, as they penetrate into the central fibrous body. The left bundle diverges from the common bundle at a 90° angle. Although, based on the ECG, the left bundle can be thought to divide into an anterior and a posterior fascicle, the true structure is quite variable. The bundle most commonly divides

FIGURE 4.2   Location of the sinus node in the right atrium.

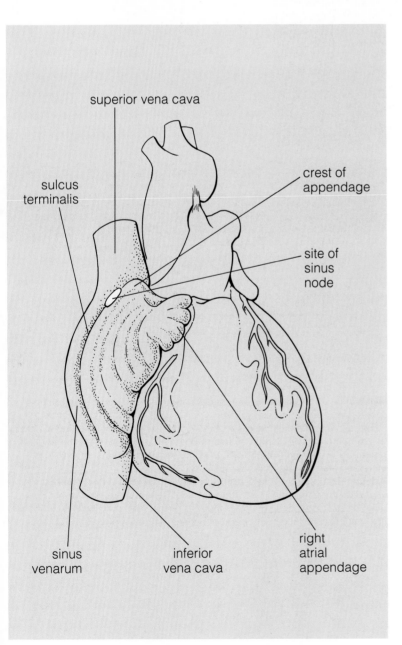

superior vena cava

sulcus
terminalis

crest of
appendage

site of
sinus
node

sinus
venarum

inferior
vena cava

right
atrial
appendage

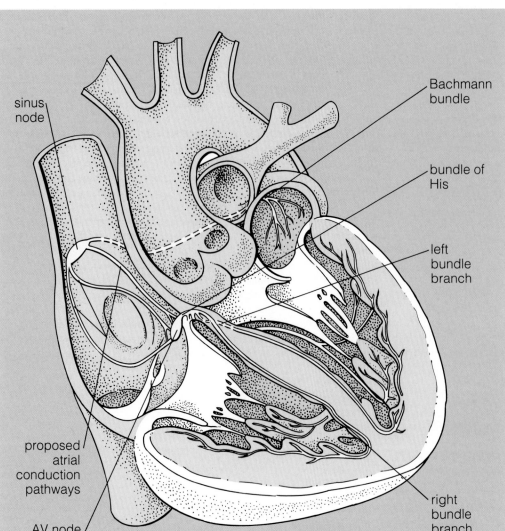

FIGURE 4.3   Normal cardiac conduction system.

sinus node

Bachmann bundle

bundle of His

left bundle branch

proposed atrial conduction pathways

AV node

right bundle branch

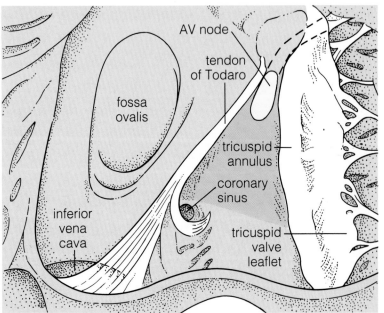

FIGURE 4.4   Triangle of Koch. The limits of the triangle are the tendon of Todaro, tricuspid valve annulus, and, posteriorly, the coronary sinus. The AV node is located at the anterior apex of the triangle.

AV node

tendon of Todaro

fossa ovalis

tricuspid annulus

coronary sinus

inferior vena cava

tricuspid valve leaflet

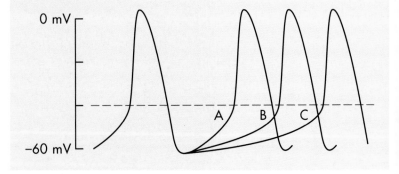

FIGURE 4.5   Transmembrane action potentials from a cell exhibiting spontaneous diastolic depolarization. The action potentials are typical of those seen in pacemaker areas of the SA node. The dashed line defines the threshold potential at which an action potential is generated. If the slope of phase 4 is decreased from B to C, the time required to reach threshold is increased and the rate of discharge slows. An increase in the slope of phase 4 depolarization from B to A results in take-off potential being reached sooner and an increase in the rate of discharge. The same process can occur in other cardiac cells, which allows them to assume the pacemaker function of the heart. (Reproduced with permission; see Figure Credits)

0 mV

−60 mV

A B C

into three separate bundles, but there is a wide variety in the structure from person to person. Ultimately, the branches of the left bundle appear to form a network of Purkinje fibers just below the endocardial surface of the left ventricular septum and the rest of the left ventricular myocardium (see Fig. 1.31). The right bundle is the continuation of the bundle of His after the separation of the left bundle, and it also appears to form a network of Purkinje fibers below the right ventricular endocardial surface. After the wave of depolarization has spread throughout the entire endocardial surface of the ventricles, the myocardium is activated simultaneously from the endocardial to the epicardial surface, which leads to the synchronized ventricular contraction. Of note is that the activation of the ventricular myocardium is responsible for the QRS complex on the standard ECG, while the intervening electrical events, including AV nodal and His–Purkinje activation, are electrically silent. The intracardiac recordings are necessary to define the depolarization of these small but essential structures.

Although definitive knowledge of the mechanisms of arrhythmias is not available, enough is known about the potential mechanisms to improve our understanding and ability to manage patients.[15-18] The current belief is that there are several basic mechanisms that account for the generation of all arrhythmias. The first mechanism is *increased automaticity*, which can occur as a normal physiologic process or as a pathologic event.

As mentioned, the sinus node is normally the dominant pacemaker for the heart, because it has faster phase 4 depolarization than the other tissues of the heart, causing a faster rate of discharge (Fig. 4.5). However, under some circumstances, other cells in the heart can depolarize at a rate faster than that of the sinus node and take over the role of pacing for the heart. This alteration can occur as an appropriate physiologic response. For example, a competitive athlete will occasionally develop a marked sinus bradycardia to the extent that the AV junction has a faster rate of spontaneous depolarization, causing a junctional escape rhythm. Such a development would be a normal response and would not require treatment.

Abnormal automaticity can also occur. For instance, a patient who has severe emphysema has high catecholamine levels in the heart. It can be hypothesized that the condition will alter the electrophysiologic properties in a different part of the atrium, causing the chamber to have a more rapid discharge rate and, consequently, producing an atrial tachycardia. This type of arrhythmia can be suppressed temporarily by pacing the heart even faster than at this site of increased automaticity, but the automatic focus will resume its role after pacing is terminated.

Another mechanism believed to account for many arrhythmias is *triggered activity*, i.e., pacemaker activity that occurs as a result of a preceding impulse or series of impulses. This is in contrast to automaticity, which occurs spontaneously. The impulse that initiates triggered activity is an afterdepolarization, which is classified as either early (EAD) or delayed (DAD), the two representing very different phenomena.

As the name suggests, EADs are episodes of depolarization of the cell membrane occurring at the terminal portion of the action potential (Phase 3) and are usually not of sufficient amplitude to reach the threshold for depolarization. EADs are felt to be responsible for episodes of the very dangerous heart rhythm known as *torsade de pointes*. This is a form of ventricular tachycardia in which the QRS axis appears to rotate on its axis (i.e., change its polarity) as it progresses (see Fig. 4.29). It is associated with quinidine toxicity, hypokalemia, and other phenomena which prolong the Q–T interval. It has been suggested that prolonged repolarization exaggerates the amplitude of these EADs, potentially allowing them to reach depolarization threshold and produce an episode of ventricular tachycardia. An EAD can be recorded with a monophasic action potential (MAP) catheter, a special catheter that takes a percutaneous recording of an action potential from the ventricular myocardium (Fig. 4.6).

DADs are very different from EADs. They also represent subthreshold depolarizations that can occur after the action potential, but DADs occur considerably after EADs, during phase 4 depolarization (Fig. 4.7). In this case spontaneously occurring premature beats or rapid ventricular pacing exaggerates the amplitude of

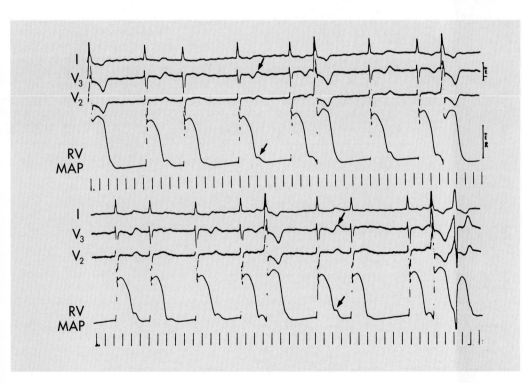

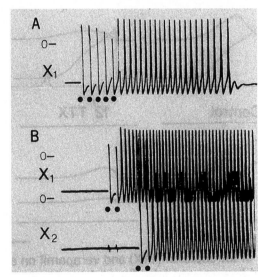

FIGURE 4.7 Triggered sustained rhythmic activity and delayed afterdepolarizations in a diseased ventricle. **(A)** Spontaneous activity triggered by a series of driven action potentials (*dots*) at the recording site X1. The size of the delayed afterdepolarizations (*arrows*) gradually increases until the afterdepolarization reaches threshold and maintains rhythmic activity after cessation of pacing. The activity ends when the last afterdepolarization fails to reach threshold (*final arrow*). **(B)** Initiation of triggered activity by intracellular current injection (*dots*) at sites X1 and X2, which lie along the same trabeculum. Although sites X1 and X2 were only 4 mm apart, the activity from one site did not propagate to the other, indicating complete dissociation between the two sites. (cycle length = 2000 msec; pulse duration = 10 msec; pulse intensity = 200 na; vertical calibration = 50 mV; horizontal calibration = 10 sec) (Reproduced with permission; see Figure Credits)

FIGURE 4.6 Monophasic action potential (MAP) recordings showing early afterdepolarizations in a patient with quinidine-induced torsade de pointes. The peak of the afterdepolarization is synchronous with the peak of the U wave, and the amplitude of both waves varies significantly with the length of the preceding R–R interval (*arrows*). (Reproduced with permission; see Figure Credits)

these DADs, such that the membrane potential achieves the threshold for depolarization. This action causes a self-perpetuating tachycardia, with each beat causing a large DAD, which in turn initiates the following beat. Some of the arrhythmias produced by digitalis toxicity are thought to occur as a result of DADs.

Re-entry is not an abnormal formation of impulses, but rather a problem with abnormal conduction. Although a variety of phenomena may account for re-entrant arrhythmias,[14] these arrhythmias have classically been described as requiring an area of slow conduction and unidirectional block (Fig. 4.8). Under normal circumstances, conduction proceeds through both normal and abnormal tissue. When a premature impulse occurs or is produced by a pacing catheter, it propagates into the re-entrant circuit. The area of slow conduction may then develop block while conduction proceeds through the other limb of the circuit. It then conducts retrograde through the area of block. Because of the slow conduction, the impulse finds the tissue remains excitable as it continues through the circuit. It therefore establishes a loop through which the wave of depolarization continuously rotates, finding an area of excitable tissue in its path. At any point in time the area just ahead in its path remains refractory from the last trip around the loop, but it will recover its excitability by the time the wave of depolarization arrives.

Re-entry is felt to be responsible for many arrhythmias, including most paroxysmal supraventricular tachycardias, atrial flutter, and sustained monomorphic ventricular tachycardia. In the electrophysiology laboratory, these arrhythmias can often be reproducibly initiated and terminated; this fact may justify the identification of re-entry as *the* mechanism of an arrhythmia. This can be concluded because although an automatic arrhythmia can generally be temporarily suppressed by overdrive pacing, it cannot be initiated or terminated by pacing.

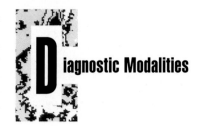

Diagnostic Modalities

Patients with arrhythmias can have an extraordinary range of symptoms, from none to a cardiac arrest, but also including palpitations, lightheadedness, syncope, presyncope, chest pain, and dyspnea. Of paramount importance in determining the diagnosis (Fig. 4.9) is an exquisitely detailed history of the events surrounding the spell that is thought to be responsible for the arrhythmia. For example, an 87-year-old man is known to have passed out on his bedroom floor, only to awaken when found by his wife. We need to know such routine information as how long he was unconscious, whether any trauma was sustained, whether any palpitations occurred prior to the spell, or whether seizure-like activity occurred. Of course, any history of cardiac disease, including prior stud-

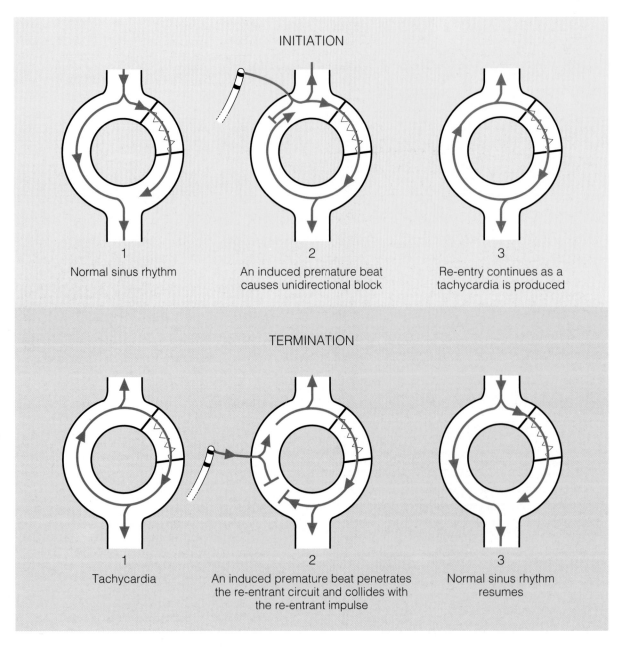

FIGURE 4.8 Mechanism of re-entry. **(A)** A common substrate could be an area of slow conduction. If a premature extrastimulus is introduced, unidirectional block can develop in one of the two limbs of the pathway. With the delay produced by the slowly conducting pathway, a re-entrant arrhythmia can then be perpetuated.
(B) Similarly, a critically timed premature beat will enter the "excitable gap" and alter the timing required for the perpetuation of the arrhythmia, thereby terminating it.

INITIATION

1
Normal sinus rhythm

2
An induced premature beat causes unidirectional block

3
Re-entry continues as a tachycardia is produced

TERMINATION

1
Tachycardia

2
An induced premature beat penetrates the re-entrant circuit and collides with the re-entrant impulse

3
Normal sinus rhythm resumes

ies of heart function, is important. But other information becomes critically important as well: had the patient recently taken any medication that could have contributed to the spell? Did he arise suddenly just before falling? Had he been feeling differently, such as episodes of chest pain or dizziness, in the days or weeks prior to the spell? The information of a witness, or of the paramedics who first attended to the patient, may provide critical information in reaching a diagnosis. On the other hand, a history of a documented arrhythmia may be misleading. It is of paramount importantance to make sure that a particular arrythmia is associated temporally with a specific symptom.

The physical examination can be helpful as well. Naturally, if the physician is present while the arrhythmia is occurring, simply palpating the pulse (if there is any!) may help in classifying the arrhythmia as either a bradyarrhythmia or tachyarrhythmia. Venous pulsations may provide insight into whether there is AV synchrony. Even when the arrhythmia is not occurring "in front of your eyes," the physical examination can provide clues to pre-existing heart disease. Likewise, the 12-lead ECG can suggest evidence of a previous myocardial infarction or perhaps demonstrate the short P–R interval and delta waves associated with the Wolff–Parkinson–White (WPW) syndrome or a long Q–T interval predisposing to torsade de pointes.

Of course, one of the primary modes of diagnosis is a direct recording of the arrhythmia while it is actually occurring. Although the information recorded is not as detailed as that obtained with direct intracardiac recordings, it is much more likely to capture an arrhythmia while the patient is riding in an ambulance, in the coronary care unit, or wearing a Holter monitor than while he is in the electrophysiology laboratory. Furthermore, even though the mechanism of an arrhythmia can be exhaustively studied in the electrophysiology laboratory, it can sometimes be difficult to determine whether the arrhythmia produced in this relatively artificial setting is the same one accounting for the patient's presenting symptoms. The arrhythmia that is directly associated with the symptoms should be the gold standard for the diagnosis!

The ability to record and analyze such an arrhythmia accurately is continually being refined. These advances have occurred both in the hospital and in the outpatient setting. More sophisticated monitoring equipment is increasingly available in the hospital setting to provide the capability of automatic recognition and recording of arrhythmias, and even the opportunity for complete recall of every heartbeat during hospitalization.

It is also often important to record the patient's cardiac rhythm while he is pursuing the normal daily routine outside of the hospital. Symptoms that occur frequently can be analyzed with the Holter monitor, which records two or three modified ECG leads continuously over 1 or more days.[8]

For unexplained arrhythmias that occur outside the hospital but are sufficiently infrequent that they are unlikely to be recorded with a 24-hour Holter monitor, there are other modalities available. Transtelephonic event monitors can be easily carried for prolonged periods of time and can be attached when an arrhythmia-related symptom occurs. When the symptom does occur, the arrhythmia can be directly transmitted by telephone, or can be recorded on tape and later transmitted by telephone to the physician for analysis. Alternatively, recording devices can be worn continuously for up to 1 month, so that they can be triggered at any time to recall an event which was too evanescent to record directly.[7,9] This can be invaluable in diagnosing a patient with unexplained syncope, often a diagnostic dilemma (Fig. 4.10). These patients can activate the device after a syncopal spell, allowing documentation of the heart rhythm prior to, during, and after the syncopal event. These devices will continue to evolve to provide increased comfort and convenience to the patient and more sophisticated recall of arrhythmias.

Other forms of electrocardiography that use sophisticated analytic techniques to collect detailed information about cardiac conduction are now available. The signal-averaged ECG is a noninvasive technique that has the ability to predict the tendency for a life-threatening ventricular arrhythmia.[6] The ECG is produced by recording and analyzing as many as several hundred beats to improve the signal-to-noise ratio and thereby improve, by several orders of magnitude, the resolution of the recording. Using this technique, one can identify an area of slow ventricular conduction that causes part of the myocardium to be depolarized later than the rest, producing a small "late potential" at the end of the QRS

FIGURE 4.9 MODALITIES USED IN DIAGNOSING ARRHYTHMIAS

- **History**
- **Physical Examination**
- **Electrocardiogram**
  12-lead
  Rhythm strip
  Holter monitor
  Event recorder
- **Electrophysiologic Studies**
- **Other**
  Signal-averaged electrocardiogram
  Head-up tilt (HUT) testing
  Esophageal electrograms
  Permanent pacing leads
  Temporary epicardial
    (postoperative only)
  Epicardial and hand-held
    (intraoperative only)
  Computerized multipolar recording
    Balloon
    Band
    Other

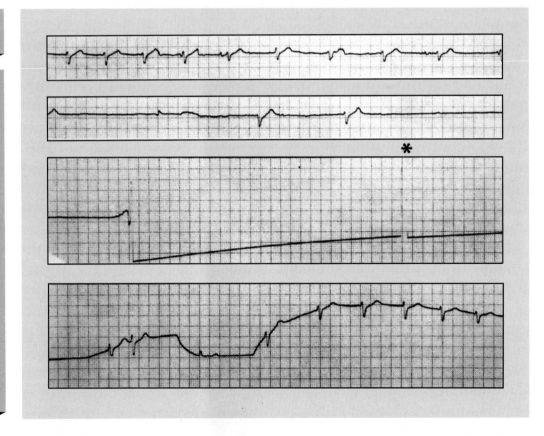

FIGURE 4.10   Loop monitor rhythm strip of 30-year-old woman with recurrent syncope and presyncope showing prolonged period of asystole. Asterisk denotes event marker initiated by observer. Of note, a subsequent electrophysiologic study was entirely normal.

in normal sinus rhythm (Fig. 4.11). At a different time, this zone of slow conduction could serve as the substrate for a re-entrant sustained ventricular tachycardia. (In fact, it is more likely that a late potential serves as a marker of a patient with areas of slow conduction who is prone to life-threatening ventricular arrhythmias. The area of slow conduction in normal sinus rhythm frequently does not correspond directly to the substrate for the tachycardia.)

Another new technique that is still being evaluated, but shows great promise in the evaluation of patients with syncope, is head-up tilt testing.[1,2] This test involves placing the patient supine on a flat table after an overnight fast and then tilting the table to a nearly upright position for a period of several minutes to 1 hour. Sometimes isoproterenol administration is used. In some patients this technique can provoke dramatic syncopal spells associated with prolonged asystole and hypotension (Fig. 4.12). It is believed that the technique reproduces the inappropriate activation of a profound vagal stimulation, which can produce a syncopal spell (Fig. 4.13). It appears to be a very useful technique for the evaluation of unexplained syncope, but its value in guiding therapy is as yet undetermined.

Electrophysiologic Study

The cardiac electrophysiologic study, although an invasive procedure, provides the most detailed information available about arrhythmias.[10] Specialized multipolar temporary pacing catheters are positioned at multiple sites in the heart by the transvenous route. These catheters are used to record and stimulate selectively to give information about intracardiac conduction and to determine the sequence of cardiac depolarization. Many arrhythmias can be reproduced in the

laboratory to determine their characteristics in order to design appropriate drug therapy. These induced arrhythmias can also be used as an index of successful drug therapy, as suppression of an arrhythmia in the laboratory implies the protection against a clinical recurrence.

The most common catheter placements for a basic study are shown in Figure 4.14. The catheters are most often inserted via the femoral vein although any large vein can be used. One catheter is placed across the tricuspid valve to the right ventricular apex to stimulate and record from that site. The intracardiac recording, or *electrogram*, occurs simultaneously with the QRS complex on the surface ECG (Fig. 4.15). A second catheter is placed in the high right atrium, which similarly is used for both pacing and recording in the atrium. As would be expected, the atrial electrogram coincides with the P wave. The third catheter is commonly placed just across the septal portion of the tricuspid valve. In this position it is used almost always just for recording. Since the electrodes straddle the tricuspid valve, they are able to record both atrial and ventricular activity. Furthermore, since they are in close proximity to the bundle of His, they record the rapid depolarization of this fiber. It is seen as a narrow spike, which in the normal patient will occur 30 to 55 msec before the beginning of ventricular activation. Since such a small amount of tissue is activated, the depolarization of the bundle of His is invisible on the surface recording. Catheters are sometimes positioned in other areas of the heart, such as the coronary sinus, which is useful for measuring activation on the left side of the heart, or the right ventricular outflow tract (not shown), which can be useful for inducing an arrhythmia that cannot be induced at a different location.

After the catheters have been positioned, the activation sequence can be analyzed in detail and a tremendous amount of information can be gained about cardiac depolarization. For instance, from the tracing in Figure 4.15 it is clear that the activation recorded in the high right atrial catheter occurs before the atrial activation near the His catheter, since the high right atrial catheter is near the sinus node, where the atrial depolarization originates. The left atrium, recorded from the coronary sinus catheter, is activated even later.

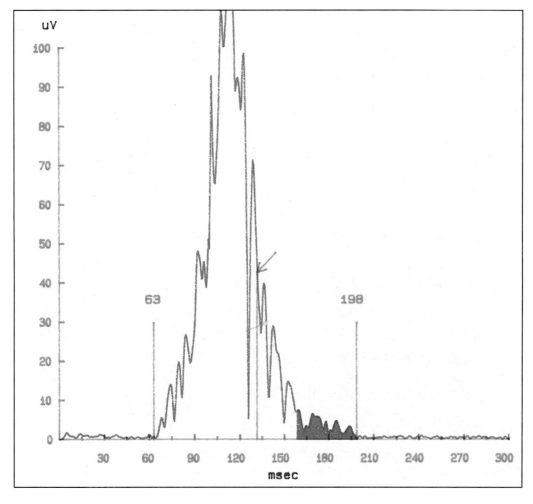

FIGURE 4.11   Signal-averaged ECG from a patient with a history of sustained monomorphic ventricular tachycardia. Note the late potential (in green), which represents an area of delayed, fractionated depolarization when the patient is in normal sinus rhythm. The area of the heart that produced this part of the tracing could potentially be the substrate for a re-entrant ventricular tachycardia in the future.

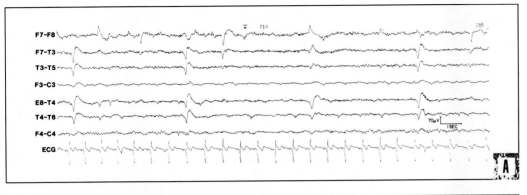

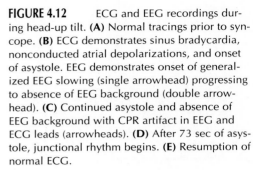

FIGURE 4.12 ECG and EEG recordings during head-up tilt. **(A)** Normal tracings prior to syncope. **(B)** ECG demonstrates sinus bradycardia, nonconducted atrial depolarizations, and onset of asystole. EEG demonstrates onset of generalized EEG slowing (single arrowhead) progressing to absence of EEG background (double arrowhead). **(C)** Continued asystole and absence of EEG background with CPR artifact in EEG and ECG leads (arrowheads). **(D)** After 73 sec of asystole, junctional rhythm begins. **(E)** Resumption of normal ECG.

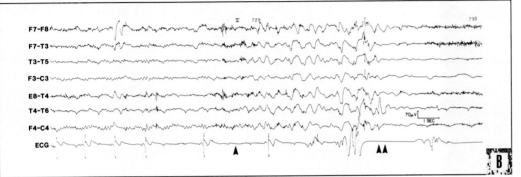

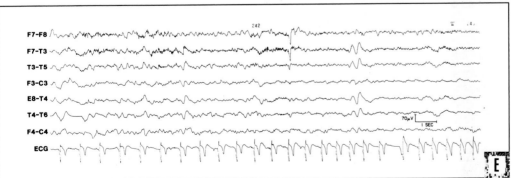

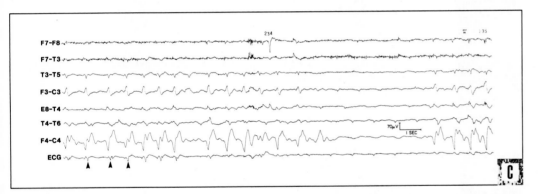

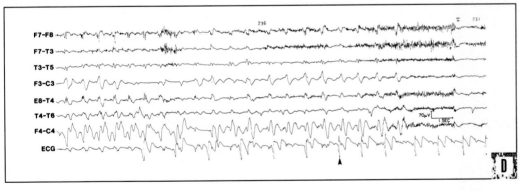

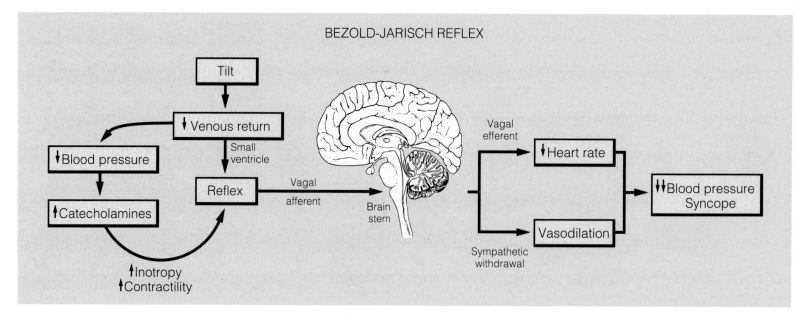

FIGURE 4.13   Bezold–Jarisch reflex, hypothesized as the mechanism of tilt table-induced hypotension and bradycardia. A head-up tilt reduces venous return, leading to a slight reduction in systolic blood pressure with a subsequent increase in serum catecholamines and a small left ventricular cavity. Vigorous contraction of a small ventricle initiates the reflex via intra-cardiac vagal mechanoreceptors. Brainstem synapses with vagal efferents lead to bradycardia, as well as to sympathetic withdrawal and peripheral vasodilatation. This results in profound hypotension and syncope. (Reproduced with permission; see Figure Credits)

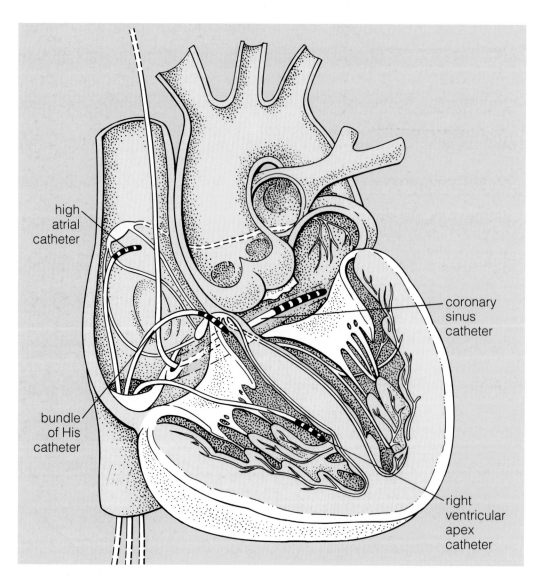

FIGURE 4.14   Positioning of catheters for a typical electrophysiologic study.

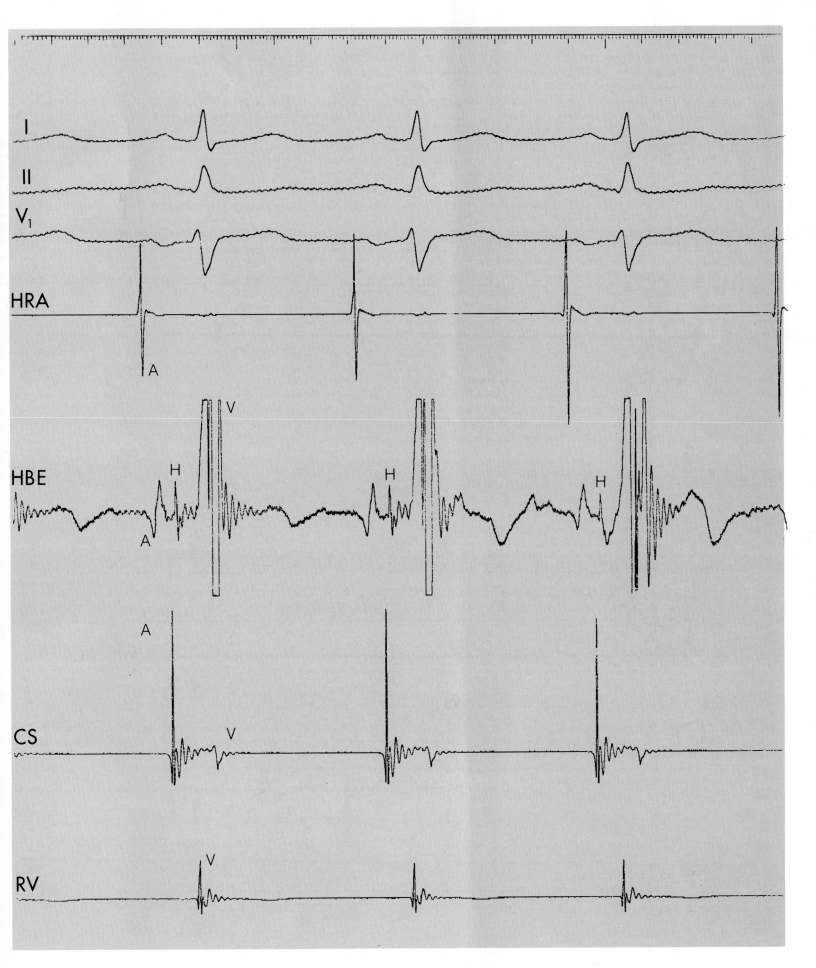

FIGURE 4.15   Typical recordings from electrode catheters (as seen in Fig. 4.14). Leads I, II, and V₁ are standard ECG leads. (HRA = high right atrium ; CS = coronary sinus; HBE = His bundle electrogram; RV = right ventricular electrogram; A = atrial electrogram; V = right ventricular electrogram)

By recording the bundle of His, one can measure the A–H interval (from the beginning of atrial activation to the beginning of the His spike), as well as the H–V interval (from the beginning of the His spike to the first evidence of ventricular activation). These are the two important components of AV conduction. As discussed later, this information can be invaluable in assessing the site of AV block and deciding whether a pacemaker is necessary.

Once the intervals have been measured, programmed stimulation is performed. Most often this involves pacing the heart at variable rates in either the atrium, with the high right atrial catheter (Fig. 4.16), or in the ventricle, with the catheter in the right ventricular apex. The second form of stimulation that is done is the insertion of premature beats. Usually up to three successive premature beats are delivered. These beats can be delivered either synchronized to the patient's own heart rhythm or following a pacing train, most often of eight beats (Fig. 4.17). The purpose of the pacing train is to establish a constant and reproducible electrophysiologic environment for evaluating the effect of the premature beats. As mentioned, often the goal is to induce an arrhythmia that has occurred clinically or that may explain the patient's symptoms. The premature beats have the best chance of reproducing the critical delay in activation necessary for establishing an area of re-entry and sustaining a tachycardia.

Once a tachycardia has been initiated there is the potential for terminating it with pacing. Again, this can be done either with pacing or by the insertion of premature beats. In either case, the goal is to alter the critical timing occurring in the area of re-entry.

Since the electrophysiology laboratory is an artificial environment, sometimes other measures are needed to induce an arrhythmia. Such provocative measures can involve the administration of medication, such as isoproterenol, to alter the conduction properties in the heart. On some occasions, altering the patient's autonomic tone can accomplish the same purpose. One technique used is carotid sinus massage, which will sometimes produce complete sinus arrest. When this occurs, it may be an indication for a permanent pacemaker (Fig. 4.18).

Reproducing an arrhythmia in the electrophysiology laboratory can provide a more accurate diagnosis of the mechanism than that obtained by routine electrocardiography. For example, with a wide-complex tachycardia, the presence of AV dissociation substantiates the diagnosis of ventricular tachycardia. But more often than not, P waves are not visible on the routine ECG. In the electrophysiology laboratory, reproduction of the tachycardia allows an analysis of the relationship between atrial and ventricular activation, which should yield a definitive diagnosis.

Very commonly, the electrophysiology laboratory is used as an index for determining whether a medication has been successful in suppressing a patient's arrhythmia. If a medication is effective at suppressing a tachycardia that was previously inducible, this is reasonable evidence that a clinical recurrence of the arrhythmia can be effectively prevented.

In the last few years, electrophysiology has been moving into the interventional realm, i.e., able not only to diagnose arrhythmias, but also to deliver treatment. In order to perform such an intervention, much more detailed information is needed in regard to the site of origin of the arrythmia or the pathways of activation. Such information is obtained by "mapping" the arrythmia. When the intervention is surgery, the mapping can be performed in the operating room, where the heart is most accessible. Alternatively, mapping can be performed in the electrophysiology laboratory, either in preparation for surgery or for direct catheter ablation.

In the operating room, mapping procedures have progressed enormously with the benefit of computer-analyzed recordings. These allow the simultaneous recording of the activation sequence of the heart from over 100 sites. The site of earliest activation of the heart will usually correspond to the target for the ablation.

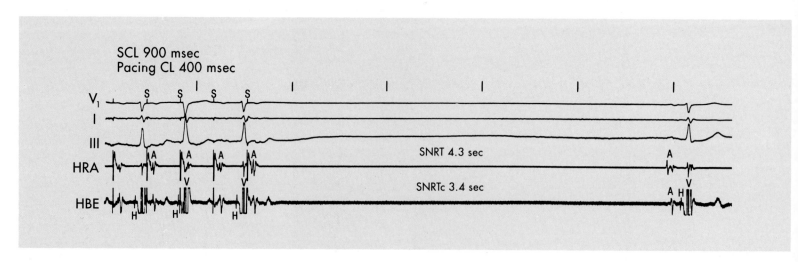

FIGURE 4.16   Prolonged pause, which was produced by the high right atrial catheter after a burst of rapid atrial pacing. This is known as the *sinus node recovery time* (SNRT). A prolonged SNRT implies sinus node dysfunction and is often an indication for a permanent pacemaker. It can be incidentally noted that there is a Wenckebach AV conduction pattern in the first few beats of the recording. (S = pacing stimulus; SCL = sinus cycle length; SNRTc = corrected sinus node recovery time, or SNRT-SCL; HRA = high right atrium; HBE = His bundle electrogram; A = atrial electrogram; V = right ventricular electrogram) (Reproduced with permission; see Figure Credits)

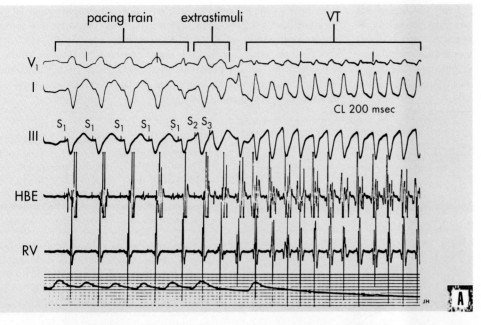

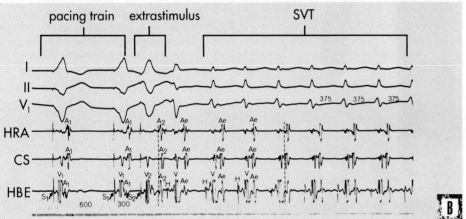

FIGURE 4.17 **(A)** Induction of sustained monomorphic ventricular tachycardia (VT) by a ventricular pacing train of eight beats (S_1) followed by two extrastimuli (S_2, S_3). Only the last five beats of the pacing train are shown. **(B)** Induction of a supraventricular tachycardia (SVT) by a ventricular pacing train followed by a single ventricular extrastimulus in a patient with WPW. (HRA = high right atrium; CS = coronary sinus; HBE = His bundle electrogram) (Reproduced with permission; see Figure Credits)

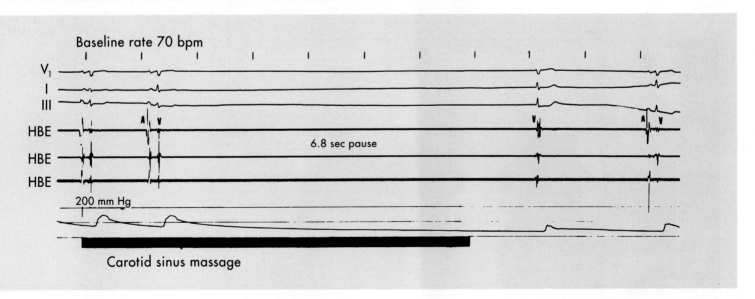

FIGURE 4.18 Evidence of carotid sinus hypersensitivity in a patient with recurrent syncope preceded by several seconds of lightheadedness. Left carotid sinus massage resulted in a 6.8-sec period of asystole. No other potential cause of syncope was found in this patient. (HBE = His bundle electrogram; A = atrial electrogram; V = ventricular electrogram) (Reproduced with permission; see Figure Credits)

For example, in the WPW syndrome a re-entrant circuit exists which produces a tachycardia involving retrograde activation of the atria from the ventricles over an accessory pathway (Fig. 4.19). By recording along the AV ring at multiple sites, a map can be drawn identifying the earliest site of activation and consequently the location of the pathway, which is the target for surgical ablation. In the operating room, this procedure is performed by placing a band along the AV ring; the band then records from all sites simultaneously.

Analogous mapping can be performed in the electrophysiology laboratory by recording from a multipolar catheter placed in the coronary sinus, which simultaneously records the atrial activation at multiple sites along the AV ring on the left side of the heart (Fig. 4.20). It is also possible to directly record the accessory pathway potential. In this case, the mapping can guide the location of an ablation catheter, which is placed near the site of earliest activation and/or the accessory pathway potential.

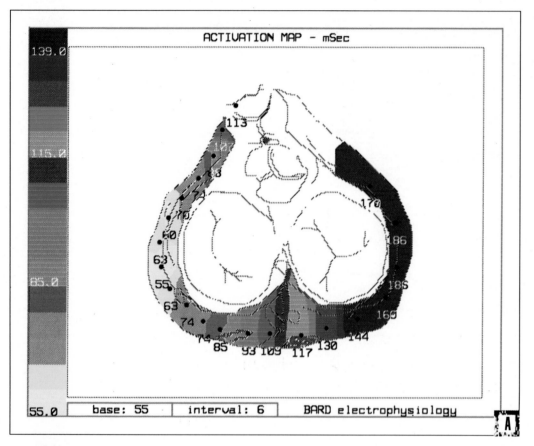

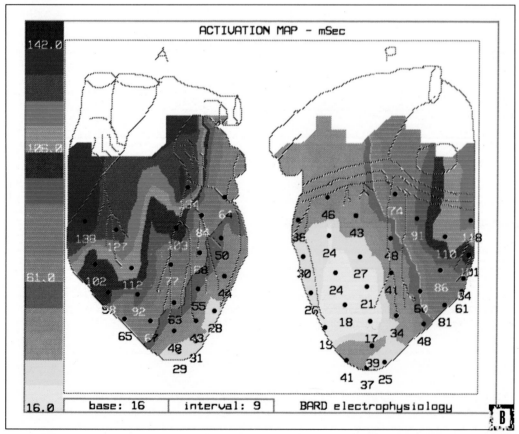

FIGURE 4.19 **(A)** Mapping of earliest atrial activation during an AV-reciprocating tachycardia in a patient with WPW. Recordings are made with a band placed on the atrial side of the AV groove during surgery. The black dots indicate the position of the recording electrodes. The numbers indicate activation times (in msec) compared to an arbitrary reference point. In this case, the earliest activation of the atrium (and hence, the location of the accessory pathway) is along the lateral wall of the mitral valve annulus (shown in yellow). **(B)** Mapping of the site of origin of sustained monomorphic ventricular tachycardia. Recordings are made after the induction of the arrhythmia from a "sock" placed around the outside of the heart during surgery. In this case, the earliest epicardial activation of the ventricle is in the inferoposterior left ventricle. (A = anterior; P = posterior; MV = mitral valve; TV = tricuspid valve; Ao = aortic valve)

Bradyarrhythmias
SINUS NODE DISEASE

Under normal awake and resting conditions, the sinus node rate should be between 60 and 100 beats per minute. The heart rate normally varies slightly with the respiratory cycle because of variation in autonomic tone. The overall sinus node rate can also alter either with variation in autonomic tone or by an abnormality in its structure or function.

Sick sinus syndrome is a general term applied to a condition in which chronic sinus node dysfunction is not associated with any clear-cut etiology, such as drug toxicity.[5,11] Pathologically, patients with the disease frequently manifest degenerative changes in the area of the sinus node. They frequently also have or develop AV nodal conduction disturbances. There are also frequently associated atrial tachyarrhythmias, such as atrial fibrillation or flutter. In this case, the condition is referred to as the *bradycardia–tachycardia syndrome*. Other common causes of sinus node dysfunction include exaggerated vagal tone, toxicity from digoxin, beta-blockers, or other drugs, and acute myocardial infarction.

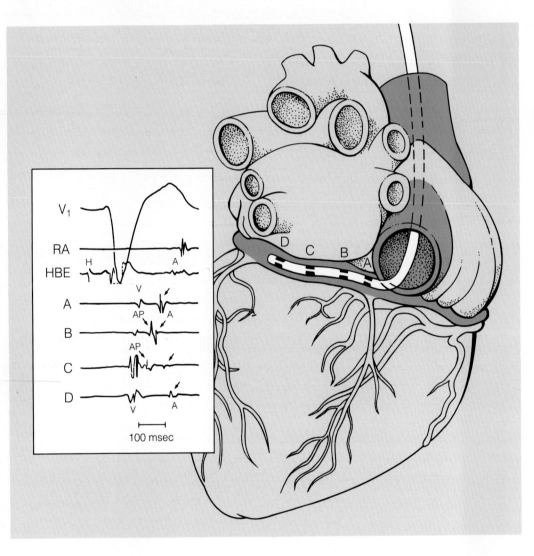

FIGURE 4.20 Multipolar coronary sinus catheter used to map the location of a left-sided accessory pathway in a patient with WPW. The criteria for the localization of the site of the accessory pathway include the earliest evidence of atrial activation during tachycardia and the presence of a large accessory pathway potential. This could be the target site for either catheter or surgical ablation. (AP = accessory pathway potential; V = ventricular electrogram; A = atrial electrogram)

SVPB   HR = 46   6:00.5A2

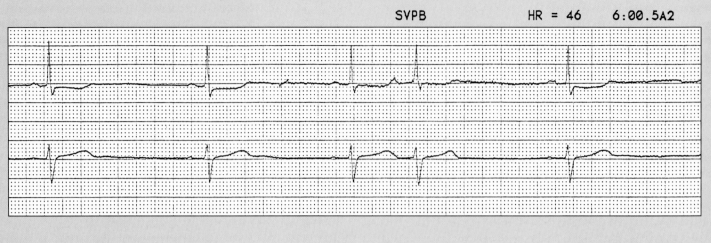

Sinus Arrest   HR = 47   6:00.6A2

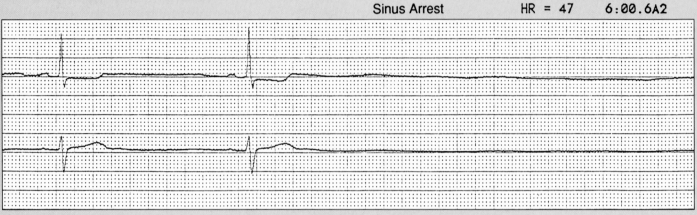

END OF EPISODE   HR = 46   6:01.1A2

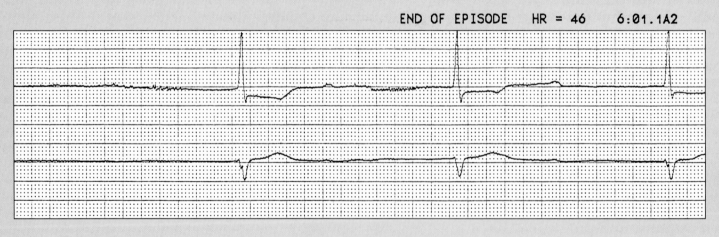

SVPB   HR = 50   6:08.5A2

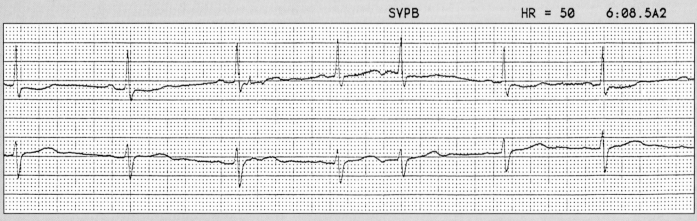

Sinus bradycardia occurs when the sinus node rate is less than 60 beats per minute and cardiac activation occurs in the normal sequence (Fig. 4.21A). The P, QRS, and T waves will therefore be unaltered and the intervals will be relatively unchanged. This can occur as an appropriate physiologic response, such as that found in the conditioned athlete, or as an inappropriate response, such as that found in the sick sinus syndrome.

Sinus node dysfunction can be manifested in other ways as well (Fig. 4.21)—one of the most common being *sinus pause*, or sinus arrest. This pause produces total absence of all electrical activity for a period of a second or more. Ultimately, conduction returns with an escape complex from the sinus node. The escape focus can, however, come from the AV node, causing a narrow QRS with no preceding P wave, or from the His–Purkinje conduction system or ventricular myocardium, causing a wide QRS-complex escape. Sinus arrest is simply a prolonged sinus pause. The pause can occur without warning, producing syncope (see Fig. 4.21A). Alternatively, the termination of a tachyarrhythmia can be followed by a pause (see Fig. 4.21B) due to a phenomenon known as *overdrive suppression*, in which the prolonged rapid rhythm temporarily suppresses the sinus node automaticity. Although this phenomenon can occur in the normal individual, a pause of greater than 2 sec after a tachycardia, a common occurrence in the *bradycardia–tachycardia syndrome*, is clear evidence of intrinsic sinus node disease.

Some patients manifest an exaggerated reflex response to stimulation of the carotid sinus (e.g., in association with tight shirt collars or sudden turning of the head). In addition to sinus pauses, these patients with hypersensitive carotid sinus syndrome can manifest AV block and/or decreased peripheral vascular resistance and hypotension.

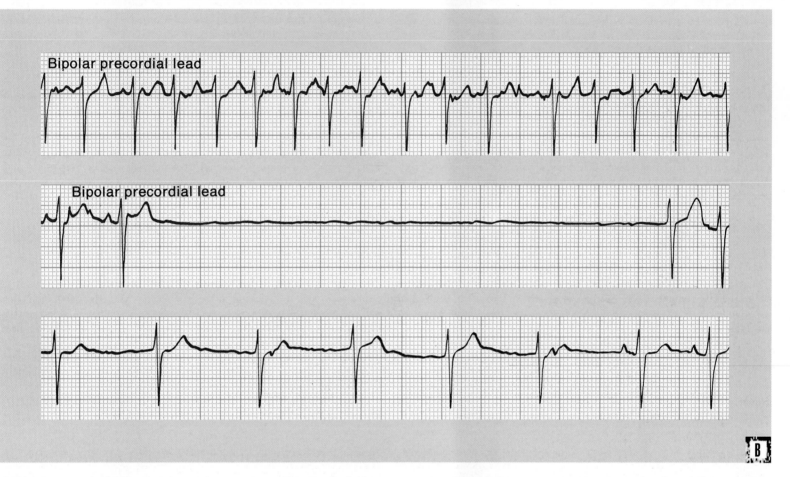

FIGURE 4.21   Manifestations of sinus node dysfunction. **(A)** (seen on the opposite page) Holter monitor recording from a 72-year-old female who experienced syncope while wearing the monitor. At the beginning of the tracing, the patient manifests a sinus bradycardia with one APC. The rate is subsequently slowed and a sinus pause lasting 23.3 sec develops (recording not shown in its entirety). **(B)** In this typical finding of sick sinus syndrome, the patient is initially in a rapid supraventricular tachycardia, which terminates abruptly. After a 5.4-sec pause, a junctional escape rhythm resumes. On the final two beats of the recording, normal sinus rhythm is restored.

AV CONDUCTION ABNORMALITIES

There are many forms of abnormal conduction between the atria and ventricles (Figs. 4.22, 4.23). However, to understand these properly, it should first be noted that AV dissociation is not the same as AV block. Sometimes the sinus node rate is selectively slowed, allowing for the AV node to serve as an escape pacemaker for the ventricle. This is called *junctional escape* (see Fig. 4.21B): there is a narrow QRS, and the P–R interval will be short, or the P wave will occur overlying or even after the QRS. The QRS complex is narrow, since ventricular conduction proceeds over the normal pathway. If there is no impairment in AV nodal conduction and, if sinus node depolarization increases for any reason, a normal P–QRS relationship will be recorded. This is an example of AV dissociation without AV block. The same phenomenon occurs when a focus below the AV node depolarizes faster than the sinus node rate, such as in sustained monomorphic ventricular tachycardia. Once again, there is no impairment of AV nodal conduction, and normal conduction will resume when the tachycardia terminates. In contrast, AV block implies abnormal function of the AV node, atrial tissue, or His– Purkinje system.

AV block most commonly occurs either in the AV node or within the His–Purkinje system. It is often difficult to tell from a standard ECG where the level of block is based, but with a His-bundle electrogram the diagnosis is easy to make (see Fig. 4.23). This distinction is important, because patients with impaired conduction in the His–Purkinje system tend to have an unreliable escape rhythm and are more likely to have related symptoms or require pacemaker implantation. It is more common to see a wide QRS with delayed conduction below the level of the AV node, but this phenomenon is not a reliable criterion on which to determine the site of the block (see Fig. 4.22).

FIRST-DEGREE AV BLOCK

First-degree AV block is recognized by a fixed, prolonged P–R interval (>200 msec), with 1:1 AV conduction (Fig. 4.23A). This condition implies abnormal conduction delay, which usually occurs either at the level of the AV node or within the His–Purkinje system. Without associated symptoms this is a benign arrhythmia, but for a patient with unexplained syncope, it can be an important clue to the diagnosis.

SECOND-DEGREE AV BLOCK

In second-degree AV block, not every atrial depolarization results in ventricular depolarization. In Mobitz Type I second-degree AV block (Fig. 4.23B) (or Wenckebach), the P–R interval prolongs progressively in each complex prior to the nonconducted P wave, and in the first P wave after the nonconducted beat the P–R interval tends to be short. The R–R interval also tends to shorten progressively in the beats prior to the nonconducted beat. Wenckebach conduction represents progressive conduction delay, which in the past was felt to occur primarily at the level of the AV node. It is now known that Wenckebach-type conduction can occur in the His–Purkinje system and, rarely, in the atrium as well. Despite these observations, when Wenckenbach-type AV block occurs with a narrow QRS, it is generally assumed that the conduction block is at the level of the AV node.

Mobitz II second-degree AV block is recognized by a nonconducted P wave when the P–R interval in the preceding complexes remains fixed (Fig. 4.23C). When it occurs in association with a wide QRS complex, it more often is felt to be associated with conduction block in the His–Purkinje system. It is important to make the distinction from Mobitz I, since patients with Mobitz II block would be at higher risk of progression to complete heart block. However, it must always be remembered that the significance of these arrhythmias should be interpreted in the context of the clinical situation.

THIRD-DEGREE AV BLOCK (COMPLETE HEART BLOCK)

Third-degree AV block implies complete blockade of AV conduction (Fig. 4.23D). When this occurs the sinus node rate is unaffected; if sinus node function is abnormal, then it has also been affected by whatever has caused the AV block or it has been affected by a separate process. The escape rhythm occurs below the level of block. When block occurs in the AV node, the escape rhythm will be from the AV node below the level of block and will therefore display a regular narrow-complex escape at 40 to 60 beats per minute. If the block occurs in the His–Purkinje system, there will be a wide-complex escape. This can occur at 30 to 40 beats per minute, but since the escape foci below the His–Purkinje conduction system are unreliable, a slower escape, or even asystole, can occur.

OTHER FORMS OF AV BLOCK

The term *2:1 AV block* refers to a sinus rhythm in which every other P wave results in a QRS. If this occurs at the level of the AV node, it will result in a narrow QRS and is an extreme form of Wenckebach conduction. If the block is below the AV node, there is generally a wide QRS; in this case there is a high rate of progression to complete heart block.

High-grade AV block occurs when more than one successive P wave is not conducted. AV block is incomplete. When this occurs with simultaneous sinus slowing in an otherwise healthy patient, it is usually due to transiently increased vagal tone and tends to be a benign condition. If there is no change in sinus rate, it could auger the progression to complete AV block.

FIGURE 4.22 CLASSIFICATION OF AV BLOCK

SURFACE ECG	SITE OF BLOCK	ECG MANIFESTATION
First-degree AV block	AVN>> HPS	Fixed P–R
Second-degree AV block		
Type I—normal QRS	AVN>>>> HPS	PR ↑ preceding nonconducted P wave
Type I—wide QRS	AVN> HPS	
Type II—normal QRS	HPS> AVN	No P–R ↑ preceding nonconducted P wave
Type II—wide QRS	HPS>>>> AVN	
2:1 Normal QRS	HPS = AVN	Every other P wave not conducted
2:1 Wide QRS	HPS>> AVN	
Complete AV block		No conducted P waves
Normal QRS	HPS = AVN	
Wide QRS	HPS>> AVN	
High-grade AV block		
Normal QRS	AVN>>> HPS	Most often P–P ↑ occurs simultaneously to AV block
Wide QRS	HPS>>>> AVN	Most often P–P interval remains fixed

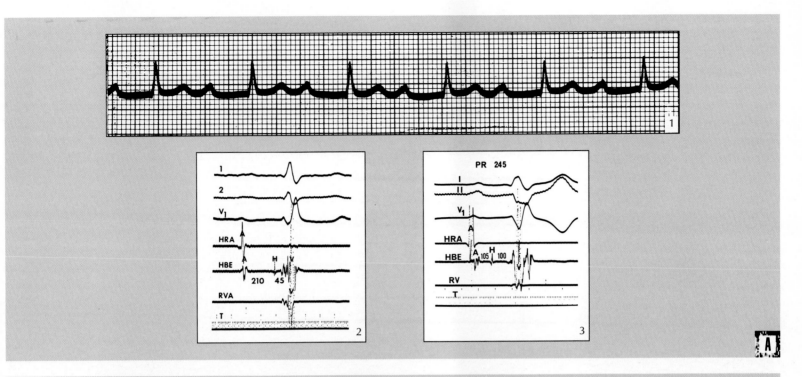

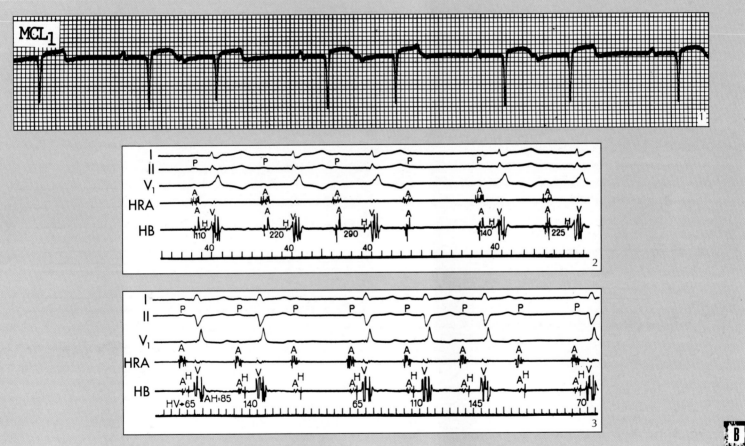

FIGURE 4.23 **(A)** Standard ECG of a patient with first-degree AV block (1), as well as intracardiac recordings of two other patients with the same conduction abnormality (2, 3). Note that the prolonged P–R interval in one of the patients (2) was due to delayed conduction in the AV node (supra-His), while the prolonged conduction in a different patient (3) was due to delay in the His–Purkinje system (infra-His). (2, 3) Note that the presence of bundle branch block on the standard ECG would not have helped identify the site of block. **(B)** Standard ECG (1) and intracardiac (2, 3) recordings for patients with second-degree AV block—Mobitz I (Wenckebach phenomenon). Note the progressive P–R interval prolongation, which terminates in a nonconducted beat. The tracings demonstrate that conduction delay and block can occur at the level of the AV node (2) or in the His–Purkinje system (3). (Reproduced with permission; see Figure Credits)

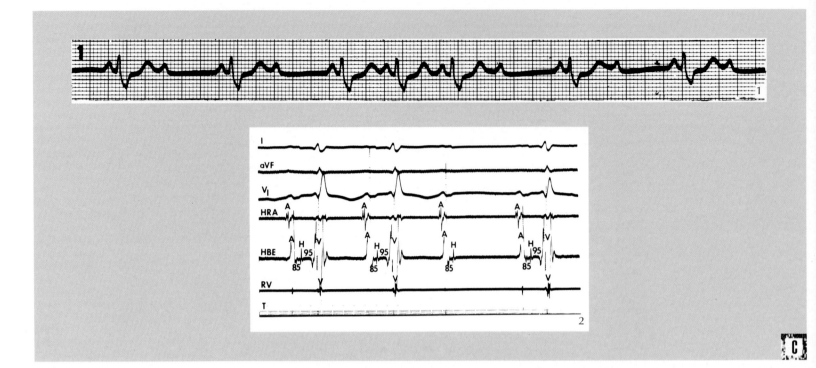

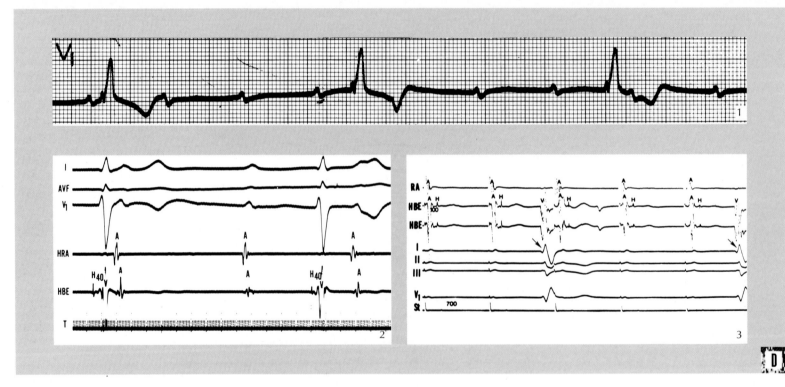

FIGURE 4.23 **(C)** Surface (1) and intracardiac (2) tracings of second-degree AV block—Mobitz II. There is no P–R prolongation prior to the non-conducted P wave. Both A–H and H–V intervals remain fixed, and there is a His bundle spike after the atrial electrogram. **(D)** ECG (1) and intracardiac (2, 3) tracings of third-degree (complete) heart block. (1) Note there is no relation between the P waves and the QRS complexes. (2) There is a block at the level of the AV node, with a His spike preceding each ventricular electrogram and an H–V interval of 40 msec. (3) Infra-His block with the His potential associated with the atrial electrogram and a coupling interval of 100 msec. In this particular recording the atrium is being paced.

Supraventricular Tachyarrhythmias

A patient with a heart rate greater than 100 beats per minute is referred to as having a tachycardia. This tachycardia is considered to be supraventricular in origin if the AV junction or the atrium participates in the arrhythmia, either as the origin of the abnormal impulse or as an essential part of the re-entrant circuit. The QRS is usually narrow. However, when the rate is fast, it is not uncommon to see aberrant ventricular conduction, which will produce a wide QRS complex and can be mistaken for ventricular tachycardia (Fig. 4.24).

TACHYARRHYTHMIAS ORIGINATING FROM THE SINUS NODE

Sinus tachycardia is, of course, the most common form of atrial tachyarrhythmia and must always be considered in the differential diagnosis. The ventricular response is greater than 100 beats per minute and P-wave morphology is normal (i.e., the P-wave axis is 0° to 90° in the frontal plane). In most cases the tachycardia occurs due to increased automaticity from the sinus node and is an appropriate response to a physiologic requirement (e.g., fever, hypoxia, decreased peripheral vascular resistance). It can of course occur as a pathologic condition (e.g., drug toxicity, hyperthyroidism).

Sinus node re-entry can also occur. It manifests normal P-wave morphology and an accelerated rate, but tends to initiate and terminate abruptly. As its name implies, it is due to re-entry occurring within the sinus node and the surrounding atrial tissue and it therefore can be initiated and terminated in the electrophysiology laboratory.

SUPRAVENTRICULAR TACHYCARDIA DUE TO RE-ENTRY

As with all arrhythmias, the cardiac history is often critically important in making the diagnosis of supraventricular tachycardia due to re-entry. But in order to classify a tachyarrhythmia correctly and manage it appropriately, it is also crucial to understand the mechanism of each type. While for any given arrythmia the mechanism is often not known with certainty, it is useful to conceptualize it by deciding whether it is due to increased automaticity or re-entry. If the cause is felt to be re-entry, knowing the site of the re-entrant loop will aid in the diagnosis as well as the subsequent management (Fig. 4.25).

FIGURE 4.24 CHARACTERISTICS OF SUPRAVENTRICULAR TACHYARRHYTHMIAS

TYPE	P-WAVE MORPHOLOGY	P-WAVE LOCATION	PRESUMED MECHANISM
Sinus Tachycardia	Normal	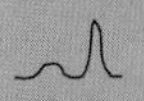	↑Automaticity
Sinus Node Re-entry	Normal	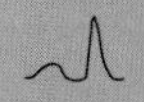	Re-entry
Automatic Atrial Tachycardia	Abnormal	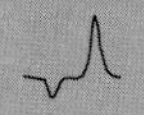	↑Automaticity
Intra-atrial Re-entry	Abnormal	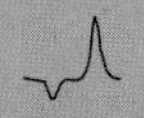	Re-entry
AV Nodal Re-entry	ABN (not seen)	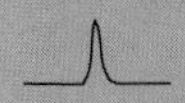	Re-entry
AV-Reciprocating Tachycardia	Abnormal	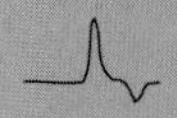	Re-entry
Multifocal Atrial Tachycardia	Varying	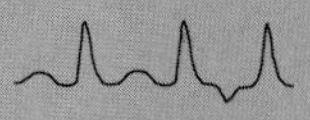	↑Automaticity
Atrial Fibrillation	Chaotic	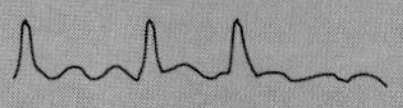	Re-entry
Atrial Flutter	Sawtooth	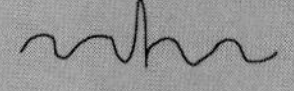	Re-entry

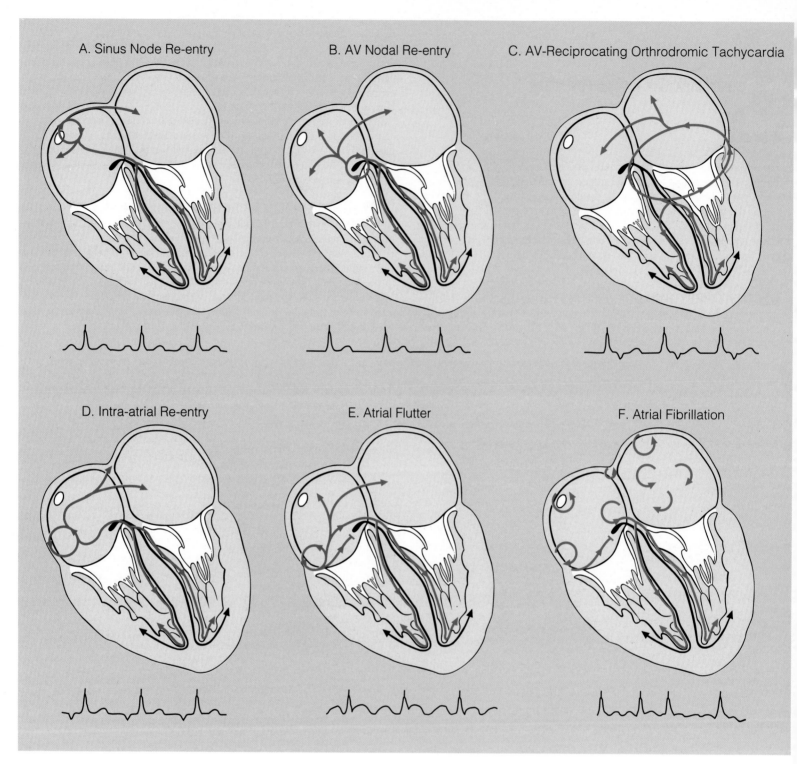

FIGURE 4.25   Supraventricular tachyarrhythmias with re-entry as the known or suspected mechanism of disease (narrow QRS complex).

The most common form of paroxysmal SVT occurring in young patients without structural heart disease is AV nodal re-entry (Fig. 4.26A). In this arrhythmia, there is a narrow QRS and the rhythm is quite regular. The re-entrant loop was previously considered to be entirely within the AV node. (It is now known that the atrium participates in the re-entrant loop to some degree.) Atrial activation generally occurs simultaneously with ventricular activation; consequently, the P wave is "buried" in the QRS and frequently is not visible.

Also occurring fairly often in young patients without organic heart disease is AV-reciprocating tachycardia, which is sometimes referred to as *circus movement tachycardia* (Fig. 4.26B). This condition also causes a regular, narrow QRS tachycardia, but in this case the P wave occurs slightly after the QRS; the R–P interval is less than that of the P–R. These patients have an accessory pathway (Kent bundle), which provides an alternate route of retrograde or ventriculoatrial conduction. In most cases this pathway does not conduct antegrade and cannot be detected on the 12-lead ECG when the patient is in normal sinus rhythm; consequently it is a "concealed" accessory pathway. The other limb of the re-entrant loop is the AV node, which conducts antegrade.

Much less common than the above tachycardias is *intra-atrial re-entry*, which occurs more frequently in patients with underlying heart disease. In this case the re-entrant loop is felt to be located entirely within the atrium. The atrial rate is generally less than 250 beats per minute. When the rate is sufficiently slow, conduction through the AV node is 1:1. The P-wave morphology is abnormal; the P waves occur before the QRS. Generally the R–P interval is greater than that of the P–R. Conduction is not always 1:1; Wenckebach conduction or even 2:1 conduction can be present.

ATRIAL FIBRILLATION AND FLUTTER
Atrial fibrillation and flutter are other arrhythmias felt to be due to re-entry. In atrial flutter, the atrial rate is 250 to 350 beats per minute, and inverted P waves are seen most commonly in the inferior leads of the ECG, producing the classical "saw-

tooth," or flutter, pattern. Ventricular conduction is rarely 1:1. In patients with normal AV conduction who are not taking antiarrhythmic medications, 2:1 conduction through the AV node is seen most often, and consequently the ventricular rate will be very regular, about 150 beats per minute. The flutter waves may be clearly seen, but at this rate every other complex might be buried in the QRS, and the T wave can also interfere with the recognition. Increasing the conduction block through the AV node may be necessary to detect the flutter waves. Variable degrees of block can sometimes be seen, which would produce an irregular ventricular response. The re-entrant loop is entirely within the atria. Atrial flutter can be distinguished from intra-atrial re-entry because the atrial rate is faster.

Atrial fibrillation does not have clearly demonstrable P waves, but rather a variable baseline representing the continuous, fragmented atrial depolarization. The ventricular response is irregular, and without medications or AV conduction abnormalities the average ventricular response can be as fast as 220 beats per minute. In atrial fibrillation there is not one re-entrant loop, but several, which are constantly moving in the atria, producing the chaotic atrial depolarization.

AUTOMATIC ATRIAL TACHYARRHYTHMIAS
In automatic atrial tachyarrhythmias there appear to be one or more areas of the atrium with an accelerated rate of depolarization, which therefore exceeds the depolarization rate of the sinus node. These tachyarrhythmias frequently occur in association with a pathologic condition, such as chronic obstructive pulmonary disease.

In an automatic atrial tachycardia the P-wave morphology is abnormal and the R–P interval is greater than that of the P–R. Conduction through the AV node can be 1:1, but can also demonstrate Wenckebach conduction or higher levels of block. An automatic atrial tachycardia is therefore indistinguishable from intra-atrial re-entry by the standard ECG; however, the two arrhythmias can be distinguished by their response to pacing and cardioversion, and by the clinical setting in which they occur.

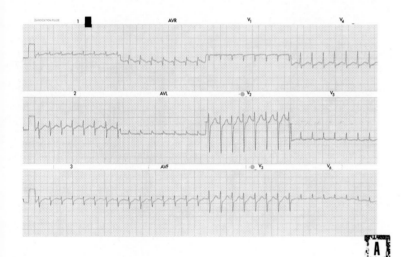
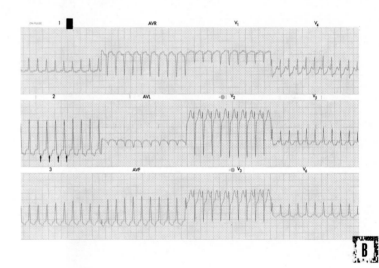

FIGURE 4.26   Standard 12-1ead ECGs from two young patients with paroxysmal palpitations. **(A)** There is a narrow complex rhythm with no visible P waves. By electrophysiologic testing, this patient was found to have an AV nodal re-entry tachycardia. **(B)** Patient with an AV-reciprocating tachycardia. Note the P waves, which occur immediately after the QRS, and are best seen in the inferior leads (*arrows*).

Paroxysmal atrial tachycardia occurring with AV block (PAT with block) is also recognized by a regular, accelerated atrial rate, but in this case there always is, as the name implies, AV block, and this can be a very high-grade block. This is a classical arrhythmia associated with digitalis toxicity, thought to be caused by triggered automaticity.

Multifocal atrial tachycardia is recognized by multiple (three or greater) P-wave morphologies and a ventricular response greater than 100 beats per minute. (If the rate is less than 100, the arrhythmia is referred to as wandering atrial pacemaker.) The ventricular response is irregularly irregular, and therefore great caution must be taken to distinguish this rhythm from atrial fibrillation. It is frequently seen in advanced chronic obstructive pulmonary disease. The mechanism is not known but, based on some of its clinical features, it has been suggested that it is caused by triggered automaticity.

TACHYARRHYTHMIAS ASSOCIATED WITH THE WPW SYNDROME

Patients with WPW syndrome display a short P–R interval and "delta" waves at the beginning of the QRS complex when they are in normal sinus rhythm (Fig. 4.27). These patients are prone to develop a variety of tachyarrhythmias.[12] They possess an accessory pathway (Kent bundle) that allows both antegrade and retrograde atrioventricular conduction independent from the AV node, which is different from the normal condition, in which the AV node is the only conduction pathway. Since antegrade conduction can occur over the accessory pathway in normal sinus rhythm, the ventricular activation will be premature and eccentric, giving rise to the typical ECG pattern.

These patients commonly have orthodromic AV-reciprocating tachycardia, which is identical to that seen in patients with concealed accessory pathways, and thus has a narrow, regular QRS. They can also (much less frequently) develop re-entry in the opposite direction, i.e., antegrade down the accessory pathway and retrograde over the AV node (antidromic AV-reciprocating tachycardia). This will cause an abnormal ventricular activation pattern and hence will always result in a regular wide-complex tachycardia.

Patients with WPW are also prone to developing atrial fibrillation and flutter. When these arrhythmias occur, the re-entrant loop, as previously discussed, is entirely in the atrium. Antegrade AV conduction can occur either through the AV node or the accessory pathway, or it can vary between the two pathways on

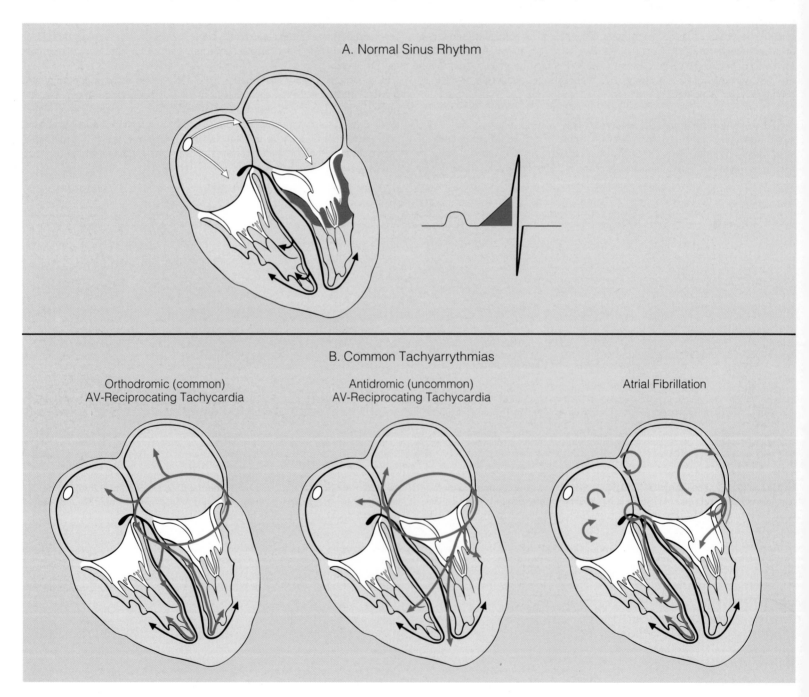

A. Normal Sinus Rhythm

B. Common Tachyarrythmias

Orthodromic (common) AV-Reciprocating Tachycardia

Antidromic (uncommon) AV-Reciprocating Tachycardia

Atrial Fibrillation

FIGURE 4.27   Wolff–Parkinson–White syndrome.

a beat-to-beat basis. Rapid conduction through the accessory pathway in atrial fibrillation is the feared complication in WPW syndrome, because this can precipitate ventricular fibrillation. It should be recalled that any of the narrow-complex tachycardias in WPW can, and not uncommonly do, develop aberrant ventricular conduction, resulting in a wide-complex morphology.

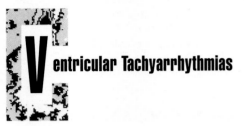

Ventricular Tachyarrhythmias

Ventricular tachyarrhythmias can frequently be diagnosed if the pattern of atrial activation is known. Since the origin of the depolarization is in the ventricle, there is often no relationship between the ventricularly based rhythm and the atrial activity; most often, normal sinus rhythm continues uninterrupted. (This is an example of AV dissociation without AV block.) Sometimes there can be retrograde conduction through the AV node, which will alter atrial depolarization, but it is uncommon to see 1:1 retrograde conduction through the AV node.

VENTRICULAR TACHYCARDIA

Ventricular tachycardia is said to be sustained if it lasts more than 30 sec or requires intervention to prevent hemodynamic collapse. It is generally classified as monomorphic if it manifests a uniform QRS morphology, and polymorphic if it does not. Nonsustained ventricular tachycardia occurs if there are three or more repetitive ventricular responses and, as the name implies, terminates spontaneously in less than 30 seconds.

Sustained monomorphic ventricular tachycardia is most often regular and almost always displays a wide QRS complex (see Fig. 4.1A). Distinguishing the rhythm from supraventricular tachycardia with aberrancy can be difficult. The importance of the medical history again comes into play. As mentioned earlier, a 55-year-old man with a history of myocardial infarction who develops a new wide-complex tachycardia will probably have ventricular tachycardia. There are many criteria for the diagnosis of ventricular tachycardias, however, that are independent of the history.

The demonstration of AV dissociation (i.e., of P waves with no relationship to the QRS) is essentially diagnostic of ventricular tachycardia. Also important is the presence of capture beats and fusion beats. Capture beats occur when an atrial depolarization is able to conduct through the AV node and "capture" the ventricle; it usually does not interrupt the ventricular tachycardia. Fusion beats are intermediate in morphology between the wide-complex rhythm and the normal QRS.

The morphology of the complexes on the 12-lead ECG can also be valuable (Fig. 4.28).[3,13] Although there is not universal agreement, criteria can be identified for diagnosing ventricular tachycardia with a fair degree of reliability. Many researchers agree that a very wide QRS (>160 msec) strongly supports the presence of ventricular tachycardia. The presence of "negative concordance" (i.e., the absence of an R wave in all of the precordial leads) is highly suggestive of ventricular tachycardia. If there are R waves present in the precordial leads, with long intervals from the beginning of the R waves to the peak of the S waves (>100 msec) this also strongly suggests the diagnosis of ventricular tachycardia. If none of these criteria, or a few other selected criteria, are satisfied,[3] supraventricular tachycardia is more likely.

Torsade de pointes is the most characteristic form of polymorphic ventricular tachycardia in the setting of Q–T prolongation. It has an unmistakeable appearance on the ECG, producing a continuously changing ECG axis (Fig. 4.29).

VENTRICULAR FLUTTER AND FIBRILLATION

When these arrhythmias occur, there is often not a great deal of time for analysis, except in retrospect once treatment has been delivered! Ventricular fibrillation produces completely disorganized ventricular depolarization, with a chaotic appearance of the baseline and without readily apparent complexes of any kind (see Fig. 4.29). When it is fine, it must be distinguished from asystole.

Ventricular flutter is an intermediate form between ventricular tachycardia and ventricular fibrillation. It is generally monomorphic, but the rate is faster than that of ventricular tachycardia, at around 300 beats per minute. The cutoff point between ventricular flutter and tachycardia is somewhat arbitrary, but it is set at a cycle length of about 220 msec (275 beats per minute).

FIGURE 4.28 CRITERIA FOR DIAGNOSIS OF VENTRICULAR TACHYCARDIA IN PATIENTS WITH WIDE QRS COMPLEX

CRITERION	RELIABILITY
AV dissociation	Excellent
Capure and fusion beats	Good–excellent
Wide QRS (>160 msec)	Fair–good
"Negative concordance"	Good–excellent
rS > 100 msec	Good

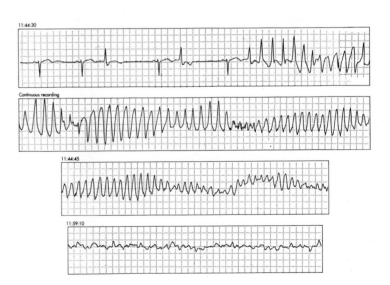

FIGURE 4.29   Tracing recorded from a 54-year-old man who collapsed and died while wearing a Holter monitor. At the beginning of the recording, the patient is in sinus bradycardia with premature ventricular beats. Then a sinus beat initiates a run of torsade de pointes. Several seconds later, the rhythm has begun to degenerate, and by 11:59, the patient is in fine ventricular fibrillation. This arrhythmia is hypothesized to be triggered from an early afterdepolarization, which is produced by the characteristic long–short sequence of two beats preceding initiation of the tachycardia. Note the prolonged Q–T interval (also associated with torsade de pointes), which was present in the first two sinus beats.

FIGURE CREDITS

Figs. 4.5, 4.17(A), 4.18 from Chatterjee K, et al: Cardiology: An Illustrated Text–Reference. Gower, New York, 1992.

Fig. 4.6 from El-Sherif N, Bekheit SS, Henkin R: Quinidine-induced long QT interval and torsade de pointes: Role of bradycardia-dependent early afterdepolarizations. J Am Coll Cardiol 14:252, 1989.

Fig. 4.7 from Gilmour RF Jr, et al: Cellular electrophysiological abnormalities of diseased human ventricular myocardium. Am J Cardiol 51:137, 1983.

Fig. 4.13 modified and redrawn from Abi-Samra F, et al: The usefulness of head-up tilt testing and hemodynamic investigations in the work-up of syncope of unknown origin. PACE 11:1202, 1988.

Fig. 4.16 from Morady F, Peters RW, Scheinman MM: Bradyarrhythmias and bundle branch block. In Scheinman MM (ed): Cardiac Emergencies. WB Saunders, Philadelphia, 1984.

Fig. 4.17(B) from Akhtar M: Electrophysiologic bases for wide QRS tachycardia. PACE 6: 81, 1983.

Fig. 4.23(B) from Akhtar M: Clinical application of electrophysiologic studies in the management of patients requiring pacemaker therapy. In Barold S (ed): Modern Cardiac Pacing. Futura Publishing Co, Mount Kisco, NY, 1985.

REFERENCES

1. Almquist A, Goldenberg IF, Milstein S, et al: Provocation of bradycardia and hypotension by isoproterenol and upright posture in patients with unexplained syncope. N Eng J Med 320:346, 1989.

2. Benditt DG, Remole S, Bailin S, et al: Tilt table testing for evaluation of neurally-mediated (cardioneurogenic) syncope: Rationale and proposed protocols. PACE 14:1528, 1991.

3. Brugada P, Brugada J, Mont L, et al: A new approach to the differential diagnosis of a regular tachycardia with a wide QRS complex. Circulation 83:1649, 1991.

4. Davies MJ, Andersen RH, Becker AE: The Conduction System of the Heart. Butterworths, Boston, 1983.

5. Dhingra RC: Sinus node dysfunction. PACE 6:1062, 1983.

6. Hall PA, Atwood JE, Myers J, et al: The signal averaged surface electrocardiogram and the identification of late potentials. Prog Cardiovasc Dis 31:295, 1989.

7. Linzer M, Prystowsky EN, Brunetti LL, et al: Recurrent syncope of unknown origin diagnosed by ambulatory continuous loop ECG recording. Am Heart J 116:1632, 1988.

8. Mandel WJ, Peter LT, Bleifer SB: Holter monitor recording. In: Mandel WJ (ed): Arrhythmias: Their Mechanisms, Diagnosis, and Management, 2nd ed. JB Lippincott, Philadelphia, 1987.

9. Manolis AS, Linzer M, Salem D, et al: Syncope: Current diagnostic evaluation and management. Ann Intern Med 12:850, 1990.

10. Ross TF, Mandel WJ: Invasive cardial electrophysiologic testing. In: Mandel WJ (ed): Arrhythmias: Their Mechanisms, Diagnosis, and Management, 2nd ed. JB Lippincott, Philadelphia, 1987.

11. Rubinstein JJ, Schulman CL, Yurchak PM, et al: Clinical spectrum of sick sinus syndrome. Circulation 46:5, 1972.

12. Waldo AL, Akhtar M, Benditt DG, et al: Appropriate electrophysiologic study and treatment of patients with the Wolff-Parkinson-White syndrome. J Am Coll Cardiol 11:1124, 1988.

13. Wellens HJ, Bar W, Lie KI: The value of the electrocardiogram in the differential diagnosis of a tachycardia with a widened QRS complex. Am J Med 64:27, 1978.

14. Wit AL, Dillon SM: Anisotropic reentry. In Zipes DP, Jalife J (eds): Cardiac Electrophysiology: From Cell to Bedside. WB Saunders, Philadelphia, 1990.

15. Zipes DP: Genesis of cardiac arrhythmias: Electrophysiological considerations. In Braunwald E (ed): Heart Disease: A Textbook of Cardiovascular Medicine, 3rd ed. WB Saunders, Philadelphia, 1988.

16. Zipes DP: Specific arrhythmias: Diagnosis and treatment. In Braunwald E (ed): Heart Disease: A Textbook of Cariovascular Medicine, 3rd ed. WB Saunders, Philadelphia, 1988.

17. Zipes DP, Akhtar M, Denes P, et al: Guidelines for clinical intracardiac electrophysiologic studies. Circulation 80:1925, 1989.

18. Zipes DP, Rahimtoola SH (Eds): State-of-the-art consensus conference of electrophysiologic testing in the diagnosis and treatment of patients with cardiac arrhythmias. Circulation 75 (suppl. III):1, 1987.

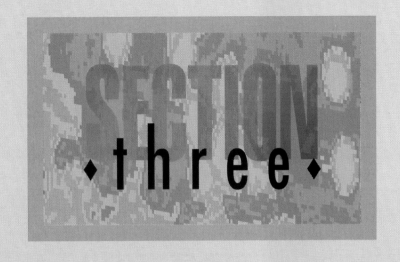

SECTION
·three·

DISEASES OF THE HEART, ARTERIES, AND VEINS

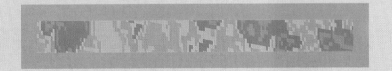

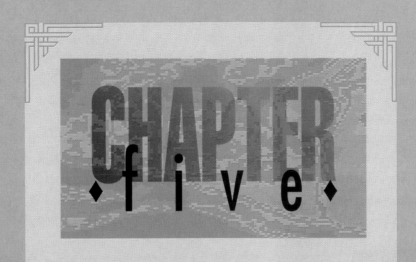

CHAPTER ·five·

CORONARY
ARTERY DISEASE

J. WILLIS HURST, MD
ANTON E. BECKER, MD
JOSEPH S. ALPERT, MD

Myocardial ischemia is due to an imbalance between myocardial oxygen consumption and oxygen supply. The most common condition underlying myocardial ischemia is obstructive coronary artery disease, which may be aggravated by additional cardiac abnormalities such as hypertrophy and dilation. Myocardial ischemia and infarction may also complicate various types of cardiac disease, such as valve abnormalities, cardiomyopathies, and congenital heart malformations.

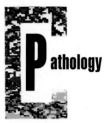
Pathology

Coronary atherosclerosis is the most common condition underlying obstructive coronary artery disease. However, other abnormalities may occur, including coronary artery spasm, coronary artery embolism, coronary ostial stenosis, coronary arteritis, coronary artery dissection and congenital artery anomaly. Coronary atherosclerosis is the most common cause of coronary disease (Fig. 5.1). The abnormality, which is confined mainly to the intima, consists of a fibrocellular proliferation with an accumulation of lipids. The latter may form a distinct mass, known as an atheroma. Usually the atheroma is delineated from the lumen by a fibrous cap (Fig. 5.2). Macrophages are dispersed throughout the atherosclerotic lesion.

The extent and severity of the obstructive atherosclerotic lesion may vary considerably. In the majority of patients the lesion is in an eccentric position, but concentric atherosclerotic lesions do occur. In advanced lesions one may often observe a layering, suggesting different episodes of growth of the plaque (Fig. 5.3). Calcification of advanced lesions is a common feature (Fig. 5.4).

The composition of atherosclerotic lesions may also differ. Occasionally the lesion is dominated by a fibrocellular proliferation (Fig. 5.5). In other instances the atherosclerotic lesion may be almost totally composed of atheroma (Fig. 5.6), or it may be almost totally fibrosed (Fig. 5.7).

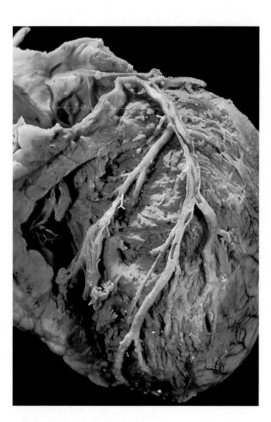

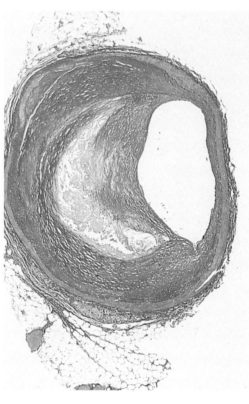

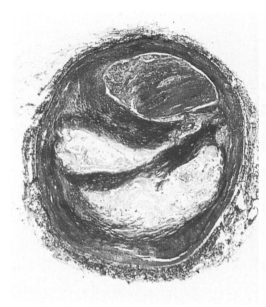

FIGURE 5.3 Histologic cross section through a coronary artery showing two distinct layers of atherosclerotic lesions. These layers suggest different episodes of growth. The lumen is obliterated by a recent thrombosis. (Reproduced with permission; see Figure Credits)

FIGURE 5.1 Multiple obstructive lesions due to atherosclerosis in the anterior descending coronary artery and major branches. (Reproduced with permission; see Figure Credits)

FIGURE 5.2 Histologic cross section through a coronary artery showing an eccentric atherosclerotic lesion. The atheroma is separated from the lumen by a fibrous cap. The medial layer is intact. (Reproduced with permission; see Figure Credits)

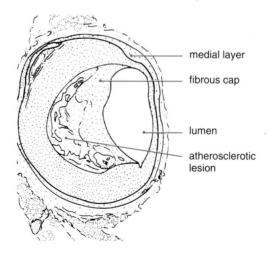

medial layer

fibrous cap

lumen

atherosclerotic lesion

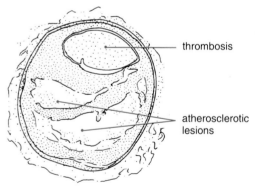

thrombosis

atherosclerotic lesions

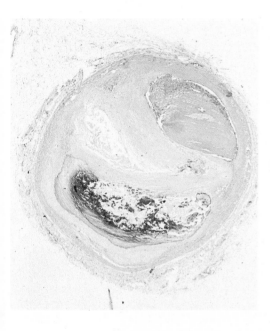

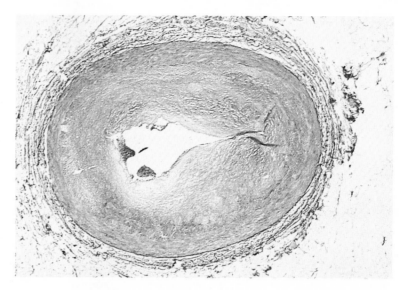

FIGURE 5.4
Calcified atheroma clearly evident by its distinct purple color. This particular stain is of the same artery shown in Figure 5.3. Calcification is a common phenomenon in advanced atherosclerotic lesions. (Reproduced with permission; see Figure Credits)

FIGURE 5.5   Concentric lesion of a coronary artery dominated by a fibrocellular proliferation. (Reproduced with permission; see Figure Credits)

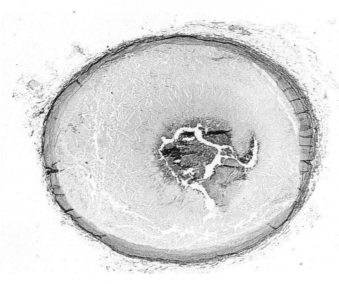

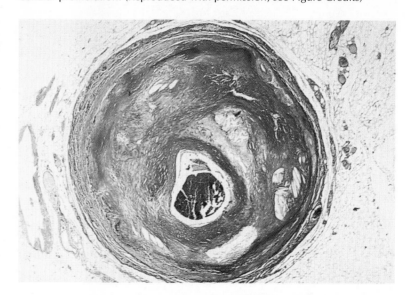

FIGURE 5.6   Cross section through a coronary artery showing an extensive atherosclerotic lesion almost totally composed of atheroma. There is hemorrhage in a crack of the atheromatous plaque. (Reproduced with permission; see Figure Credits)

FIGURE 5.7   Cross section through a coronary artery showing an atherosclerotic lesion almost totally composed of fibrosed tissue. There is a thrombus in the lumen. (Reproduced with permission; see Figure Credits)

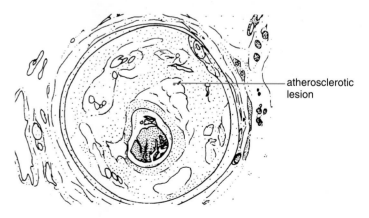

atherosclerotic lesion

Coronary thrombosis is an important complication, which may be initiated by plaque fissure (Fig. 5.8). Various bypass grafts may be occluded by thrombi (Figs. 5.9, 5.10) or fibrocellular intimal proliferation (Fig. 5.11).

The muscular media of the affected coronary artery is usually intact, providing a morphologic substrate for vasospasm. Thus, in the majority of cases, the fixed stenosis caused by the atherosclerotic lesion can be aggravated by contraction of the intact muscular wall. Coronary arteries with early atherosclerotic lesions appear to be particularly sensitive to this phenomenon.[16,19]

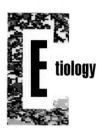

Etiology

The etiology of atherosclerosis is not known. The condition is more common in males, and in individuals who smoke tobacco, have hypertension, are obese, have elevated serum cholesterol, eat a high-fat diet, have diabetes, or are inac-

tive. These risk factors or markers seem to regulate the acceleration rate of the disease in individuals who have a genetically determined tendency toward the disease (Figs. 5.12–5.15). The response-to-injury theory is considered one of the best hypotheses to explain how the lesion develops in patients with or without risk factors (Fig. 5.16).

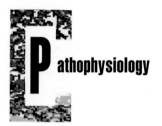

Pathophysiology

An adequate amount of blood carrying a proper amount of oxygen must reach the myocardial cells so that they can contract and relax 60 to 90 times per minute for as long as one lives. Blood flow is determined by pressure gradients. The left ventricular myocardium in the normal heart is perfused during diastole when the pressure in the coronary arteries is about 80 mmHg and the pressure within the left ventricle is 0 to 5 mmHg. There is less myocardial perfusion during systole because the systolic pressure in the coronary epicardial arteries is

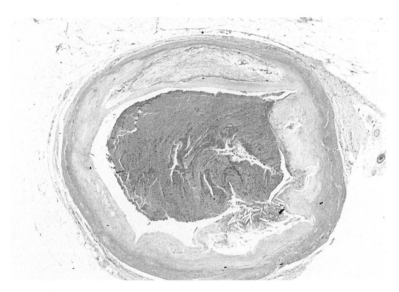

FIGURE 5.8   Cross section through a coronary artery demonstrating a plaque fissure and adherent thrombus occluding the lumen. (Reproduced with permission; see Figure Credits)

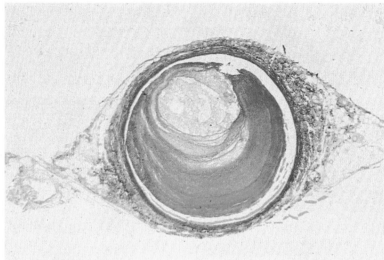

FIGURE 5.9   Venous bypass graft occluded by a recent thrombus. (Reproduced with permission; see Figure Credits)

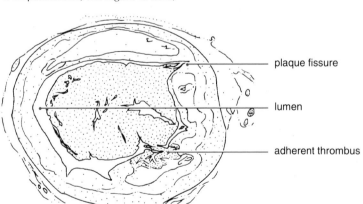

plaque fissure

lumen

adherent thrombus

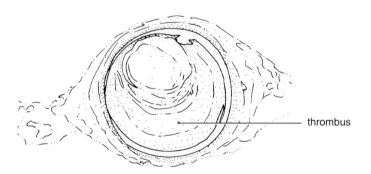

thrombus

about equal to the systolic pressure within the left ventricle. The myocardial perfusion of the right ventricle is different from that of the left ventricle and septum. It occurs during diastole and systole, because the pressure in the coronary arteries during diastole and systole is always higher than that within the right ventricle. It is easy to understand why tachycardia, with consequent short diastoles, influences myocardial perfusion of the left ventricle and septum. Furthermore, the amount of blood delivered to the myocardium must be regulated so that more blood can be delivered during exercise than during rest. Although the epicardial coronary arteries can change their size, they do not control coronary flow as much as the small intramyocardial coronary branches, which are called *resistance arterioles*. Considerable research is now underway in an effort to understand the factors that control the resistance vessels. One of these factors is the effect of end-diastolic ventricular pressure on myocardial perfusion (see Fig. 2.11).

Coronary blood flow is not impeded until an obstructing lesion occludes about 50% of the luminal diameter of the artery, equivalent to 75% cross-sectional obstruction (Fig. 5.17). This degree of stenosis may permit adequate myocardial perfusion when the individual is at rest but not during exercise. This leads to consideration of the supply–demand concept of myocardial perfusion. The supply end of the system includes the coronary artery pressure, size of the coronary artery lumen, and oxygen content of the blood, while the demand end of the system includes the work of the myocardium and myocardial cellular metabolism. Certain clinical syndromes, discussed later in this chapter, can be analyzed in terms of this concept: Is the myocardial ischemia due to a problem in the supply end of the myocardial perfusion system, in the demand end of the myocardial perfusion system, or in both ends of the system? At times specific therapy can be linked to the pathophysiologic fault that is deduced to be present. This approach has ushered in a new era in which it is possible to think in pathophysiologic terms about the basic mechanisms responsible for clinical syndromes.

The clinical syndromes associated with atherosclerotic coronary disease are listed in Figure 5.18. These syndromes and their subsets are defined later in this

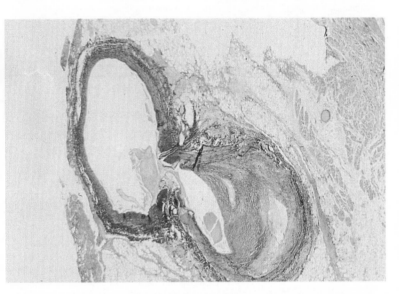

FIGURE 5.10   Venous bypass graft sutured at the site of a significant preexistent atherosclerotic lesion in the major coronary artery. This often leads to early graft thrombosis. (Reproduced with permission; see Figure Credits)

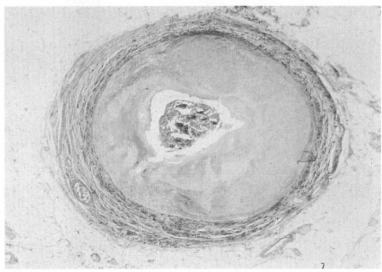

FIGURE 5.11   Fibrocellular intimal proliferation of a venous bypass graft. This development is a complication that eventually may lead to total obliteration of the graft. (Reproduced with permission; see Figure Credits)

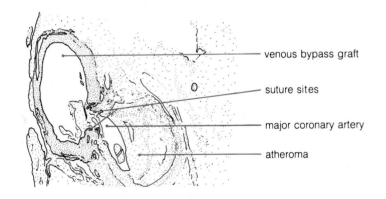

venous bypass graft

suture sites

major coronary artery

atheroma

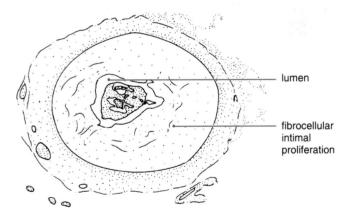

lumen

fibrocellular intimal proliferation

FIGURE 5.12 RISK FACTORS FOR ATHEROSCLEROSIS

Hypertension	Menopause/birth control pills
Smoking	Gout
Old age	Obesity
Diabetes	Arterial irradiation
Hyperlipidemia	Cardiac transplantation
Family history	Trace metals
Male gender	Decrease in physical activity
Type A personality	

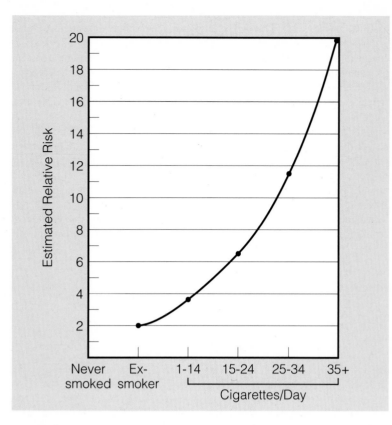

FIGURE 5.13   Relative risk of myocardial infarction due to cigarette smoking in women under 50 years of age. (Reproduced with permission; see Figure Credits)

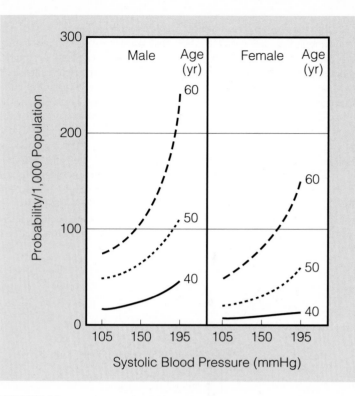

FIGURE 5.14   Risk of developing cardiovascular disease over an 8-year period according to the level of systolic blood pressure in men and women. (Reproduced with permission; see Figure Credits)

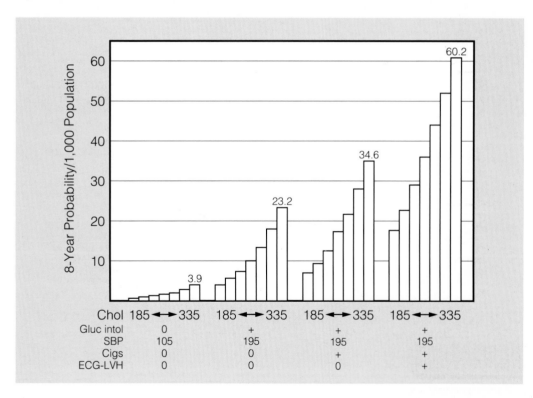

FIGURE 5.15   Risk of developing cardiovascular disease over an 8-year period according to serum cholesterol levels and other risk factors in 35-year-old men. (Chol = cholesterol; Gluc intol = glucose intolerance; SBP = systemic blood pressure; Cigs = cigarette smoking; LVH = left ventricular hypertrophy by ECG) (Reproduced with permission; see Figure Credits)

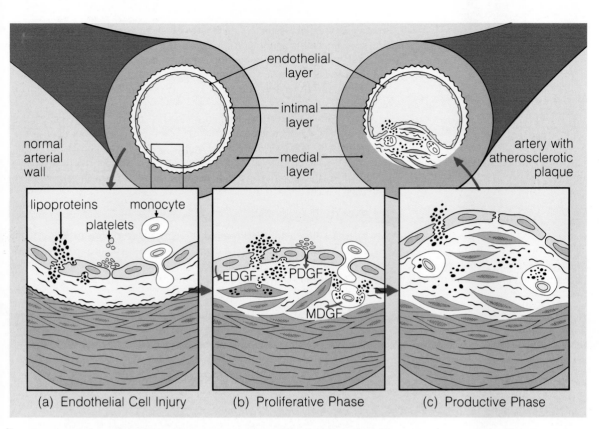

FIGURE 5.16 Genesis of an atherosclerotic plaque. Endothelial cell injury **(a)** leads to excessive influx of lipoproteins, invasion of monocytes/macrophages, and adherence of platelets. This leads to a proliferative phase **(b)** in which a macrophage reaction and release of growth factors (EDGF, MDCF, PDGF) set in motion a process of smooth muscle proliferation. This eventually results in a productive phase **(c)** in which connective tissue elements are formed leading to distinct plaque formation. (Reproduced with permission; see Figure Credits)

(a) Endothelial Cell Injury   (b) Proliferative Phase   (c) Productive Phase

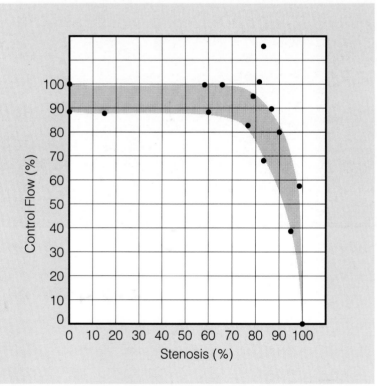

FIGURE 5.17 Reduction in myocardial blood flow plotted against stenosis of the coronary arterial lumen. Myocardial blood flow is maintained at essentially control levels until the arterial lumen is reduced by approximately 80% or more. At this point, myocardial blood flow falls rapidly as stenosis increases. (Redrawn with permission; see Figure Credits)

Clinical Manifestations

chapter and, when possible, the pathophysiology responsible for each is stated, along with the prognosis and treatment. Initially it is necessary to discuss the methods of identifying the various syndromes.

CLINICAL SETTING

Coronary atherosclerosis is more common in males than in females. In either sex it occurs more frequently in individuals who: are in a certain age range (30 to 70 years); smoke tobacco; are hypertensive; have hyperlipidemia; are obese; have a carotid artery bruit, abdominal aneurysm, or peripheral arterial disease; have diabetes; are inactive; have hyperuricemia; have certain electrocardiographic abnormalities; have a Type A personality; have a family history of premature atherosclerotic coronary disease; have xanthoma; have had mediastinal irradiation; are undergoing renal dialysis; or have had a cardiac transplant. In females the use of contraceptive pills is an additional risk factor.

Coronary atherosclerosis is common even when the factors listed above are absent. Conversely the disease may not be present when several of the risk factors are present. However, the disease is more common in a population of subjects with risk factors than in a population of subjects without risk factors. Data other than risk factors are required to diagnose the presence of the disease in an individual patient.

PATIENT HISTORY

The patient with serious and advanced coronary atherosclerosis may display no symptoms. Sudden death from the disease may occur without preceding symptoms. The patient may even have objective evidence of repeated bouts of myocardial ischemia with no symptoms; this is called *silent ischemia.*

FIGURE 5.18 CLINICAL SPECTRUM OF ATHEROSCLEROTIC CORONARY ARTERY DISEASE*

CORONARY ATHEROSCLEROSIS WITHOUT ANGINA OR OTHER EVIDENCE OF ISCHEMIA
CORONARY ATHEROSCLEROSIS WITH REVERSIBLE MYOCARDIAL ISCHEMIA
    Stable syndromes
        Stable angina pectoris
        Positive exercise test
        Anginal equivalents
    Unstable syndromes
        Unstable angina pectoris and equivalents
        Postinfarction angina pectoris
        Prinzmetal's angina pectoris
        Prolonged myocardial ischemia without
           objective evidence of infarction

CORONARY ATHEROSCLEROSIS WITH IRREVERSIBLE MYOCARDIAL ISCHEMIA AND NECROSIS
    Very early profound ischemia
    Early evolving infarction
    Uncomplicated completed infarction
    Complicated infarction
SUDDEN DEATH †
SYNCOPE †
CARDIAC ARRHYTHMIAS †
ISCHEMIC CARDIOMYOPATHY ‡
ATHEROSCLEROTIC CORONARY ARTERY DISEASE IN COMBINATIONS WITH OTHER CONDITIONS

*This classification of atherosclerotic coronary artery disease permits the linkage of pathophysiology, clinical syndromes, prognosis, and specific treatment. Clear definitions of the syndromes and their treatment are discussed in the text. (Reproduced with permission; see Figure Credits)
†Sudden death may occur in patients with reversible myocardial ischemia. It may also occur in patients who have had infarction due to irreversible myocardial ischemia. The mechanism for syncope may be similar to the mechanism for sudden death. Cardiac arrhythmias occurring in patients with coronary atherosclerotic artery disease may be, but are not always, due to myocardial ischemia.
‡The heart of patients with ischemic cardiomyopathy have areas of infarction due to irreversible ischemia. The same patients may also experience episodes of reversible ischemia.

In patients who experience *angina pectoris* due to myocardial ischemia the discomfort is usually located in the retrosternal area. Patients often use a variety of adjectives to describe the discomfort: tightness, indigestion, burning, aching, pain, or simply a "bad" feeling in the chest. Angina pectoris may be described as any unpleasant feeling in the retrosternal area that has not been noted previously. The discomfort may radiate into the left arm, right arm, throat, mandible, or upper back. It is occasionally located in the precordial area. The duration of the discomfort is usually 1 to 3 minutes, rarely lasting longer than 10 minutes. The discomfort is usually precipitated by effort, emotional distress, exposure to cold, or eating. Angina pectoris is usually relieved by nitroglycerin.[3,11]

The chest discomfort thought to be angina pectoris due to atherosclerotic heart disease must be differentiated from discomfort associated with other diseases, such as emotional disturbances, esophageal reflux, esophageal spasm, esophageal rupture, peptic ulcer, gallbladder disease, herpes zoster, Tietze's syndrome, chest wall syndromes, thoracic outlet syndrome, pneumothorax, mediastinal emphysema, pulmonary emboli, pericarditis, other causes of myocardial ischemia such as aortic valve disease and cardiomyopathy, and other causes of coronary disease such as coronary spasm, coronary anomalies, and pulmonary hypertensive pain. It is important to remember that angina pectoris due to coronary atherosclerosis is common, as are many of the other causes of chest discomfort. Accordingly, the coexistence of two conditions, each causing chest discomfort, is also common. The identification of one cause of chest discomfort does not exclude another cause.

There are several different types of angina pectoris (see Fig. 5.18). The effort necessary to produce angina can be graded according to the guidelines established by The Canadian Cardiovascular Society (Fig. 5.19). The predictive value of the history of angina pectoris depends upon the type of history obtained (Fig. 5.20).

Patients may experience chest discomfort that lasts longer than angina pectoris. This symptom is designated as *prolonged chest discomfort due to myocardial*

FIGURE 5.19 GRADING OF EFFORT REQUIRED TO PRODUCE ANGINA*

CLASS 1: Ordinary physical activity does not cause angina, such as walking and climbing stairs. Angina with strenuous or rapid or prolonged exertion at work or recreation.

CLASS 2: Slight limitations of ordinary activity. Walking or climbing stairs rapidly; walking uphill; waking or stair climbing after meals, in cold, in wind, under emotional stress, or only during the few hours after awakening. Walking more than two level blocks and climbing more than one flight of ordinary stairs at a normal pace and in normal conditions.

CLASS 3: Marked limitation of ordinary physical activity. Walking one to two level blocks and climbing one flight of stairs in normal conditions and at normal pace.

CLASS 4: Inability to carry on any physical activity without discomfort. Anginal syndrome may be present at rest.

*Established by The Canadian Cardiovascular Society. (Reproduced with permission from the American Heart Association, Inc. and the author; see Figure Credits)

FIGURE 5.20 PREDICTIVE VALUE OF THE HISTORY INDICATING ARTHEROSCLEROTIC CORONARY ARTERY DISEASE

TYPE 1	TYPE 2	TYPE 3
Male or female, aged 45 and over; brief* retrosternal chest discomfort produced by effort; history easily obtained. —predictive value >90%.	Male or female, aged 45 and over; brief* retrosternal chest discomfort not always produced by effort and often occurring at rest; history difficult to obtain. —predictive value 75%.	Female, aged 40–45 years; brief* retrosternal chest discomfort produced by effort or occurring at rest; history easily obtained or obtained with difficulty. —predictive value 50%.

*Brief chest discomfort: defined as lasting 1 to 3 minutes (up to 10 minutes)
(Modified with permission; see Figure Credits)

ischemia. The discomfort is similar to angina pectoris but lasts from 10 to 20 minutes up to several hours, usually occurring while the patient is at rest. Cardiac muscle may or may not be permanently damaged; when it is, *myocardial infarction* is diagnosed. The condition must be differentiated from many of the same conditions listed under angina pectoris.

There are several subsets of both angina pectoris and prolonged myocardial ischemia (see Fig. 5.18). These are discussed in the section on various subsets of coronary atherosclerotic heart disease.

Anginal equivalents are due to ischemia but are not associated with chest pain (see Fig. 5.18). The patient may have palpitation, dyspnea on effort, or exhaus-tion. *Palpitation* may occur at rest or with effort. Palpitation due to a cardiac arrhythmia is usually not caused by ischemia except under certain circum-stances. *Dyspnea* on effort or at rest as a new symptom in a patient without lung disease may be due to transient global myocardial ischemia, which results in an elevation of left ventricular diastolic pressure, left atrial pressure, and pulmonary venous pressure. *Exhaustion* on effort or at rest in a middle-aged person who has no other cause for the symptom may be due to global ischemia secondary to coronary atherosclerosis, which results in decreased cardiac output during exer-cise. Anginal equivalents have less predictive value than angina, but they pro-vide important clues to pursue.

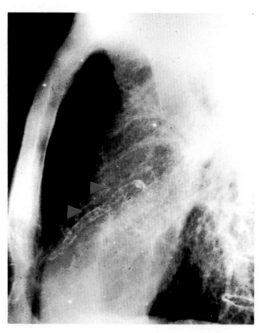

FIGURE 5.21 Lateral chest x-ray of calcification of left anterior descending coronary artery. Coron-ary artery calcification appears radiographically as linear, parallel densities that move during the cardiac cycle. (Reproduced with permission; see Figure Credits)

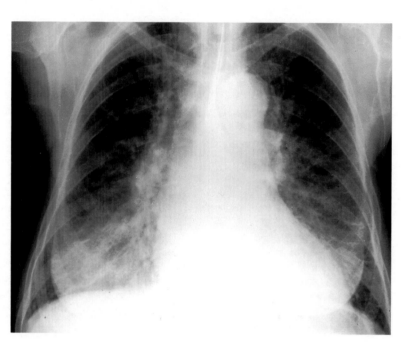

FIGURE 5.22 Posteroanterior chest film of a patient with longstanding angina pectoris and severe coronary artery disease. Cardiomegaly with left ventricular enlargement and pulmonary venous hypertension are evident. (Reproduced with permission; see Figure Credits)

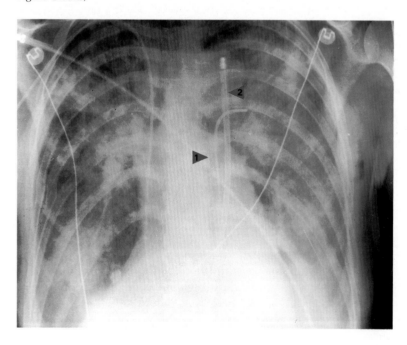

FIGURE 5.23 Portable chest x-ray of a patient with extensive myocardial infarction and cardio-genic shock. The film shows a normal-size heart and bilateral pulmonary alveolar edema. Note the Swan-Ganz catheter *(arrow 1)* and intra-aor-tic balloon catheter *(arrow 2)*. (Reproduced with permission; see Figure Credits)

PHYSICAL EXAMINATION

On physical examination, the patient with coronary atherosclerosis is often found to be normal. Carotid artery bruit, abdominal aneurysm, or peripheral arterial disease is an indicator that the patient is likely to have coronary atherosclerosis. Examination during an attack of angina pectoris may reveal pallor and an atrial or ventricular gallop sound.

The patient with septal rupture due to infarction may have a systolic murmur that is heard to the left of the midsternal area or occasionally at the apex. Rupture of a papillary muscle due to infarction may produce a systolic murmur at the apex. Such a murmur may not be present when the systolic pressure is low.

The patient with ischemic cardiomyopathy may exhibit an abnormally prolonged apex impulse and atrial and ventricular gallop sounds, as well as other physical signs of heart failure. A myocardial aneurysm may produce an abnormal pulsation of the precordium; such a pulsation may be seen and felt.

LABORATORY STUDIES
CHEST RADIOGRAPHY

The chest film of a patient with coronary atherosclerosis is usually normal. The heart may be large when there is ischemic cardiomyopathy or when multiple myocardial infarcts have occurred; evidence of heart failure may be found in such patients. A ventricular aneurysm may be noted. On rare occasion calcification of the coronary arteries or of the myocardium due to an old infarction may be seen (Figs. 5.21–5.25).

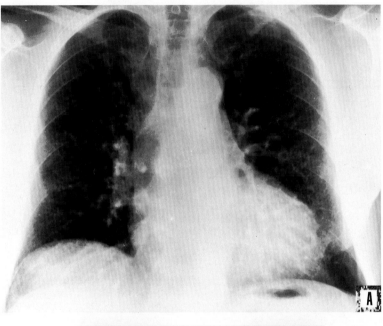

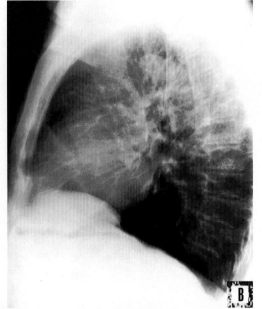

FIGURE 5.24
Posteroanterior (A) and lateral (B) chest projections of a patient with rupture of the interventricular septum secondary to myocardial infarction. The left and right ventricles are only slightly enlarged. The pulmonary vascularity is plethoric, and there is evidence of pulmonary venous hypertension. The pulmonary trunk is not enlarged. (Reproduced with permission; see Figure Credits)

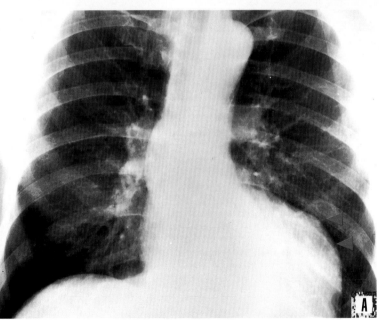

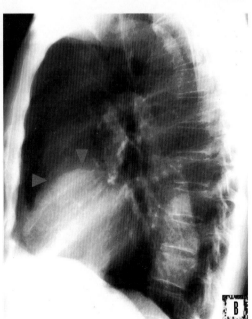

FIGURE 5.25
Posterior (A) and lateral (B) chest projections of a patient with an aneurysm of the anterolateral wall of the left ventricle. The left ventricle is enlarged and there is a deformity of the left lower border of the cardiac silhouette. Note the double density in the area immediately beneath the aortic valve on lateral view. (Reproduced with permission; see Figure Credits)

The resting electrocardiogram (ECG) is usually normal in patients with angina pectoris due to coronary atherosclerosis. A small percentage of patients show ST-segment displacement (mean ST vector directed away from the cardiac apex) or T-wave abnormalities.

The ECG may be normal or nondiagnostic in about 20% of patients with other evidence of myocardial infarction. The abnormalities, when present, include the

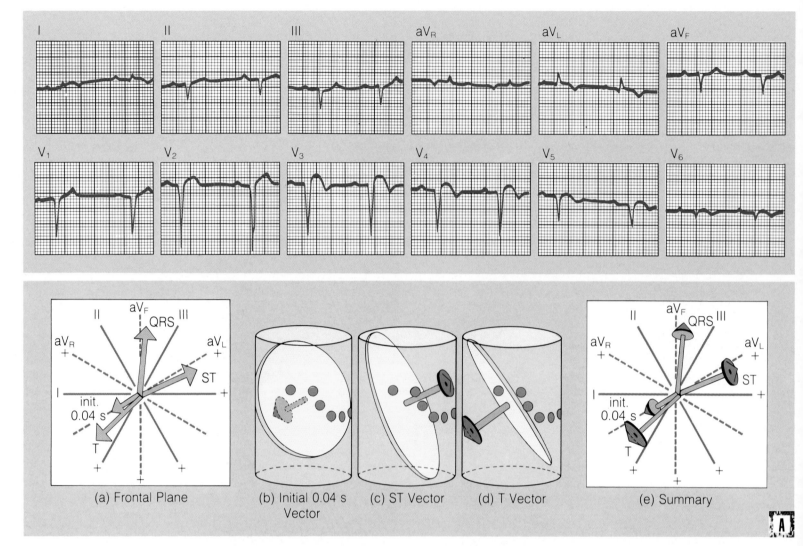

FIGURE 5.26 **(A)** ECG of a 48-year-old patient with an extensive anterior myocardial infarction. **(a)** The QRS complexes are resultantly negative in leads II and III and slightly positive in lead I; this can be represented by a mean vector directed relatively parallel with the negative limb of lead aV$_F$ but directed so that a small positive quantity will be projected on lead I. The initial 0.04 second portion of the QRS cycle is negative in leads I and aV$_L$ and positive in lead III and can be represented by a small mean vector directed perpendicular to lead II. The T wave is large and positive in lead III and slightly positive in lead aV$_R$ and can be represented by a mean vector directed just to the right of the positive limb of lead III. The ST segment is elevated in leads I, II, and aV$_L$ and slightly depressed in leads III, aV$_R$, and aV$_F$. Accordingly the mean ST vector is directed relatively parallel with the positive limb of aV$_L$ but directed so that a small positive quantity will be projected on lead II. **(b,c,d)** The mean initial 0.04 second vector is rotated markedly posteriorly and deviated from the frontal plane approximately 80° because

the initial 0.04 second is negative in all the precordial leads. The mean ST vector is rotated at least 45° anteriorly because the ST segment is elevated in all the precordial leads but is less elevated in leads V$_1$ and V$_6$. The mean T vector is approximately flush with the frontal plane because the T wave is upright in lead V$_1$, and inverted in leads V$_2$–V$_6$. **(e)** The spatial arrangement of the vectors. The mean spatial initial 0.04 second vector is located abnormally to the right and is posteriorly directed. This vector is directed away from a large area of anterior dead zone. The mean ST vector is directed toward an area of epicardial injury located in the anterolateral portion of the left ventricle. The mean T vector is rotated away from an area of anterolateral epicardial ischemia. It is interesting that the tracing was made 3 months after the acute infarction and that the abnormal ST vector is still present, suggesting the possibility of ventricular aneurysm at the site of infarction. (Reproduced with permission; see Figure Credits)

following: the mean vector for the initial 0.04 second of the QRS complexes points away from the infarction; and the mean ST vector points toward the area of infarction; the mean T vector points away from the area of infarction. ECGs showing anterior and inferior myocardial infarctions are shown in Figure 5.26.

When the method of vector electrocardiography is understood, it is easy to predict the electrocardiographic signs of infarction of different areas of the left ventricle and septum (Fig. 5.27). All three abnormalities may not be present in every patient. There may be only T-wave abnormalities or ST-T abnormalities, or there may be abnormalities of the initial 0.04 second of the QRS complex, T waves, and ST segments.

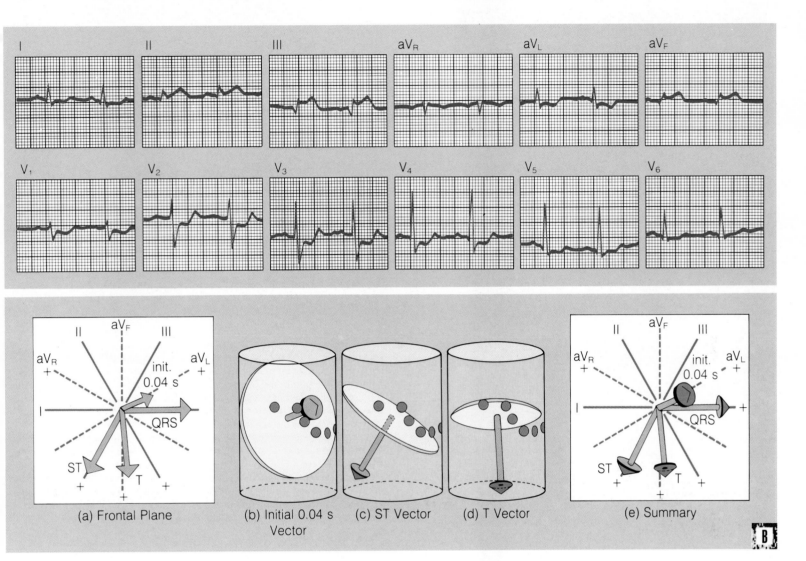

(a) Frontal Plane (b) Initial 0.04 s Vector (c) ST Vector (d) T Vector (e) Summary

FIGURE 5.26 **(B)** ECG of a 62-year-old patient with an acute posterior myocardial infarction. **(a)** The frontal plane projection shows the mean QRS, ST, T, and initial 0.04 second vectors. The mean QRS vector is directed perpendicular to lead aV_F because the QRS complex is resultantly zero in lead aV_F. The ST-segment displacement is greatest in lead III and least in lead aV_R and can be represented by a mean vector directed parallel with the positive limb of lead III. The mean T vector is directed just to the left of the positive limb of lead aV_F. The initial 0.04 second of the QRS complex is negative in lead III and aV_F and resultantly slightly positive in lead II. The initial 0.04 second of the QRS cycle can be represented by a mean vector directed relatively perpendicular to lead II, but it is located so that a small positive quantity will be projected on lead II. **(b,c,d)** The mean spatial initial 0.04 second vector is rotated approximately 80° anteriorly because the initial 0.04 second of the QRS complex is resultantly positive in lead V_1–V_4. (The Q wave in V_5

is 0.02 second in duration and the transitional pathway for the mean pathway for the mean initial 0.04 second vector lies near V_6.) The mean spatial ST vector is rotated posteriorly since the ST segment is depressed in all the precordial leads. The mean spatial T vector is tilted at least 15° anteriorly since all the precordial leads record upright T waves. **(e)** The mean spatial initial 0.04 second vector is abnormal in position because it is located too far to the left of the horizontally directed mean spatial QRS vector. The mean spatial ST vector is directed toward the area of inferoposterior epicardial injury and the mean spatial initial 0.04 second vector is directed away from the area of posterior myocardial necrosis. The infarction is clinically only 3 hours old and the mean T vector has not yet assumed the position of being directed away from the ischemia surrounding an area of necrosis. (Reproduced with permission; see Figure Credits)

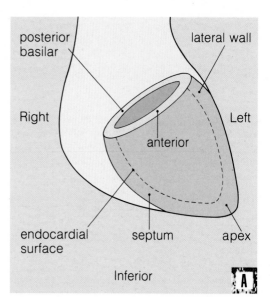

posterior basilar

lateral wall

Right

Left

anterior

endocardial surface

septum

apex

Inferior

A

FIGURE 5.27

(A) Frontal view of the left ventricle as seen within the cardiac silhouette. The dashed lines indicate the endocardial surface. Various regions of the left ventricle are identified. (Reproduced with permission; see Figure Credits)

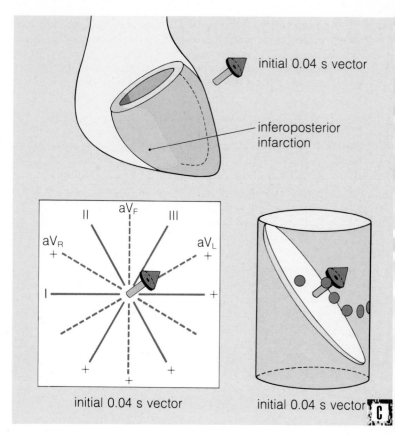

initial 0.04 s vector

inferoposterior infarction

aV_R II aV_F III aV_L

I +

+ + +

initial 0.04 s vector

initial 0.04 s vector

C

FIGURE 5.27   **(C) (a)** Myocardial infarction located on the inferoposterior surface of the left ventricle. The electrical forces generated by the diametrically opposite part of the heart dominate the electrical field during the initial 0.04 second of the QRS cycle, and the mean initial 0.04 second vector is directed away from the area of infarction. **(b)** The mean initial 0.04 second vector is treated as though it originates in the center of the chest and the hexaxial reference system has been superimposed. This enables one to study the projection of the mean initial 0.04 second vector on the frontal lead axes. In this case a Q wave will be recorded in leads II, III, aV$_F$, and aV$_R$, and an R wave will be recorded in leads I and aV$_L$. **(c)** The influence of the mean initial 0.04 second vector on the precordial leads. In this case initial R waves will be recorded in all the precordial leads. (Reproduced with permission; see Figure Credits)

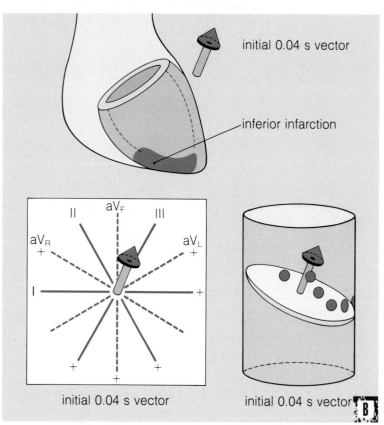

initial 0.04 s vector

inferior infarction

aV_R II aV_F III aV_L

I +

+ + +

initial 0.04 s vector

initial 0.04 s vector

B

FIGURE 5.27   **(B) (a)** Myocardial infarction located in the inferior wall of the left ventricle. The electrical forces generated by the muscle of the diametrically opposite wall dominate the electrical field during the initial 0.04 second of the QRS cycle, and the mean initial 0.04 second vector is directed away from the area of infarction. **(b)** The mean initial 0.04 second vector is treated as though it originates in the center of the chest and the hexaxial reference system has been superimposed. This enables one to study the projection of the mean initial 0.04 second vector on the frontal lead axes. In this case a Q wave will be written in leads II, III, and aV$_F$, and an R wave will be written in leads I, aV$_R$, and aV$_L$. This type of myocardial infarction is usually called an inferior infarction. **(c)** The influence of the mean initial 0.04 second vector on the precordial leads. In this case there will be initial R waves in all the precordial leads. (Reproduced with permission; see Figure Credits)

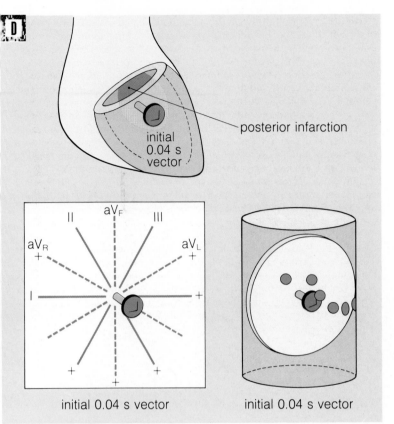

FIGURE 5.27 **(D) (a)** Myocardial infarction located on the posterior wall of the left ventricle—a true posterior infarct. The electrical forces generated by the anterior surface of the heart dominate the electrical field during the initial 0.04 second of the QRS cycle. **(b)** The mean initial 0.04 second vector is treated as though it originates in the center of the chest and the hexaxial reference system has been superimposed. This enables one to study the projection of the mean spatial 0.04 second vector on the frontal lead axes. In this case the frontal plane projection of the vector is quite small, producing an R wave in leads I, II, aV$_F$, and aV$_L$, and a Q wave in lead aV$_R$. The mean 0.04 second vector is perpendicular to lead III, and therefore the initial 0.04 second of the QRS complex in lead II will be resultantly zero. **(c)** The influence of the mean initial 0.04 second vector on the precordial leads. In this case initial R waves will be recorded in all the precordial leads, and the R wave in the right precordial leads will be quite large. (Reproduced with permission; see Figure Credits)

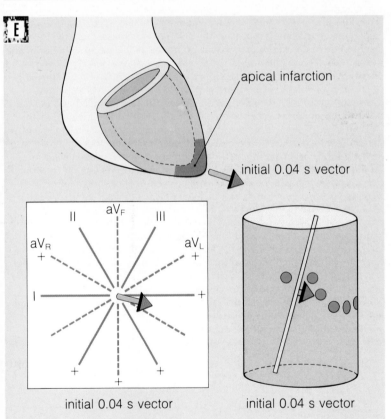

FIGURE 5.27 **(E) (a)** Myocardial infarction located in the apical portion of the left ventricle. If the infarcted area is relatively small, there may be little change in the QRS contour other than reduced magnitude. This is because a large number of normal initial QRS forces can still be generated by the intact muscle. In addition, there may be little ventricular muscle opposite the area of infarction located at the apex and therefore few opposing forces are generated. **(b)** The mean initial 0.04 second vector is treated as though it originates in the center of the chest, and the hexaxial reference system is imposed. This enables one to study the projection of the mean initial 0.04 second vector on the frontal lead axes. In this case the initial 0.04 second vector is quite small and is directed in a normal manner. A small Q wave will be recorded in lead III, but leads I, II, aV$_L$, and aV$_F$ will record a resultantly positive deflection for the first 0.04 second of the QRS cycle. **(c)** The influence of the mean 0.04 second vector on the precordial leads. In this case an initial Q wave will be recorded in lead I, and positive R waves will be recorded in leads V2–V6. (Reproduced with permission; see Figure Credits)

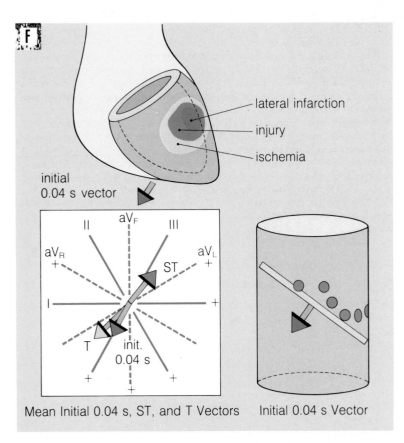

Mean Initial 0.04 s, ST, and T Vectors | **Initial 0.04 s Vector**

FIGURE 5.27 **(F) (a)** Myocardial infarction located in the lateral portion of the left ventricle. The electrical forces generated in the opposite portion of the heart dominate the electrical field during the initial 0.04 second of the QRS cycle, and the mean initial 0.04 second vector is directed away from the infarction. The area of infarcted tissue is surrounded by an area of myocardial injury located predominantly in the epicardial region of the left ventricle. The mean ST vector will be directed toward the area of epicardial injury. The area of dead and injured tissue is surrounded by an area of epicardial ischemia. The mean T vector will be directed away from the area of epicardial ischemia. **(b)** The mean initial 0.04 second, ST, and T vectors are treated as though they originate in the center of the chest and the hexaxial reference system has been superimposed. This enables one to study the projection of the vectors on the lead axes. In this case a Q wave will be recorded in leads I and aV_L, and an R wave will be recorded in leads II, III, and aV_F. The mean initial 0.04 second vector is perpendicular to lead aV_R, and therefore the initial 0.04 second of the QRS complex in lead aV_R will be resultantly zero. The ST segment will be elevated in leads I and aV_L and depressed in leads II, III, aV_F, and aV_R. The T wave will be inverted in leads I and aV_L and upright in leads II, III, aV_F; and aV_R. **(c)** The influence of the mean initial 0.04 second vector on the precordial leads. In this case a Q wave will be recorded in leads V_2–V_6. Although it is not illustrated, the ST segment would be elevated in leads V_2–V_6 and depressed in lead V_1. The T wave would be inverted in V_2–V_6, and upright in lead V_1. (Reproduced with permission; see Figure Credits)

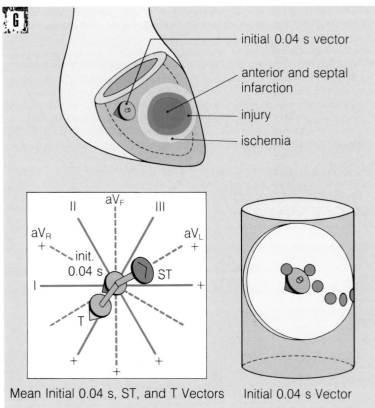

Mean Initial 0.04 s, ST, and T Vectors | **Initial 0.04 s Vector**

FIGURE 5.27 **(G) (a)** Myocardial infarction located in the anterior and septal region of the left ventricle. The electrical forces generated in the opposite portion of the ventricular muscle dominate the electrical field during the initial 0.04 second of the QRS cycle, and the mean initial 0.04 second vector is directed away from the infarcted area. The area of infarction is surrounded by an area of epicardial myocardial injury. The mean ST vector will be directed toward the area of epicardial injury. The area of dead and injured tissue is surrounded by a zone of epicardial ischemia. The mean T vector will be directed away from the area of epicardial ischemia. **(b)** The mean initial 0.04 second, ST, and T vectors are treated as though they originate in the center of the chest, and the hexaxial reference system has been superimposed. This enables one to study the projection of the vectors on the frontal lead axes. In this case the frontal plane projection of the mean initial 0.04 second vector is quite small, producing a Q wave in leads I and aV_L and an R wave in leads III, aV_F, and aV_R. The mean 0.04 second vector is perpendicular to lead II, and therefore the initial 0.04 second of the QRS complex in lead II will be resultantly zero. The ST segment will be elevated in leads I and aV_L and will be depressed in leads III, aV_F; and aV_R. There will be no ST-segment displacement in lead II. The T wave will be inverted in leads I and aV_L and will be upright in leads II, III, aV_F, and aV_R. **(c)** The influence of the mean initial 0.04 second vector on the precordial leads. In this case a Q wave will be recorded in all the precordial leads. Although it is not illustrated, the ST segment would be elevated and the T waves would be inverted in all the precordial leads. (Reproduced with permission; see Figure Credits)

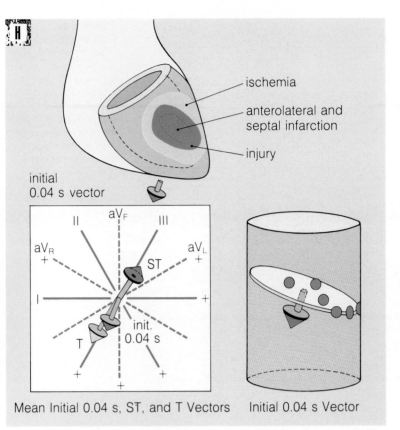

Mean Initial 0.04 s, ST, and T Vectors | **Initial 0.04 s Vector**

FIGURE 5.27 **(H) (a)** Myocardial infarction located in the anterolateral and septal portion of the left ventricle. The electrical forces generated in the opposite portion of the heart dominate the electrical field during the initial 0.04 second of the QRS cycle, and the mean initial 0.04 second vector is directed away from the infarcted area. The area of dead tissue is surrounded by an area of epicardial myocardial injury, and the ST vector will be directed toward the area of epicardial injury. Surrounding the latter area is an area of epicardial myocardial ischemia. The mean T vector will be directed away from the area of epicardial ischemia. **(b)** The mean initial 0.04 second, ST, and T vectors are treated as though they originate in the center of the chest, and the hexaxial reference system has been superimposed. This enables one to study the projection of the vectors on the frontal lead axes. In this case a Q wave will be recorded in leads I, aV_L, and aV_R, and an R wave will be recorded in leads II, III, and aV_F. The ST segment will be elevated in leads I and aV_L and depressed in leads II, III, aV_F, and aV_R. The T wave will be inverted in leads I and aV_L, resultantly zero in lead aV_R, and upright in leads II, III, and aV_F. **(c)** The influence of the mean initial 0.04 second vector on the precordial leads. In this case a Q wave will be recorded in leads V_1–V_3, and the initial 0.04 second of the QRS cycle will be resultantly zero in leads V_4—V_6. Although it is not illustrated, the ST segment would be elevated in leads V_1–V_3, and isoelectric in leads V_4–V_6. The T waves would be inverted in leads V_1–V_3 and flat in leads V_4–V_6. (Reproduced with permission; see Figure Credits)

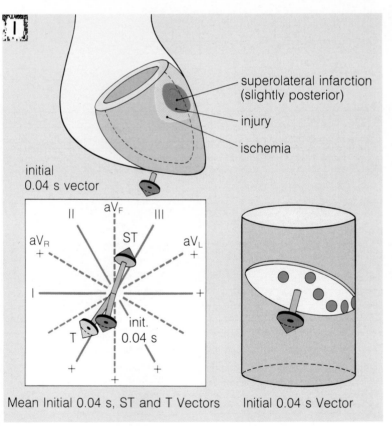

Mean Initial 0.04 s, ST and T Vectors | **Initial 0.04 s Vector**

FIGURE 5.27 **(I) (a)** Myocardial infarction located in the superolateral wall of the left ventricle and slightly posteriorly. The electrical forces generated in the opposite portion of the ventricular muscle dominate the electrical field during the initial 0.04 second of the QRS cycle, and the mean initial 0.04 second vector is directed away from the infarcted area. The area is surrounded by a zone of epicardial injury, and the mean ST vector will be directed toward the area of epicardial injury. The zone of injury is surrounded by a zone of epicardial ischemia, and the mean T vector will be directed away from the zone. **(b)** The mean initial 0.04 second, ST, and T vectors are treated as though they originate in the center of the chest, and the hexaxial reference system has been superimposed. This enables one to study the projection of the vectors on the frontal lead axes. In this case a Q wave will be recorded in leads I, aV_L, and aV_R and an R wave will be recorded in leads II, III, and aV_F. R waves will be written in the precordial leads because the infarct is located in a slightly posterior position. The ST segment will be elevated in leads I, aV_L, and aV_R and depressed in leads II, III, and aV_F. The T wave will be inverted in leads I and aV_L and upright in leads II, III, aV_F, and aV_R. **(c)** The influence of the mean initial 0.04 second vector on the precordial leads. Initial R waves will be recorded in all the precordial leads. Although it is not illustrated, the ST segment would be slightly depressed and the T waves would be upright in all the precordial leads. (Reproduced with permission; see Figure Credits)

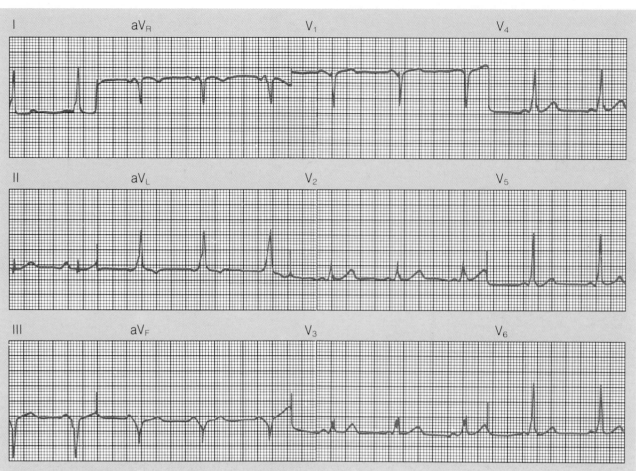

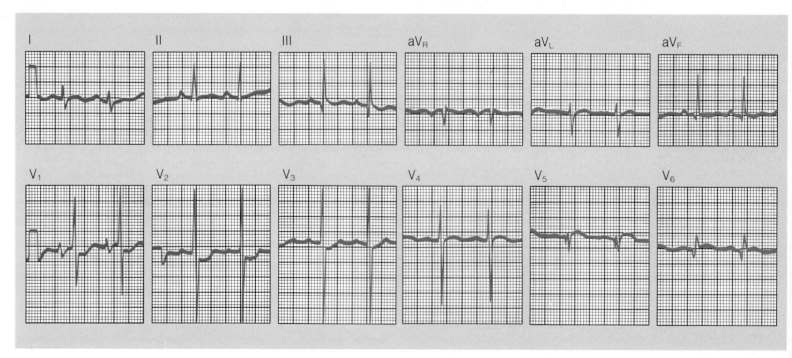

FIGURE 5.29 ECG of a 10-year-old boy with muscular dystrophy. The boy was on digitalis, sodium restriction, and diuretics for heart failure. The abnormal Q waves and ST segment in leads V_5 and V_6 could be mistaken for myocardial infarction. (Reproduced with permission; see Figure Credits)

There are several conditions that may be mistaken for myocardial infarction. The ECG of a patient with the Wolff-Parkinson-White (WPW) syndrome may simulate infarction (Fig. 5.28). The ECGs of patients with hypertrophic cardiomyopathy or dilated cardiomyopathy (including neuromuscular disorders) may mimic infarction (Fig. 5.29). The ECGs of patients with acute pulmonary embolism may suggest myocardial infarction (Fig. 5.30). Patients with complex congenital lesions, myocardial abnormalities due to sarcoid, amyloid, or neoplastic disease, and acute myocarditis may all exhibit ECGs that resemble the tracings of myocardial infarction due to coronary atherosclerosis (Figs. 5.31, 5.32).

Right or left bundle branch block may occur, but these abnormalities are also seen with many other forms of heart disease. This is also true for atrial fibrillation, ventricular rhythm disturbances, and atrioventricular block.

The ECG obtained during an exercise stress test may reveal abnormalities that are not seen in the tracing made while the patient is at rest (Fig. 5.33).

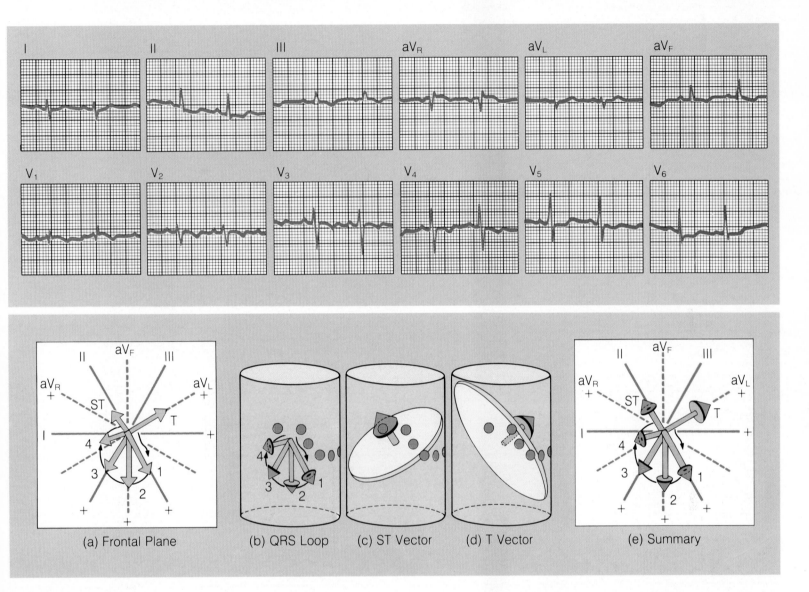

(a) Frontal Plane   (b) QRS Loop   (c) ST Vector   (d) T Vector   (e) Summary

FIGURE 5.30   ECG of a 54-year-old patient made shortly after pulmonary embolism. **(a)** The frontal plane projection shows the mean spatial QRS loop and ST and T vectors. **(b)** The QRS loop is broken down into four successive spatial instantaneous vectors. Each of these instantaneous vectors is oriented in space, producing a rough outline of the mean spatial QRS loop. **(c)** The mean ST vector is rotated 40° anteriorly because the ST segment is elevated in V_1–V_3 and depressed in V_5 and V_6. **(d)** The mean T vector is rotated approximately 20° posteriorly because the T wave is inverted in V_1–V_4 and upright in V_5 and V_6. Note that when the mean T vector, or any vector, is in this position, only a small amount of posterior rotation is necessary to produce inverted T waves in several of the precordial leads. **(e)** The spatial arrangement of the vectors. The QRS loop is rotund and is inscribed in a clockwise manner. The initial forces are to the left and are rotated anteriorly, producing an initial R wave in lead V_1. Vector 4, illustrating the terminal QRS vectors, is directed to the right and anteriorly, producing an S wave in leads 1 and V_1–V_6, and an R wave in V_1. The mean ST vector is directed toward the right shoulder and indicates subendocardial injury, while the mean T vector is directed to the left and posteriorly, indicating right ventricular ischemia. These findings are typical of acute cor pulmonale secondary to pulmonary embolism. At times only right ventricular ischemia may be present. The inverted T waves in leads V_1–V_4 may lead the physician to believe they are due to the ischemic effects of myocardial infarction due to atherosclerotic coronary artery disease, whereas they are actually due to acute pulmonary embolism. (Reproduced with permission; see Figure Credits)

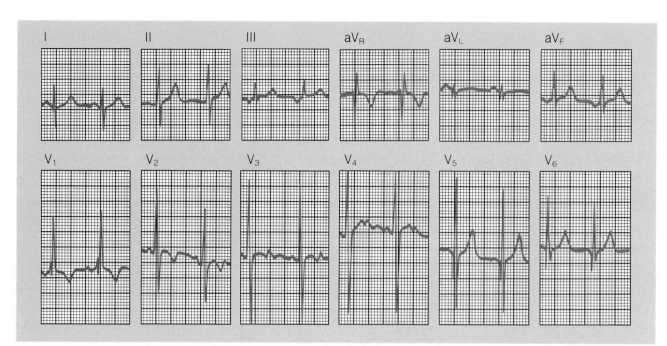

FIGURE 5.31
ECG of a 7-year-old male with aortic septal defect. The large Q waves in leads aV_L, V_5 and V_6 could be misinterpreted as myocardial infarction. They are probably related to septal hypertrophy in this patient with congenital heart disease. (Reproduced with permission; see Figure Credits)

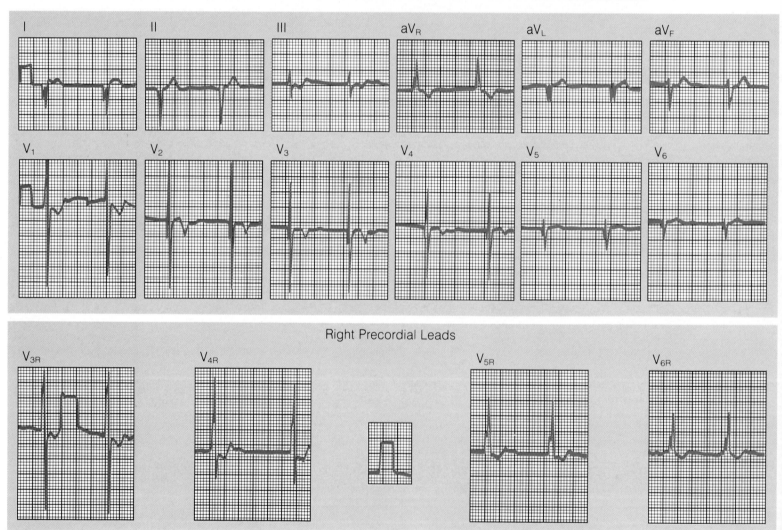

FIGURE 5.32   ECG of a 9-year-old boy with congenital heart disease. The diagnostic studies were compatible with isolated dextrocardia, transposition of the great vessels, and intracardiac shunt. The Q wave in leads I, II, aV_L, and V_2–V_6 could be misinterpreted as being due to myocardial infarction. (Reproduced with permission; see Figure Credits)

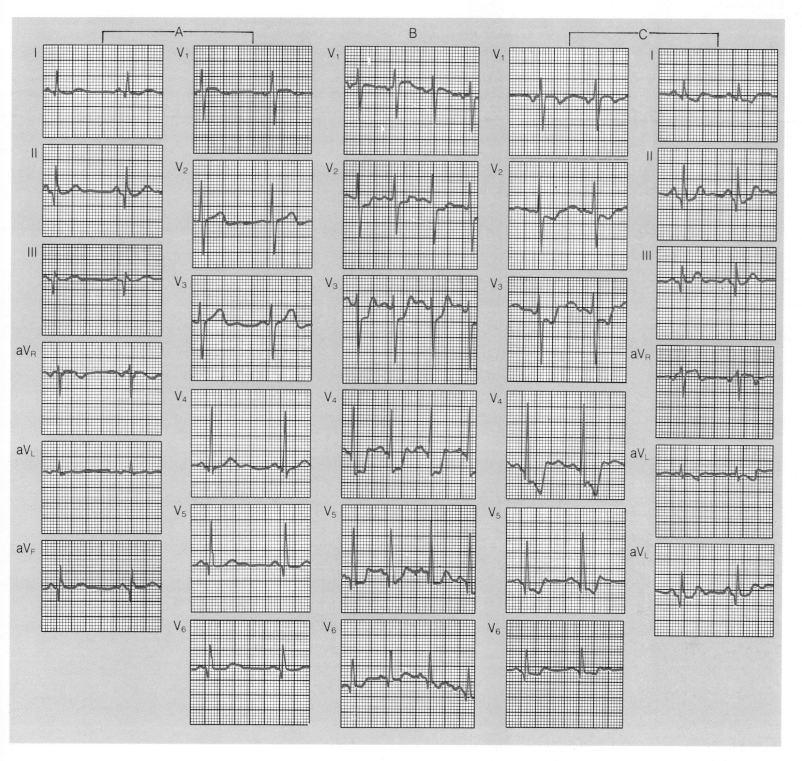

FIGURE 5.33 Rest **(A)**, exercise **(B)**, and recovery **(C)** ECGs recorded on a 59-year-old man. The patient underwent treadmill testing to evaluate increasingly severe angina pectoris in the previous 6 months. Inferior myocardial infarction had occurred 6 years previously. The resting ECG demonstrates old inferolateral infarction and left atrial abnormality. Excercise was terminated by exertional angina pectoris at a peak heart rate of 110 beats per minute (bpm) and peak workload of 6 METs. !schemic ST-segment depression is noted during exercise in leads V_2–V_5, maximally (0.5 mV) in lead V_4. Post-exertional T-wave inversion is noted m V_2–V_5, accompanied by ischemic ST depression maximally (0.4 mV) in lead V_4. Major lesions in the three major coronary arteries were bypassed surgically. The patient had been largely asymptomatic and without recurrent infarction during the 6 years following initial infarction; an exercise test performed 6 months previously demonstrated similar ST-segment abnormalities at a peak heart rate of 145 bpm and peak workload of 9 METs. Beta blockers were withdrawn 72 hours prior to testing. (Reproduced with permission; see Figure Credits)

Exercise is employed to increase myocardial oxygen demand, thereby producing myocardial ischemia (Fig. 5.34). The Bruce protocol is commonly used as the standard test. One millimeter or more of downward displacement of the ST segment at the J point that continues for 0.08 second is considered to be a positive response (Figs. 5.35–5.37). The predictive value of a positive response in a middle-aged male is about 80%. Therefore, a false-positive response occurs in 10% to 20% of male patients. The predictive value of a negative response in a middle-aged male, excluding coronary disease, is about 90%. The predictive value of a positive response in a female 40 to 50 years of age is about 50%. Therefore, a false-positive, response is common in females. The predictive value of a negative response, excluding coronary disease, in a woman 40 to 50 years of age, is 90% or more.

The exercise ECG is not indicated for diagnostic reasons when the history of stable angina pectoris has a predictive value of 90% (see Fig. 5.20). An exercise test should not be done routinely in patients thought to have unstable angina. The exercise test rarely clarifies the diagnosis of chest pain in women who are 40 to 50 years of age. A negative test in such patients is helpful but in practice

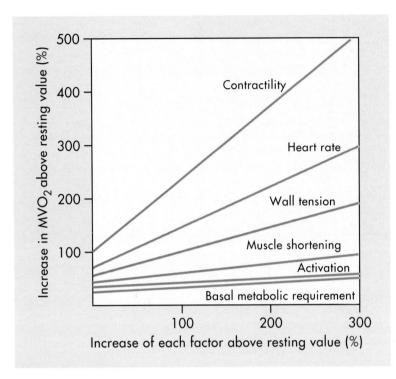

FIGURE 5.34 Changes in various factors contributing to myocardial oxygen requirements during exercise. (Reproduced with permission; see Figure Credits)

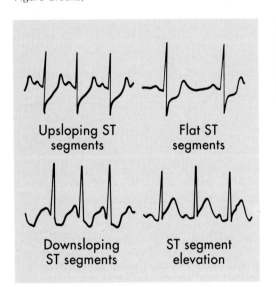

FIGURE 5.35 ST-segment changes seen with ischemia. (Reproduced with permission; see Figure Credits)

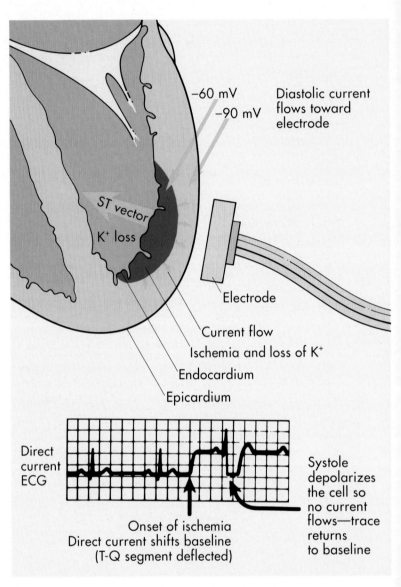

FIGURE 5.36 Mechanism of ST-segment depression as the subendocardium becomes ischemic. The loss of potassium from the cells causes a diastolic current flow toward the epicardium and the monitoring electrode. This deflects the baseline upward during diastole, which is unmasked by the total depolarization at the time of the R wave, returning the baseline to zero during the ST interval. (Reproduced with permission; see Figure Credits)

the number of false-positives makes the test less useful. Other information is obtained from an exercise test, including angina or a fall in blood pressure during the test, and the degree of exercise tolerance. Nuclear exercise tests (discussed below) are helpful when a false-positive electrocardiographic exercise test is anticipated (Fig. 5.38).

Long-term monitoring of the ECG is indicated when the physician suspects cardiac arrhythmia after myocardial infarction. Artifacts may occur in such recordings and the physician must be aware of their appearance. Episodic myocardial ischemia can also be detected by ambulatory ECG monitoring.

ECHOCARDIOGRAPHY

Most patients with coronary atherosclerosis have normal echocardiograms prior to the development of cardiac muscle damage. The echocardiogram (Fig. 5.39) can be used to detect left ventricular thrombi, right ventricular thrombi, or wall-motion abnormalities including a left ventric-ular aneurysm; it is also used to calculate the ejection fraction and to show pericardial effusion. Other conditions may also be identified. This is important because coronary disease may coexist with many other conditions or other diseases may mimic coronary disease (Figs. 5.40–5.44).

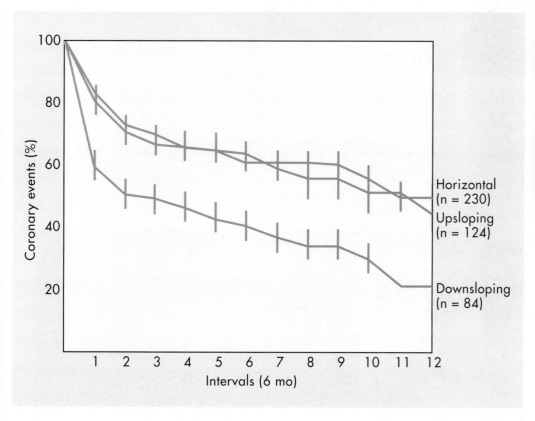

FIGURE 5.37   Prevalence of coronary events per year in subjects with upsloping, horizontal, and downsloping ST-segment depression. Note the more serious implications in those with downsloping STs. (Reproduced with permission; see Figure Credits)

FIGURE 5.38 CAUSES OF A FALSE-POSITIVE OR UNINTERPRETABLE ECG EXERCISE TEST

Digitalis therapy
LVH
LBBB
Female sex
Hypothyroidism
Hypokalemia

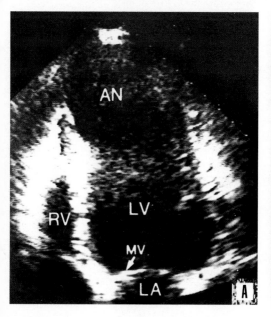
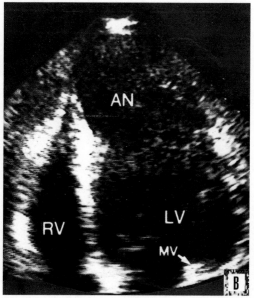
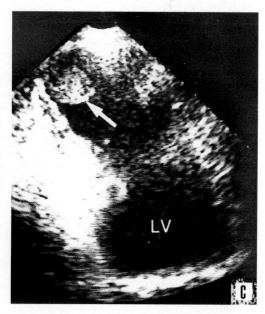

FIGURE 5.39   Cross-sectional echocardiograms obtained in a patient with a recent anterior myocardial infarction. The systolic frame of the apical four-chamber view (A) and diastolic frame of the same view (B) show a large apical aneurysm (AN). The left ventricle (LV) is moderately dilated at its base, but there is extensive thinning of the apical wall. The aneurysm has a wide neck and fundus. (C) Apical two-chamber view shows a round mass (arrow) partially filling the aneurysm as it extends from the surface of the akinetic wall, indicative of a mural thrombus. (RV = right ventricle; LA = left atrium; MV = mitral valve). (Reproduced with permission; see Figure Credits)

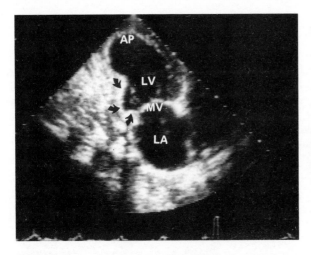

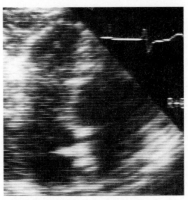

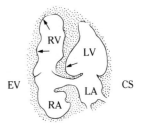

FIGURE 5.40 Two-chamber echocardiogram of the left ventricle (LV) in a patient with a moderate-to-large inferior myocardial infarction. Note the basal location (*arrow*) of the area of infarction and the preserved apical (AP) geometry. (LA = left atrium; MV = mitral valve) (Reproduced with permission; see Figure Credits)

FIGURE 5.41 Echocardiogram of right ventricular (RV) infarction. A cause of RV dilation is RV infarction. This condition is distinguished from others by a history of recent inferior wall left ventricular (LV) infarction. Note in this example that the RV is apex-forming. However, unlike other causes of RV volume overload, real-time imaging shows dyskinesis (*arrows*). Furthermore, there is remodelling or diastolic deformity of the inferior interventricular septum (LV, *arrow*). This image was taken with the proper inferior angulation to detect an abnormality in the inferior septum. Inferior angulation of the four-chamber view is documented when the coronary sinus (CS) and eustacian valve (EV) are imaged at the base of the heart. The cavity labelled RA probably represents the mouth of the inferior vena cava as it enters the RA. (Reproduced with permission; see Figure Credits)

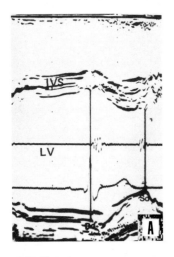

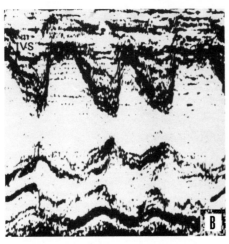

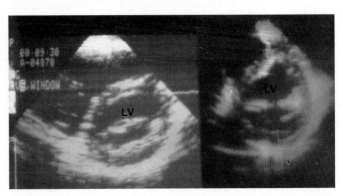

FIGURE 5.43 Normal short-axis view (left) contrasted with short-axis view (right) in a patient with an anteroseptal infarction. Note the rather striking remodelling at the anteroseptal junction. (Reproduced with permission; see Figure Credits)

FIGURE 5.42 Mitral regurgitation complicating myocardial infarction. **(A)** M-mode of a normal left ventricle. Note that the motion of the septum (IVS) and the motion of its opposite posterior wall are fairly symmetric. **(B)** Severe mitral insufficiency arising from ischemic damage to the interior base of the LV. This damage has undermined the support of the posteromedial papillary muscle. The resulting mitral insufficiency has exaggerated the motion of the septum. The damaged inferior wall has only poor inward motion, in marked contrast to the IVS. (Reproduced with permission; see Figure Credits)

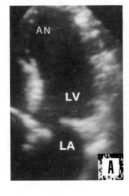

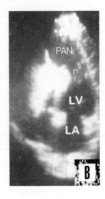

FIGURE 5.44 **(A)** Aneurysm (AN) of the left ventricular (LV) apex seen in the apical four-chamber view. **(B)** Pseudo-aneurysm (PAN) identified by its connection to the LV across a narrow neck (n). (Reproduced with permission; see Figure Credits)

Coronary arteriography and left ventriculography are now routine since it became obvious that both types of studies are necessary in the majority of patients in whom coronary atherosclerosis is suspected. The risk of the procedure is about 0.01%. Coronary arteriography and left ventriculography are used for diagnostic purposes and to determine if coronary bypass surgery or coronary angioplasty are needed for proper treatment (Figs. 5.45–5.50).

Coronary arteriography and left ventriculography are indicated in the following cases:

1. Patients with a positive exercise ECG or thallium stress test
2. Young patients with stable angina pectoris
3. Elderly patients with disabling stable angina pectoris

4. Patients with unstable angina (unless they are elderly and have other reasons why angioplasty or surgery should not be employed)
5. Several days after successful thrombolytic treatment for myocardial infarction
6. Early in infarction when emergency angioplasty or surgery is to be used in therapy
7. Following infarction when angina continues or occurs for the first time
8. Following infarction when the submaximal ECG stress test or the thallium stress test is positive
9. Patients in whom surgery is planned for abdominal aneurysm or peripheral arterial disease and the dipyridamole ^{201}thallium (^{201}Tl) test is abnormal
10. Patients undergoing cardiac catheterization for valve disease.

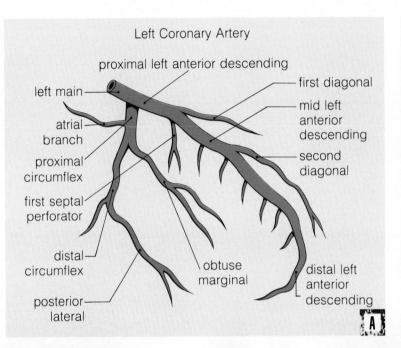

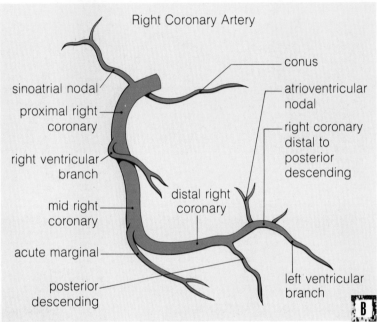

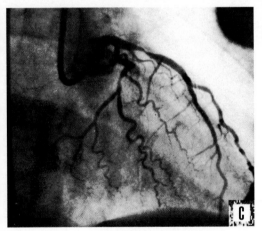

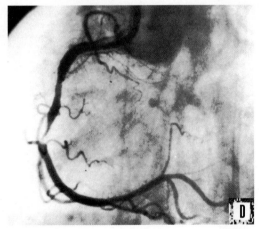

FIGURE 5.45 **(A)** Anatomy of the left coronary artery as seen in the right anterior oblique view. **(B)** Anatomy of the right coronary artery as seen in the left anterior oblique view. **(C)** Right anterior oblique view of the left coronary artery shows high-grade stenosis of the left anterior descending branch proximal to the first septal perforating branch. **(D)** Left anterior oblique view of the right coronary artery shows a high-grade lesion in its midportion. (Reproduced with permission; see Figure Credits)

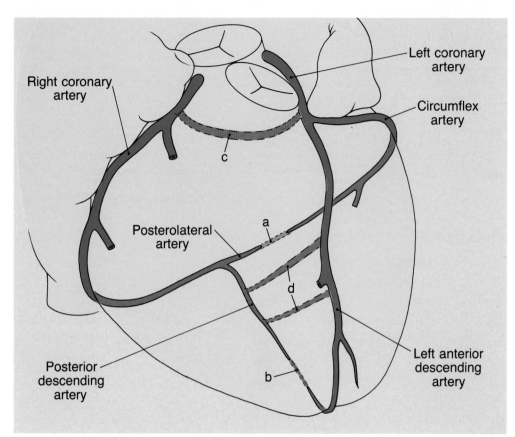

FIGURE 5.46 The most common collateral pathways between the right and left coronary arteries. **(A)** Connection between the posterolateral and distal circumflex arteries. **(B)** Connection between the distal left anterior descending and posterior descending arteries. **(C)** Connection between the right coronary and left anterior descending arteries via the conus artery. **(D)** Connection between the left anterior descending and posterior descending arteries via septal branches. (Reproduced with permission; see Figure Credits)

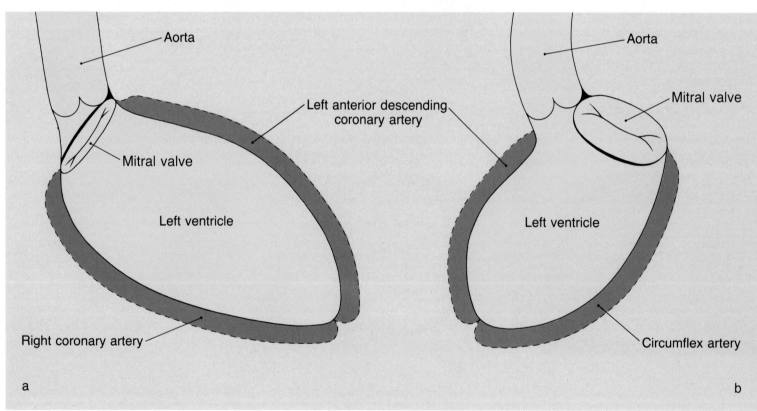

FIGURE 5.47 Vascular territories of the left ventricle. **(A)** Right anterior oblique projection of a left ventriculogram. **(B)** Left anterior oblique projection of a left ventriculogram. The apex is an area of overlapping circulation, served by both the left anterior descending and the circumflex arteries. (Reproduced with permission; see Figure Credits)

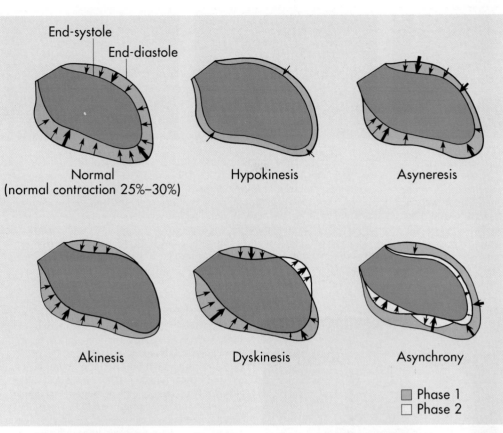

End-systole

End-diastole

Normal
(normal contraction 25%–30%)

Hypokinesis

Asyneresis

Akinesis

Dyskinesis

Asynchrony

☐ Phase 1
☐ Phase 2

FIGURE 5.48   Patterns of left ventricular contraction in the right anterior oblique projection. Arrows indicate wall motion and shaded areas indicate end-systole. Asyneresis describes localized hypokinesis. (Reproduced with permission; see Figure Credits)

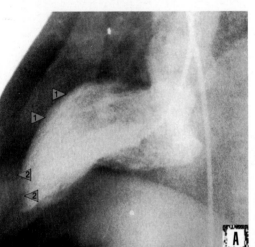

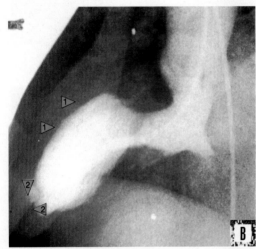

FIGURE 5.49   Right anterior oblique projections of a left ventriculogram in diastole (**A**) and systole (**B**) in a patient with an anterolateral left ventricular aneurysm. Note the prominence of the anterolateral wall of the left ventricle in diastole (*arrows 1 in* A), which is even more conspicuous during systole (*arrows 1 in* B). The filling defect at the apex (*arrows 2*) represents a mural thrombus. (Reproduced with permission; see Figure Credits)

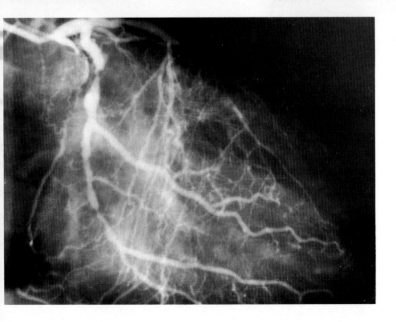

FIGURE 5.50   Left coronary arteriogram showing occlusion of the left anterior descending and circumflex arteries and severe stenosis of the marginal 1 (diagonal) artery. There is collateral circulation from the left anterior descending artery to the posterior descending artery via the septal artery, and from the circumflex artery to the posterolateral artery. (Reproduced with permission; see Figure Credits)

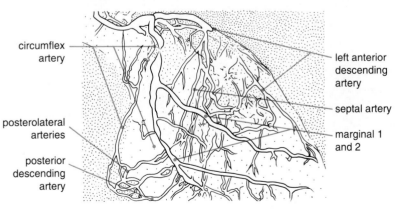

circumflex artery

left anterior descending artery

septal artery

marginal 1 and 2

posterolateral arteries

posterior descending artery

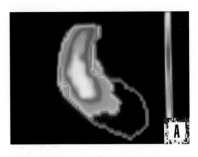
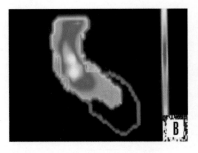
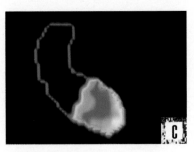
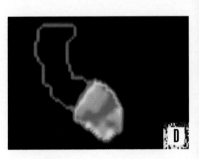

FIGURE 5.51 First-pass ⁹⁹ᵐTc scan of a 45-year-old man with coronary arteriographic evidence of a 48% diameter narrowing of the left anterior descending artery. The abnormal test result influenced the physicians to conclude that the borderline lesion in the left anterior descending artery was significant. **(A)** In this scan, taken at rest, the blue line represents the end-diastolic contour; the outer limit of the purple area represents the end-systolic contour. **(B)** In this image, taken during exercise, the blue line represents the end-diastolic contour; the outer limit of the purple area represents the end-systolic contour. Note that the purple area is larger and the distance between it and the blue line is smaller after exercise. This abnormality represents anterior hypokinesis after exercise. **(C,D)** These images reveal that the regional ejection fraction is diminished in the outer myocardial wall during exercise. The left ventricular ejection infraction at rest was 69% and during exercise it declined to 66%; this is abnormal. The left ventricular end-diastolic volume at rest was 122 mL and during exercise it was 151 mL; this is abnormal. The left ventricular end-systolic volume at rest was 38 mL and during exercise it was 51 mL; this is abnormal. (Reproduced with permission; see Figure Credits)

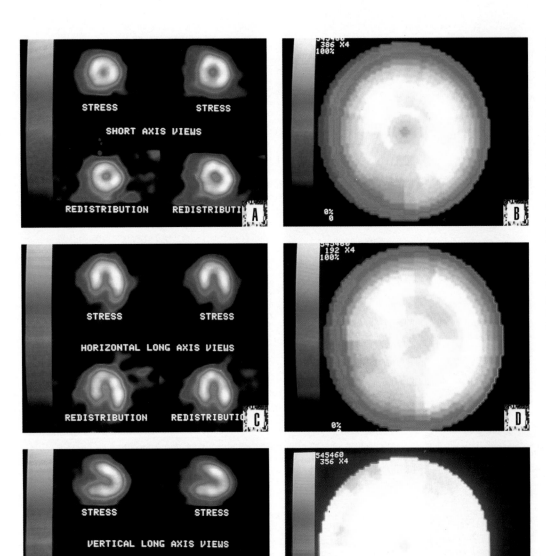

FIGURE 5.52 **(A–F)** Normal tomographic ²⁰¹T1 studies obtained using a rotating gamma scintillation camera. Selected tomographic slices are shown at stress and redistribution in the short axis **(A)**, horizontal long axis **(C)**, and vertical long axis **(E)**. Note the uniform homogeneous uptake of ²⁰¹T1 in the myocardium. **(B,D,F)** Functional quantitative images ("bull's-eye displays") are also shown. Each short-axis tomographic slice from apex to base is subjected to maximal count circumferential profile analysis. These profiles then are displayed as a series of concentric circles with the apex at the center and the base at the periphery. They are positioned in the same way as are the short-axis tomographic slices shown in **(A)**. The bull's-eye displays in **(B)** and **(D)** were obtained from stress and delayed images. **(F)** The bull's-eye for ²⁰¹T1 washout. Note that there is uniform uptake of ²⁰¹T1 at stress and redistribution and that the washout bull's-eye also is uniform with no abnormal zones depicted. (Reproduced with permission; see Figure Credits)

The technetium-99m (^{99m}Tc) ventriculogram, gated and first pass, can be used to measure the ejection fraction at rest and with exercise (Fig. 5.51). The normal resting ejection fraction is 50% to 70% and normally should increase with exercise. Patients with myocardial ischemia due to coronary atherosclerosis may have a low resting ejection fraction or one that may not increase with exercise. Patients with cardiomyopathy or elderly subjects who are unaccustomed to exercise may have similar findings.

The exercise ^{201}T1 scan with resting reperfusion studies may demonstrate evidence of infarction or exercise-induced ischemia (Fig. 5.52). Dipyridamole ^{201}Tl scans demonstrate areas of potentially ischemic myocardium in patients who are incapable of exercise (Fig. 5.53). Left bundle branch block may give false-positive evidence indicating ischemia. Recent technological improvements such as tomographic ^{201}T1 (SPECT) scanning (Fig. 5.54) have increased the accuracy of this test for the diagnosis of obstructive coronary arterial lesions.

Nuclear studies do not identify nonobstructive coronary atheroclerosis. Such studies do not become abnormal until the coronary obstruction is sufficiently severe to interface with coronary blood flow. Even when the coronary disease is sufficiently severe to produce myocardial ischemia, the nuclear tests are only about 85% sensitive and about 90% specific. Nuclear studies have their greatest value as screening tests in patients whose pretest probability of coronary disease is in the intermediate to low range. The T1 scan may be used following coronary arteriography as a means of judging the significance of borderline lesions (Fig. 5.55)

A recently developed nuclear diagnostic technique employs short-lived, positron-emitting radionuclides and tomographic imaging. Positron-emission tomography (PET) scan images are generated using a variety of elements and compounds that are said to reflect myocardial blood flow and various aspects of myocardial metabolism (e.g., radiolabelled glucose and fatty acids). Abnormal myocardial blood flow with preserved metabolic activity implies that the myocardium is still viable. Abnormal myocardial blood flow and metabolism imply that the affected zone is necrotic (Fig. 5.56).

Pyrophosphate molecules labelled with ^{99m}Tc are avidly taken up by necrotic myocardium. A "hot-spot" scan results with the radionuclide concentrated in the zone of infarcted myocardium. This technique can be employed to demonstrate and localize infarcted myocardium in patients with left bundle branch block or delayed admission to the hospital following a clinical event suggestive of myocardial infarction (Fig. 5.57).

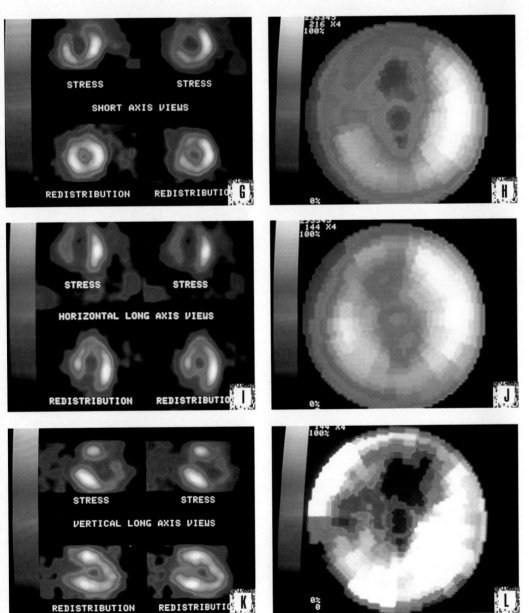

FIGURE 5.52 (continued) **(G–L)** Tomographic ^{201}T1 images in a patient with critical disease of the left anterior descending coronary artery. Shown in the same format as that for **(A–F)**. A large perfusion defect is demonstrated in the anterior wall, septum, and apex. Complete redistribution is demonstrated. The bull's eye displays show abnormal ^{201}T1 uptake at stress with virtually complete normalization at delayed imaging **(H-J)**. In the bull's-eye shown in **(L)**, there is abnormal ^{201}T1 washout depicted as dark blue and black, defining the precise zone of myocardial ischemia. (Reproduced with permission; see Figure Credits)

FIGURE 5.53 T1-201 IMAGE INTERPRETATION*

STRESS OR DIPYRIDAMOLE INFUSION	REST/REDISTRIBUTION	INTERPRETATION
Normal	Normal	No infarction or "ischemia"
Abnormal	Normal	Stress-induced "ischemia"
Abnormal	Abnormal—less than stress	"Ischemia" and infarction
Abnormal	Abnormal—no change	Infarction without apparent "ischemia"

*General pattern for interpretation of perfusion scintigrams. (Reproduced with permission; see Figure Credits)

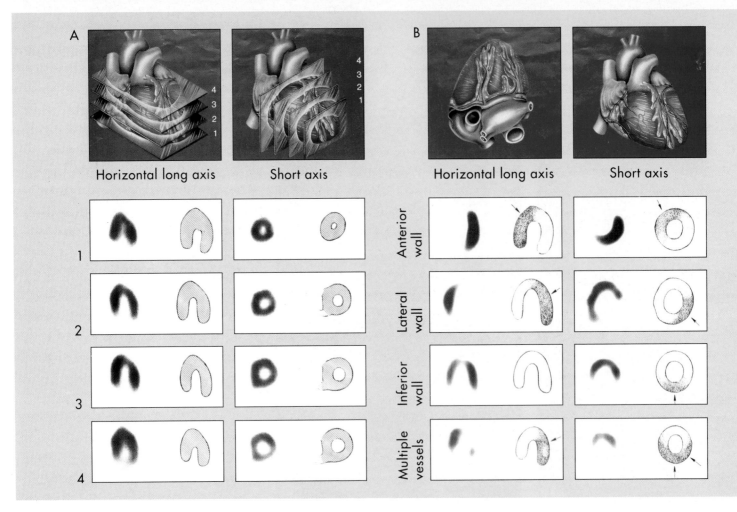

FIGURE 5.54 **(A)** Long- and short-axis SPECT reconstructions of a normal perfusion scintigram. **(B)** SPECT 201Tl images with a variety of perfusion abnormalities illustrated in long and short axes. (Reproduced with permission; see Figure Credits)

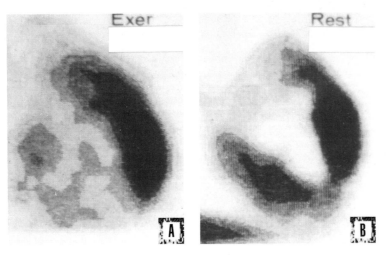

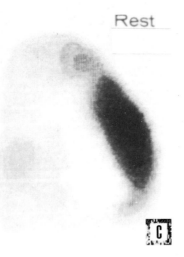

FIGURE 5.55 Myocardium at ischemic risk. Stress **(A)** and rest **(B)** myocardial perfusion scintigrams in a patient with right coronary stenosis estimated to be 40% . The scintigram clearly reveals evidence of reversible inferior ischemia. Subsequently, the patient went on to have a spontaneous infarction in the same region as shown on the rest image **(C)**. This study illustrates the difference between angiographic anatomy and scintigraphic pathophysiology, while providing one form of evidence for the ability of scintigraphy to identify myocardium at ischemic risk. (Reproduced with permission; see Figure Credits)

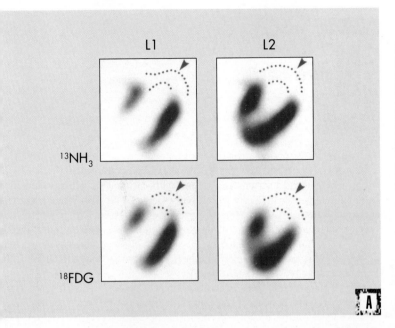

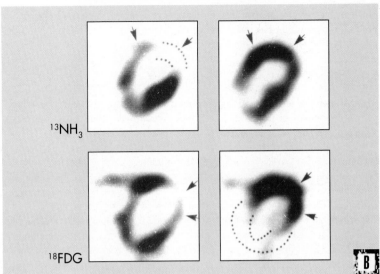

FIGURE 5.56 **(A)** Positron-emission tomogram at two levels through the left ventricle showing the myocardial distribution of nitrogen-13 ammonia (13NH3), a perfusion marker, and fluorine-18 fluorodeoxyglucose (18FDG), a marker of glucose uptake. In this patient with a prior anterior wall infarct there are matched perfusion and metabolic defects. **(B)** Mismatched pattern in another patient with prior infarction shows a perfusion (13NH3) defect, but persistent glucose (18FDG) uptake in the anterior wall, suggesting that viable myocardium persists in the infarct zone. (Reproduced with permission; see Figure Credits)

FIGURE 5.57 Extensive 99mTc pyrophosphate (TcPYP) uptake. **(A)** The extensive pattern of TcPYP uptake demonstrated in multiple projections is related to a poor prognosis. In surviving patients, it indicated a widespread subendocardial or shell infarction. **(B)** The related ECG shows widespread ST-segment depression without Q waves. (Reproduced with permission; see Figure Credits)

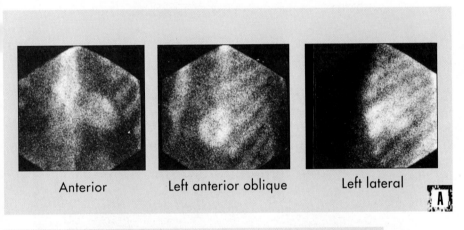

Anterior Left anterior oblique Left lateral

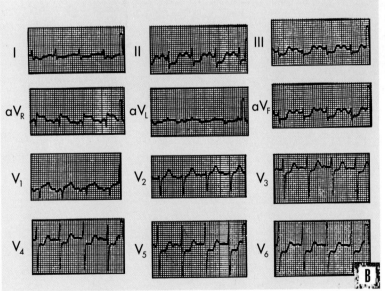

Nuclear magnetic resonance images demonstrate various aspects of the pathophysiology of myocardial infarction, including infarct size, aneurysm, pseudoaneurysm, and mural thrombus (Figs. 5.58–5.60).

CARDIAC ENZYMES

The MB band of serum creatine phosphokinase (CK) becomes elevated when a sufficient number of myocardial cells die. Accordingly, the test is used when myocardial infarction is suspected.

In general the larger the infarct, the higher the CK and MB band. The prognosis becomes poorer as the levels of CK and MB band increase. It is important to remember, however, that a patient with infarction who has only a little rise in CK and MB band due to a small infarction may have a poor prognosis if there has been a previous infarction. The total amount of myocardial damage determines the prognosis.

It should also be emphasized that there are many serious coronary events that are not associated with permanent myocardial damage. Therefore the failure of the CK and MB band to rise does not imply that an episode of chest pain due to myocardial ischemia is harmless.

OTHER LABORATORY TESTS

Determinations of the fasting blood sugar and lipid profile are often indicated in patients with coronary atherosclerosis.

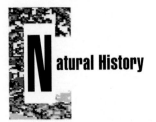

Natural History

The prognosis of patients with asymptomatic coronary atherosclerosis who exhibit no other evidence of myocardial ischemia is not known.

The average annual mortality of patients with *stable angina pectoris* who do not have left main coronary artery obstruction is about 3% to 4%. When hypertension and abnormal Q waves or ST-segment displacement are present in the ECG, the annual mortality is 8%. The prognosis of patients with stable angina cannot be accurately determined by the severity of the symptoms. Ventricular ectopy probably worsens prognosis, but it is difficult to separate this abnormality from other determinants of survival.

Individuals with excellent exercise tolerance have a better prognosis than those who do not. If a person can reach a heart rate of 160 beats per minute or attain stage 4 on the Bruce protocol, his or her annual mortality rate will be about 1% to 2%. The inability to attain stage 2 due to a cardiac cause is associated with an annual mortality rate of 6% to 10%. This predictor is independent of displacement of the ST segment since the absence of ST change does not guarantee prolonged survival. Also, in patients who have as much as 2 mm of

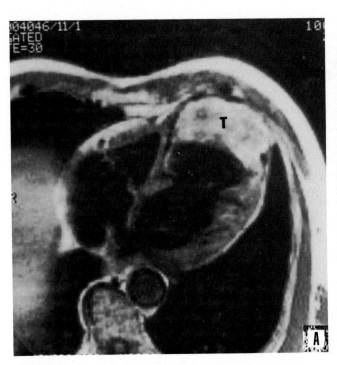

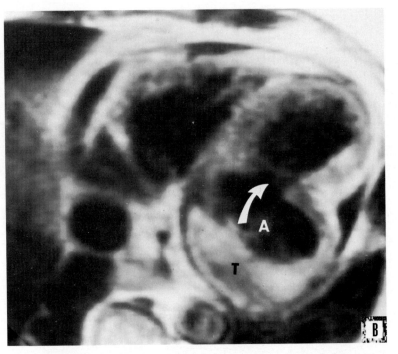

FIGURE 5.58 **(A)** ECG-gated spin-echo images in transverse plane demonstrating complications of myocardial infarctions. True aneurysm involves the anteroapical region and contains mural thrombus (T). **(B)** False aneurysm (A) involves posterior region and contains throm-

bus (T). True aneurysm has a wide ostium while the false aneurysm has a narrow ostium *(curved arrow)*. (Reproduced with permission; see Figure Credits)

ST-segment displacement in the ECG with exercise, there is a good correlation between the duration of exercise and the five-year survival. The shorter the exercise period required to produce the ECG change, the poorer the prognosis. The development of angina during an exercise test may be an independent marker, while the development of hypotension indicates a poor prognosis.

Kent and co-workers[6] reported on patients who currently had little or no angina but had a history of previous angina or infarction. They found that the patients who entered the study with triple-vessel disease and poor exercise performance had a 9% annual mortality. In contrast, patients with triple-vessel disease who had excellent exercise performance had an annual mortality of 4%.

Staniloff and colleagues[13] reported a group of 819 patients who were referred to them for ^{201}Tl diagnostic studies. They found that 17% of patients with a severe thallium reperfusion defect had a coronary event during the following years, compared with 1% of patients with no abnormalities. A large reperfusion defect, more than one defect, and increased thallium in the lungs imply a poor prognosis.

The ejection fraction, determined by radionuclide ventriculography, gives useful information regarding prognosis. Patients with a diminished ejection fraction at rest (or the failure of the ejection fraction to rise with exercise) are in a poor-risk group compared with those with normal ejection fractions at rest that become higher with exercise. There are, of course, other causes of these abnormalities besides coronary disease and this limits the value of the test to some degree. However, ejection fraction as an estimate of ventricular function is a more valuable prognostic marker than the extent of arteriographic narrowing (Fig. 5.61).

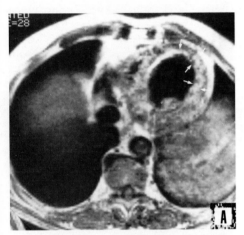

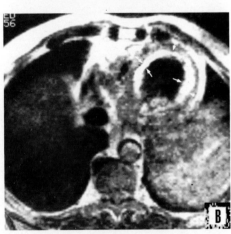

FIGURE 5.59   Transverse images through the apical portion of the left ventricle in a patient with acute infarction. **(A)** First echo image. **(B)** Second echo image. The increased intensity of the infarcted myocardium *(small arrows)* is more evident of the second image. (Reproduced with permission; see Figure Credits)

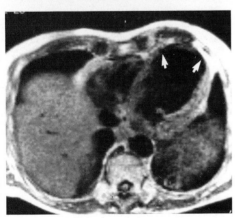

FIGURE 5.60   Gated reverse image through the middle of the left ventricle of a patient with a chronic anteroseptal myocardial infarction. MR image shows thinning of the anterior portion of the septum and the anterior segment *(arrows)*. (Reproduced with permission; see Figure Credits)

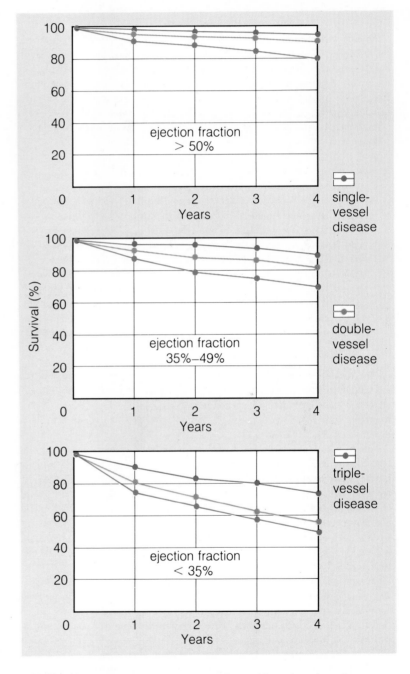

FIGURE 5.61   Data on the 4-year survival in stable patients from the Coronary Artery Surgery Study (CASS) registry. The study involved 6791 patients, 73% with typical angina pectoris. The importance of left ventricular performance, judged on the basis of ejection fraction, is illustrated. Regional wall-motion abnormalities showed a similar trend (i.e., worsening prognosis with increasing wall-motion abnormalities for all grades of coronary arteriosclerosis). (Reproduced with permission; see Figure Credits)

Workers at the Cleveland Clinic were the first to present evidence that the anatomic location of the coronary lesions influenced the survival of patients with coronary disease (Fig. 5.62).

Friesinger has summarized the prognostic implications of angiographic findings in patients with stable angina pectoris as follows:

> ...Prognosis worsens as the extent of arteriographic abnormality increases. The outlook for so-called single-vessel disease and good ventricular function is good, less than 1% to 2% mortality rate per year. Disease localized to the left anterior descending artery carries a poorer prognosis than a similar degree of disease localized to the right coronary artery. Left main coronary artery lesions carry a very poor prognosis. So-called double- and triple-vessel disease are intermediate....
>
> (From Hurst JW (ed): The Heart, 6th ed., McGraw-Hill, New York, p. 922. Used with permission.)

Patients with *unstable angina pectoris* or prolonged myocardial ischemia without evidence of infarction have a poorer prognosis than patients with stable angina pectoris. The National Cooperative Study[9] revealed that patients with unstable angina assigned to medical therapy had, at 30 months, a 10% mortality rate, a 19% incidence of infarction, and a 36% cross-over to surgery for unacceptable angina.

Friesinger has summarized the prognostic implication of unstable angina as follows:

> ...Prompt attention to evaluation and therapy are of critical importance in patients with new onset or a change in symptoms since the incidence of sudden cardiac death and myocardial infarction in the 3 to 6 months following onset of an unstable anginal syndrome is higher than in stable patients.... Several studies have reported a 10% to 15% incidence of left main coronary artery obstruction which is higher than it is in most reports of stable angina pectoris. Patients who experience ST-segment elevation during episodes or whose episodes persist despite excellent drug therapy or who have had previous symptomatic ischemic heart disease tend to have a worse prognosis than those without such features. Left ventricular function is an important prognostic factor....
>
> (From Hurst JW (ed): The Heart, 6th ed., p. 923–924. Used with permission.)

Patients with *prolonged myocardial pain due to ischemia* without evidence of myocardial infarction may be viewed in another way. Patients with prolonged chest discomfort may not all have coronary disease. If they do, as shown by arteriography, the 1- to 2-year prognosis is similar to that of patients who have objective evidence of infarction.

Patients with *Prinzmetal's variant angina* usually have obstructive disease of the epicardial arteries and in addition have coronary artery spasm. A few patients have coronary spasm without coronary atherosclerosis. Waters and colleagues[17] reported that 18% of patients die during the first 3 months following the onset of variant angina. Patients with severe coronary atherosclerosis and left ventricular dysfunction who respond poorly to treatment have the worst prognosis.

Myocardial infarction can be divided into four phases: (1) early myocardial ischemia; (2) evolving infarction; (3) completed infarction; and (4) complicated infarction.

Patients may die with an arrhythmia during the early minutes of an episode of myocardial ischemia; this early phase of infarction is called *very early profound ischemia*. Patients succumbing in this period do not live long enough for infarction to develop. About one fifth of patients with an acute coronary event die within 1 to 2 hours.

The period occurring 1 to 6 hours after the onset of chest discomfort is designated as the phase of *evolving myocardial infarction*. This distinction is important because early intervention with thrombolytic therapy, coronary angioplasty, or coronary bypass surgery is associated with reduced mortality. The prognostic determinants of an evolving infarct are shown in Figure 5.63.

Completed myocardial infarction is defined as the period after the first 6 hours following the onset of chest pain due to ischemia. In general there is a 6% to 10% mortality during the first year after infarction, with more deaths occurring during the first 6 months than the second 6 months. The mortality is 3% to 4% per year in the second and third year after infarction. In order to identify subsets of patients who are at greater-than-usual risk, it is necessary to perform either a submaximal exercise ECG, a radionuclide study, or coronary arteriography and ventriculography.

The submaximal exercise ECG stress test performed before the patient with myocardial infarction is discharged from the hospital can be used to determine prognosis. Angina, ST-segment displacement, or poor exercise performance are used as end points in the test. One study of 210 patients revealed that patients who had no ST-segment displacement had a 2.1% mortality the first year after infarction and patients with abnormal ST-segment displacement had a 27% mortality the first year after infarction.[15] Patients with a positive response should have a coronary arteriogram because bypass surgery or angioplasty may be needed.

Gibson and collaborators[4] showed that the results of ^{201}Tl studies in patients after myocardial infarction had higher predictive value for future cardiac events than the results of submaximal exercise ECG testing or arteriography. Leppo and co-workers[7] used dipyridamole ^{201}Tl scintigraphy in patients prior to discharge after infarction. They noted a much higher mortality in a mean follow-up period of 19 months for patients with transient defects as compared with patients who had no transient defects.

Patients who have complications such as angina or ventricular arrhythmias following infarction should have coronary arteriography rather than noninvasive tests performed. Many physicians believe that coronary arteriography should be performed in most patients following myocardial infarction. Others believe that the procedure should be done only on those patients who are found to be at poor risk by noninvasive means. The ejection fraction is a more powerful predictor of survival than the extent of the coronary disease because most patients with infarction have multivessel disease. The clinician, of course, uses several factors to determine prognosis after infarction (Fig. 5.64).

A *complicated infarction* is defined as one in which certain events occur that alter the prognosis and treatment of the patient. Friesinger's comments highlight the problem of predicting the prognosis of patients with a complicated infarction:

> ...Several investigators have attempted to utilize the multiplicity and complexity of features involved in estimating prognosis in acute infarction by developing a prognostic index which incorporates those factors that have greatest importance and are additive. In such analyses, objective data are given preference over subjective data (e.g., ECG changes in preference to pain), quantitative information over semiquantitative information (congestion on chest x-ray, or wedge pressure, in preference to rales), and permanent findings over transient figures (e.g., the presence of bundle branch block over rhythm disturbances)....
>
> (From Hurst JW (ed): The Heart, 6th ed., p. 927–928. Used with permission.)

Patients who have angina pectoris, heart failure, shock, or certain arrhythmias after infarct are in a high-risk group. Patients with papillary muscle or septal rupture are at great risk of dying unless surgery is performed without delay. A few patients with external rupture of the heart may be saved by emergency surgery but the number is small. A ventricular aneurysm may develop and be responsible for heart failure, arrhythmias, and systemic emboli.

Sudden death is usually due to an arrhythmia rather than an infarction. The one-year mortality of the survivors of sudden death who do not have infarction is 4%, whereas the one-year mortality of the survivors of sudden death associated with infarction is 26%. Ventricular fibrillation occurring in the coronary care unit is not associated with an extremely poor prognosis if it is treated promptly. Such data indicate that ventricular fibrillation that results in early death occurs in a pathophysiologic setting that is different from the arrhythmia occurring some hours after infarction.

Patients who have cardiac arrest and are resuscitated outside the hospital should have coronary arteriography. The procedure should also be performed on those patients who had ventricular fibrillation in the coronary care unit. Electrophysiologic study is also indicated in these patients.

Heart failure as a result of *ischemic cardiomyopathy* is a serious complication. Half the patients die within 3 years. Survival rates of patients with a ventricular aneurysm, mitral regurgitation due to papillary muscle rupture or dysfunction, and even septal rupture may improve with surgery. In contrast, patients with diffuse myocardial disease rarely benefit from bypass surgery. Cardiac transplantation may be indicated in some patients with severe ischemic cardiomyopathy.

Prevention of Atherosclerotic Coronary Heart Disease

There is evidence to support the view that the elimination or management of risk factors may decelerate or even occasionally reverse the atheromatous process. Many individuals have the disease even when known risk factors are not apparent. This fact suggests that the etiology of the disease may be genetically determined and that the known risk factors are accelerators.

It seems prudent to alter the risk factors, when possible, even though they may only be accelerators. Accordingly tobacco smoking should be curtailed or stopped; hypertension should be controlled; obesity should be avoided; a low-fat, low-cholesterol diet is desirable; a serum cholesterol level of 200 mg dL or lower should be attained with drugs if dietary control is not successful; diabetes should be controlled; type A personality traits should be altered if possible; and an active exercise program should be pursued.

Syndromes of Atherosclerotic Coronary Artery Disease

PATIENTS WITHOUT ANGINA OR OBJECTIVE EVIDENCE OF MYOCARDIAL ISCHEMIA

These patients are identified when a coronary arteriogram, performed because the patient has valve disease, reveals evidence of coronary atherosclerosis.

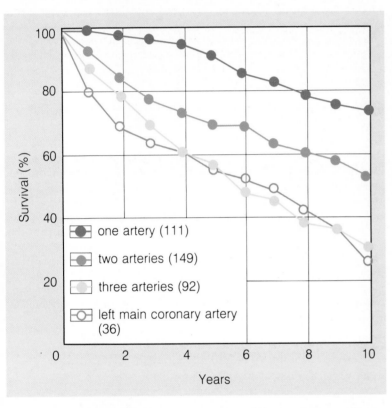

FIGURE 5.62 Survival curves of medically treated patients. These subjects could have had coronary bypass surgery but chose not to. (Reproduced with permission; see Figure Credits)

Legend:
- one artery (111)
- two arteries (149)
- three arteries (92)
- left main coronary artery (36)

FIGURE 5.63 PROGNOSTIC DETERMINANTS: EVOLVING MYOCARDIAL INFARCTION

Infarct size and residual ventricular function	Angina pectoris of more than 3-months' duration
Clinical manifestations (especially left ventricular dysfunction)	Age
ECG changes (especially location of infarct and conduction defects)	Infarct extension
	Heart size (and left ventricular hypertrophy)
Peak enzyme levels	Associated diseases
Blood pressure	Diabetes
Previous infarction and scarring	Hypertension
	Pulmonary disease

(Reproduced with permission; see Figure Credits)

N = 764

- four factors (2%)
- three factors (7%)
- two factors (19%)
- one factor (39%)
- no factor (33%)

FIGURE 5.64 Risk stratification was graphed for 764 (of 866) patients with completed myocardial infarction. Mortality 2 years following myocardial infarction varied from 3% for those with none of the factors to 60% if all four factors were present. The four risk factors were (old) New York Heart Association function classes II–IV before admission, pulmonary rales in the upper lung zones during evolving infarction, occurrence of 10 or more ventricular ectopic depolarizations per hour, and a radionuclide ejection fraction below 0.40. The data were obtained during the convalescence period and prior to hospital discharge. The numbers in parentheses denote the percentage of the population with the specific number of factors. (Reproduced with permission; see Figure Credits)

STABLE ANGINA PECTORIS

The adjective *stable* is used when angina has been present and unchanging for 60 days or more. The frequency of attacks, duration of episodes, and precipitating causes must not have changed during that period. The physician must be certain that the patient has not decreased his or her activity during the period as a means of controlling the angina, because this could signify that the exercise tolerance has decreased and would therefore be an indication that the angina is increasing.

The pathophysiology of stable angina pectoris is usually related to an increase in the demand side of the myocardial supply–demand system. An increase in the work of the myocardium increases the oxygen requirements of the heart cells.

The patient's angina must be categorized as class 1, 2, 3, or 4 using the Canadian Cardiovascular Society recommendations (see Fig. 5.19).

Many patients under age 70 with stable angina will have a coronary arteriogram and left ventriculogram to be certain of the diagnosis and to determine the need for coronary angioplasty or surgery.

Exceptions are patients whose history has a predictive value of 70% to 80% and have negative or minimally positive results in exercise ECGs, ^{201}Tl scans, or exercise ^{99m}Tc tests; who are over the age of 75 and have class 1 or 2 stable angina; or who have another disease that prevents further workup.

POSITIVE EXERCISE TEST IN ASYMPTOMATIC PATIENTS

The asymptomatic patient may develop angina during the treadmill test, because the test demands more effort than the patient expends during his or her daily activities. The patient may, however, develop an abnormal ST-segment displacement, hypotension, or a cardiac arrhythmia during the test but may not develop angina. Most males who exhibit these responses with or without angina should have a coronary arteriogram. Since it is not useful to perform exercise ECGs in middle-aged women because of the high false-positive response, ^{201}Tl scans are indicated when these patients are asymptomatic.

ANGINAL EQUIVALENTS

Anginal equivalents are nonanginal signals of myocardial ischemia, including dyspnea on effort, abrupt dyspnea at rest, exhaustion with effort, chronic fatigue, and cardiac arrhythmias. Whereas the predictive value of these symptoms is not as high as it is with angina, such symptoms should not be dismissed without considering myocardial ischemia due to coronary disease.

Patients with anginal equivalents should be considered for coronary arteriography. A ^{201}Tl stress test may be diagnostic in some patients, but many times it is unwise to exercise such patients, especially those with dyspnea or arrhythmia.

UNSTABLE ANGINA PECTORIS

The adjective *unstable* signifies that angina pectoris has made its first appearance, has been present for less than 60 days, has increased in frequency or duration, or has occurred with less provocation, or at rest when it did not formerly do so.

The pathophysiology of unstable angina is usually related to further obstruction of the supply end of the myocardial oxygen supply–demand system. Such patients have an ulcerated atherosclerotic plaque, coronary thrombosis, coronary spasm, or some other cause for the acceleration of the obstructive process. They are more likely to have sudden death or myocardial infarction within the near future than patients with stable angina.

Unless there is some contraindication, the patient with unstable angina pectoris should have coronary arteriography and left ventriculography. Exercise tests are usually contraindicated.[18]

POSTINFARCTION ANGINA PECTORIS

This is a form of unstable angina. The term *immediate* postinfarction angina pectoris refers to episodes that occur during the first few days after infarction. The term *delayed* postinfarction angina pectoris refers to episodes that occur days to weeks after infarction. Because dead muscle cannot produce pain, the appearance of postinfarction angina pectoris despite medical treatment is a serious matter, often presaging a more serious coronary event. Most patients with this syndrome should have coronary arteriography.

PRINZMETAL'S ANGINA (VARIANT ANGINA)

This is another form of unstable angina. Prinzmetal's angina is due to coronary artery spasm. Patients usually have coronary spasm superimposed on atherosclerotic lesions, but a small percentage have coronary artery spasm only. The angina usually takes place when the patient is at rest, and it tends to occur at the same time each day. Tobacco, alcohol, and cocaine have been incriminated as precipitating agents. The ECG recorded during an attack of angina may show ST-segment elevation in contrast to the downward ST-segment displacement seen with ordinary angina (Fig. 5.65). Transient Q waves, atrioventricular block, and ventricular arrhythmias may occur during an episode.

Stress tests are seldom indicated in such patients. Coronary arteriography is indicated, and intravenous ergonovine may be used to provoke spasm during the procedure. The drug may precipitate persistent coronary spasm, but it does not provoke spasm in all patients with the syndrome.

PROLONGED MYOCARDIAL ISCHEMIA WITHOUT OBJECTIVE EVIDENCE OF INFARCTION

Angina pectoris produced by effort usually lasts 1 to 5 minutes after the activity is discontinued. Whenever the chest discomfort is more prolonged, lasting 20 to 30 minutes, and especially when it occurs at rest, it is highly likely that the pathophysiologic mechanism involved is related to further narrowing of a coronary artery, either by spasm, thrombosis, or both. The ECG may show downward displacement of the ST segment and/or T-wave inversion that persists for hours or days. The ST segment may be elevated during the episode of pain; this is referred to as Prinzmetal's phenomenon.

Myocardial necrosis is not evident as measured by serum cardiac enzymes. It is likely, however, that a few myocardial cells die when ischemia persists for 20 minutes.

Stress tests in such patients are usually contraindicated, and coronary arteriography should be performed unless other conditions contraindicate it.

CORONARY ATHEROSCLEROSIS WITH IRREVERSIBLE MYOCARDIAL ISCHEMIA AND NECROSIS
VERY EARLY PROFOUND ISCHEMIA

This term is used to designate the first phase of myocardial infarction. The patient may be at home, at work, or participating in other events when the pain occurs. The spouse or bystander decides that emergency help is indicated and calls the rescue squad or physician. Although the ECG and the results of the serum cardiac enzymes test are not available, the patient is treated for myocardial infarction. This stage of infarction is similar to the syndrome of prolonged myocardial ischemia without infarction (see above) and shifts into the stage of early evolving infarction (see below).

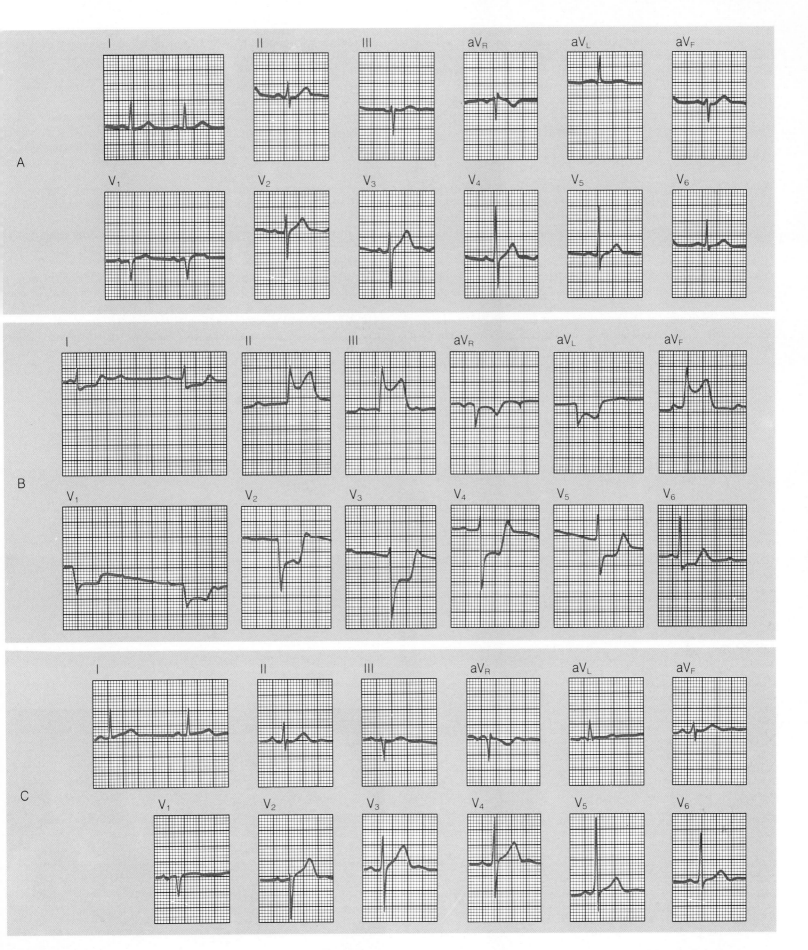

FIGURE 5.65   ECGs of a 59-year-old male with Prinzmetal's angina pectoris who was experiencing repeated bouts of anterior chest discomfort at rest. **(A)** This ECG was recorded at 10 AM; the patient was having no chest pain at the time. **(B)** In an ECG recorded at 5 PM during an episode of chest pain, note the high degree of atrioventricular block and marked ST-segment displacement. The mean ST vector is directed inferoposteriorly. **(C)** The ECG recorded at 6:15 PM the same day is similar to the one recorded at 10 AM. Coronary arteriography revealed a discrete lesion (95% obstruction) in the right coronary artery. Left ventricular function was normal. The patient illustrates destructive coronary disease plus coronary artery spasm. (Reproduced with permission; see Figure Credits)

In early and profound ischemia the first noticeable changes are depletion of enzymes and disturbances in the functional characteristics of the cells. At a light-microscopic level the Z bands of myofibrils are further apart. Hydropic cell swelling indicates the loss of ability to control osmolality of the cell (Fig. 5.66). This process still may be reversible, but in the early stages it most likely renders the cell vulnerable to reperfusion. The latter may lead to contraction band changes (see Fig. 5.66), most likely due to excessive calcium influx.

EARLY EVOLVING MYOCARDIAL INFARCTION

This term is used to designate the first 3 to 6 hours after the onset of chest pain due to myocardial ischemia. It is well established that after a 6-hour period most of the myocardial cells that were initially ischemic have either died or returned to normal. Accordingly, any intervention designed to save myocardial cells must be instituted during the first 3 hours—the sooner the intervention the better.

The ECG may show ST–T wave abnormalities and may or may not reveal abnormal Q waves. The result of the determination of serum cardiac enzymes is usually not available when an intervention is implemented.

The earliest changes of myocardial necrosis are eosinophilia of the cell cytoplasm due to an increased acidity within the cells, accompanied by pyknosis of nuclei. Occasionally a wavy appearance of myofibrils can be observed as an indication of overstretched injured cells (Fig. 5.67). An inflammatory response is not yet present. Enzyme staining techniques may reveal the infarct (Fig. 5.68).

UNCOMPLICATED COMPLETED MYOCARDIAL INFARCTION

Myocardial infarction is characterized by chest pain due to myocardial ischemia that usually lasts longer than 20 minutes, the development of Q waves and/or ST-T wave abnormalities in the ECG, and elevation of the serum cardiac enzymes. All of these features may not be present in all cases and the infarction may be discovered at arteriography and ventriculography or at autopsy.

The term *completed* signifies that most of the ischemic myocardium has become necrotic or has returned to normal. As a rule this occurs within 6 hours after the onset of pain. *Uncomplicated* signifies that complications such as cardiac arrhythmias, heart failure, or shock have not developed. The designation of uncomplicated should not be made until after the fourth day following the onset of chest pain.

A reactive response to the afflicted injury is seen depending on the time of irreversible ischemic myocardial cell change. Early invasion of polymorphonuclear granulocytes appears at approximately 12 hours following onset of infarction with a maximal concentration seen at about 3 days (Fig. 5.69). The first signs of macrophage activity appear at approximately 3 to 5 days, while the first signs of onset of fibrotic repair occur approximately 1 week following onset of infarction (Figs. 5.70, 5.71).

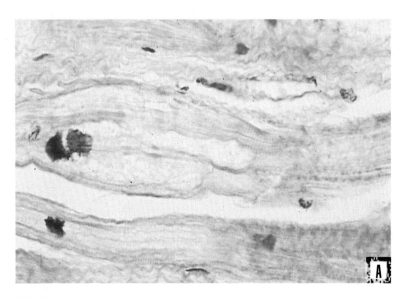
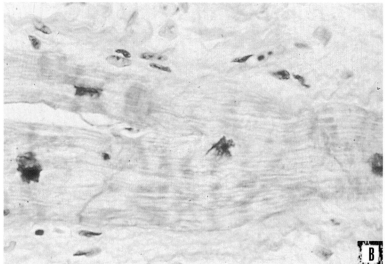

FIGURE 5.66   Early ischemic changes: hydropic cell swelling **(A)** and additional contraction band changes **(B)**. (Reproduced with permission; see Figure Credits)

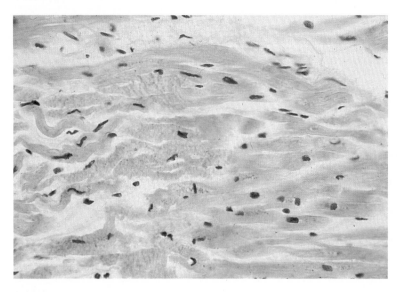
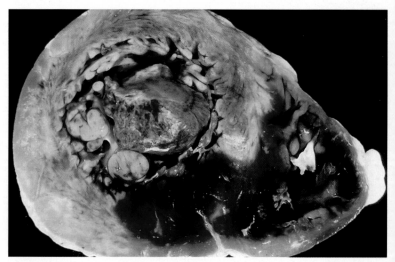

FIGURE 5.67   Eosinophilia of the myocytes: the earliest indication of myocardial necrosis. Nuclear pyknosis and so-called wavy appearance of the cells dominate the histology. (Reproduced with permission; see Figure Credits)

FIGURE 5.68   Cross section of a heart with an acute myocardial infarction. Using the macroenzyme technique, the area containing viable myocardial cells stains dark purple. The infarct is characterized by absent staining. (Reproduced with permission; see Figure Credits)

It appears that during the first week following onset of infarction, the myocardium is edematous, and hence prone to mechanically induced complications.

COMPLICATED COMPLETED MYOCARDIAL INFARCTION

The complications of myocardial infarction include cardiac arrhythmias and conduction disturbances, persistent or recurrent chest pain due to myocardial ischemia, heart failure, hypotension, shock, cardiac arrest, pericarditis, pulmonary embolism, systemic embolism, rupture of the ventricular septum, papillary muscle dysfunction and rupture, cardiac rupture, and emotional turmoil.[7]

Cardiac Arrythmias and Conduction Disturbances Arrhythmias occurring *early* in the course of myocardial infarction include the following:

1. Sinus tachycardia, which may be ominous because it is often associated with, or precedes the development of, left ventricular dysfunction
2. Sinus bradycardia, which, when treated properly, does not alter hospital mortality to a significant degree
3. Sinus node dysfunction, which occurs in a small percentage of patients and may require treatment

4. Atrial premature depolarizations, which occur in about half of patients with myocardial infarction
5. Atrial tachycardia, which is defined as three or more ectopic P waves occurring at a rate greater than 100 beats per minute, and is seen in about 20% of patients
6. Atrial flutter, which occurs in about 5% of the patients
7. Atrial fibrillation, which is a common complication of myocardial infarction
8. Accelerated atrioventricular junctional rhythm and atrioventricular tachycardia
9. Premature ventricular depolarizations, which occur in 80% of patients
10. Ventricular tachycardia and ventricular fibrillation
11. First- and second-degree atrioventricular block, varying atrioventricular block, and complete heart block
12. Right and left bundle branch block and bifascicular block.

Arrhythmias may also occur *late* in the course of myocardial infarction. Premature ventricular depolarizations, ventricular tachycardia, ventricular fibrillation, and cardiac arrest may develop days, weeks, or months after the patient has been discharged from the hospital.

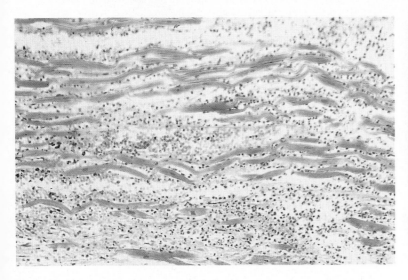

FIGURE 5.69 Necrosis of myocardial cells, with edema and a heavy infiltration of polymorphonuclear leukocytes, in this myocardial infarct of 3 to 5 days' duration. (Reproduced with permission; see Figure Credits)

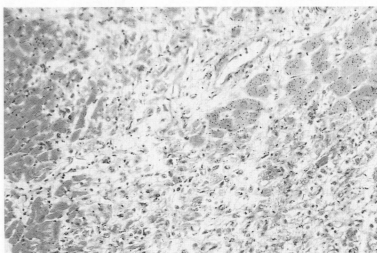

FIGURE 5.70 Abundance of macrophages and early fibroblastic proliferation during the early stages of repair following myocardial infarction. The changes are in accord with an infarction of approximately 7 to 10 days' duration. (Reproduced with permission; see Figure Credits)

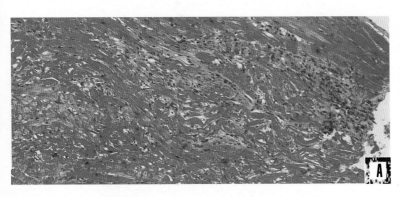

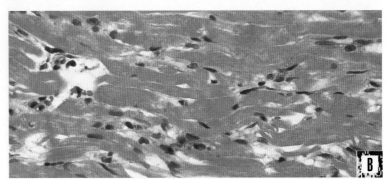

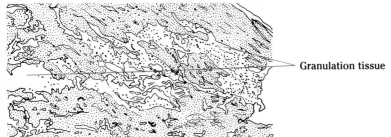

Granulation tissue

FIGURE 5.71 **(A)** Low-power photomicrograph of an endomyocardial biopsy from a 61-year-old woman showing features of an organizing infarct. There is early granulation tissue at the edge of the infarct. **(B)** The higher power shows that the myocytes in the center of the infarct have lost nuclei and cross striations; these features are characteristic of ischemic damage. (Reproduced with permission; see Figure Credits)

Postinfarction Angina Pectoris   When unstable angina pectoris occurs *early* after myocardial infarction, it signifies that myocardial ischemia is continuing, since dead tissue does not produce pain. When drug therapy fails to relieve recurrent angina, it is a signal for the physician to obtain a coronary arteriogram and left ventriculogram. If suitable coronary anatomy is found, it may be necessary to have coronary bypass surgery or coronary angioplasty.[10]

When unstable angina pectoris occurs *late* in the course of infarction, weeks or months after discharge from the hospital, the patient should have coronary arteriography and left ventriculography. In addition, when suitable anatomy is identified, the patient should have coronary bypass surgery or coronary angioplasty.

Ventricular Dysfunction   About two thirds of patients with acute myocardial infarction have elevations of left ventricular filling pressure but may exhibit no clinical signs of heart failure. About one half of patients with acute infarction have a decrease in resting cardiac output. The stroke volume and ejection fraction decrease and the end-systolic volume increases when there is considerable myocardial destruction.

The patient with left ventricular infarction may have mild to severe dyspnea. A left ventricular gallop (S_3) is associated with a pulmonary wedge pressure more than 12 mmHg. Abnormal neck vein distention or pulsation may be present when the pulmonary arterial wedge pressure is normal in patients with right ventricular infarction or severe lung disease. In contrast these signs may not be seen when there is early left ventricular dysfunction. Rales may not be heard in patients with interstitial pulmonary edema. Because of this, physical examination of the lungs is not as useful as the chest x-ray film in identifying heart failure with pulmonary congestion.

Echocardiography and/or radionuclide ventriculography can be used to study ventricular function in patients with acute infarction. Furthermore, it can be used to determine serial changes. The procedure is not used routinely but may be indicated when complicated infarction is suspected.

It is not necessary to insert a Swan-Ganz catheter into the pulmonary artery of patients with uncomplicated myocardial infarction, but patients with heart failure, right ventricular infarction, persistent pain, hypotension, and shock should have continuous hemodynamic monitoring.

Right ventricular infarction may occur in patients with inferior wall infarction of the left ventricle that extends beyond the crux into the right ventricular wall (Fig. 5.72). Isolated right ventricular infarction is rare, but when it occurs, it usually presents in the setting of chronic lung disease with resultant right ventricular hypertrophy and dilation.

The clinical picture is that of "right heart failure" with abnormal neck veins and is characterized by distention of the external jugular veins and abnormal pulsations of the internal jugular veins because of a large V wave and rapid Y descent; right ventricular S_3 and S_4 gallop sounds; arterial hypotension; clear lung fields on the chest film; and evidence of an inferior infarction with elevation of the ST segments in lead V_{4R}. The right-sided filling pressures are greater than the left sided filling pressures, and the systolic pressure in the right ventricle and pulmonary arteries is about normal. The clinical picture resembles constrictive pericarditis, including the equalization of diastolic pressures and a diastolic dip and plateau in the right ventricular pressure curve. Cor pulmonale may be clinically similar, but the systolic and diastolic pulmonary artery pressures are elevated with a normal wedge pressure.

Physicians now realize that evidence of myocardial dysfunction may be identified by hemodynamic measurements, echocardiography, and radionuclide ventriculography in patients without clinical symptoms. The clinician must also exclude ventricular aneurysm whenever heart failure is detected by using echocardiography.

Reversible Hypotensive States   The *bradycardia-hypotensive syndrome* is usually seen in patients with an inferoposterior infarction. The ischemic area stimulates the vagal afferent fibers and produces bradycardia and hypotension. The skin is warm, and at least early in the course the signs of systemic hypoperfusion are not present.

Cardiogenic Shock   Many patients have all the signs of shock when they reach the hospital. Systolic blood pressure is usually below 100 mmHg and sinus tachycardia is present. Pulmonary edema is usually evident. The skin is pale and moist, and urine output is diminished. There is evidence of massive infarction, the cardiac output is low, and the pulmonary wedge pressure is high. Most patients do not survive.

Some patients develop shock more gradually as a result of a slow and steady increase in myocardial destruction. Surgical intervention may be needed when papillary muscle or interventricular septal rupture is present. Unfortunately the prognosis is poor.

Nonarrhythmic Cardiac Arrest   Sudden death in patients with acute myocardial infarction is usually the result of ventricular fibrillation, although asystole may occur. Sudden death may also occur as a result of electromechanical dissociation. These patients have such feeble contractions of the heart due to global myocardial ischemia than no heart sounds are produced and no blood pressure is generated. The ECG, however, shows QRS complexes. Treatment is unsatisfactory because resuscitative measures usually fail.

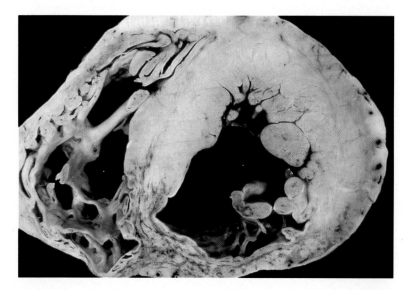

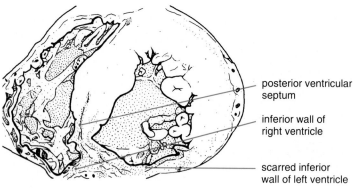

posterior ventricular septum

inferior wall of right ventricle

scarred inferior wall of left ventricle

FIGURE 5.72   Scarred inferior wall infarction of the left ventricle, extending onto the posterior ventricular septum and inferior wall of the right ventricle. (Reproduced with permission; see Figure Credits)

Pericarditis   Acute pericarditis may occur during the first few days after the onset of myocardial infarction (Fig. 5.73). The pain of pericarditis is aggravated by inspiration, and a pericardial rub may or may not be heard. Alternately a pericardial rub may be heard without associated pain. The ECG may not reveal the usual signs of pericarditis.

Dressler's syndrome may develop several weeks or months after myocardial infarction. The condition is characterized by fever, chest pain aggravated by inspiration, pericardial rub, left pleural effusion, and pleural rub. Cardiac tamponade is rare. The syndrome is considered to be the result of an immunologic response to the damaged myocardium.[14]

Pulmonary Embolism   About 30% of patients with acute myocardial infarction have thrombi in the veins of their calves as determined by ^{125}I-labeled fibrinogen scanning. Pulmonary embolism is unlikely unless the thrombi are located in veins that are proximal to the calf (Fig. 5.74). Leg exercise and early ambulation decrease the thrombi in the leg veins and also decrease pulmonary emboli. Pulmonary emboli are responsible for about 1% of deaths.

Pulmonary emboli may produce episodes of dyspnea, tachycardia, cyanosis, and, as pulmonary infarction develops, a pleural friction rub. The Pao_2 may diminish and the $Paco_2$ may remain normal. A definite diagnosis may not be established without a pulmonary scan, but it may not be wise to move the patient from the coronary care unit to the radiology department in order to perform the examination. An echocardiogram should be performed on patients with pulmonary emboli to determine if the thrombi from the legs have been retained in the right ventricle.

Systemic Arterial Embolism   Although the incidence of systemic emboli has decreased in recent years, new data obtained using cross-sectional echocardiography have stimulated a new approach to this problem.

Systemic emboli following myocardial infarction are the result of thrombi located in the left ventricle (Fig. 5.75). The thrombi are more likely to form in akinetic or dyskinetic areas of the left ventricle of patients who have had a large anterior myocardial infarction. Accordingly, it seems wise to obtain a cross-sectional echocardiogram on such patients.

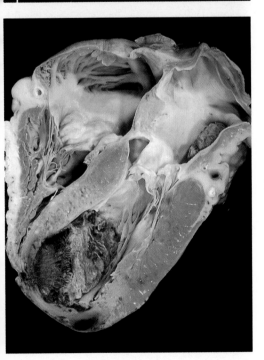

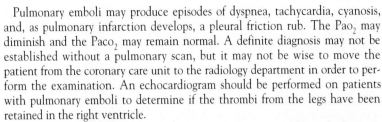

FIGURE 5.73 Fibrinous pericarditis in a case of acute myocardial infarction. (Reproduced with permission; see Figure Credits)

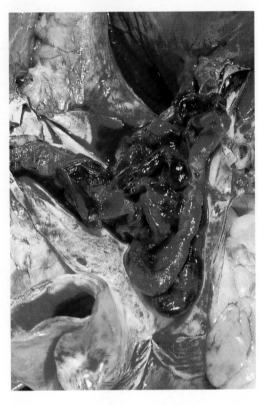

FIGURE 5.74 Saddle thromboembolus in the bifurcation of the pulmonary trunk. This condition is a complication of deep vein thrombosis of the legs. (Reproduced with permission; see Figure Credits)

FIGURE 5.75 Longitudinal section through a heart with intracavitary left ventricular thrombosis complicating myocardial infarction. (Reproduced with permission; see Figure Credits)

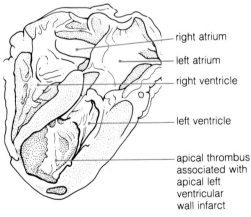

right atrium

left atrium

right ventricle

left ventricle

apical thrombus associated with apical left ventricular wall infarct

Ventricular Septal Rupture   This complication occurs in about 2% of patients with myocardial infarction (Fig. 5.76). It usually occurs during the first week in patients who have experienced their first transmural infarction.

Septal rupture is usually recognized by the appearance of a systolic murmur located in the third and fourth intercostal space near the sternum, although the murmur may occasionally be louder at the apex. The event usually is associated with pulmonary edema and shock. The bedside use of the Swan-Ganz catheter has made it possible to identify the presence and magnitude of a left-to-right shunt and to separate it from mitral regurgitation due to rupture of a papillary muscle.[1]

Papillary Muscle Dysfunction   This condition is due to infarction or ischemia of a papillary muscle of the mitral valve (Fig. 5.77). The associated segment of the ventricular wall is usually infarcted. The condition is recognized by the development of a new, systolic murmur at the apex, either holosystolic or mid- to late systolic in duration. A V wave may be noted in the pressure curve recorded when the Swan-Ganz catheter is in the pulmonary artery wedge position. Cross-sectional echocardiography may differentiate between papillary muscle dysfunction and rupture.[12]

Papillary Muscle Rupture   Complete rupture of the belly of a papillary muscle produces severe mitral regurgitation, pulmonary edema, shock, and death. If the infarction does not produce complete severance of the muscle or if there is rupture of one or two of the heads of the muscle, the situation may be less serious, allowing time for surgical correction. The posteromedial papillary muscle is more commonly involved than the anterolateral one (Fig. 5.78). About one third or more patients with papillary muscle rupture have single-vessel coronary disease.

The condition is recognized by the identification of a new systolic murmur at the apex, pulmonary congestion, and hypotension. A systolic murmur may not be heard if the patient is in shock, myocardial contractility is markedly dimin-

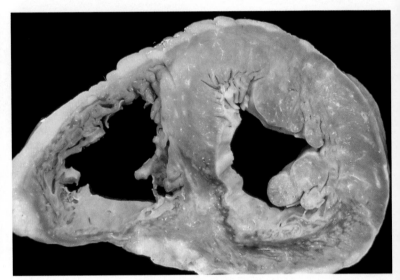

FIGURE 5.76   Ventricular septal rupture complicating acute myocardial infarction. (Reproduced with permission; see Figure Credits)

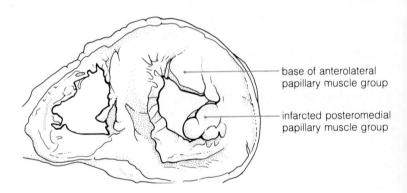

FIGURE 5.77   Papillary muscle dysfunction due to extensive myocardial infarction involving the area at the base of the posteromedial papillary muscle group of the left ventricle. (Reproduced with permission; see Figure Credits)

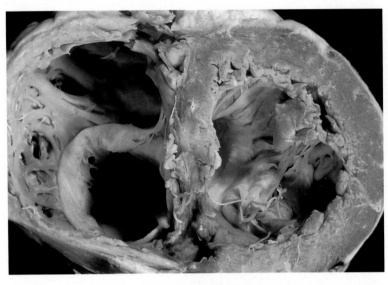

ventricular septal rupture

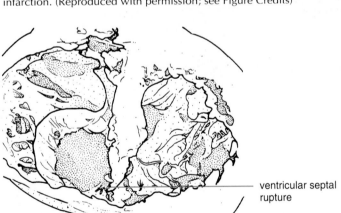

base of anterolateral papillary muscle group

infarcted posteromedial papillary muscle group

ished, or there is complete separation of the muscle from the ventricular wall. An abnormal V wave may be seen in the pressure curve recorded with the Swan-Ganz catheter in the pulmonary wedge position. The cross-sectional echocardiogram may detect a flail leaflet of the mitral valve leaflets.

External Cardiac Rupture   Rupture of the myocardial wall is responsible for about 10% of deaths due to myocardial infarction (Fig. 5.79). Patients with cardiac rupture are usually in their 60s and have a transmural infarction with poor collateral circulation, as well as hypertension.

External rupture of the heart produces sudden death, signs of cardiac tamponade due to hemorrhage into the pericardial space, and abrupt severe pericardial pain and rub. The ECG may show no new changes from those of myocardial infarction.

Emotional Responses   Patients with coronary disease, especially those with an acute event such as myocardial infarction, may pass through several identifiable phases of emotional reaction: denial, acceptance, fear and anxiety, depression, and realistic adaptation. The physician must be able to recognize each of these stages, even when minor diagnostic clues are present.

Ventricular Aneurysm   Ventricular aneurysms are usually associated with transmural infarction of the anterior and apical region of the heart (Fig. 5.80). Common complications include ventricular arrhythmias, congestive heart failure, or peripheral emboli. A ventricular aneurysm rarely ruptures.

The aneurysm may produce an abnormal ectopic pulsation on the surface of the chest or a large apical impulse. A systolic murmur and ventricular gallop may be heard at the apex. The ECG usually shows the Q waves of anterior infarction and persistent shift of the ST segments. An abnormal bulge of the myocardium may be seen on the chest radiograph, and calcium may be noted in the wall of the aneurysm. It is surprising, however, how often the chest film reveals no abnormality. A ventricular aneurysm and thrombus may be detected by cross-sectional echocardiography.

A nuclear ventriculogram can also be used to identify the presence and extent of a ventricular aneurysm, as well as determine the ejection fraction.

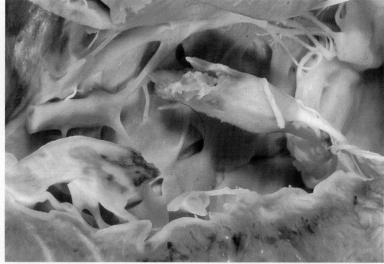

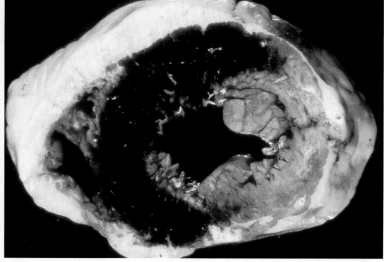

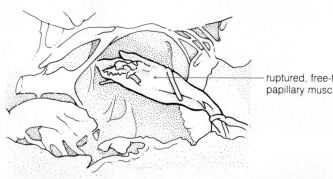

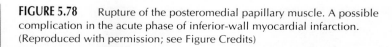

FIGURE 5.78   Rupture of the posteromedial papillary muscle. A possible complication in the acute phase of inferior-wall myocardial infarction. (Reproduced with permission; see Figure Credits)

ruptured, free-floating papillary muscle

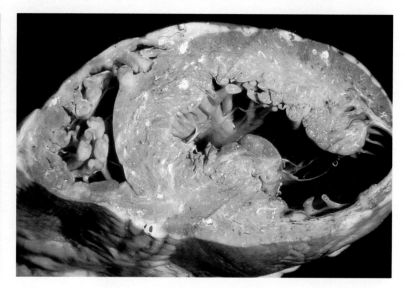

FIGURE 5.79   Cardiac rupture of the left ventricular lateral free wall. In an acute myocardial infarction, the rupture causes sudden death. The macroenzyme stain of the cross section of the heart shows the infarcted area as a pale-brown zone; the dark-purple area represents viable myocardium. (Reproduced with permission; see Figure Credits)

FIGURE 5.80   Ventricular aneurysm of the left ventricular lateral free wall located between both papillary muscle groups. (Reproduced with permission; see Figure Credits)

A ventricular aneurysm is best studied by left ventriculography (Fig. 5.81). The size, location, and presence of a thrombus can be detected with this technique. A coronary arteriogram can be performed at the same time, and a decision can be made regarding cardiac surgery.

A *false aneurysm* of the left ventricle may result from myocardial infarction when there is a small rupture and slow leakage of blood into the pericardial space (Fig. 5.82). The pericardium adheres to the infarct and contains the hematoma. False aneurysms may be detected by cross-sectional echocardiography. True aneurysms have a wide neck connecting them to the ventricle; false or pseudoaneurysms are connected by a narrow neck (Fig. 5.83).

Shoulder–Hand Syndrome The shoulder–hand syndrome has almost disappeared since patients with myocardial infarction are permitted to perform more physical acts including the use of their arms early after the event. Formerly patients developed pain, stiffness, and decreased motion of the shoulders and arms because of inactivity. In this syndrome the skin of the fingers becomes shiny and swollen.

SUDDEN DEATH

Atherosclerotic coronary artery disease is the most common cause of sudden death, usually due to ventricular fibrillation. Cardiac asystole and electrical-mechanical dissociation may also be causes. Less than 50% of patients who experience cardiac arrest and are resuscitated give a history of angina pectoris; the death or the episode resulting in resuscitation is the first evidence of disease.

When resuscitation is successful, coronary arteriography should be performed. Following coronary arteriography, an electrophysiologic study should be performed.

SYNCOPE

Some of the mechanisms responsible for sudden death may produce syncope or near-syncope. Patients with atherosclerotic coronary heart disease may have

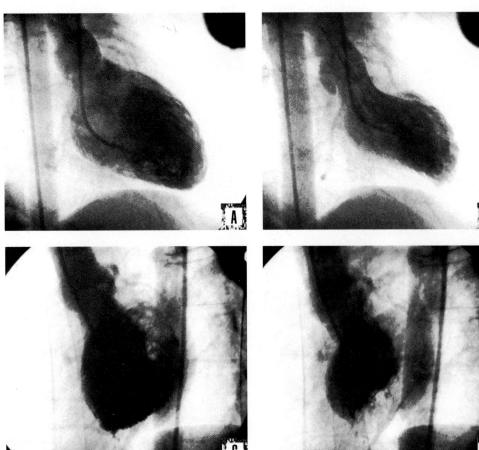

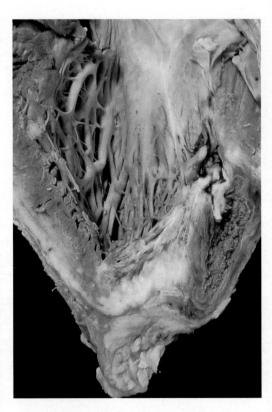

FIGURE 5.82 Pseudoaneurysm of the left ventricle due to incomplete rupture in the setting of an acute myocardial infarction. (Reproduced with permission; see Figure Credits)

FIGURE 5.81 Left ventriculography performed by biplane technique for this case of ventricular aneurysm. Right anterior oblique views show the left ventricle at end diastole (**A**) and at end systole (**B**). Note the contraction abnormality of the anterior wall. Left anterior oblique views show the left ventricle at end diastole (**C**) and at end systole (**D**). (Reproduced with permission; see Figure Credits)

syncope due to ventricular arrhythmias. Ischemia is often the cause of arrhythmias, but nonischemic ventricular re-entry is also a common cause of ventricular tachycardia. Some patients with Prinzmetal's syndrome may have a combination of atherosclerotic obstruction plus spasm of the right coronary artery, which may produce high-grade atrioventricular block and syncope.

CARDIAC ARRHYTHMIAS

Cardiac arrhythmia may occur with all types of heart disease and may be seen in patients with no other evidence of heart disease. All arrhythmias and conduction disturbances may be seen in patients with atherosclerotic coronary artery disease. It is not always possible to determine whether the arrhythmia is actually due to the ischemia and ventricular scarring secondary to atherosclerotic coronary disease or due to an unrelated disease such as Lenegre's or Lev's disease. In addition an abnormal rhythm such as atrial fibrillation may be due to hemodynamic alterations produced by complications of atherosclerotic coronary artery disease rather than by ischemia itself. It should be obvious that the difference among syncope, sudden death, and cardiac arrhythmias without symptoms is determined by the type of arrhythmia and its duration.

The arrhythmia may be discovered on routine ECG, but Holter monitoring is often necessary.

ISCHEMIC CARDIOMYOPATHY

Atherosclerotic coronary heart disease is a major cause of cardiomyopathy (Fig. 5.84); heart failure is the usual consequence. It is often difficult to separate other causes of cardiomyopathy from ischemic cardiomyopathy. Ischemic and nonischemic cardiomyopathies may produce heart failure, arrhythmias, peripheral emboli, angina pectoris, or ECG signs suggesting infarction. Ischemic cardiomyopathy due to coronary disease and idiopathic cardiomyopathy may occur in the same patient.

The presence of ischemic cardiomyopathy is determined with certainty by coronary arteriography and left ventriculography.

FIGURE 5.83   Differences between a pseudoaneurysm and a true aneurysm. (Reproduced with permission; see Figure Credits)

Mural thrombus

Thinned out myocardial scar

Infarcted segment

Transmural infarct with rupture

Pericardium

Thrombus

TRUE ANEURYSM
1. Wide base
2. Walls composed of myocardium
3. Low risk of free rupture

PSEUDOANEURYSM
1. Narrow base
2. Walls composed of thrombus and pericardium
3. High risk of free rupture

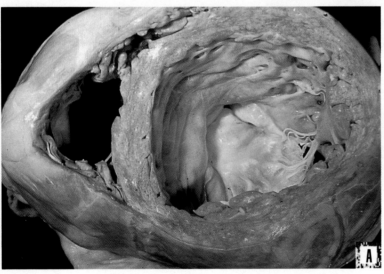

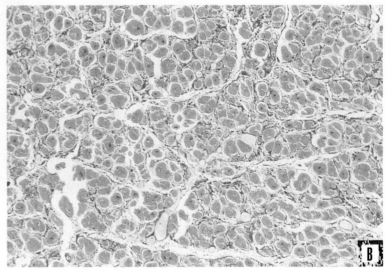

FIGURE 5.84   Ischemic cardiomyopathy. **(A)** The left ventricular cavity may be widely dilated with a hypertrophic wall. **(B)** Histologically there is extensive lacelike myocardial fibrosis. (Reproduced with permission; see Figure Credits)

Atherosclerotic Coronary Artery Disease in Patients With Other Diseases

CHEST PAIN FOLLOWING CORONARY BYPASS SURGERY

Nonischemic chest pain often appears after bypass surgery. The pain may be due to pericarditis, chest wall problems, sternal infection, or anxiety. The discomfort is usually easy to separate from angina pectoris or prolonged pain due to myocardial ischemia. At times, however, the pain is clearly due to myocardial ischemia or cannot be differentiated from it. Then it is necessary to consider the possibilities of graft closure or progression of atherosclerosis in the native coronary arteries.

An exercise ECG or a ^{201}T1 stress test may solve the diagnostic problem. A coronary arteriogram is usually indicated when the probability for cardiac ischemia is high.

CAROTID ARTERY DISEASE WITH CORONARY ARTERY DISEASE

A male patient with a carotid bruit due to carotid artery disease (Fig. 5.85) is likely to have coronary atherosclerosis as well. It is important to question a patient with coronary disease for symptoms of transient ischemic attacks and to listen for carotid bruits that may be related to occlusive carotid disease. It is equally important to question patients who are to undergo carotid artery surgery for symptoms of coronary disease such as angina pectoris.

Rigid guidelines for patients with carotid artery disease who also have evidence of atherosclerotic coronary artery disease have not been developed. Asymptomatic carotid bruits in patients who are to undergo coronary bypass surgery are usually investigated with noninvasive tests of the carotid arteries. If these studies show that the carotid arteries are not occluded to a significant degree, coronary bypass surgery is performed without carotid artery surgery. The patient with transient ischemic attacks should usually have additional studies of the carotid arteries, including a carotid arteriogram, prior to coronary bypass surgery.

ABDOMINAL AORTIC ANEURYSM OR PERIPHERAL VASCULAR DISEASE WITH ATHEROSCLEROTIC CORONARY ARTERY DISEASE

Workers at the Cleveland Clinic have performed the best clinical study of patients who have coronary artery disease and peripheral vascular disease.[5] Patients who have an atherosclerotic abdominal aortic aneurysm or have intermittent claudication due to atherosclerotic lesions of the peripheral arteries usually have atherosclerotic coronary artery disease even if they are asymptomatic (Fig. 5.86).

It is wise to perform a stress ECG or a ^{201}T1 scan in patients without angina before surgery for an abdominal aortic aneurysm or obstructive arterial disease of

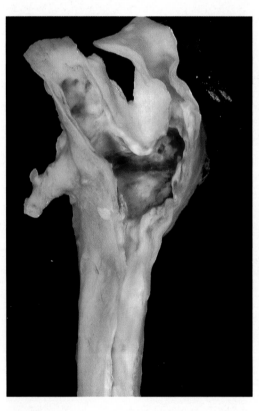

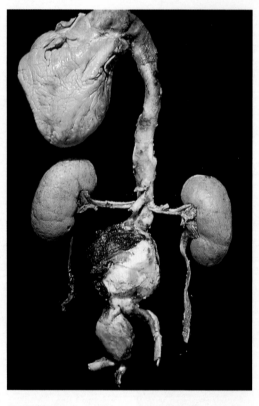

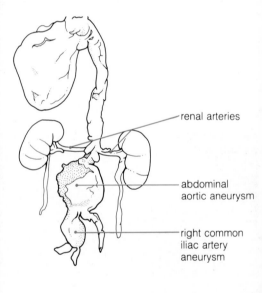

FIGURE 5.85   Obstructive atherosclerosis of the carotid artery found at the site of the bifurcation of internal and external arteries. (Reproduced with permission; see Figure Credits)

FIGURE 5.86   Atherosclerotic aneurysm of the abdominal aorta located distal to the renal arteries. There is an additional aneurysm in the right common iliac artery. The atherosclerosis of the

aorta is associated with obstructive atherosclerotic coronary artery disease. (Reproduced with permission; see Figure Credits)

the lower extremities is performed. Patients who have angina or positive stress tests should have a coronary arteriogram prior to surgery for an abdominal aortic aneurysm or atherosclerotic disease of the arteries to the legs. Patients who cannot exercise may require the dipyridamole [201]T1 test.[2]

Patients with concomitant coronary artery and peripheral vascular disease are at high risk for the occurrence of myocardial infarction during the perioperative period associated with surgery for the aneurysm or obstructive disease of the arteries to the legs.

CARDIAC VALVE DISEASE WITH ATHEROSCLEROTIC CORONARY ARTERY DISEASE

Many patients with cardiac valve disease also have coronary atherosclerosis, and some have angina pectoris without coronary atherosclerosis. This is common in patients with aortic valve disease (Fig. 5.87). Some patients with valve disease

also have significant asymptomatic coronary disease. It is not possible without a coronary arteriogram to determine the contribution that valve or coronary disease makes to produce myocardial ischemia. Accordingly all adult candidates for valve surgery should have a coronary arteriogram.

ATHEROSCLEROTIC CORONARY ARTERY DISEASE AND NONCARDIOVASCULAR PROBLEMS REQUIRING SURGERY

It is not uncommon for patients with atherosclerotic coronary artery disease to require surgery for noncardiovascular problems. Common examples are patients with angina or objective evidence of myocardial ischemia who need cholecystectomy or prostate surgery. Coronary arteriography may be indicated in such patients; when the coronary arterial anatomy is favorable, it is usually wise for coronary bypass surgery to precede nonurgent surgery on the gallbladder or prostate.

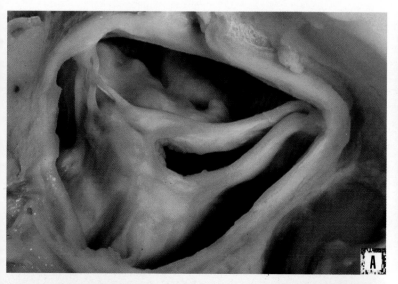

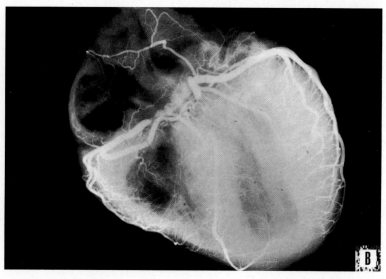

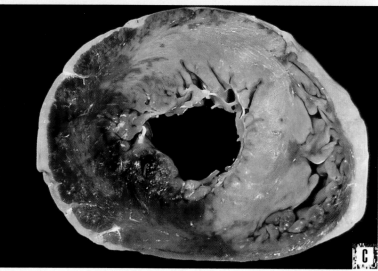

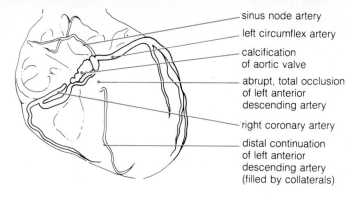

sinus node artery
left circumflex artery
calcification of aortic valve
abrupt, total occlusion of left anterior descending artery
right coronary artery
distal continuation of left anterior descending artery (filled by collaterals)

FIGURE 5.87   Isolated calcific aortic stenosis **(A)** associated with atherosclerotic coronary artery disease. **(B)** Postmortem coronary arteriogram shows calcifications at the aortic valve level and abrupt total occlusion of the left anterior descending coronary artery. **(C)** Macroenzyme technique in a cross section of the heart shows recent transmural myocardial infarction of the anterior wall of the left ventricle and the ventricular septum, which corresponds with the occluded anterior descending artery seen on the arteriogram. (Reproduced with permission; see Figure Credits)

ACKNOWLEDGMENT

Acknowledgment: This chapter is based in part on Chapter 45 (pp. 882–1008) in The Heart, 6th edition, McGraw-Hill, New York, 1986. Chapter 45 was written by JW Hurst, SB King III, GC Friesinger, PF Walter, and DC Morris. Additional contributions were made by Theodore Hersh, MD, Robert B. Smith, MD, and Burton Sobel, MD. Some of the text has been abstracted and used with the permission of the authors and publisher.

FIGURE CREDITS

Figs. 5.1–5.4, 5.6, 5.7, 5.9–5.11, 5.16, 5.18–5.20, 5.26–5.32, 5.46, 5.47, 5.51, 5.52, 5.61–5.68, 5.70, 5.72–5.82, 5.84–5.87 from Hurst JW (ed): Atlas of the Heart. Gower, New York, 1988.

Figs. 5.5, 5.8, 5.66, 5.67, 5.69–5.72, 5.79 from Becker AE, Anderson RH: Cardiac Pathology. Raven Press, New York, 1983.

Fig. 5.13 drawn from data in Sloan D: Relation of cigarette smoking to myocardial infarction in young women. N Engl J Med 798:1273, 1978.

Fig. 5.14 redrawn from Kannel WB, et al: Hypertension as an ingredient of a cardiovascular risk profile. Br J Hosp Med 11:508, 1974.

Fig. 5.15 redrawn from Kannel WB: Cholesterol in the prediction of atherosclerotic disease. New perspectives based on the Framingham Study. Ann Intern Med 90:85, 1979.

Fig. 5.16 adapted and redrawn from Becker AE, Hoedemaeker PJ: Pathologie. Wetenschappelijke Uitgeverij Bunge, Utrecht, 1984.

Fig. 5.17 from May AG, Deweese JA, Rob CG: Hemodynamic effects of atrial stenosis. Surgery 53(4):513, 1963.

Figs. 5.18, 5.28, 5.33, 5.39, 5.45, 5.52, 5.63, 5.81 from Hurst JW (ed): The Heart, 6th ed. McGraw-Hill, New York, 1986. Fig. 5.39 courtesy of Joel M. Felner, MD, Atlanta, GA. Fig. 5.52A–I courtesy of the Department of Radiology, Emory University School of Medicine, Atlanta, GA.

Fig. 5.19 from Campeau L: Letter to the editor. Circulation 54:522, 1976.

Figs. 5.21–5.25, 5.46, 5.47, 5.49, 5.50 from Kassner EG: Atlas of Radiologic Imaging. Gower, New York, 1989.

Figs. 5.26, 5.27, 5.30 redrawn from Hurst JW, Woodson GC: Atlas of Spatial Vector Electrocardiography. The Blakiston Co., New York, 1952.

Fig. 5.28 redrawn from Castellanos A, Myerberg RJ: The resting electrocardiogram. In Hurst JW (ed): The Heart, 6th ed., McGraw-Hill, New York, 1986.

Fig. 5.33 redrawn from DeBusk RF: Technique of exercise testing. In: Hurst JW (ed): The Heart, 6th ed., McGraw-Hill, New York, 1986.

Figs. 5.29, 5.31, 5.32 redrawn from Hurst JW, Wenger NK (eds): Electrocardiographic Interpretation. McGraw, New York, 1963.

Fig. 5.34–5.37, 5.40–5.44, 5.48, 5.53, 5.60, 5.71, 5.83 from Chatterjee K, et al: Cardiology: An Illustrated Text–Reference. Gower, New York, 1992. Fig. 5.44B courtesy of Ralph Clark, MD, Pacific Medical Center, San Francisco, CA. Fig. 5.54 courtesy of R. VanHeertum, St. Vincent's Hospital, New York, NY, and The General Electric Co., Milwaukee, WI. Fig. 5.55 courtesy of M. Goris, MD, Stanford University, Stanford, CA. Fig. 5.56 courtesy of Heinrich Schelbert, MD, UCLA, Los Angeles, CA.

Fig. 5.45, 5.48 redrawn and modified from Grossman W: Cardiac Catheterization and Angiography, 2nd ed. Lea & Febiger, Philadelphia, 1980.

Fig. 5.51 courtesy of Gordon DePuey, MD, Atlanta, GA.

Fig. 5.57 from Botvinick E, et al: Acute myocardial infarction: Clinical application of technetium 99m stannous pyrophosphate infarct scintigraphy. Circulation 59:257, 1979.

Fig. 5.59 from McNamara MT, et al: Detection and characterization of acute myocardial infarctions in man using gated magnetic resonance imaging. Circulation 71:717, 1985.

Fig. 5.61 redrawn from Mock MB, et al: Survival of medically tested patients in the Coronary Artery Surgery Study (CASS) Registry. Circulation 6:562, 1982.

Fig. 5.62 redrawn from Proudfit WL, Bruschke AVG, Sones FM Jr: Natural history of obstructive coronary artery disease: Ten-year study of 601 nonsurgical cases. Prog Cardiovasc Dis XXI (1): 61, 1978.

Fig. 5.63 from Friesinger GC: Prognosis of atherosclerotic coronary heart disease. In Hurst JW (ed): The Heart, 6th ed., McGraw-Hill, New York, 1986.

Fig. 5.64 redrawn from Multicenter Postinfarction Research Group: Risk Stratification and Survival of Myocardial Infarction (Arthur J. Moss, MD, Principal Investigator), N Engl J Med 1983:308–331.

Figs. 5.65 from Hurst JW, King SB III, Friesinger GC, Walter PF, Edwards JE: Atherosclerotic coronary heart disease: Angina pectoris, myocardial infarction, and other manifestations of myocardial ischemia. In Hurst JW (ed): The Heart, 4th ed. McGraw-Hill, New York, 1982: 1090. ECG provided by Joel M. Felner, MD, Atlanta, GA.

Fig. 5.81 from Franch RH, King SB III, Douglas JS Jr: Techniques of cardiac catheterization. In Hurst JW (ed): The Heart, 6th ed., McGraw-Hill, New York, 1986.

REFERENCES

1. Barzilai B, Davis VG, Stone PH, et al: Prognostic significance of mitral regurgitation in acute myocardial infarction. Am J Cardiol 65:1169, 1990.

2. Boucher CA, Brewster DC, Darling RC, et al: Determination of cardiac risks by dipyridamole-thallium imaging before peripheral vascular surgery. N Engl J Med 312:389, 1985.

3. Francis GS, Alpert JS: Modern Coronary Care. Little Brown, Boston, 1990.

4. Gibson RS, Watson DD, Crampton RS, et al: Pre-discharge 201-thallium scintigraphy to identify post-infarction patients at high risk for future cardiac events. Circulation 68(2):321, 1983.

5. Hertzer NR, Beven EG, Young JR, et al: Coronary artery disease in peripheral vascular patients: A classification of 1000 coronary angiograms and results of surgical management. Ann Surg 199(2):223, 1984.

6. Kent KM, Rosing DR, Ewels CJ, et al: Prognosis of asymptomatic or mildly symptomatic patients with coronary artery disease. Am J Cardiol 49(8):1823, 1982.

7. Lavie CJ, Gersh BJ: Mechanical and electrical complications of acute myocardial infarction. Mayo Clin Proc 65:709, 1990.

8. Leppo JA, O'Brien J, Rothendler JA, et al: Dipyridamole-thallium-201 scintigraphy in the prediction of future cardiac events after myocardial infarction. N Engl J Med 310:1014, 1984.

9. National Cooperative Study Group to Compare Medical and Surgical Therapy: Unstable angina pectoris. I. Report of protocol—patient population. Am J Cardiol 42:839, 1978.

10. Qiao JH, Fishbein MC: The severity of coronary atherosclerosis at sites of plaque rupture with occlusive thrombosis. J Am Coll Cardiol 17:1138, 1991.

11. Schaper W, Schaper J: Adaptation to and defense against myocardial ischemia. Cardiology 77:367, 1990.

12. Smyllie JH, Sutherland GR, Geuskens R, et al: Doppler color flow mapping in the diagnosis of ventricular septal rupture and acute mitral regurgitation after myocardial infarction. J Am Coll Cardiol 15:1449, 1990.

13. Staniloff H, Diamond G, Forrester J, et al: Prediction of death, infarction, and worsening chest pain with exercise electrocardiography and thallium scintigraphy. Am J Cardiol 49:967,1982.

14. Sugiura T, Iwasaka T, Takayama Y, et al: Factors associated with pericardial effusion in acute Q wave myocardial infarction. Circulation 81:4477, 1990.

15. Theroux P, Waters DD, Helphen C, et al: Prognostic value of exercise testing soon after myocardial infarction. N Engl J Med 30(7):341, 1979.

16. Tousoulis D, Kaski JC, Bogaty P, et al: Reactivity of proximal and distal angiographically normal and stenotic coronary segments in chronic stable angina pectoris. Am J Cardiol 67:1195, 1991.

17. Waters DD, Szlachcic J, Miller D, et al: Clinical characteristics of patients with variant angina complicated by myocardial infarction or death within 1 month. Am J Cardiol 49:658, 1982.

18. Zalewski A, Shi Y, Nardone D, et al: Evidence for reduced fibrinolytic activity in unstable angina at rest. Clinical, biochemical, and angiographic correlates. Circulation 83:1685, 1991.

19. Zeiher AM, Schachinger V, Weitzel SH, et al: Intracoronary thrombus formation causes focal vasoconstriction of epicardial arteries in patients with coronary artery disease. Circulation 83:1519, 1991.

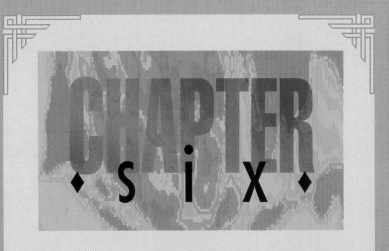

CHAPTER
◆ S I X ◆

VALVULAR
HEART DISEASE

J. WILLIS HURST, MD

CHARLES E. RACKLEY, MD

ANTON E. BECKER, MD

JOSEPH S. ALPERT, MD

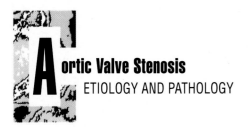

Aortic Valve Stenosis
ETIOLOGY AND PATHOLOGY

Aortic valve stenosis may result from a variety of conditions.[12] Congenital abnormalities, such as bicuspid aortic valve with a small annulus or unicuspid aortic valve, usually produce symptoms early in life (see Chapter 7). Occasionally such malformations may become manifest in adulthood (Fig. 6.1). In older patients rheumatic heart disease (Fig. 6.2) and isolated calcific disease of the elderly (Fig. 6.3) are the most common pathologic conditions. In the latter situation approximately half of patients have an underlying congenitally bicuspid aortic valve without hypoplasia (Fig. 6.4), while the remainder have a trifoliate aortic valve (Figs. 6.5). Calcification of the valve eventually occurs in all types of stenosis, including the congenital forms that first become symptomatic in adulthood.[16,50]

PATHOPHYSIOLOGY

The size of the aortic orifice is normally 2 to 3 cm². Stenosis of the aortic valve creates resistance to ejection, and a pressure gradient develops during systole between the left ventricle and the aorta. The elevated left ventricular pressure produces a pressure overload on the left ventricle, which remodels itself by increasing the thickness of the left ventricular wall—a process known as concentric hypertrophy.[36] Dilation of the left ventricular cavity does not occur

until myocardial contractility is depressed.[55,56] The left ventricular end-diastolic pressure becomes elevated in patients with aortic stenosis. Atrial contraction then contributes to the left ventricular diastolic volume of blood that is subsequently ejected during left ventricular systole.[70] Left ventricular diastolic compliance decreases, thus contributing to elevated left ventricular end diastolic pressure. This eventually leads to left atrial enlargement.

Eventually the sustained left ventricular pressure load leads to dilation of the left ventricle and decreased contractility of the myocardium (Fig. 6.6).[13] Myocardial ischemia may occur due to restricted coronary blood flow to the hypertrophied myocardium. Concomitant coronary artery disease occurs in 50% of older adults with aortic stenosis.

CLINICAL MANIFESTATIONS

Aortic stenosis is more common in males than in females. A congenital origin should be considered in young patients with isolated aortic stenosis. Middle-aged patients who have aortic stenosis in association with mitral valve disease usually have a rheumatic etiology, regardless of a history of rheumatic fever. Middle-aged patients with isolated aortic stenosis may have congenital biscuspid aortic valve disease. Elderly patients may have nonrheumatic, noncongenital, calcific aortic stenosis.

SYMPTOMS

Patients experience symptoms late in the course of the disease, including angina pectoris, dyspnea due to heart failure, syncope, and sudden death.

Angina Pectoris   Angina pectoris is the most common symptom of aortic stenosis. Life expectancy in the afflicted is about 5 years after the development of myocardial ischemia. Coronary atherosclerosis is often pre-

FIGURE 6.1   Aortic valve stenosis in an adult due to a congenitally malformed valve, most likely unicuspid in nature. (Reproduced with permission; see Figure Credits)

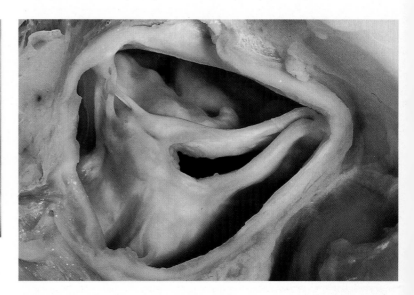

FIGURE 6.2   Rheumatic aortic valve stenosis with marked commissural fusion and fibrotic leaflets with calcifications. In such instances, pathologic studies almost always reveal an affected mitral valve, which is not necessarily clinically manifest. (Reproduced with permission; see Figure Credits)

sent in adult patients with aortic stenosis even when no symptoms are present. Myocardial ischemia occurs due to restriction of myocardial blood flow by the stenosis combined with a left ventricular oxygen consumption that is greater than normal due to the increase left ventricular muscle mass and left ventricular systolic pressure. Oxygen availability is also decreased at the left ventricular subendocardial level as a result of an increase systolic wall stress.[31]

Dyspnea   The survival period is about 2 years for adults with aortic stenosis who have dyspnea due to heart failure.[2]

Syncope   Syncope is a common symptom in patients with aortic stenosis. It may be the first symptom noted by the patient, often occurring after exertion.[19] Survival is about 3 to 4 years in patients with syncope.

Sudden Death   Sudden death is the feared event in patients with severe aortic stenosis; it occurs in about 3% to 5% of asymptomatic patients. The mechanisms responsible for syncope are undoubtedly responsible for sudden death; the final pathophysiologic pathway is usually a cardiac arrhythmia.

PHYSICAL EXAMINATION

In severe aortic stenosis the pulse pressure becomes narrowed and the upstroke of the arterial pulse is slow. This diminished amplitude with delayed pulse peak has been described as *pulsus parvus et tardus*.

While the apex impulse may not be displaced laterally, the duration of the impulse may be prolonged. The left atrial contribution to left ventricular filling may be detected, and a systolic thrill may be felt in the second intercostal space near the sternum and in the neck.

The auscultatory findings in valvular aortic stenosis include a diamond-shaped systolic murmur, a decrease in intensity of aortic valve closure (A_2), faint aortic regurgitation, and paradoxical splitting of the second sound. In young patients a systolic ejection sound may be heard at the apex.[24] The systolic murmur may be higher pitched at the apex in older patients; it usually radiates into the neck or laterally to the apical area. Accordingly, it may be difficult to separate the murmur of aortic stenosis from carotid artery bruits, which occur commonly in the elderly (Crawley et al, 1978). The murmur may not be heard, or it may be misjudged as unimportant, in patients with severe pulmonary emphysema, severely diminished cardiac output, or mitral stenosis.

LABORATORY STUDIES

Chest Radiography   Early in the course of the disease the chest film may show a normal-sized heart,[40] although later the heart may become enlarged. Post-stenotic dilation of the aorta, calcification of the aortic valve (best seen on the lateral view), and a slightly enlarged left atrium may be seen on the radiograph (Fig. 6.7).

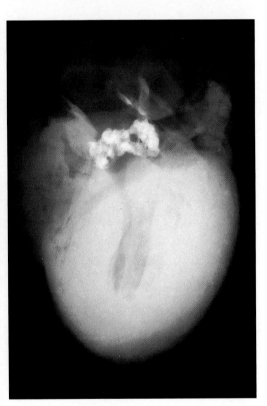

FIGURE 6.3
Postmortem x-ray film of a heart with isolated calcific aortic stenosis. (Reproduced with permission; see Figure Credits)

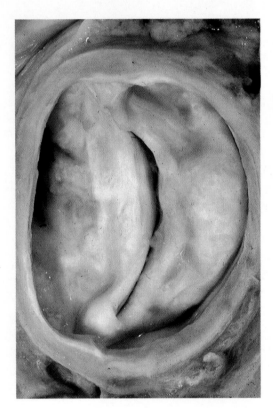

FIGURE 6.4
Isolated calcific stenosis in association with a congenitally bicuspid aortic valve. (Reproduced with permission; see Figure Credits)

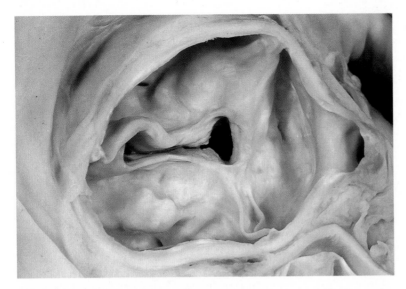

FIGURE 6.5   Isolated aortic valve stenosis caused by a trileaflet aortic valve. It is the result of an atherosclerotic/calcific degeneration within the valve itself. (Reproduced with permission; see Figure Credits)

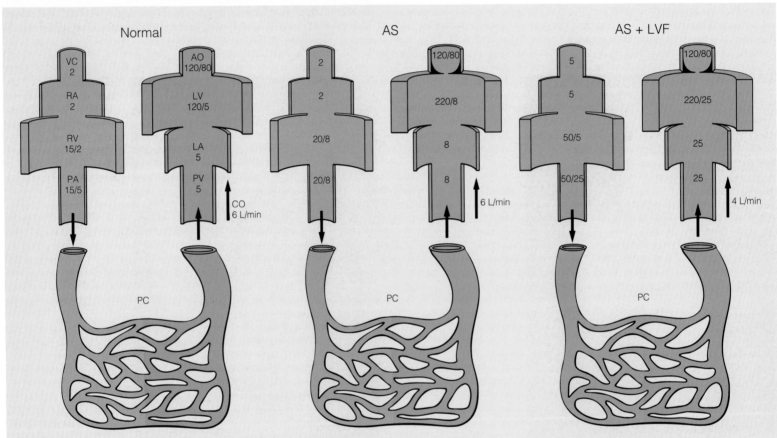

FIGURE 6.6   Pathophysiology of aortic stenosis (AS). The top panel presents normal hemodynamics, and the middle panel demonstrates severe AS and a well-compensated left ventricle (LV). The LV is hypertrophied because of the increase in pressure work. LV systolic pressure is 220 mmHG and AS pressure is 120 mmHg, causing a l00-mm gradient across the aortic valve. LV diastolic pressure is slightly increased at 8 mmHg; this small increase in LV diastolic pressure is transmitted to the pulmonary capillaries (PC). Cardiac output (CO) is normal at 6 L/min. In the bottom panel, severe AS and left ventricular failure (LVF) are depicted . The gradient across the aortic valve is the same as that in the middle panel, but LVF in the bottom panel has caused elevation of LV diastolic pressure to 25 mmHg. As a result, left atrial, pulmonary venous, and PC pressures also rise to 25 mmHg. LV stroke volume falls and systemic cardiac output is reduced to 4 L/min. There is a secondary rise in pulmonary arterial and right ventricular pressures as a result of the increase in pulmonary venous pressure. (VC = vena cava; RA = right atrium; RV = right ventricle; PA = pulmonary artery; PV = pulmonary veins; LA = left atrium; AO= aorta) (Redrawn with permission; see Figure Credits)

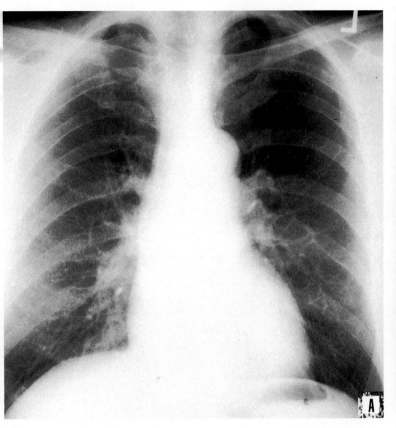

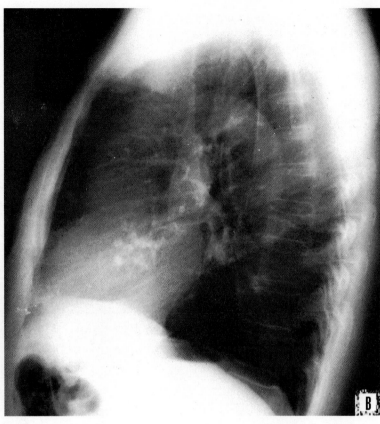

FIGURE 6.7   **(A)** Posteroanterior chest x-ray of a 62-year-old male with calcific aortic stenosis. Note a normal-sized heart with a slightly enlarged ascending aorta. **(B)** Lateral view reveals considerable calcification of the aortic valve. (Reproduced with permission; see Figure Credits)

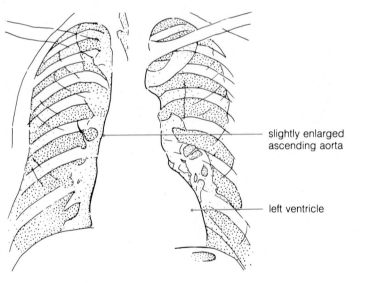

slightly enlarged
ascending aorta

left ventricle

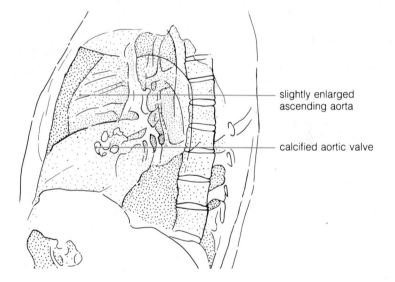

slightly enlarged
ascending aorta

calcified aortic valve

Electrocardiography The electrocardiogram (ECG) shows evidence of left ventricular hypertrophy. The QRS voltage is often increased, and the mean T vector eventually comes to lie 180° away from the mean QRS vector (the so-called LVH with strain). There may be a left atrial abnormality (Fig. 6.8).

Echocardiography Aortic valve stenosis may be differentiated by echocardiography from nonvalvar types of left ventricular outflow tract obstruction, such as idiopathic hypertrophic subaortic stenosis.[61] Thickening, calcification, decreased mobility of the aortic valve leaflets, and the degree of left ventricular hypertrophy can all be detected on the echocardio-

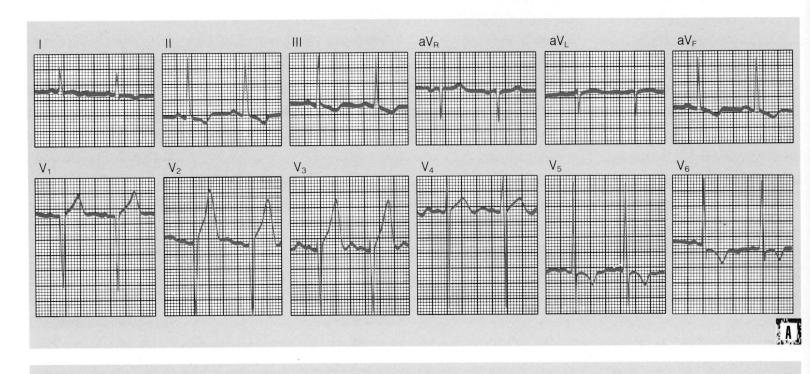

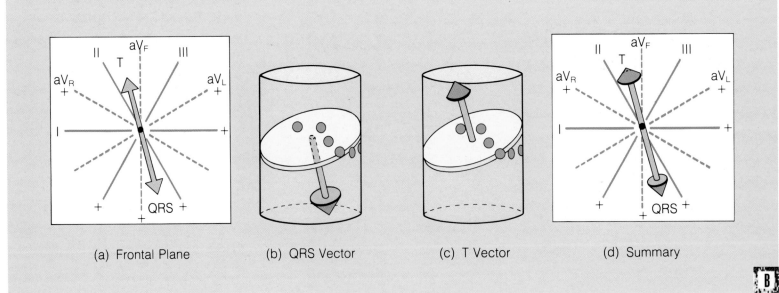

(a) Frontal Plane   (b) QRS Vector   (c) T Vector   (d) Summary

FIGURE 6.8 **(A)** ECG of a 32-year-old with calcific aortic stenosis and left ventricular hypertrophy. **(B)** (a) The QRS complex is largest in lead II, slightly positive in lead I, and negative in lead aV$_L$. QRS complexes of this nature can be represented by a mean vector directed to the right of the positive limb of lead II. The T wave is slightly negative in lead I, large and negative in leads II, III, and aV$_F$, and positive in lead aV$_L$. Accordingly the mean T vector is directed to the right of the negative limb of lead aV$_F$, but to the left of a perpendicular to lead aV$_L$. (b,c) The spatial orientation of the mean QRS and T vectors. The mean QRS is rotated 50° posteriorly, because the transitional pathway passes between the V$_4$ and V$_5$ positions. The mean T vector is

tilted 50° anteriorly, because the transitional pathway passes between the V$_4$ and V$_5$ positions. Note the increased magnitude of the QRS complexes. (d) The spatial arrangement of the vectors. The mean QRS vector is directed downward and posteriorly, and the mean T vector is directed to the right and anteriorly; the spatial QRS–T angle is 180°. These findings are characteristic of left ventricular hypertrophy associated with an abnormally wide QRS–T angle. The mean QRS vector is vertically directed and may be related to the thin, long-chested torso of the patient. (Reproduced with permission; see Figure Credits)

gram (Fig. 6.9). Left ventricular function can be estimated from chamber dimensions, estimates of end-diastolic and end-systolic volumes, and the ejection fraction. A bicuspid aortic valve can also be identified.[58] A systolic separation of the aortic leaflets of less than 8 mm detected by cross-sectional echocardiography in long-axis sections is predictive of severe aortic stenosis.[23]

The systolic pressure gradient across the aortic valve can be determined using the Doppler technique (Fig. 6.10). This is an excellent method of following the pressure gradient across the aortic valve, although the results may not be as accurate as determining the gradient by cardiac catheterization. The Doppler technique is more accurate when it is used to determine the mean systolic gradient across the aortic valve rather than the peak-to-peak systolic gradient across the valve. A reasonably accurate estimate of aortic valve area may be obtained by employing the continuity equation.

Cardiac Catheterization

The purpose of cardiac catheterization is to confirm the presence of aortic valve stenosis, measure its severity, and exclude or identify the presence of other cardiac disease, especially coronary disease.

The normal valve area is 2–3 cm². A reduction of 75% or more, resulting in an orifice size less than 0.8 cm², is necessary to produce significant impairment of flow and cardiac output.[25] This degree of stenosis is usually accompanied by a left ventricular–aortic systolic pressure gradient exceeding 50 mmHg (Figs. 6.11, 6.12). A gradient must always be assessed in relationship to the cardiac output (Fig. 6.13); for example, a gradient of 30 mmHg may be very significant if the cardiac output is low.

Quantitative angiography provides measurements of end-diastolic and systolic volumes, the ejection fraction, and left ventricular mass.[52]

Coronary arteriography in adults reveals a 50% prevalence of coronary atherosclerosis regardless of reported angina.[8]

Radionuclide Studies

Radionuclide ventriculography using technetium-99m (^{99m}Tc) is often used to determine the resting and the exercise ejection fractions and thallium-201 (^{201}Tl) scanning at rest and with exercise may identify areas of myocardial scarring or ischemia. However, exercise testing in patients with severe aortic valvar stenosis may be dangerous; accordingly radionuclide tests are usually performed at rest.

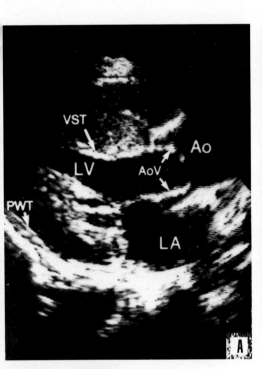
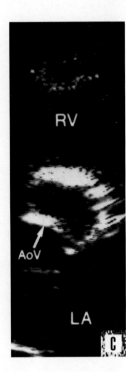
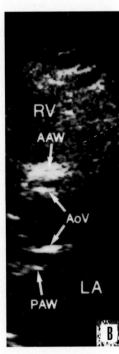
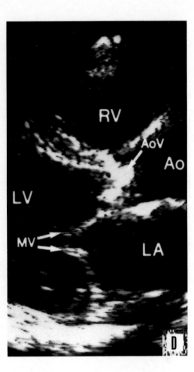

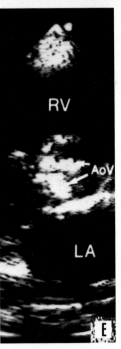

FIGURE 6.9 Cross-sectional echocardiograms of two patients with severe aortic stenosis, one with bicuspid valve (A–C), the other with a calcified trileaflet valve (D,E). **(A)** Parasternal long-axis view shows systolic doming of the anterior and the posterior cusps of the aortic valve (AoV). During diastole (not shown) the aortic cusps prolapse into the left ventricular outflow tract. Left ventricular hypertrophy is present, and the left atrium (LA) is dilated. **(B)** Parasternal short-axis view at the level of the aortic valve in systole shows only two aortic cusps that are parallel to the anterior (AAW) and the posterior (PAW) aortic walls. **(C)** In the parasternal short-axis view at the level of the aortic valve in diastole the closure of the aortic valve is represented by an abnormal, dominant, single echo, which appears S-shaped. **(D)** Parasternal long-axis view in systole shows a dense mass of calcium totally obscuring the leaflets and the orifice of the aortic valve. **(E)** Parasternal short-axis view at the level of the aorta in systole shows a heavily calcified trileaflet aortic valve with markedly reduced opening. (VST = ventricular septal thickness; PWT = posterior wall thickness; Ao = aorta; LV = left ventricle; RV = right ventricle; MV = mitral valve) (Reproduced with permission; see Figure Credits)

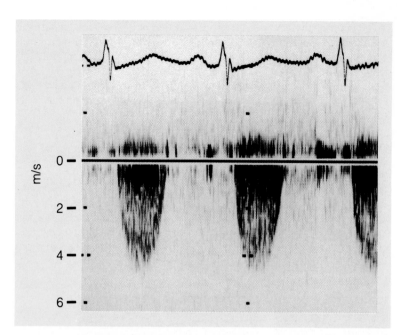

FIGURE 6.10 Severe aortic stenosis evaluated from the apical approach using a nonimaging, continuous-wave Doppler. The waveform shows flow away from the transducer, with a peak velocity of approximately 4.6 m/sec, predicting a peak pressure gradient of 86 mmHg. (Reproduced with permission; see Figure Credits)

FIGURE 6.11 Left ventricular and aortic pressures from a patient with aortic valve stenosis. Note a peak-to-peak pressure gradient of about 48 mmHg between the left ventricular systolic pressure and the aortic pressure. (Reproduced with permission; see Figure Credits)

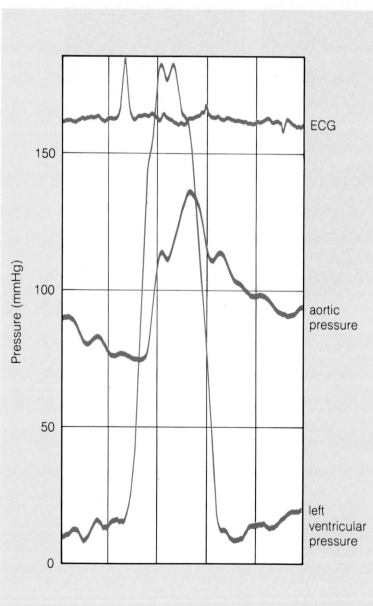

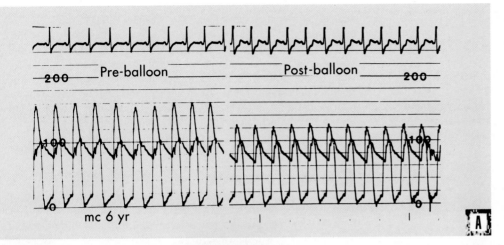

mc 6 yr

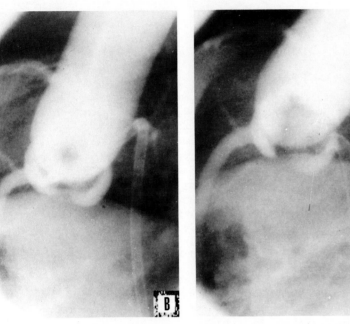

FIGURE 6.12   **(A)** Pressure tracings obtained before and after balloon dilation of a congenitally stenotic aortic valve. The predilation gradient was 60 mmHg (left ventricular pressure 160/0,18; aortic presure 100/78). After balloon dilation, the gradient was reduced to 20 mmHg (left ventricular pressure 120/0,18; aortic pressure 100/65). **(B)** Angiographic appearance of stenotic valve before dilation (left), with the negative jet of blood passing through the narrowed orifice. After dilation (right), a wider stream of nonopacified blood is seen, with apparent enlargement of the orifice. (Reproduced with permission; see Figure Credits)

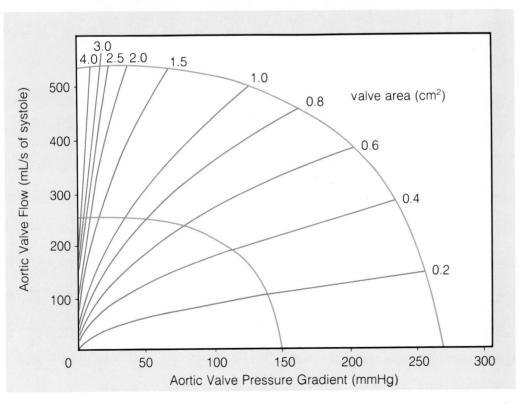

FIGURE 6.13   The relationship of cardiac output to the pressure gradient across the aortic valve in patients with aortic stenosis. When the valve area remains the same, the transaortic valve gradient increases as the cardiac output increases. (Reproduced with permission; see Figure Credits)

Adults with aortic stenosis have an average mortality of 9% per year. The survival time is often less than 5 years once symptoms develop; then the incidence of sudden death is 15 to 20%.[20] Angina is associated with an average life expectancy of 5 years; less than 5% of patients with this symptom survive for 10 to 20 years.[74] The survival time after syncope is 3 to 4 years, and the survival time after the development of left ventricular failure is about 2 years.[2] The actuarial survival of patients with aortic stenosis treated medically is depicted from the time of diagnosis in Figure 6.14.

In a subset of adult patients with accelerated aortic stenosis a rather rapid acceleration of the narrowing of the valve may occur. The aortic valve gradient in such cases may increase from 40 mmHg to 75 mmHg within 2 years.

Aortic Valve Regurgitation
ETIOLOGY AND PATHOLOGY

In past decades rheumatic fever and syphilis were the major causes of aortic valve regurgitation; however, with the decline in incidence and prevalence of these diseases other etiologies should be considered (Fig. 6.15). The pathology of this condition is diverse; acute or chronic pathological processes may be responsible. Basically, abnormalities of the valve leaflets and/or the aortic root may result in aortic regurgitation.

In chronic regurgitation the valve may show fibrosis of the leaflets with retraction and immobilization with or without accompanying calcification. The sequelae of rheumatic fever typify the chronic condition (Fig. 6.16), but most other types of abnormalities that affect the connective tissue core of the leaflets can also produce these changes (see Fig. 6.15). Congenitally bicuspid aortic valve is an important condition, particularly in the setting of a large conjoined cusp; prolapse toward the left ventricular cavity may occur with or without dystrophic calcification (Fig. 6.17). Conditions affecting the aortic root are manifold; Marfan's syndrome may be the best example (Fig. 6.18). An important abnormality of uncertain origin is aorticoannuloectasia (Fig. 6.19). Acute regurgitation is generally due to sudden disruption of the integrity of the aortic valve; infective endocarditis is by far the most common cause (Figs. 6.20, 6.21).

PATHOPHYSIOLOGY

Chronic aortic valve regurgitation causes a gradual increase in end diastolic volume of the left ventricle. As a result of this volume load the heart remodels itself by left ventricular dilation and increased thickness of the left ventricular wall. The left ventricular stroke volume is also increased. The increase in end-diastolic volume may be associated with a minimal increase in diastolic pressure in the early stages of the condition. The diastolic compliance of the left ventricle is increased, and compensatory left ventricular hypertrophy normalizes systolic wall stress or after load. Forward cardiac output remains normal during rest and exercise.

In the late stages of chronic aortic valve regurgitation primary myocardial factors or secondary lesions, such as coronary disease, may depress the contractile state of the left ventricular myocardium, producing an increase in end-systolic volume and a decrease in the ejection fraction. This is associated with an increase in end-diastolic pressure due to a decrease in compliance, leading to elevation of left atrial pressure and, hence, to pulmonary venous hypertension (Fig. 6.22).

The hemodynamic changes of acute aortic valve regurgitation differ from the chronic condition if the acute damage occurs in a patient with no previous regurgitation. The left ventricle does not have sufficient time to adapt to considerable aortic regurgitation. Accordingly an abrupt rise in left ventricular end-

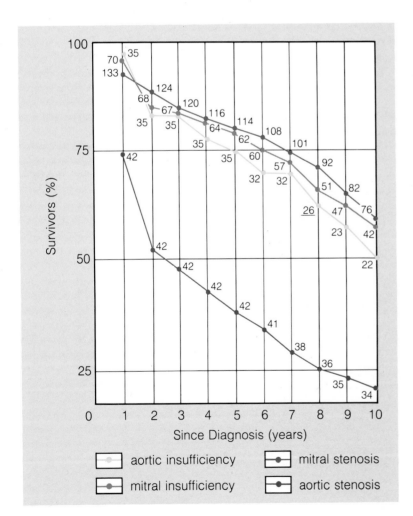

FIGURE 6.14   The actuarial survival of patients with valvular heart disease treated medically from the time of diagnosis. (The numbers at each of the dots indicate the number of patients known to be dead or alive at a point in time. The percentage survival figures have been corrected accordingly to reflect the actual number of patients in the series at that time.) (Reproduced with permission; see Figure Credits)

diastolic pressure may occur with little ventricular dilation. The left ventricular end-diastolic pressure may rise and approach, or even exceed, left atrial pressure, prematurely closing the mitral valve. These sudden changes may produce pulmonary venous hypertension and pulmonary edema.

If acute regurgitation is superimposed on chronic aortic valve regurgitation, the hemodynamic and clinical consequences depend on the summation of the chronic and the acute hemodynamic changes.

CLINICAL MANIFESTATIONS
SYMPTOMS

The patient may notice prominent pulsations in the carotid artery and at the apex of the heart when lying on the left side. The patient may be aware of premature heart beats, since the stroke volume is quite large after the long diastole.

Symptoms due to Heart Failure   Patients with long-standing chronic aortic valve regurgitation develop symptoms of heart failure, including dyspnea with effort, orthopnea, paroxysmal nocturnal dyspnea, pulmonary edema, and fatigue.

Angina Pectoris   The angina associated with aortic valve regurgitation tends to occur at rest when bradycardia is present and lasts longer than angina due to coronary disease alone. The exact cause of the angina, however, cannot be determined by an analysis of the symptoms.

Other Symptoms   Patients with severe aortic valve regurgitation may have carotid sheath pain, abdominal pain, postural dizziness, and excessive sweating.[27] Patients with acute aortic valve regurgitation may develop abrupt pulmonary edema, hypotension, and even shock.

PHYSICAL EXAMINATION

The etiology of aortic valve regurgitation may be immediately evident upon physical examination if it is associated with Marfan's syndrome, osteogenesis imperfecta, or ankylosing spondylitis.

A rapid carotid upstroke and a wide pulse pressure may result in a hyperdynamic state with a pulsus bisferiens. When the regurgitation is severe, it produces a profound effect on the peripheral arterial pulsation. When heart failure is severe, however, the systemic diastolic blood pressure may be normal because of the elevation of the diastolic pressure in the left ventricle.

The heart may be normal in size when chronic aortic valve regurgitation is slight or when the regurgitation is acute. Patients with moderately severe chronic regurgitation have enlarged hearts; the apex impulse is displaced inferolaterally, and is hyperdynamic and larger than normal.

The first heart sound at the apex may be diminished in intensity especially if the P–R interval is long. A systolic ejection sound may be heard along the left sternal border due to abrupt distention of the aorta. Secondary to aortic valve regurgitation there may be a systolic aortic murmur in the second right intercostal space, a systolic murmur at the apex, a diastolic rumble (Austin Flint murmur) at the apex, and a systolic tricuspid murmur.[59]

The characteristic diastolic murmur of aortic valve regurgitation is high-pitched. It is best heard along the left sternal border, using the diaphragm of the stethoscope with firm pressure; the patient should be leaning forward after exhaling. When there is aortic root disease, the murmur may be best heard to the right of the sternum. A high-pitched, cooing diastolic murmur may be heard when an aortic leaflet is lacerated or retroverted or when a hole develops

---

FIG. 6.15 ETIOLOGY OF CHRONIC AND ACUTE AORTIC REGURGITATION*

CHRONIC AORTIC REGURGITATION

Rheumatic fever
Syphilis
Aortitis (Takayasu)
Heritable disorders of connective tissue
  Marfan's syndrome
  Ehlers–Danlos syndrome
  Osteogenesis imperfecta
Congenital heart disease
  Bicuspid aortic valve
  Interventricular septal defect
  Sinus of Valsalva aneurysm
Arthritic diseases
  Ankylosing spondylitis
  Reiter's syndrome
  Rheumatoid arthritis
  Lupus erythematousus

Aortic root disease
Dissection of the aorta
Hypertension
Arteriosclerosis
Myxomatous degeneration of valve
Infective endocarditis
Following prosthetic valve surgery
Associated with aortic stenosis
Ergot toxicity

ACUTE AORTIC REGURGITATION

Rheumatic fever
Infective endocarditis
Congenital (rupture of sinus of Valsalva)

Acute aortic dissection
Following prosthetic valve surgery
Trauma

*Note that certain disorders are capable of producing both acute and chronic regurgitation.
(Reproduced with permission; see Figure Credits)

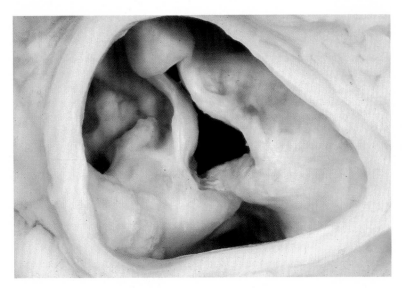

FIGURE 6.16 Rheumatic aortic valve with commissural fusion and leaflet fibrosis. The pathology suggests stenosis and regurgitation as a functional consequence. (Reproduced with permission; see Figure Credits)

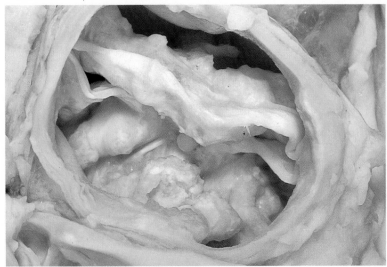

FIGURE 6.17 Bicuspid aortic valve from an adult with evidence of fibrosis and calcification; prolapse of the conjoined leaflet results in aortic valve regurgitation. (Reproduced with permission; see Figure Credits)

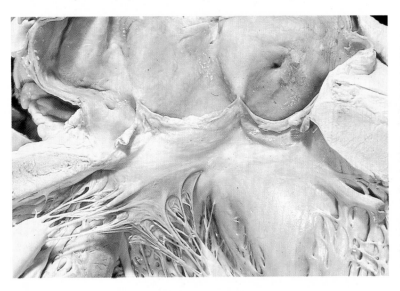

FIGURE 6.18 Aortic root dilation in a patient with Marfan's disease resulting in aortic regurgitation. (Reproduced with permission; see Figure Credits)

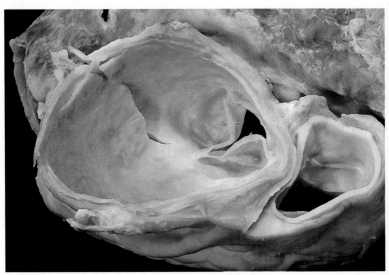

FIGURE 6.19 Aorticoannuloectasia with a markedly dilated ascending aorta resulting in chronic aortic regurgitation. (Reproduced with permission; see Figure Credits)

FIGURE 6.20 Infective endocarditis of the aortic valve with extensive destruction of leaflet tissue. This condition leads to acute regurgitation. (Reproduced with permission; see Figure Credits)

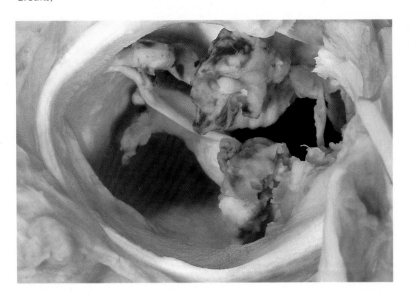

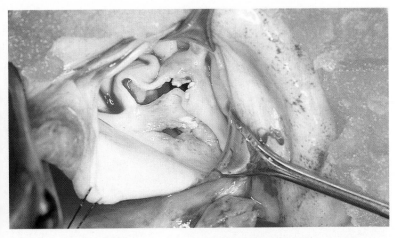
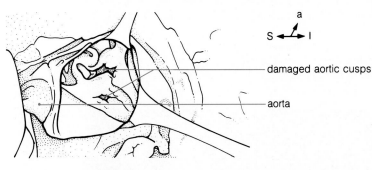

damaged aortic cusps

aorta

FIGURE 6.21 Operative view of a severely damaged aortic valve secondary to bacterial endocarditis. Urgent surgical intervention was required due to intractable heart failure, which was aggravated by the presence of an aortic–right atrial fistula. (Reproduced with permission; see Figure Credits)

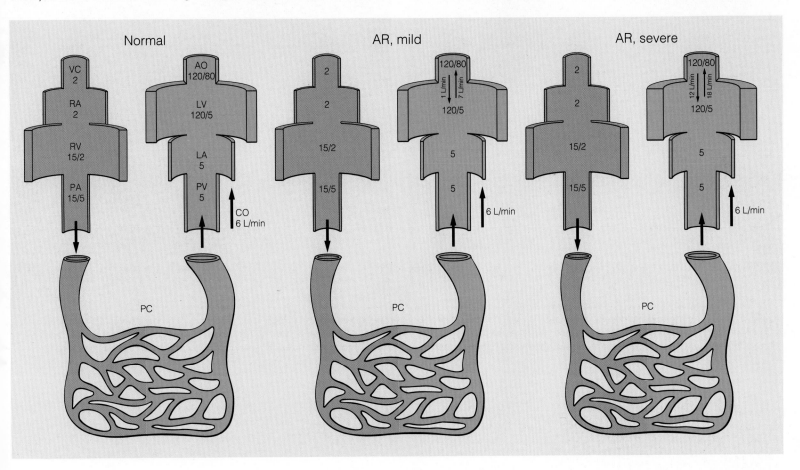

FIGURE 6.22 Pathophysiology of aortic regurgitation (AR). The top panel presents normal hemodynamics and the middle panel depicts mild AR. There is a regurgitant flow of 1 L/min from the aorta (AO) into the left ventricle (LV). LV pressures are unchanged because the volume of the regurgitant flow is so small. In the bottom panel, severe AR is depicted, with a 12 L/min flow back into the LV across the insufficient aortic valve. The LV is hypertrophied and dilated and pumps 18 L/min -12 of regurgitant flow and 6 of normal systemic forward cardiac output (CO). LV failure has not developed and LV diastolic pressure is normal. (VC = vena cava; RA = right atrium; RV = right ventricle; PA = pulmonary artery; PC = pulmonary capillaries PV = pulmonary veins) (Redrawn with permission; see Figure Credits)

because of endocarditis. This type of murmur is often heard with acute aortic regurgitation. The first sound is usually faint in such cases because of premature closure of the mitral valve. A ventricular gallop sound heard at the apex is usually a sign of left ventricular dysfunction.

The Austin Flint diastolic rumble heard at the apex is due, in part, to the impingement of aortic regurgitant flow on the anterior leaflet of the mitral valve, thereby producing functional mitral stenosis.

Chest Radiography　　Chronic aortic valve regurgitation produces a dilated left ventricle, an enlarged left atrium, and a dilated aortic root (Fig. 6.23). The heart size or shape may not be altered in acute regurgitation, but pulmonary edema may be present.

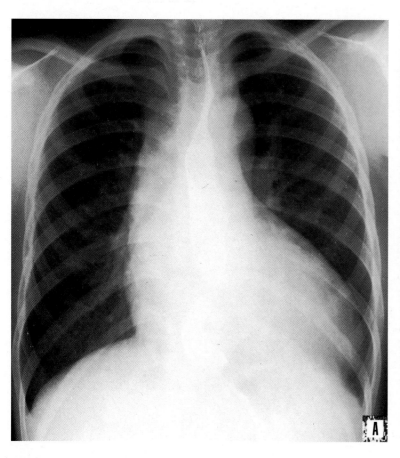

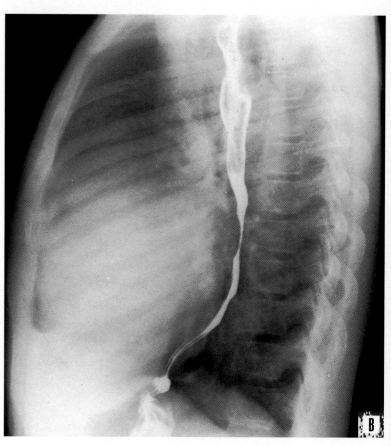

FIGURE 6.23　　Barium opacifies the esophagus on the chest films of a patient with aortic regurgitation. (**A**) Posteroanterior view reveals marked enlargement of the left ventricle with dilation of the aorta beginning in the root and extending through the distal arch. The lung fields are normal. (**B**) Lateral projection demonstrates posterior displacement of the esophagus by an enlarged left atrium. (Reproduced with permission; see Figure Credits)

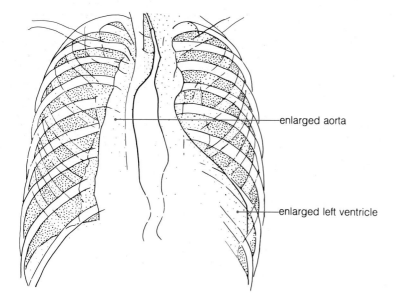

enlarged aorta

enlarged left ventricle

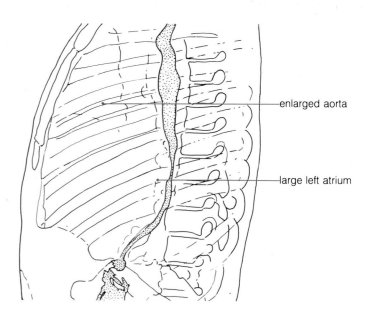

enlarged aorta

large left atrium

Electrocardiography   The ECG shows left ventricular hypertrophy.[67] The QRS voltage is increased, and the ST–T wave may be of the diastolic overload type, that is, the mean vector representing the large ST and T waves is parallel to the mean QRS vector. The pattern of left ventricular strain may also be present when the mean ST–T vector is pointed in a direction that is opposite to the mean QRS vector (Fig. 6.24). The P–R interval may be prolonged.

Echocardiography   The echocardiogram can provide anatomic information about the aortic root and the aortic valve, including vegetations. It can also give measurements of ventricular function. An increase in aortic dimension suggests chronic regurgitation. Left ventricular stroke volume and the ejection fraction can be calculated at rest and during supine exercise.

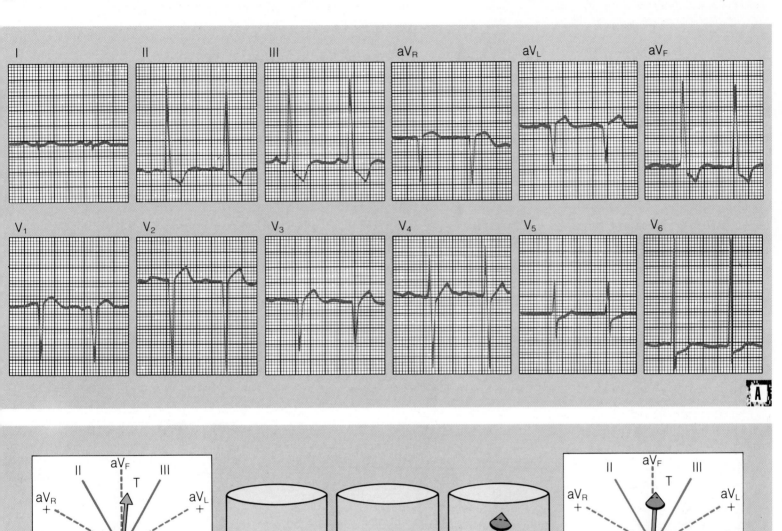

FIGURE 6.24   **(A)** ECG of a 16-year-old girl with Marfan's syndrome and severe aortic regurgitation. **(B)** (a) Frontal plane projection shows the mean QRS, initial 0.04 second, and T vectors. (b) The initial 0.04 second vector is slightly positive in lead I and negative in aV_R and aV_L; therefore it is just to the left of aV_F. There are Q waves in leads V_1 to V_3, and R waves in leads V_4 to V_6. (c) The mean QRS vector is resultantly negative in lead I and slightly more positive in lead III compared with lead II. The vector must be just to the right of aV_F. The mean QRS vector is transitional between V_4 and V_5. (d) The mean T vector is opposite the mean QRS vector; and since it is positive in lead I, it is drawn slightly to the left of the perpendicular to lead I. (e) The spatial arrangement of the vectors. The striking ventricular forces and the vertical mean QRS axis are common in young people with left ventricular hypertrophy. Decreased anterior forces and ST-segment elevation in V_1 and V_2 are common findings with severe left ventricular hypertrophy. (Reproduced with permission; see Figure Credits)

Mitral valve abnormalities recognized on the echocardiogram include diastolic fluttering of the anterior mitral valve leaflet and rapid early closure of a thickened mitral valve (Fig. 6.25).[51] In acute aortic regurgitation a flail aortic leaflet may be seen, and aortic dissection can often be recognized.[72]

Pre- and postoperative studies suggest that a left ventricular end-systolic dimension greater than 55 mm may identify a patient at high risk for the development of heart failure. The aortic valve should be replaced before irreversible left ventricular damage has occurred. The echocardiogram is useful in identifying such patients.

The diastolic flow across the aortic valve can be determined and roughly quantitated by the Doppler technique (Figs. 6.26–6.28).

Cardiac Catheterization   Cardiac catheterization is indicated to assess the severity of aortic regurgitation in patients thought to have moderately severe to severe regurgitation (Figs. 6.29), to determine left ventricular function, and to identify other cardiac abnormalities, such as mitral valve disease or coronary artery disease.

Cardiac catheterization results may easily be misinterpreted. A dilated left ventricular chamber may dilute the contrast medium, giving the impression of minimal regurgitation, whereas regurgitation into normal-sized left ventricular chamber may create an impression of severe aortic regurgitation.[33] Left ventricular end-diastolic pressure cannot be used as an index of left ventricular function in patients with chronic aortic regurgitation, because there may be an increase in the diastolic compliance and the end-diastolic wall stress with a normal preload. This measurement is more useful in patients with acute aortic regurgitation. The ejection fraction is useful, but this value is artificially preserved in the volume overload of chronic aortic regurgitation, since systolic ejection begins at a lower than normal level of left ventricular pressure.

Contractility should be estimated from angiographic and echocardiographic measures of left ventricular end-systolic volume and ejection fraction in patients with chronic aortic regurgitation. Contractility is more depressed in patients with heart failure than in asymptomatic patients (Fig. 6.30).[48]

Coronary arteriography should be performed in adults who are undergoing cardiac catheterization for aortic regurgitation, since coronary disease may produce angina and left ventricular dysfunction.

Radionuclide Studies   Technetium-99m ventriculograms at rest and during exercise can be used to quantify the amount of regurgitant flow and to determine the ejection fraction.[5] With normal cardiac function the ejection fraction should be in the normal range, increasing with exercise. A fall in ejection fraction with exercise indicates poor myocardial contractility, which can occur before the patient becomes symptomatic. The test is often used in following patients to establish the optimum time for aortic valve replacement.

Thallium-201 scintigraphy can identify perfusion defects in the myocardium that suggest the presence of associated coronary disease.

Other Imaging Modalities   Gated MR images demonstrate the aortic regurgitant jet with considerable clarity. Semiquantitative estimates of regurgitant volume can be obtained (Fig. 6.31).

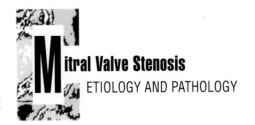

NATURAL HISTORY

Seventy-five percent of patients with significant chronic aortic valve regurgitation survive 5 years, and 50% survive for 10 years after the diagnosis has been made. Patients with mild-to-moderate aortic regurgitation are likely to survive 10 years.[60] Many patients with trivial aortic regurgitation live a normal life span, but they are predisposed to infective endocarditis. Patients who develop heart failure often expire within 2 years; the average survival after the onset of angina is 5 years.

Patients with a preoperative ejection fraction of 45% and cardiac indices greater than 2.5 L/min/m² have a greater long-term survival after surgery than do patients with less than 45% ejection fractions and cardiac indices of less than 2.5 L/min/m².[22] The actuarial survival of patients with chronic aortic regurgitation treated medically from the time of diagnosis is shown in Figure 6.14. Patients with acute aortic regurgitation and pulmonary edema have a very poor prognosis; surgical intervention is usually necessary.

Mitral Valve Stenosis
ETIOLOGY AND PATHOLOGY

Mitral valve stenosis is usually caused by scarring of the valve following rheumatic fever. Fibrosis affects the valve leaflets and the commissures restricting valve mobility. Retraction may eventually lead to a funnel-type valve (Fig. 6.32), cordal fibrosis, and obliteration of the intercordal spaces (Fig. 6.33), thus

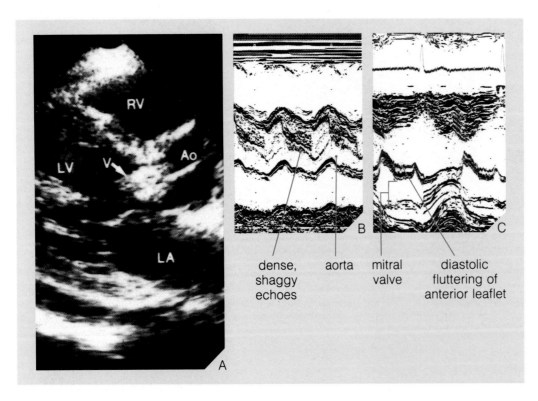

FIGURE 6.25   Cross-sectional and M-mode echocardiograms from a patient with aortic regurgitation due to infective endocarditis. **(A)** Cross-sectional echocardiogram in the long axis parasternal view reveals a large aortic vegetation (V). **(B)** M-mode echocardiogram of the aortic valve shows dense, shaggy echoes visible on the aortic leaflets during diastole consistent with an aortic valve vegetation. **(C)** M-mode echocardiogram of the mitral valve shows high-frequency diastolic fluttering of the anterior leaflet of the mitral valve consistent with aortic regurgitation. (Ao = aortic valve; LA = left atrium; LV = left ventricle; RV = right ventricle) (Reproduced with permission; see Figure Credits)

dense, shaggy echoes   aorta   mitral valve   diastolic fluttering of anterior leaflet

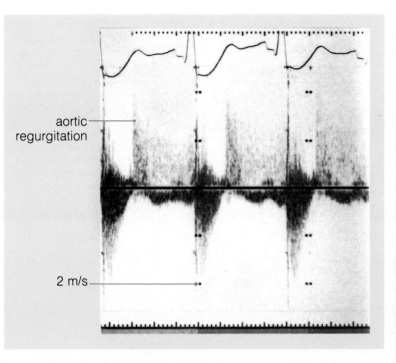

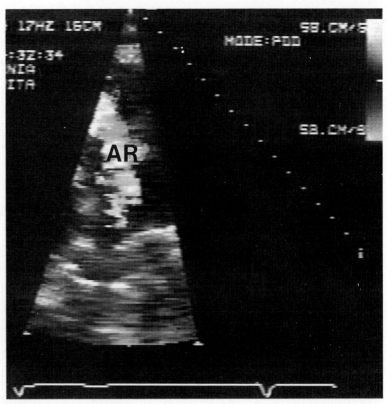

FIGURE 6.26 Continuous-wave Doppler recording from the apex toward the aortic valve depicting high-velocity diastolic flow jet due to aortic regurgitation. (Reproduced with permission; see Figure Credits)

FIGURE 6.27 Apical four-chamber view with color-flow Doppler. A turbulent aortic regurgitation jet (AR) originates in the aortic valve and penetrates all the way into the apex of the left ventricle. (Reproduced with permission; see Figure Credits)

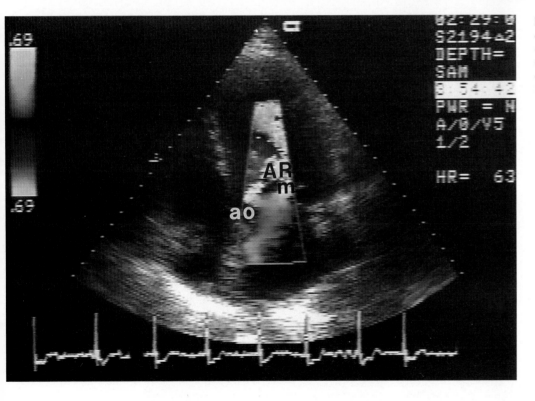

FIGURE 6.28 Apical four-chamber view with color-flow Doppler. An aortic regurgitation jet (AR) can be seen emanating from the aortic valve (ao) and mixing with mitral inflow (m) to form a combined jet. (Reproduced with permission; see Figure Credits)

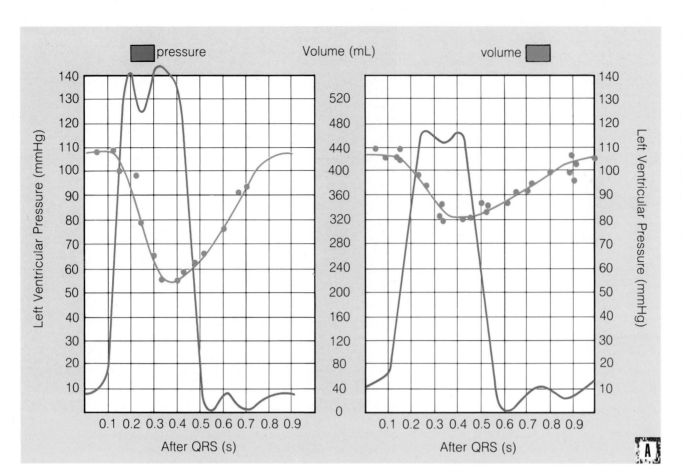

FIGURE 6.29
(A) Left ventricular pressure and volume from two patients with aortic regurgitation. The patient on the left enjoyed unrestricted activity without symptoms, whereas the patient on the right was extremely limited by left ventricular failure. (B) Acutal measurements during unrestricted activity. (Reproduced with permission; see Figure Credits)

Unrestricted Activity		Restricted Activity
436	end-diastolic volume (mL)	430
219	end-systolic volume (mL)	329
217	left ventricular stroke volume (mL)	101
97	forward stroke volume (mL)	67
120	aortic regurgitation (mL)	34
217/436 = 50	ejection fraction (%)	101/430 = 23
474	left ventricular weight (g)	561
8	left ventricular end-diastolic pressure (mmHg)	13

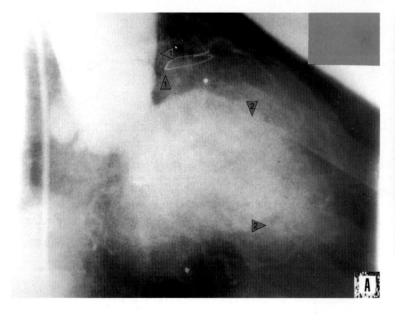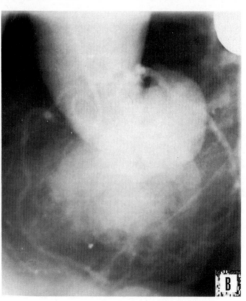

FIGURE 6.30
Thoracic aortogram of severe aortic insufficiency. Right anterior (A) and lateral (B) views show reflux of contrast material from the dilated ascending aorta (arrows 1) into the left ventricle (arrows 2), which is completely opacified. (Reproduced with permission; see Figure Credits)

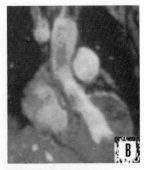
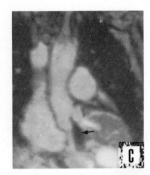
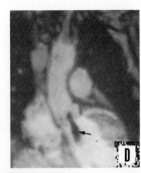

FIGURE 6.31   Cine 11R MR images in the coronal plane of aortic regurgitation. Images acquired in systole **(A,B)** and diastole **(C,D)**. Note the signal void (arrow) emanating from the closed aortic valve. (Reproduced with permission; see Figure Credits)

FIGURE 6.32
Long-axis cross section through a heart with a rheumatic mitral valve showing funnel-like stenosis. (Reproduced with permission; see Figure Credits)

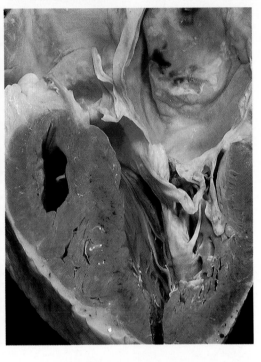

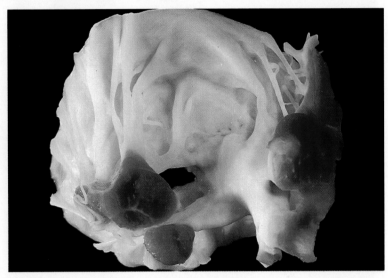

FIGURE 6.33   Resected rheumatic mitral valve with extensive obliteration of intercordal spaces and leaflet fibrosis—features underlying mitral stenosis. (Reproduced with permission; see Figure Credits)

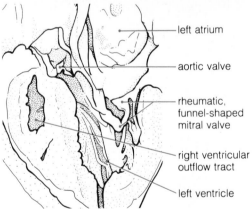

- left atrium
- aortic valve
- rheumatic, funnel-shaped mitral valve
- right ventricular outflow tract
- left ventricle

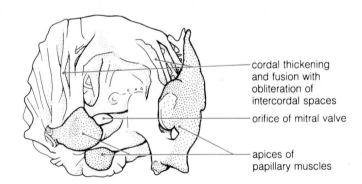

- cordal thickening and fusion with obliteration of intercordal spaces
- orifice of mitral valve
- apices of papillary muscles

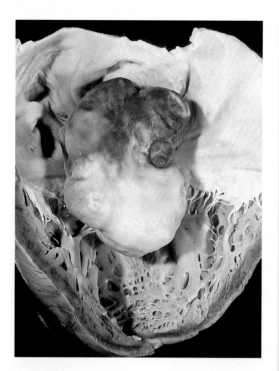

FIGURE 6.34 Left atrial myxoma obstructing the mitral orifice. (Reproduced with permission; see Figure Credits)

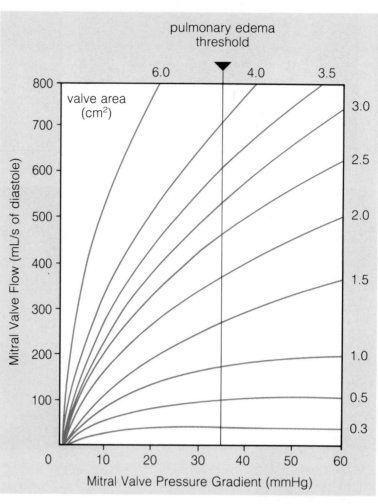

FIGURE 6.35 Relationship between the mean diastolic gradient across the mitral valve and rate of flow across the mitral valve per second of diastole, as predicted by the Gorlin and Gorlin formula. When the mitral valve area is 1.0 cm² or less, very little additional flow can be achieved by an increased pressure gradient. Transudation of fluid from the pulmonary capillaries and the development of pulmonary edema begin when pulmonary capillary pressure exceeds the oncotic pressure of plasma, which is about 25 to 35 mmHg. It is also apparent that severe mitral regurgitation is incompatible with very tight mitral stenosis. (Reproduced with permission; see Figure Credits)

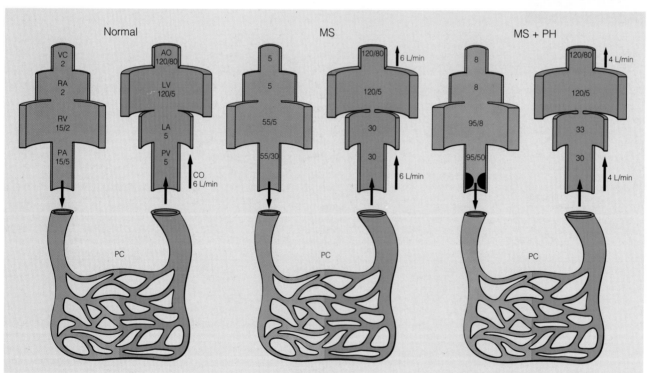

FIGURE 6.36 Pathophysiology of mitral stenosis (MS). The top panel presents normal hemodynamics and the middle panel shows severe MS without reactive pulmonary hypertension (PH). Left atrial pressure is 30 mmHg and there is a 25-mm gradient M across the mitral valve during diastole. The increased left atrial pressure is transmitted to the pulmonary capillaries (PC) and pulmonary artery (PA) and results in an increase in pulmonary arterial pressure to 55/30 mmHg. Right ventricular systolic pressure must therefore increase to 55 mmHg as well. There is slight dilation and hypertrophy of the right ventricle (RV) and left atrium (LA). In the bottom panel, severe reactive PH is depicted, but the MS is not more severe than that depicted in the middle panel. The RV is hypertrophied and dilated and has failed, with right atrial and central venous pressures rising to 8 mmHg and cardiac output (CO) falling to 4 L/min. (VC = vena cava; RA = right atrium; PV = pulmonary veins; LV = left ventricle; AO= aorta) (Redrawn with permission; see Figure Credits)

contributing markedly to the inflow obstruction. Congenital mitral valve stenosis is almost always part of a more complex cardiac malformation; usually the patient becomes symptomatic at an early age.

Other conditions, such as methysergide maleate (Sansert) toxicity causing mitral stenosis are rare. Left atrial myxoma may obstruct the orifice (Fig. 6.34). Occasionally endocarditis may present with signs of mitral stenosis due to excessive thrombotic vegetations occluding the orifice. A malfunctioning mitral prosthesis may also produce stenosis of the mitral orifice, and the large papillary muscles of idiopathic cardiac hypertrophy may impede the flow of blood into the ventricle. A calcified mitral ring usually produces regurgitation rather than stenosis.

PATHOPHYSIOLOGY

Significant mitral valve blockade produces a decrease in diastolic blood flow through the valve, resulting in a pressure gradient between the left atrium and the left ventricle. The relationship of the mean diastolic pressure gradient and flow across the mitral valve is shown in Figure 6.35. The mean diastolic gradient is determined by the cardiac output and the time required for diastole. As the left atrial pressure rises, it produces an elevation of pulmonary venous pressure (Fig. 6.36). This leads to compensatory dilation of the lymphatics and the bronchial veins due to pulmonary bronchial venous shunting (Fig. 6.37); soon medial hypertrophy and arterialization of the pulmonary veins occur (Fig. 6.38). The muscular pulmonary arteries and arterioles become hypertrophic, and inti-

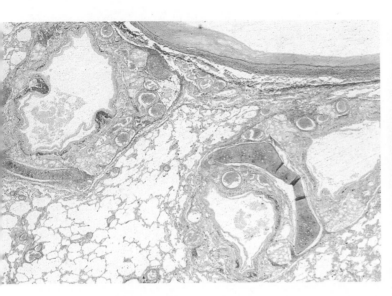

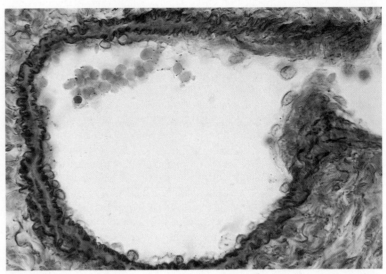

FIGURE 6.37   Histologic section of lung tissue from a patient with chronic pulmonary venous hypertension. Note the dilated bronchial venous plexus. (Reproduced with permission; see Figure Credits)

FIGURE 6.38   Arterialization of the pulmonary vein in a patient with congenital mitral valve stenosis. A distinct muscular media is formed, sandwiched between an inner and outer elastic lamina. (Reproduced with permission; see Figure Credits)

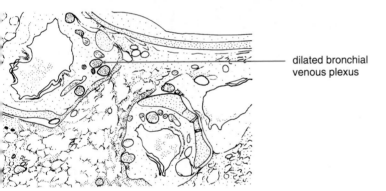

dilated bronchial venous plexus

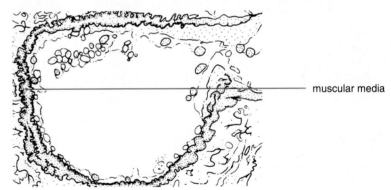

muscular media

mal fibrosis develops (Fig. 6.39); the resulting pulmonary hypertension causes right ventricular hypertrophy.[37]

CLINICAL MANIFESTATIONS

About 50% of patients with mitral stenosis due to rheumatic fever provide a history of rheumatic fever.[63] This condition occurs more often in women; symptoms begin to appear in the early 30s or older, although mitral stenosis due to rheumatic fever may occur at a younger age in women from Third-World countries. Congenital mitral stenosis may produce symptoms at an early age.

SYMPTOMS

Patients complain of dyspnea on effort, fatigue, palpitation, hemoptysis, and hoarseness. The symptoms that result from embolic events and the symptoms that accompany infective endocarditis are also noted.[65]

Dyspnea   Patients may be asymptomatic for many years, and then gradually develop dyspnea on effort. They may walk less rapidly and, by limiting their activity, avoid dyspnea. Such patients may then deny dyspnea, although the mitral valve obstruction may be gradually increasing.

Patients with slight or no dyspnea may develop severe dyspnea and pulmonary edema when atrial fibrillation develops. Left ventricular filling is compromised by the rapid rate and the short diastoles in such patients. Pulmonary edema may develop during pregnancy.[71]

Fatigue   Fatigue usually accompanies dyspnea in patients with mitral stenosis, but occasionally it dominates the clinical picture.

Palpitation   Atrial fibrillation, either paroxysmal or persistent, is a common complication of mitral stenosis. The patient usually detects tumultuous heart action and develops dyspnea and weakness. Patients with mitral stenosis and atrial fibrillation are highly prone to arterial embolization.

Hemoptysis   Hemoptysis may occur as a result of an increase in pulmonary venous pressure, pulmonary emboli, or recurrent bronchitis. At times hemoptysis may be severe enough to require emergency valve surgery.[64]

Hoarseness

Hoarseness occasionally occurs when the recurrent laryngeal nerve is trapped between the enlarged left pulmonary artery and the aorta or aortic ligament.

Peripheral Emboli   Emboli to the brain may produce strokes and seizures; peripheral emboli to the arms, legs, spleen, and kidneys may also occur.[3]

PHYSICAL EXAMINATION

The patient may exhibit a malar flush, and the internal jugular veins may pulsate abnormally due to tricuspid regurgitation.

The heart rhythm may be normal, or it may reveal the signs of atrial fibrillation. The apex impulse is normal or diminished in patients with isolated mitral stenosis. There may be a sustained anterior lift of the precordium, signifying right ventricular hypertrophy. A diastolic rumble may be palpated at the apex, and the first heart sound may be easily palpated. The second heart sound may be felt when there is pulmonary hypertension.

The auscultatory features of mitral stenosis are a loud first heart sound, the opening snap of the mitral valve, a diastolic rumble with presystolic accentuation, and a loud pulmonary valve closure sound (Fig. 6.40).[75] The pulmonary closure component of the second sound may increase in intensity due to pulmonary hypertension; it is heard best in the second and third left intercostal spaces. The murmur of pulmonary regurgitation may be present with advanced disease.

The examiner must listen for the murmur of mitral stenosis with the patient in the left lateral recumbent position after exercise. The opening snap, the loud

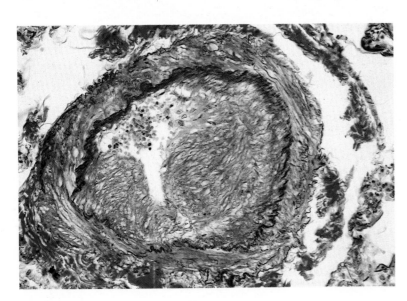

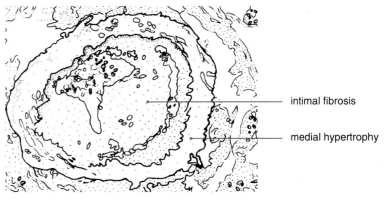

FIGURE 6.39   Histologic section of lung tissue from a patient with chronic pulmonary venous hypertension. Note the muscular pulmonary artery with medial hypertrophy and cushion-like intimal fibrosis. (Reproduced with permission; see Figure Credits)

first sound, and the loud pulmonary component of the second sound are heard best by using the diaphragm of the stethoscope applied with firm pressure. These abnormalities are distributed over a wide area on the chest. The diastolic rumble, which is heard in a localized area at the apex, is best heard with the bell of the stethoscope applied with light pressure.

Other conditions may produce a diastolic rumble at the apex, including mitral regurgitation, aortic regurgitation causing an Austin Flint rumble, patent arterial duct, interventricular septal defect, left atrial myxoma, the Carey Coombs murmur of acute rheumatic fever and, rarely, calcification of the mitral valve annulus. A tricuspid valve rumble secondary to atrial septal defect may be mistaken for a mitral valve rumble.

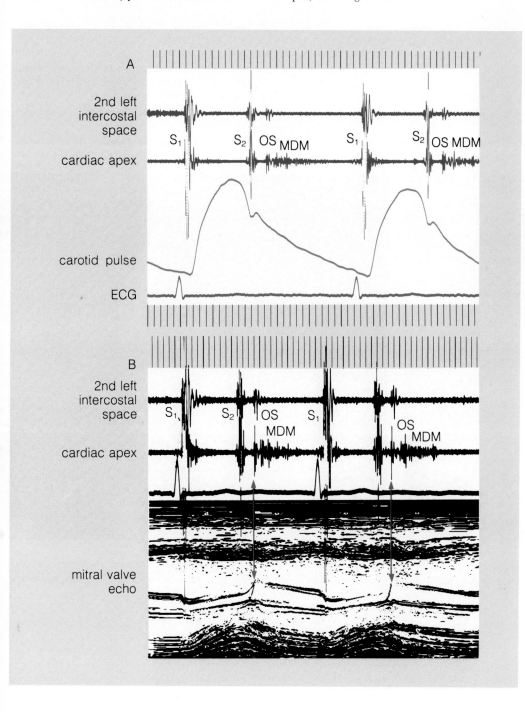

FIGURE 6.40   Phonocardiographic tracings, obtained at the second left intercostal space and cardiac apex, and carotid pulse tracing from a patient with mitral stenosis and atrial fibrillation. **(A)** A loud first sound (S_1) and the opening snap (OS) of the mitral valve occurs 0.11 sec after the second heart sound (S_2) which is in turn followed by a low frequency mid-diastolic murmur (MDM) at the cardiac apex. **(B)** Phonocardiogram, obtained at a slower paper speed (50 mmls), and M-mode echocardiogram showing a relation between the first heart sound and the completion of the closing movement of the mitral valve and, similarly, the opening snap accompanying the termination of the opening movement of the valve. (Reproduced with permission; see Figure Credits)

VALVULAR HEART DISEASE

Chest Radiography   On the chest film of a patient with mitral stenosis, the pulmonary arterial trunk, the left atrial appendage, the large left atrium, and Kerley B lines are all prominent (Figs. 6.41, 6.42). [18] Calcification of the mitral valve leaflets is often seen.

Electrocardiography   The ECG of a patient with mitral stenosis reveals broad and notched P waves when there is normal rhythm (Figs. 6.43, 6.44). The mean QRS vector may be normal or directed to the right; it may show right ventricular hypertrophy. Atrial fibrillation is frequently present.[44]

Echocardiography   The M-mode echocardiogram of a patient with mitral stenosis shows a decrease in the E-F slope of the anterior leaflet of the mitral valve, and failure of the posterior leaflet to move downward (Fig. 6.45). A thickened, calcified, and immobile valve is usually seen in the two-dimensional echocardiogram (Figs. 6.46, 6.47). Doppler recordings are employed to measure the valvular gradient and estimate the mitral valve area.[13]

Cardiac Catheterization   The mitral valve pressure gradient, the mitral valve area, and the pulmonary artery pressure can be calculated from data acquired at cardiac catheterization (Fig. 6.48).[21] The normal mitral valve area is 4 to 6 cm^2. Hemodynan abnormalities develop when the valve area is reduced to 1.5 to 2.5 cm^2; pulmonary congestion develops when the valve area is 1.1 to 1.5 cm^2. Symptoms such as dyspnea usually indicate a valve area of 1.0 cm^2 or less.

Patients with dyspnea due to mitral stenosis usually exhibit a pulmonary arterial wedge pressure greater than 15 to 20 mmHg.[32] The pulmonary arterial pressure and the pulmonary arteriolar resistance become elevated in patients with mitral stenosis. The pressure may almost reach systemic levels in some patients. In some symptomatic patients with normal pulmonary wedge pressures it is necessary to measure the pulmonary arterial pressure after exercise.

Segmental and global wall abnormalities may be detected by left ventriculography (Fig. 6.49).[28] Angiography is also used to detect mitral regurgitation and left atrial tumor (Fig. 6.50). Coronary arteriography is used to detect coronary

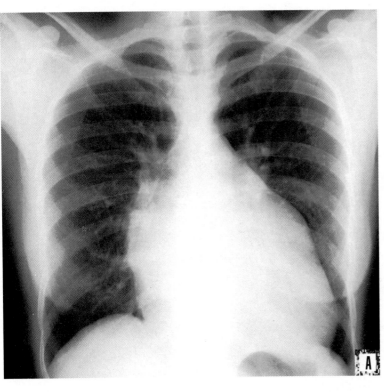

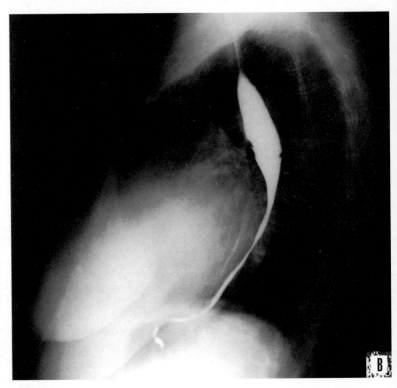

FIGURE 6.41   (A) Posteroanterior chest x-ray of a patient with rheumatic mitral stenosis. Note the enlarged left atrium that can be seen as a double density through the heart shadow. The superior pulmonary veins are distended, while the inferior pulmonary veins are not prominent. (B) Lateral view of the barium-filled esophagus shows an enlarged left atrium. (Reproduced with permission; see Figure Credits)

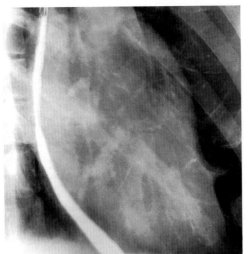

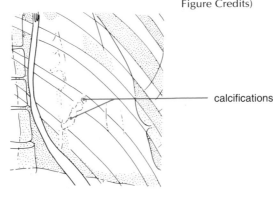

calcifications

FIGURE 6.42   Mitral valve calcification on lateral chest x-ray. There is barium in the esophagus. (Reproduced with permission; see Figure Credits)

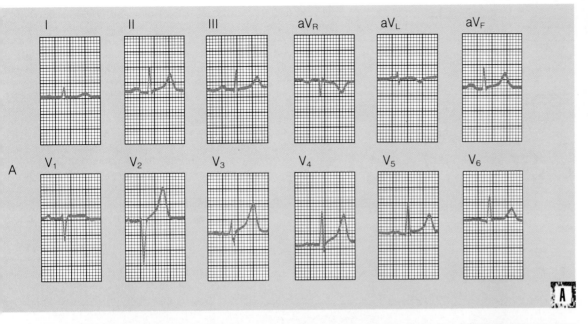

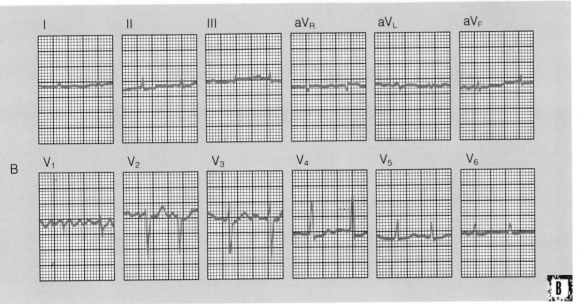

FIGURE 6.43   ECG recordings from patient with mitral stenosis made 7 years apart; during this time the patient's symptom and hemodynamic findings had progressed. **(A)** The first ECG shows a left atrial abnormality and a + 60° frontal mean QRS vector. **(B)** The recording obtained 7 years later shows atrial fibrillation with coarse fibrillatory waves and a + 85° mean QRS vector. (Reproduced with permission; see Figure Credits)

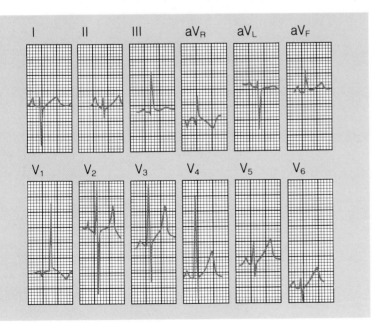

FIGURE 6.44   ECG obtained from a two-year-old girl with congenital mitral stenosis. Tall, peaked P waves of right atrial abnormality are present in leads I, II, and V_2. The QRS electrical axis is directed markedly to the right. The tall, monophasic R wave in lead V_1 and the deep S wave in V_6 reflect right ventricular hypertrophy. The large RS complexes in V_2 and V_3 suggest biventricular hypertrophy, possibly caused by coexisting coarctation of the aorta. (Reproduced with permission; see Figure Credits)

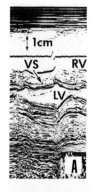
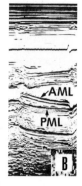
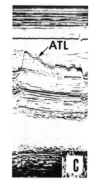
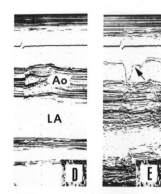
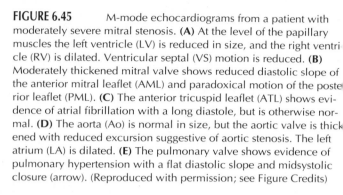

FIGURE 6.45   M-mode echocardiograms from a patient with moderately severe mitral stenosis. **(A)** At the level of the papillary muscles the left ventricle (LV) is reduced in size, and the right ventricle (RV) is dilated. Ventricular septal (VS) motion is reduced. **(B)** Moderately thickened mitral valve shows reduced diastolic slope of the anterior mitral leaflet (AML) and paradoxical motion of the posterior leaflet (PML). **(C)** The anterior tricuspid leaflet (ATL) shows evidence of atrial fibrillation with a long diastole, but is otherwise normal. **(D)** The aorta (Ao) is normal in size, but the aortic valve is thickened with reduced excursion suggestive of aortic stenosis. The left atrium (LA) is dilated. **(E)** The pulmonary valve shows evidence of pulmonary hypertension with a flat diastolic slope and midsystolic closure (arrow). (Reproduced with permission; see Figure Credits)

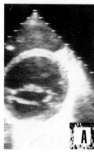
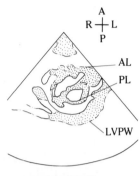
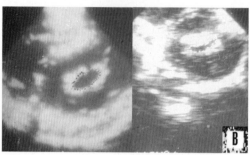

FIGURE 6.46   **(A)** Two-dimensional echocardiography used to estimate the severity of mitral stenosis by obtaining a short-axis image through the limiting orifice. **(B)** Planimetric method used to outline the maximal area of the limiting orifice. The echocardiogram in A superficially resembles those in B, but its opening is reduced by low flow. Note that while the mitral stenotic valves have central openings, the low-flow valve opens along the entire diameter of the chamber. (Reproduced with permission; see Figure Credits)

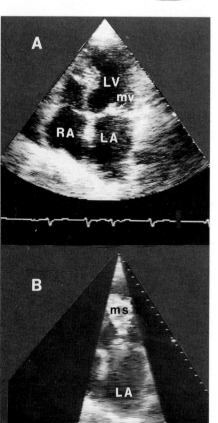

FIGURE 6.47   Apical four-chamber view of rheumatic mitral stenosis. **(A)** Two-dimensional imaging shows decreased mobility and thickening of mitral valve (mv) leaflets. **(B)** Color-flow Doppler indicates turbulent mitral stenosis jet (ms). (LA = left atrium; LV = left ventricle; RA = right atrium) (Reproduced with permission; see Figure Credits)

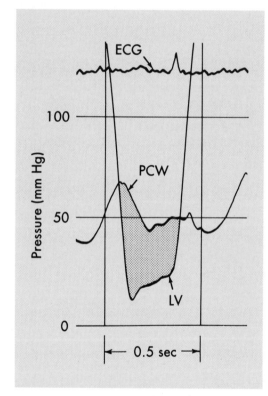

FIGURE 6.48   Pulmonary capillary wedge (PCW) and left ventricular diastolic pressure (LV) tracings from a patient with severe mitral stenosis. The gradient between left atrium and left ventricle in diastole is depicted by the stippled area. (Reproduced with permission; see Figure Credits)

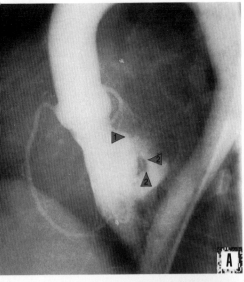
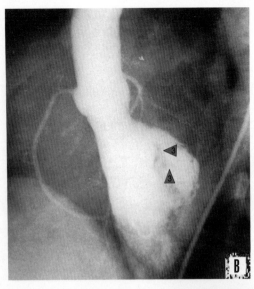

FIGURE 6.49 Left ventriculogram in long-axis view of mitral stenosis. **(A)** In diastole, movement of the mitral leaflets is restricted. The abnormal anterior leaflet (*arrow 1*) is outlined by contrast material along most of its surface. The mitral orifice (*arrows 2*) is smaller than normal. **(B)** In systole, the heads of the papillary muscles are projected close to the margin of the mitral orifice. The filling defect (*arrows 3*) represents thickening of the margins of the mitral leaflets due to fibrosis. (Reproduced with permission; see Figure Credits)

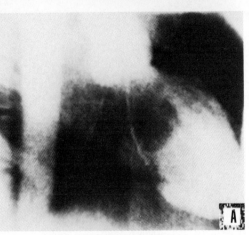
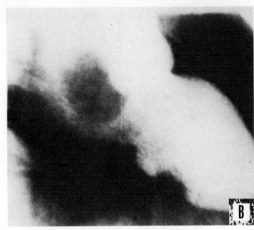

FIGURE 6.50 **(A)** Left ventriculogram in the right anterior oblique projection. A mobile left atrial myxoma is seen as a space-filling defect within the mitral valve in diastole. **(B)** Sufficient mitral regurgitation is present to delineate the myxoma in the left atrium in systole. (Reproduced with permission; see Figure Credits)

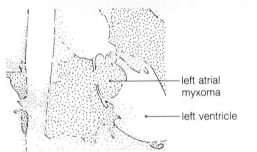
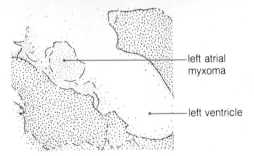

left atrial myxoma

left ventricle

left atrial myxoma

left ventricle

atherosclerosis in all adult patients undergoing cardiac catheterization for mitral stenosis.[9]

Radionuclide Studies   The [99mTc] ventriculogram can be used to determine left ventricular function. It is possible to measure the left ventricular ejection fraction, the end-diastolic volume, the cardiac output, and the stroke volume at rest and after exercise. Right ventricular function can also be assessed.[45]

NATURAL HISTORY

While rheumatic fever usually occurs between ages 8 and 12 years, mitral stenosis is usually detected about 20 years later. Symptoms usually occurring by ages 40 to 50 years include dyspnea, fatigue, and palpitation (atrial fibrillation). Of patients with mitral stenosis, atrial fibrillation occurs in about 50%, and systemic emboli occur in about 10% to 20%.[1,69]

FIG. 6.51 ETIOLOGY OF CHRONIC AND ACUTE MITRAL REGURGITATION

CHRONIC REGURGITATION

Mitral leaflet prolapse (congenital, myxomatous degeneration)
Coronary artery disease
Left ventricular dilation (numerous causes)
Rheumatic fever
Calcified mitral annulus
Heritable disorders of connective tissue (Marfan's syndrome,
   Ehlers–Danlos syndrome, osteogenesis imperfecta)
Papillary muscle dysfunction (infarction)
Lupus erythematosus

ACUTE REGURGITATION

Rupture of tendinous cords (myxoma, endocarditis, trauma)
Rupture of papillary muscle (infarction, trauma)
Perforation of leaflet (endocarditis)

(Reproduced with permission; see Figure Credits)

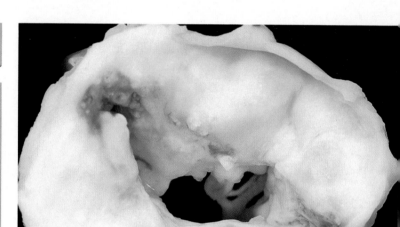

FIGURE 6.52   Resected mitral valve with leaflet retraction due to scarring secondary to rheumatic fever. Leaflet retraction is the dominant clinical feature in mitral value regurgitation. (Reproduced with permission; see Figure Credits)

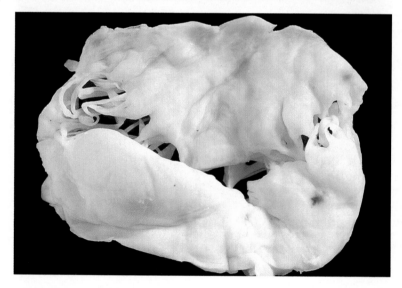

FIGURE 6.53   Resected mitral valve with prolapse of the middle scallop of the posterior leaflet due to myxomatous degeneration of the mitral valve and tendinous cords. (Reproduced with permission; see Figure Credits)

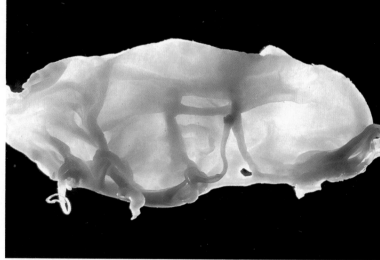

FIGURE 6.54   Undersurface of a prolapsing mitral valve leaflet demonstrating the middle scallop with ruptured cords. (Reproduced with permission; see Figure Credits)

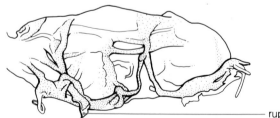

ruptured cord

Bacterial endocarditis may develop in patients with mitral stenosis. It is less frequent in patients with isolated severe stenosis than it is in those with milder degrees of stenosis associated with mitral regurgitation.

The average age of patients who are treated medically is 48 years. The survival curve of patients with mitral stenosis is shown in Figure 6.14.

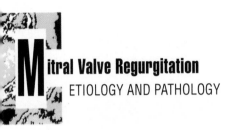

Mitral Valve Regurgitation
ETIOLOGY AND PATHOLOGY

The causes of chronic and acute mitral regurgitation are listed in Figure 6.51. Rheumatic fever is the most common cause of chronic mitral valve regurgitation; in these cases leaflet retraction usually dominates the pathologic state

(Figs. 6.52). In the Western world, mitral valve prolapse has become an important cause of regurgitation. The underlying pathology is a floppy valve characterized by myxomatous degeneration of the leaflets and tendinous cords, accompanied by dilation of the valve annulus (Fig. 6.53). Cordal rupture is a frequent complication, leading to abrupt onset of signs of left heart failure (Fig. 6.54).[15] Patients with coronary disease and its complications may have mitral regurgitation because of papillary muscle dysfunction (Fig. 6.55). Patients with cardiomyopathy may also develop mitral regurgitation as a result of left ventricular and mitral annular dilation. Acute mitral regurgitation may be due to infarction of the papillary muscle due to coronary disease, particularly when this is complicated by partial or complete rupture of the muscle (Fig. 6.56). Mitral regurgitation may also be caused by infective endocarditis (Fig. 6.57) or ruptured tendinous cords due to trauma.

PATHOPHYSIOLOGY

The amount of the left ventricular stroke volume that is ejected into the left atrium determines the extent of left atrial and left ventricular dilation.[7] Chronic mitral regurgitation produces a volume overload on the left ventricle and the

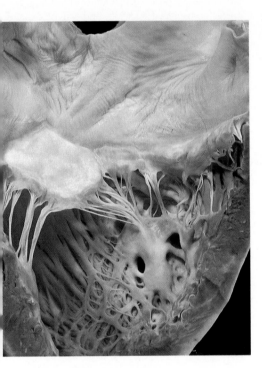

FIGURE 6.55
Scarred myocardium in the area of the posteromedial papillary muscle due to obstructive coronary heart disease. Papillary muscle dysfunction is the cause of mitral regurgitation in this case. (Reproduced with permission; see Figure Credits)

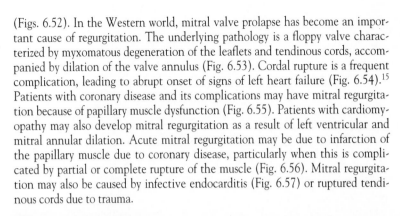

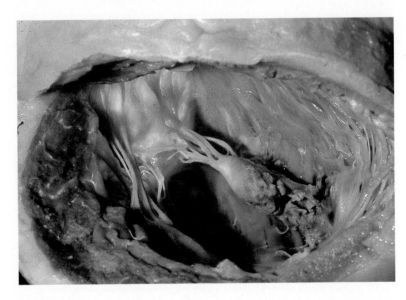

FIGURE 6.56   Acute mitral regurgitation resulting from a ruptured anterolateral papillary muscle as a complication of acute myocardial infarction. (Reproduced with permission; see Figure Credits)

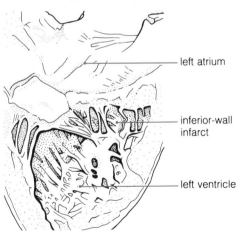

left atrium

inferior-wall infarct

left ventricle

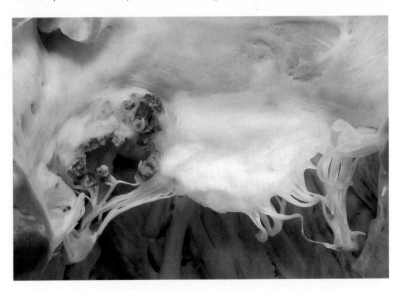

FIGURE 6.57   Infective endocarditis of the mitral valve, localized in the area of the anterolateral commissure, resulting in mitral regurgitation. (Reproduced with permission; see Figure Credits)

left atrium; the pressure also gradually rises in the left atrium, the pulmonary veins, and the pulmonary capillaries (Figs. 6.58, 6.59).

The left ventricle dilates to accommodate the increase in diastolic volume that occurs as a result of regurgitation.[53] In addition, the left ventricle remodels itself by increasing its wall thickness (see Fig. **2.6A**). During the remodeling the alignment of the tendinous cords and the papillary muscles becomes deranged, which may increase the mitral regurgitation. The left ventricular compliance increases, and the left ventricular end-diastolic pressure remains normal or slightly elevated for a long period of time.

Mitral valve prolapse is associated with large, thin leaflets, elongated cords, dilation of the valve annulus, and abnormal systolic contraction patterns of the left ventricle ranging from hyperkinesis to akinesis.[47] Regurgitation may be slight, moderate, or severe.

The magnitude of chronic regurgitation is related predominantly to the position of the valve leaflets during systole.

Patients with coronary disease may have chronic mitral regurgitation, usually due to a combination of papillary muscle dysfunction, dilation of the left ventricle, and dyskinetic motion of the posterior myocardial wall.[54]

Mitral regurgitation occurs in patients with dilated cardiomyopathy; the left ventricle dilates, and the tendinous cords and the papillary muscles have a new physical relationship to the valve leaflets.[5] The dilation of the left ventricle seems to have more influence on the amount of regurgitation than the degree of dilation of the valve annulus.

The altered physiology that results from acute mitral valve regurgitation is quite different from that produced by chronic incompetence of the valve. The abrupt development of mitral regurgitation is not associated with abrupt dilation of the atrium or the left ventricle.[42] These structures have inadequate time to adjust to the increased volume; because of this, the end-diastolic pressure of the left ventricle, the left atrial pressure, and the pulmonary artery pressure become markedly elevated. A severe pressure load is created, which is in marked contrast to the volume overload that is secondary to chronic mitral regurgitation. As stated earlier, the causes of acute mitral regurgitation are rupture of the tendinous cords due to myxomatous degeneration, infective endocarditis, trauma, and papillary muscle rupture due to myocardial infarction.

CLINICAL MANIFESTATIONS

The clinical picture that results from mitral regurgitation is determined by the amount of regurgitation, whether it is chronic, acute, or a combination of the two, and other abnormalities that may be present in the heart.

SYMPTOMS

Patients with chronic but mild mitral valve regurgitations have no symptoms.[66] Severe chronic regurgitation produces symptoms associated with heart failure, such as fatigue and dyspnea on effort.[35] Palpitation may be related to atrial fibrillation. Some patients with mitral valve prolapse have atrial and ventricular arrhythmias, chest pain of uncertain etiology, and anxiety.[73]

Patients with acute mitral regurgitation may experience the symptoms associated with abrupt and severe pulmonary edema and shock.

PHYSICAL EXAMINATION

Palpation of the precordium may be normal in patients with mild chronic regurgitation. More severe regurgitation may produce a palpable thrill at the apex, a hyperdynamic apical impulse that is displaced leftward, and a hyperdynamic anterior lift of the precordium located to the left of the sternum, secondary to abrupt dilation of the left atrium.

The murmur secondary to rheumatic mitral regurgitation is usually holosystolic; it begins with the first sound, which may be diminished in intensity because the valve leaflets may not coapt properly. The increased volume of blood entering the left ventricle during diastole produces a ventricular gallop sound. When the volume of blood is large, it causes a low-pitched, diastolic rumbling murmur at the apex. The second sound may be split abnormally, because ventricular systole is shortened and aortic valve closure occurs earlier than usual.

Patients with mitral valve prolapse have additional anomalies. Abnormalities of the chest wall may be apparent; the anteroposterior diameter of the chest may be narrow, or pectus excavatum or scoliosis may be present. Evidence of Marfan's syndrome may be obvious. The murmur may appear after an early systolic click. A change in the size of the left ventricular cavity produced by standing causes the click and the murmur to occur earlier in systole (Fig. 6.60).

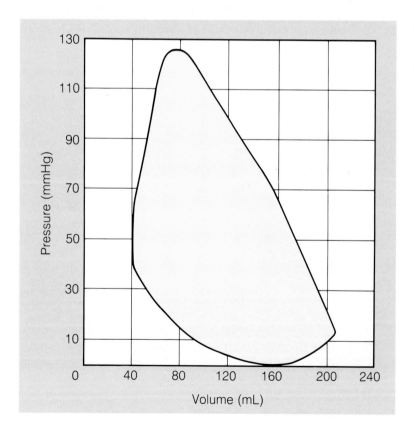

FIGURE 6.58   Left ventricular pressure–volume recording from a patient with mitral regurgitation. There is a loss of the isovolumic contraction phase on the right side of the pressure–volume loop due to the mitral valve regurgitation. The early diastolic filling is initiated by the 40 mmHg V wave in the left atrium. (Reproduced with permission; see Figure Credits)

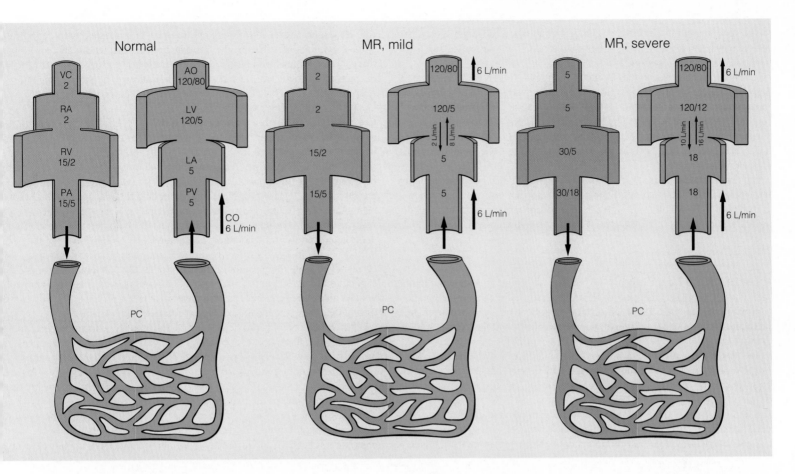

| Normal | MR, mild | MR, severe |

FIGURE 6.59 Pathophysiology of mitral regurgitation (MR). The top panel presents normal hemodynamics and the middle panel shows mild MR. There is regurgitant flow across the mitral valve of 2 L/min. Consequently, during diastole 8 L/min flow into the left ventricle—6 L/min represent right ventricular cardiac output (CO) arriving in the left atrium and 2 L/min represent the regurgitant flow that has entered the left atrium (LA) during left ventricular systole. Left-sided pressures are still normal. In the bottom panel, severe MR is depicted, with 10 L/min flowing from the left ventricle (LV) to the LA during systole. Left atrial and pulmonary venous pressures are increased to 18 mmHg. As a result, right ventricular systolic and pulmonary arterial pressures must also increase. LV end-diastolic pressure is slightly higher because of LV hypertrophy and dilation. (VC = vena cava; RA = right atrium; RV = right ventricle; PA = pulmonary artery; PC = pulmonary capillaries; PV = pulmonary veins; AO = aorta) (Redrawn with permission; see Figure Credits)

FIGURE 6.60

Phonocardiograms recorded near the apex in a patient with mitral valve prolapse. Note that a late systolic click (x) moves to a position early in systole when the patient is standing. (Reproduced with permission; see Figure Credits)

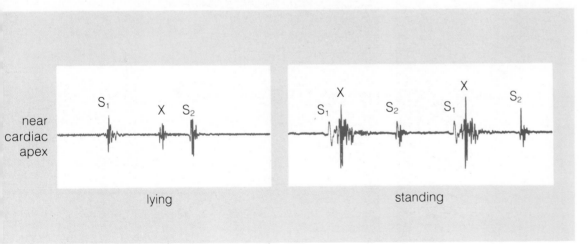

near cardiac apex

lying   standing

The systolic murmur produced by chronic regurgitation secondary to coronary disease may begin in early, mid-, or late systole, and is often associated with atrial and ventricular gallop sounds.[29]

Patients with acute regurgitation due to rupture of the tendinous cords or the papillary muscle usually exhibit signs of pulmonary edema.[62] The heart is not large, unless it was large before cordal rupture. The apical systolic murmur of ruptured tendinous cords is usually loud, radiating laterally or toward the base of the heart. It is often heard over the cervical and the thoracic areas of the spine, and it may even be heard on the top of the head and over the sacrum. An atrial gallop is usually heard.

Papillary muscle rupture due to myocardial infarction may not produce a murmur, because the infarcted ventricular muscle may not be capable of vigorous contraction.[68] A systolic murmur is usually heard as well as an atrial gallop sound. The patient may display signs of shock and pulmonary edema.

LABORATORY STUDIES

Chest Radiography   The chest film may show no abnormality when mitral regurgitation is slight. Moderate and severe mitral regurgitation may produce evidence of left atrial enlargement, left ventricular enlargement, calcification of the mitral annulus or the leaflets, and signs of heart failure (Fig. 6.61).

Electrocardiography   The ECG may be normal. When mitral regurgitation is moderately severe, the ECG usually reveals left ventricular hypertrophy, left atrial abnormality when normal rhythm is present, or atrial fibrillation.

Echocardiography   The echocardiogram may show evidence of mitral valve prolapse, calcification, increased diastolic dimensions of the left ventricle, systolic wall-motion abnormalities, and an increase in size of the left atrium. Acute mitral regurgitation may be associated with echocardiographic abnormalities that can be attributed to ruptured tendinous cords, a papillary muscle rupture, or a perforated valve leaflet. The cross-sectional echocardiogram of a patient with mitral regurgitation may reveal a prolapsing anterior mitral leaflet (Fig. 6.62). Mitral regurgitation can also be detected by the Doppler technique (Figs. 6.63–6.65).

Cardiac Catheterization   Cardiac catheterization is used to assess ventricular function, to identify other cardiac abnormalities, and to determine the presence or absence of coronary disease.

An abnormal V wave may be seen in the pulmonary wedge pressure tracing. Left ventricular function can be determined by measuring the end-diastolic pressure and the ejection fraction and estimating the amount of blood that is regurgitated (Fig. 6.66). Quantitative angiography may be used to measure left ventricular stroke volume, which is identified as the difference between end-diastolic and end-systolic volumes. The end-diastolic volume may be increased but the ejection fraction may be normal until left ventricular dysfunction occurs. Eventually the pressure in the left atrium, the pulmonary veins, and the capillaries becomes elevated. The ratio of end-systolic wall stress to end-systolic volume index can be computed; this measure of left ventricular function can be used to determine the likelihood of postoperative improvement.

Left ventriculography also detects mitral valve prolapse and associated anomalies, such as wall-motion abnormalities (Fig. 6.67). It must be emphasized that minor degrees of mitral valve prolapse are not detected with this technique.

Mitral regurgitation secondary to coronary artery disease is usually associated with left ventricular dilation and abnormal posterior wall motion usually located at the base of the papillary muscle.

The left atrial V wave may be huge; it is often identified during the insertion of a Swan–Ganz catheter to the wedge position in patients with acute mitral regurgitation.[42] The left ventricular angiogram reveals a large amount of regurgi-

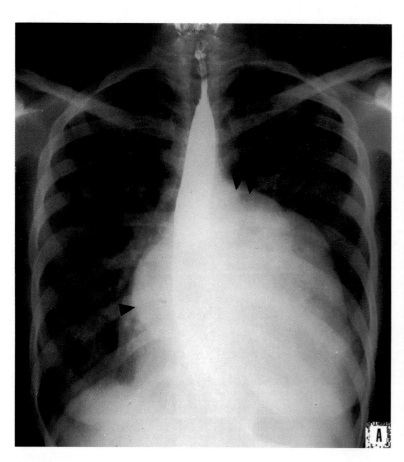
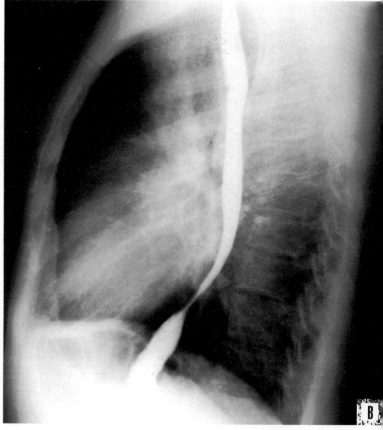

FIGURE 6.61   **(A)** Posteroanterior chest radiograph of the barium-filled esophagus of a patient with rheumatic mitral regurgitation. Cardiomegaly is present, with the left ventricle extending toward the lateral chest wall. The enlarged left atrium can be seen as a double density (*single arrow*), and the pulmonary artery segment (*double arrows*) is prominent. **(B)** Lateral view reveals the large left atrium. (Reproduced with permission; see Figure Credits)

tation into the left atrium and the pulmonary veins when there is severe mitral valve regurgitation.

Radionuclide Studies Radionuclide ventriculography can used to identify the resting (Fig. 6.68) and exercise ejection fractions.

Thallium scans can be used to exclude myocardial ischemia in patients with mitral valve prolapse, since stress exercise ECGs often yield false positive results for ischemia.

NATURAL HISTORY

The natural history and prognosis depend on the etiology of the condition. Patients with chronic mitral regurgitation may have no symptoms for many years. The pressure in the pulmonary veins may not rise and the ejection fraction may be normal, because left atrial compliance remains normal, protecting the lungs. The left atrium may actually become "giant-sized" and the patient may not be severely disabled. Atrial fibrillation may develop and systemic emboli may occur, although not as often as with mitral stenosis. Endocarditis may occur, producing further valve damage. The survival curve of patients with chronic mitral regurgitation is shown in Figure 6.14.

Patients with mitral valve prolapse may have atrial and ventricular arrhythmias that do not correlate with the severity of the anatomic abnormality. The prognosis is excellent in most patients with prolapse; a small percentage have sudden death, ruptured tendinous cords, endocarditis, or heart failure.

The prognosis of patients with mitral valve regurgitation due to coronary disease depends on the state of the myocardium, the degree of coronary disease, and the amount of regurgitation.[66]

Acute mitral valve regurgitation is serious and may lead to shock, pulmonary edema, and death. Although the majority of patients die, an increasing number have improved prognoses through surgery.

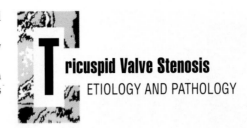

Tricuspid Valve Stenosis

ETIOLOGY AND PATHOLOGY

Tricuspid valve stenosis may be congenital in origin. Usually it is part of a more complex cardiac malformation, leading to symptoms early in life (see Chapter 7). An exception is Ebstein's malformation, which can occasionally produce tricuspid stenosis, although regurgitation more commonly dominates. While rheumatic fever may affect the tricuspid valve, it is extremely uncommon that this progresses to valve stenosis.[10] Other rare conditions, such as the carcinoid syndrome, may affect the tricuspid valve to such an extent that stenosis occurs (Fig. 6.69). Blockade of the tricuspid valve may be due to right atrial myxoma (Fig. 6.70), other neoplasms, or thrombi. Tricuspid valve stenosis may be the result of the thrombotic obstruction of a tricuspid valve prosthesis.

PATHOPHYSIOLOGY

The normal area of the tricuspid valve is 7 cm². The flow of blood from the right atrium into the right ventricle is impeded when the valve area is reduced to 1.5 cm². An elevation of the right atrial pressure to 10 mmHg is usually associated with peripheral edema (Fig. 6.71). The cardiac output falls with significant tricuspid stenosis.[17] When the condition is due to rheumatic fever, it is usually associated with mitral valve disease, which may also play a role in the altered hemodynamics.

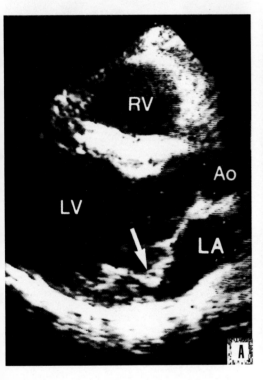
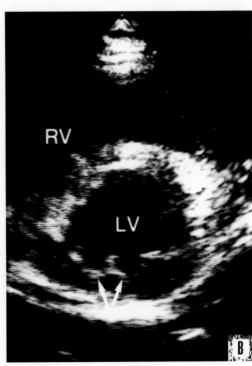
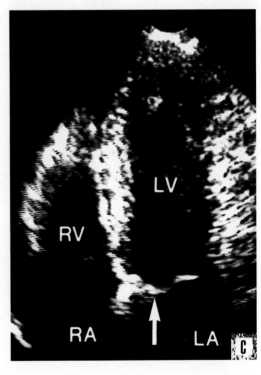

FIGURE 6.62 **(A)** Cross-sectional echocardiogram from a patient with severe mitral valve prolapse. (Most cases are mild.) On the parasternal long-axis view in systole, the anterior and posterior leaflets arch posteriorly (arrow), above the level of the atrioventricular groove and behind the normal coaptation point into the left atrium. **(B)** Parasternal short-axis view at the level of the mitral valve and the left ventricular outflow tract in systole shows the anterior leaflet buckling posteriorly (arrows). **(C)** The apical four-chamber view in systole shows the classic image of a prolapsing anterior mitral leaflet (arrow). (RV = right ventricle; LV = left ventricle; Ao = aorta; RA = right atrium; LA = left atrium) (Reproduced with permission; see Figure Credits)

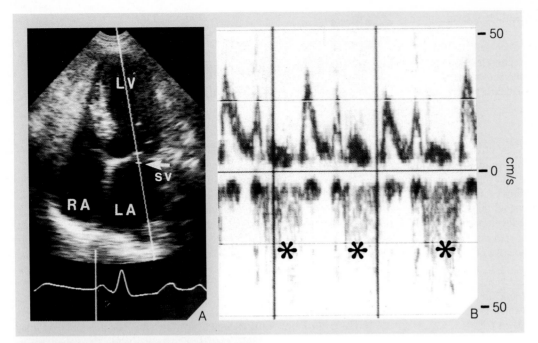

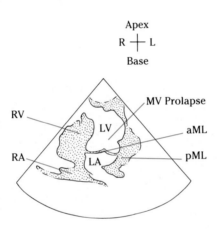

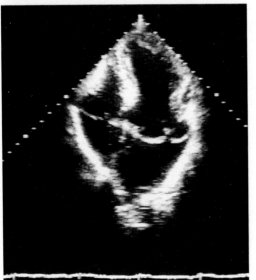

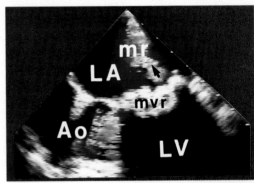

FIGURE 6.63 Mitral regurgitation examined from the apical approach in Doppler recording. **(A)** The sample volume (SV, arrow) is positioned just to the left of the left atrial (LA) side of the closed mitral leaflets in systole. **(B)** The flow waveform shows the laminar diastolic emptying of the left atrium; a systolic flow disturbance (asterisks) is diagnostic of mitral regurgitation. (LV = left ventricle; RA = right atrium) (Reproduced with permission; see Figure Credits)

Apex
R ┼ L
Base

FIGURE 6.65 Transesophageal echocardiogram demonstrating paravalvular mitral regurgitation (*arrow*, mr) emanating from the sewing ring of a tilting-disc prosthesis (mvr). (Ao = aortic valve; LA = left atrium; LV = left ventricle) (Reproduced with permission; see Figure Credits)

FIGURE 6.64 Four-chamber echocardiographic view of patient with both mitral and tricuspid prolapse. Note that the posterior mitral valve leaflet (pML) is elongated. Since both the anterior and posterior leaflets (aML, pML) prolapse, the valve has a moustache appearance. (Reproduced with permission; see Figure Credits)

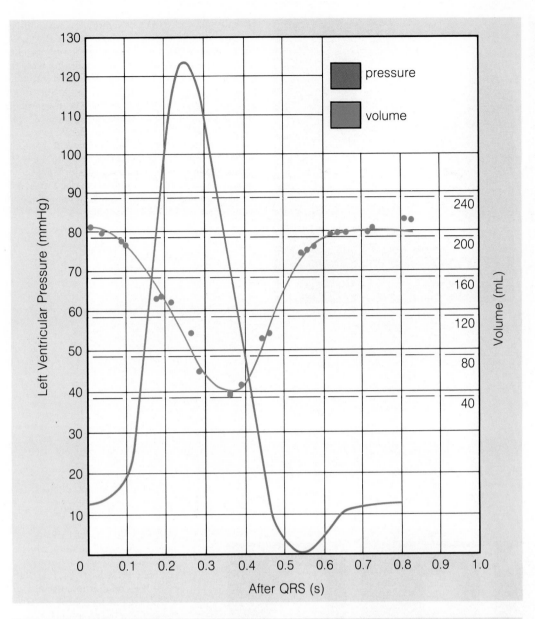

FIGURE 6.66   Left ventricular pressure and volume in a patient with mitral regurgitation. (Reproduced with permission; see Figure Credits)

end-diastolic volume	208 mL
end-systolic volume	42 mL
left ventricular stroke volume	166 mL
forward stroke volume	30 mL
regurgitant stroke volume	136 mL
ejection fraction	166/208 = 80%
left ventricular weight	247 g
left ventricular end-diastolic pressure	14 mmHg

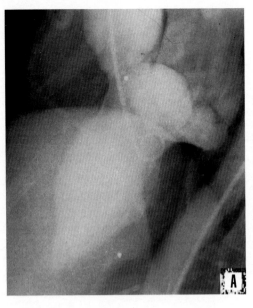

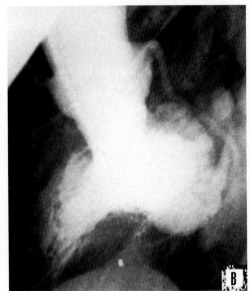

FIGURE 6.67 **(A)** Left ventriculogram in the left anterior oblique view of a prolapsed mitral valve with mitral insufficiency. The anterior and posterior mitral leaflets protrude into the left atrium. Note the opacification of the left atrium, indicating insufficiency of the mitral valve. The density of the left atrium is less than that of the left ventricle. **(B)** Left ventricular angiogram in the left anterior oblique view of a prolapsed mitral valve without mitral insufficiency (shown in the systolic phase). The anterior and posterior mitral leaflets prolapse superiorly into the left atrium. (In this projection, the posterior leaflet appears as a semicircular collection of contrast material surrounding the anterior leaflet.) (Reproduced with permission; see Figure Credits)

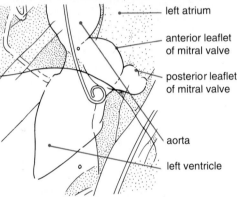

left atrium

anterior leaflet
of mitral valve

posterior leaflet
of mitral valve

aorta

left ventricle

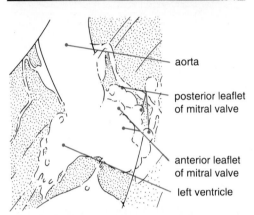

aorta

posterior leaflet
of mitral valve

anterior leaflet
of mitral valve

left ventricle

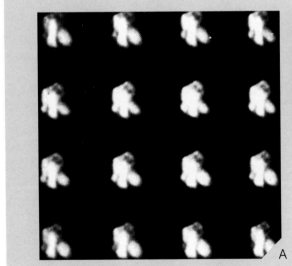

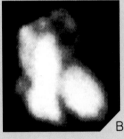

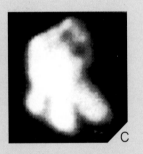

left ventricular ejection fraction 29%
right ventricular ejection fraction 7%

FIGURE 6.68 **(A)** Sixteen frames of a gated equilibrium radionuclide angiogram from a patient with severe mitral regurgitation. The end-diastolic **(B)** and end-systolic **(C)** images show left ventricular and right ventricular dysfunction. The pulmonary artery wedge pressure in the patient was 29 mmHg, and the pulmonary artery pressure was 60/30 mmHg. The pulmonary artery, the right atrium, and the left atrium are prominent. (Reproduced with permission; see Figure Credits)

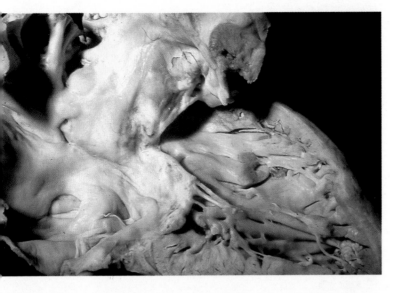

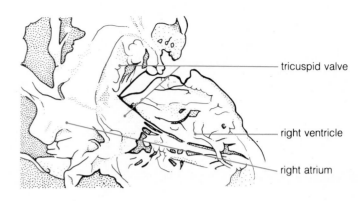

tricuspid valve

right ventricle

right atrium

FIGURE 6.69   Carcinoid syndrome affecting the tricuspid valve. Valve thickening and partial immobilization may cause regurgitation and often stenosis. (Reproduced with permission; see Figure Credits)

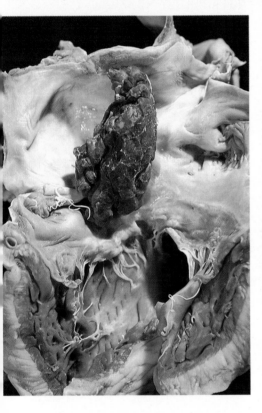

FIGURE 6.70   A right atrial myxoma obstructing the tricuspid orifice. (Reproduced with permission; see Figure Credits)

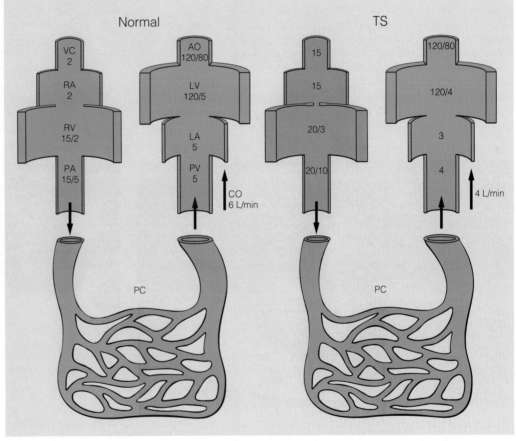

FIGURE 6.71   Pathophysiology of tricuspid stenosis (TS). The upper panel presents normal hemodynamics and the lower panel demonstrates severe TS. During diastole, there is a 12-mm gradient (right atrial pressure of 15 mmHg; right ventricular pressure of 3 mmHg) across the tricuspid valve. The marked increase in right atrial pressure is transmitted to the central veins. Pulmonary areterial and left-sided pressures are normal. The stenotic lesion results in a decrease in right ventricular filling and a resultant decrease in forward cardiac output (CO to 4 L/min). (VC = vena cava; RA = right atrium; RV = right ventricle; PA = pulmonary artery; PC = pulmonary capillaries; PV = pulmonary veins; LV = left atrium; left ventricle; AO= aorta) (Redrawn with permission; see Figure Credits)

CLINICAL MANIFESTATIONS
SYMPTOMS

Patients with significant tricuspid stenosis experience fatigue and dyspnea. Tricuspid stenosis may, to some degree, protect the lungs in patients with mitral stenosis.[39] The patient may notice large a waves in the internal jugular venous pulse.

PHYSICAL EXAMINATION

A large a wave may be detected by the examiner in the internal jugular venous pulse. The right ventricle is not palpable. Respiratory variation in splitting of the second heart sound may be absent, since right ventricular filling remains fairly constant throughout the respiratory cycle.

The tricuspid component of the first sound may be louder than normal. A diastolic rumble that becomes louder with inspiration may be heard at the end of the left sternal border. An opening snap may also be heard.

The physical signs of aortic and/or mitral valve disease are often present and may in fact mask the physical signs of tricuspid stenosis.

LABORATORY STUDIES

Chest Radiography The right atrium may be large, and calcium may be seen in the tricuspid valve leaflets or annulus.[49]
Electrocardiography The P waves may become large, or atrial fibrillation may be present. Congenital tricuspid atresia may produce left ventricular hypertrophy in the ECG, but acquired isolated tricuspid stenosis is not associated with right or left ventricular hypertrophy.
Echocardiography The echocardiogram (Figs. 6.72, 6.73) and the Doppler technique (Fig. 6.74) may be used to identify tricuspid stenosis.
Cardiac Catheterization The pressure gradient between the right ventricle and the right atrium is normally less than 1 mmHg.[38] The gradient is elevated in patients with tricuspid stenosis; however, small gradients may not be detected. The tricuspid valve area in patients with tricuspid stenosis is less than 1.5 cm². (Congenital tricuspid atresia is discussed in Chapter 7. An atrial septal defect is always present in such patients.)

NATURAL HISTORY

The natural history depends on the etiology of the tricuspid valve blockade. Rheumatic tricuspid valve disease is usually associated with mitral stenosis, and the natural history depends more on the severity of the mitral valve disease. Some observers believe that pulmonary congestion is less and that peripheral edema dominates the clinical picture when both mitral and tricuspid stenosis are present. The presence of tricuspid stenosis may lead one to underestimate the degree of mitral stenosis.

The natural history of tricuspid stenosis in patients with carcinoid syndrome is determined by the other aspects of the syndrome and the degree of stenosis of the valve, which, in general, progresses slowly.

Tricuspid Valve Regurgitation
ETIOLOGY AND PATHOLOGY

Tricuspid valve regurgitation is usually secondary to right ventricular dilation and heart failure caused by disease of the left side of the heart.

Bacterial endocarditis, particularly in drug addicts, is the most common cause of isolated regurgitation of the tricuspid valve (Fig. 6.75). Other causes include myocardial infarction, which may cause right ventricular overload leading to regurgitation or, rarely, rupture of the septal papillary muscles to the tricuspid valve (Fig. 6.76), carcinoid syndrome (see Figs. 6.69, 6.73), prolapse of the tri-

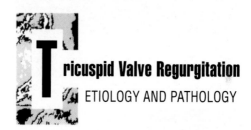

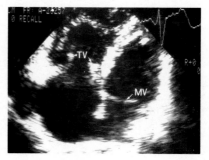

FIGURE 6.73
Echocardiogram of carcinoid heart disease and tricuspid insufficiency/tricuspid stenosis. Note that the right ventricle is apex-forming and that the right atrium dwarfs the left. The tricuspid (TV) is thickened. The characteristic of this stubby, thickened, and practically immobilized valve is that it has greatly limited mobility and remains partially opened during systole. (Reproduced with permission; see Figure Credits)

FIGURE 6.72 Cross-sectional echocardiogram in the apical four-chamber view from a child with a severely stenotic tricuspid valve. The tricuspid annulus (T) is smaller than the mitral annulus (M). The right ventricle (RV) is diminutive; the tricuspid leaflets open down-wise. The right atrium (RA) is enlarged. (LV = left ventricle) (Reproduced with permission; see Figure Credits)

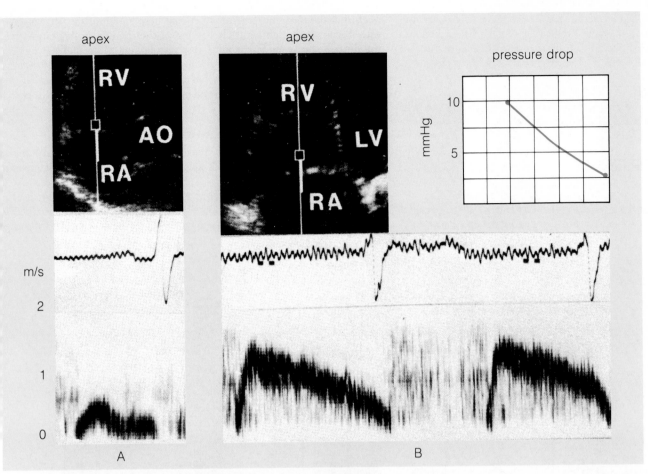

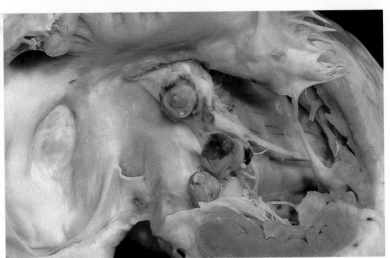

FIGURE 6.75   Infective endocarditis in a drug addict leading to isolated tricuspid valve regurgitation. (Reproduced with permission; see Figure Credits)

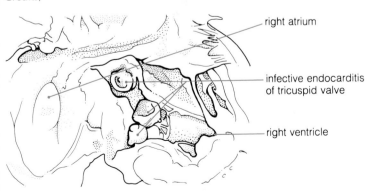

- right atrium
- infective endocarditis of tricuspid valve
- right ventricle

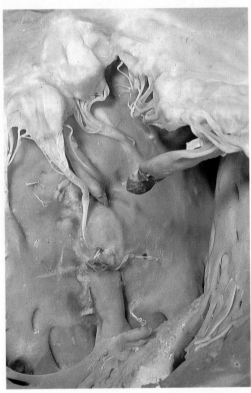

cuspid valve particularly in patients with Marfan's syndrome, and congenital heart disease, such as ostium primum atrioventricular septal defect or Ebstein's malformation. Trauma with laceration of the tricuspid valve apparatus or a faulty prosthetic tricuspid valve may also cause tricuspid valve regurgitation.

PATHOPHYSIOLOGY

Tricuspid valve regurgitation during systole produces an increase in the right atrial pressure and a large V wave in the right atrial pressure curve and in the internal jugular vein (Fig. 6.77).[26]

CLINICAL MANIFESTATIONS
SYMPTOMS

Tricuspid regurgitation that is secondary to right ventricular dilation related to left-sided heart disease is associated with dyspnea and fatigue. Paroxysmal nocturnal dyspnea and pulmonary edema may be diminished in patients with disease of the left ventricle because of the tricuspid regurgitation, but the decrease in symptoms is more likely to be due to an increase in pulmonary arteriolar resistance. Patients who have bacterial endocarditis involving the tricuspid valve may have fever and fatigue. Patients with the carcinoid syndrome have flushing and other features of this unusual disease.

PHYSICAL EXAMINATION

Atrial fibrillation is often present. Tricuspid regurgitation produces a large V wave in the internal jugular venous pulse. The liver may be large and pulsate with each systole.

A holosystolic murmur may be heard at the lower end of the sternum; it may increase in intensity with inspiration. An opening snap of the tricuspid valve may be heard on rare occasion. The pulmonary component of the second sound

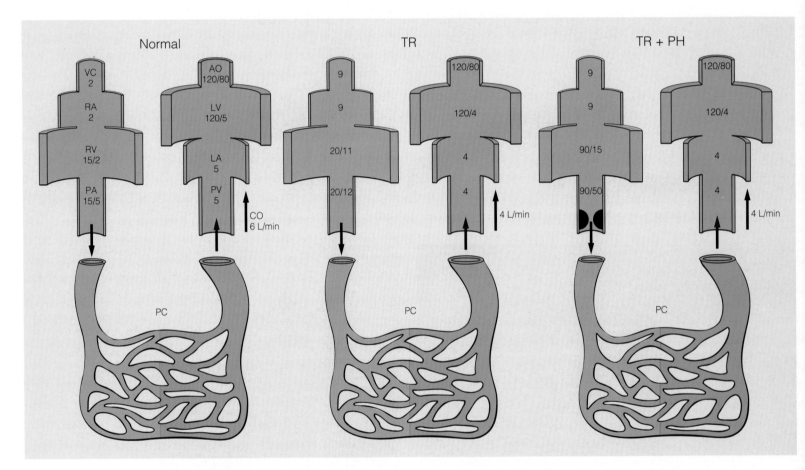

FIGURE 6.77 Pathophysiology of tricuspid regurgitation (TR). The top panel presents normal hemodynamics and the middle panel demonstrates a case of TR without PH. There is severe regurgitation across the tricuspid valve during right ventricular systole. Consequently, right atrial and central venous pressures are elevated. Right ventricular diastolic pressure increases, the right ventricle (RV) dilates, and forward cardiac output (CO) is reduced to 4 L/min. In the bottom panel, TR secondary to PH is depicted. Severe PH is present, and the RV has dilated and hypertrophied in response to the remarkable increase in pulmonary arterial pressure. Severe TR results with consequent elevation in central venous and right atrial pressures. Forward CO is reduced to 4 L/min. Left heart pressures are unaltered. (VC = vena cava; RA = right atrium; PA = pulmonary artery; PC = pulmonary capillaries; PV = pulmonary veins; LA = left atrium; LV = left ventricle; AO= aorta) (Redrawn with permission; see Figure Credits)

may be louder than normal, and the murmur of pulmonary regurgitation may be heard in patients with tricuspid regurgitation associated with pulmonary hypertension. Signs of additional valve disease or myocardial disease are usually evident in patients with tricuspid valve regurgitation.

LABORATORY STUDIES

Chest Radiography   Chest films of patients with secondary tricuspid regurgitation reveal the abnormalities of the primary heart disease, including right atrial enlargement. The chest film of a patient with tricuspid regurgitation due to endocarditis may show only right atrial enlargement (Fig. 6.78).

Electrocardiography   The ECG of a patient with secondary tricuspid regurgitation may reveal abnormal P waves and right, left, and combined ventricular hypertrophy that reflects the primary heart disease. Right or left bundle branch block may be present in patients with severe heart disease. Atrial fibrillation may be detected.

The ECG of a patient with primary tricuspid regurgitation may show a right atrial abnormality.

Echocardiography   Systolic prolapse of the tricuspid valve may be detected on the echocardiogram. Valvular calcification and an increase in the left and right ventricular dimensions may be noted. Vegetations on the tricuspid valve may also be identified by echocardiography in patients with endocarditis (Fig. 6.79). Doppler studies reveal the extent of the regurgitant jet (Fig. 6.80).

Cardiac Catheterization   A prominent V wave in the right atrial pressure curve indicates tricuspid regurgitation.

Catheterization may reveal abnormalities of the aortic and the mitral valves, evidence of dilated cardiomyopathy including ischemic cardiomyopathy, and coronary disease.

Angiographic evidence of tricuspid regurgitation is difficult to demonstrate, unless it is severe, since the catheter itself may produce an incompetent tricuspid valve (Fig. 6.81).

NATURAL HISTORY

Secondary tricuspid regurgitation is a marker of severe, advanced heart disease; the natural history is that of the causative disease of the left side of the heart.

The natural history of primary tricuspid regurgitation due to endocarditis is that of endocarditis plus the associated hemodynamic alteration. The condition is lethal unless antibiotic and surgical therapy is implemented in a timely fashion.

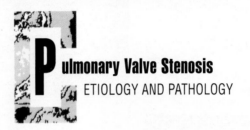

Pulmonary Valve Stenosis
ETIOLOGY AND PATHOLOGY

Pulmonary valve stenosis is almost always due to congenital heart disease (see Chapter 7), although it may be related to the carcinoid syndrome.[34] When due to carcinoid, the leaflets become immobilized due to a proliferation of connective tissue on the arterial side of the cusps (Fig. 6.82).

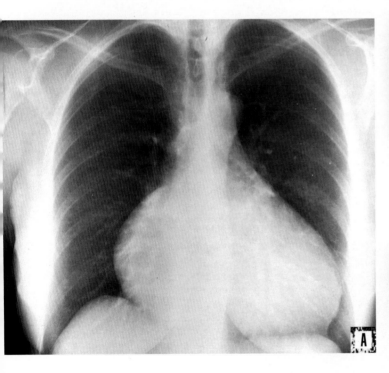

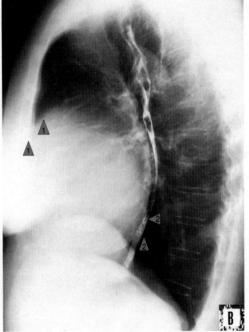

FIGURE 6.78
Posteroanterior (**A**) and lateral (**B**) chest x-rays of severe tricuspid insufficiency. Note the markedly enlarged right atrium, which projects to the right and anteriorly (*arrows 1, B*). The enlarged right ventricle displaces the left ventricle posteriorly (*arrows 2, B*), mimicking left ventricular enlargement. (Reproduced with permission; see Figure Credits)

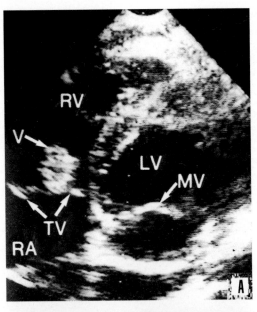
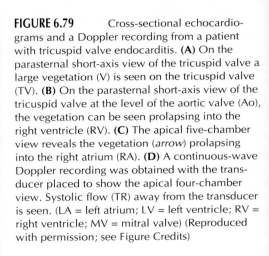

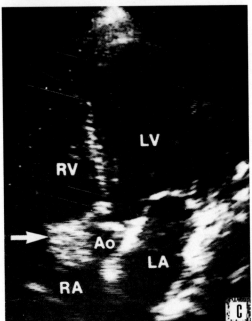
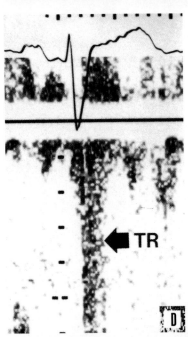

FIGURE 6.79 Cross-sectional echocardiograms and a Doppler recording from a patient with tricuspid valve endocarditis. **(A)** On the parasternal short-axis view of the tricuspid valve a large vegetation (V) is seen on the tricuspid valve (TV). **(B)** On the parasternal short-axis view of the tricuspid valve at the level of the aortic valve (Ao), the vegetation can be seen prolapsing into the right ventricle (RV). **(C)** The apical five-chamber view reveals the vegetation (*arrow*) prolapsing into the right atrium (RA). **(D)** A continuous-wave Doppler recording was obtained with the transducer placed to show the apical four-chamber view. Systolic flow (TR) away from the transducer is seen. (LA = left atrium; LV = left ventricle; RV = right ventricle; MV = mitral valve) (Reproduced with permission; see Figure Credits)

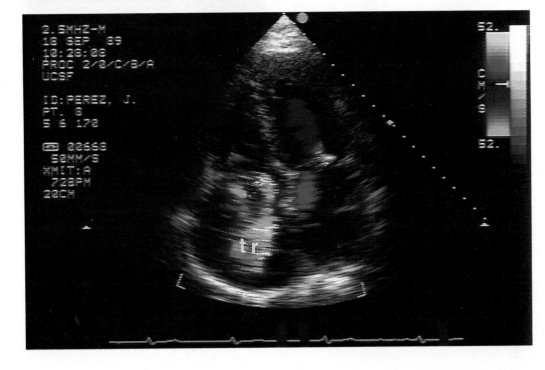

FIGURE 6.80 Severe tricuspid regurgitation (tr) shown through colorflow Doppler. The blue jet emanates from two different sites on the tricuspid valve and fills most of the enlarged right atrium. (Reproduced with permission; see Figure Credits)

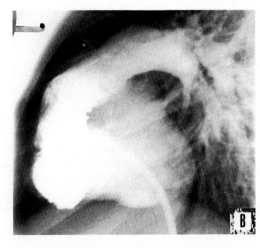

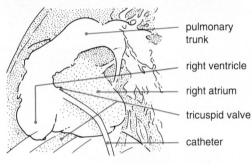

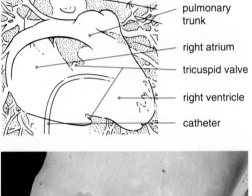

FIGURE 6.81 Frontal **(A)** and lateral **(B)** projections of right ventriculogram showing severe tricuspid insufficiency. Note the complete, dense opacification of the right atrium, indicating the severe condition. Because the catheter, which is advanced from the right atrium, may interfere with valve closure, the degree of tricuspid insufficiency is often exaggerated on venous angiograms. (Reproduced with permission; see Figure Credits)

pulmonary trunk

right atrium

tricuspid valve

right ventricle

catheter

pulmonary trunk

right ventricle

right atrium

tricuspid valve

catheter

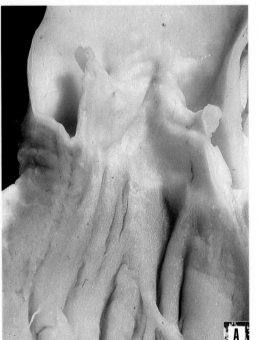

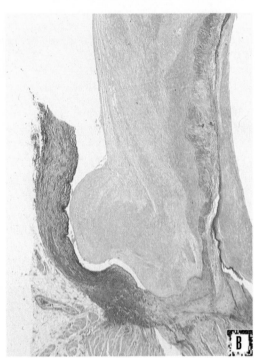

FIGURE 6.82 **(A)** Pulmonary valve stenosis due to carcinoid syndrome. The pulmonary valve shows marked thickening. **(B)** Histologic section shows the deposition of collagenous material on the arterial side of the valve cusp, underlying immobilization and stenosis (elastic tissue stain counterstained with van Gieson's stain). (Reproduced with permission; see Figure Credits)

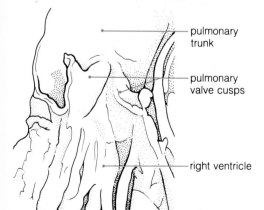

pulmonary trunk

pulmonary valve cusps

right ventricle

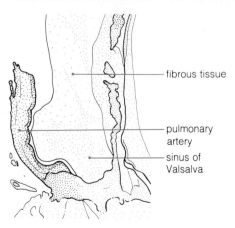

fibrous tissue

pulmonary artery

sinus of Valsalva

PATHOPHYSIOLOGY

A discussion of the abnormal physiology of pulmonary valve stenosis can be found in the relevant section under "Pulmonary Stenosis" in Chapter 7 (Fig. 6.83).

CLINICAL MANIFESTATIONS
SYMPTOMS

Patients with the carcinoid syndrome and pulmonary valve stenosis exhibit episodes of flushing, and less commonly diarrhea and asthma. (The symptoms associated with congenital pulmonary valve stenosis are discussed in Chapter 7.)

PHYSICAL EXAMINATION

The patient with carcinoid syndrome may have telangiectasia, and enlarged liver, flushing, wheezing, and systolic murmur heard in the second intercostal space to the left of the sternum. The pulmonary component of the second sound may be delayed and decreased in intensity.(The abnormalities associated with congenital pulmonary valve stenosis are discussed in Chapter 7.)

LABORATORY STUDIES

Chest Radiography   The pulmonary trunk may be prominent on chest radiographs of patients with pulmonary valve stenosis due to the carcinoid syndrome. (For the chest film in patients with congenital pulmonary valve stenosis see Chapter 7.)
Electrocardiography   The ECG of a patient with pulmonary valve stenosis associated with the carcinoid syndrome may show prominent right atrial P waves and right-axis deviation of the mean QRS vector. (For the ECG of patients with congenital pulmonary stenosis, see Chapter 7.)
Echocardiography   The echocardiogram may reveal pulmonary valve stenosis in patients with the carcinoid syndrome.
  (For the echocardiogram of a patient with congenital pulmonary valve stenosis, see Chapter 7.)
Cardiac Catheterization   Pulmonary valve stenosis is identified when there is a pressure gradient across the pulmonary valve. Angiographic studies on patients with the carcinoid syndrome may reveal decreased contractility of the right ventricle.
Special Laboratory Tests   When the carcinoid syndrome is suspected, the urine should be examined for the presence of 5-hydroxyindoleacetic acid.

NATURAL HISTORY
The natural history of the patient with the carcinoid syndrome depends on the site of the tumor, the extent of metastases, and the degree of heart damage. (The natural history of a patient with congenital pulmonary valve stenosis is discussed in Chapter 7.)

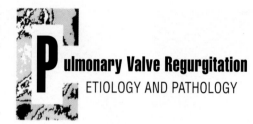

Pulmonary Valve Regurgitation
ETIOLOGY AND PATHOLOGY

Pulmonary valve regurgitation may be associated with congenital pulmonary valve stenosis (see Chapter 7) or pulmonary hypertension. Primary pulmonary hypertension occurs without obvious cause. Pulmonary hypertension may be due to congenital heart disease, including ventricular or atrial septal defect, or a patent arterial duct. Acquired causes of pulmonary hypertension include rheumatic mitral stenosis (in which the murmur of pulmonary regurgitation is referred to as a Graham Steell murmur), severe chronic lung disease, pulmonary emboli, and primary pulmonary hypertension. Pulmonary valve regurgitation may be associated with an atrial septal defect when the pulmonary blood flow is large and the pulmonary pressure is only slightly elevated. The murmur of pulmonary valve regurgitation may be heard in patients who undergo chronic renal dialysis. Pulmonary valve regurgitation may be caused by carcinoid involvement of the pulmonary valve or by previous surgery on the valve. Bacterial endocarditis may involve the pulmonary valve, producing incompetence.

PATHOPHYSIOLOGY
Pulmonary valve regurgitation produces a volume overload of the right ventricle; this alone can usually be tolerated without producing heart failure.[29] Since most of the causes of pulmonary valve regurgitation are associated with right ventricular hypertension, the volume load is superimposed on the pressure load, which is the cause of right ventricular hypertrophy (Fig. 6.84).

CLINICAL MANIFESTATIONS
SYMPTOMS

Pulmonary valve regurgitation itself rarely causes any symptoms. When present, symptoms are usually related to the causative disease and to pulmonary arteriolar disease. Patients with pulmonary hypertension may experience dyspnea, syncope, and even sudden death.

PHYSICAL EXAMINATION

When pulmonary valve regurgitation is secondary to some other type of heart disease, the abnormalities found on physical examination are those of the primary disease.

When pulmonary valve regurgitation is caused by pulmonary hypertension, the second component of the second heart sound is louder than normal. A high-pitched, decrescendo, diastolic murmur may be heard along the left sternal border. The murmur immediately follows the second heart sound. It is difficult to differentiate this murmur from the murmur of aortic valve regurgitation.

When pulmonary valve regurgitation is due to heart disease that is associated with normal or low pulmonary arterial pressure, it produces a low-pitched, descrescendo, diastolic murmur, which is heard along the left sternal border. The pulmonary component of the second sound may be normal or decreased in intensity. The murmur may not immediately follow the second heart sound.

LABORATORY STUDIES

Chest Radiography The chest films of patients with secondary pulmonary valve regurgitation reveal the characteristics of the primary disease. The chest films of patients with primary pulmonary valve regurgitation may be normal, or they may reveal a large pulmonary trunk with or without enlargement of the right ventricle and right atrium.

Electrocardiography The ECG reveals the abnormalities associated with the heart disease responsible for secondary pulmonary regur-

gitation. The ECG of a patient with pulmonary regurgitation due to primary pulmonary hypertension may show right atrial abnormality and other features signifying right ventricular hypertrophy.

Echocardiography M-mode and cross-sectional echocardiograms of a patient with pulmonary hypertension and valve regurgitation are shown in Figure 6.85. The Doppler technique is an excellent method of identifying pulmonary regurgitation (Figs. 6.86, 6.87); mild regurgitant flow may be recorded in normal subjects.[43]

Cardiac Catheterization Pulmonary valve regurgitation cannot be detected by pressure measurements, but the features of the heart disease that is responsible for pulmonary valve regurgitation may be detected. It is also difficult to demonstrate pulmonary valve regurgitation by angiography.

NATURAL HISTORY

The natural history of patients with secondary pulmonary valve regurgitation is that of the heart disease responsible for it. The natural history of patients with primary pulmonary valve regurgitation due to endocarditis or carcinoid is also that of the primary disease.

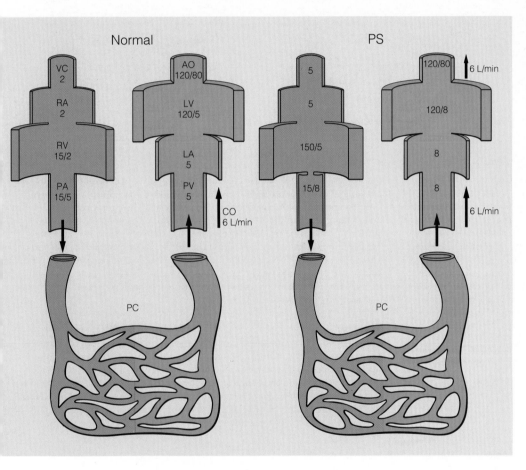

FIGURE 6.83 Pathophysiology of pulmonary valve stenosis (PS). The upper panel presents normal hemodynamics and the lower panel depicts severe PS. Thre is a 135-mm gradient across the pulmonic valve (right ventricular systolic pressure of 150 mmHg; pulmonary arterial systolic pressure of 15 mmHg). This marked increase in right ventricular pressure work results in dilatation and hypertrophy of that chamber. There is a modest increase in right ventricular diastolic pressure (5 mmHG), which is transmitted to the right atrium (RA) and central vein. Left-sided pressures are normal. The right ventricle (RV) has not failed and therefore forward cardiac output (CO) remains normal at 6 L/min. (VC = vena cava; PA = pulmonary artery; PC = pulmonary capillaries; PV = pulmonary veins; LA = left atrium; LV = left ventricle; AO = aorta) (Redrawn with permission; see Figure Credits)

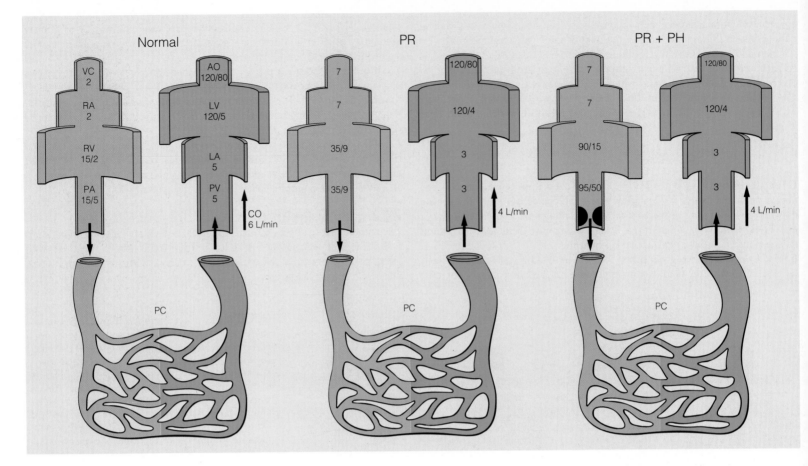

FIGURE 6.84   Pathophysiology of pulmonic regurgitation (PR). The top panel presents normal hemodynamics and the middle panel depicts PR without pulmonary hypertension (PH). Right ventricular diastolic and pulmonary arterial diastolic pressures are equal because of the communication between these two chambers during diastole. There is moderate dilatation and hypertrophy of the right ventricle (RV), with subsequent elevation in right ventricular diastolic pressure. Increased right ventricular diastolic pressure is transmitted to the right atrium (RA) and central veins. Right ventricular systolic output and pressure are increased because of the increase in diastolic filling from the regurgitation. Left-sided pressures are normal. There is a modest decrease in forward cardiac output (CO). The bottom panel depicts PR sec-ondary to severe PH. A variety of conditions may result under such severe circumstances. Marked right ventricular hypertrophy and dilatation result from the marked pressure and volume overload. The pulmonic valve is insufficient as a result of the marked increase in pulmonary artery pressure. Right ventricular diastolic pressure is elevated and this elevation is transmitted to the RA and central veins. Left-sided pressures are normal. Forward CO is reduced because of the reduction in right ventricular stroke volume. (VC = vena cava; PC = pulmonary capillaries; PV = pulmonary veins; PA = pulmonary arteries; LA = left atrium; LV = left ventricle; AO = aorta) (Redrawn with permission; see Figure Credits)

FIGURE 6.85   Cross-sectional **(A)** and M-mode **(B)** echocardiograms from a patient with pulmonary valve regurgitation due to primary pulmonary hypertension. **(A)** The parasternal short-axis view of the pulmonary valve (PV) shows a dilated main pulmonary artery (PA). **(B)** An M-mode tracing of the pulmonary valve demonstrates the absence of the a **AU: "A" INSTEAD?** wave and premature closing of the pulmonary valve referred to as a "notch" (*arrow*). (Ao = aorta) (Reproduced with permission; see Figure Credits)

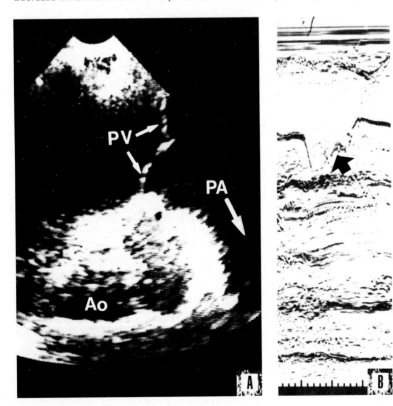

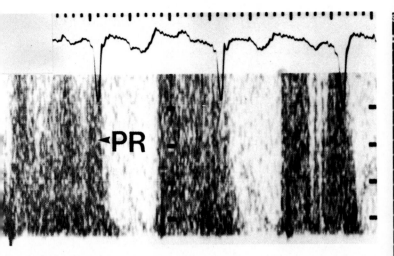

FIGURE 6.86 Parasternal short-axis view of a continuous-wave Doppler recording from a patient with pulmonary regurgitation. Diastolic flow (PR) is recorded flowing toward the transducer. (Reproduced with permission; see Figure Credits)

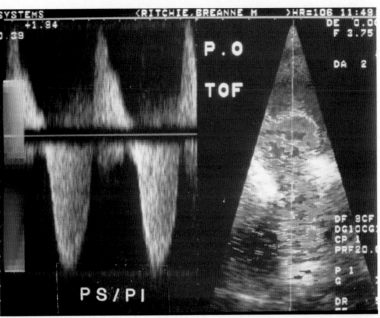

FIGURE 6.87 Color-flow mapping demonstrating flow acceleration and turbulence in an extracardiac conduit with moderate residual pulmonary outflow obstruction and pulmonary insufficiency. This is characteristic of an adequate result after tetralogy repair. (Reproduced with permission; see Figure Credits)

ACKNOWLEDGEMENT

This chapter is based in part on Rackley CE, Edwards JE, Wallace RB, et al: Aortic valve disease; Rackley CE, Edwards JE, Karp RB: Mitral valve disease; Rackley CE, Edwards JE, Wallace RB, et al: Tricuspid and pulmonary valve disease. In Hurst JW (ed): The Heart, 6th ed. McGraw-Hill, New York, 1986.

FIGURE CREDITS

Figs. 6.1–6.3, 6.5, 6.17, 6.19, 6.20, 6.21, 6.23, 6.33, 6.37–6.39, 6.52, 6.53–6.55, 6.57, 6.70, 6.76, 6.85 from Hurst JW: Atlas of the Heart. Gower, New York, 1988.

Figs. 6.4, 6.16, 6.18, 6.32, 6.34, 6.56, 6.69, 6.75, 6.82B from Becker AE, Anderson RH: Cardiac Pathology. Raven, New York, 1983.

Fig. 6.6, 6.22, 6.36, 6.59, 6.71, 6.77, 6.83, 6.84 redrawn from Selzer A: Principles of Clinical Cardiology: An Analytic Approach. WB Saunders, Philadelphia, 1975.

Figs. 6.7, 6.41, 6.61 courtesy of Robert G. Sybers, MD, and Wade H. Shuford MD, Atlanta, GA; Hurst JW: Atlas of the Heart. Gower, New York, 1988.

Fig. 6.8 redrawn from Hurst JW, Goodson GC Jr: Atlas of Spatial Vector Electrocardiography. The Blakiston Co., New York, 1952; Hurst JW: Atlas of the Heart. Gower, New York, 1988.

Figs. 6.9, 6.10, 6.15, 6.40, 6.43, 6.45, 6.50, 6.51, 6.58, 6.60, 6.62, 6.63, 6.66 from Hurst JW: The Heart, 6th ed. McGraw-Hill, New York, 1986. Figs. 6.40, 6.60 courtesy of Ernest Craige, MD. Fig. 6.43 redrawn and courtesy of I. Sylvia Crawley, MD, Atlanta, GA.

Figs. 6.9, 6.25, 6.26, 6.45, 6.62, 6.79, 6.85A, B, 6.86 courtesy of Joel M. Felner, MD, Atlanta, GA; from Hurst JW: Atlas of the Heart. Gower, New York, 1988.

Fig. 6.11 redrawn and courtesy of Robert H. Franch, MD, Atlanta, GA; from Hurst JW: Atlas of the Heart. Gower, New York, 1988.

Figs. 6.12, 6.27, 6.28, 6.31, 6.46, 6.47, 6.64, 6.65, 6.73, 6.80, 6.87 from Chatterjee K, et al: Cardiology: An Illustrated Text–Reference. Gower, New York, 1992.

Fig. 6.13 redrawn from Grossman W: Cardiac Catheterization and Angiography. Lea & Febiger, Philadelphia, 1980; from Hurst JW: Atlas of the Heart. Gower, New York, 1988.

Fig. 6.14 redrawn from Rapaport E: Natural history of aortic and mitral valve disease. Am J Cardiol 35:221, 1975; from Hurst JW: Atlas of the Heart. Gower, New York, 1988.

Fig. 6.24 redrawn from Silverman ME, Myerburg RJ, Hurst JW: Electrocardiography: Basic Concepts and Clinical Applications. McGraw-Hill, New York, 1983; from Hurst JW: Atlas of the Heart. Gower, New York, 1988.

Fig. 6.29 redrawn from Rackley CE, et al: Quantitation of myocardial function in valvular heart disease. In Brewer LA (ed): Prosthetic Heart Valves. Charles C Thomas, Springfield, IL 1969; from Hurst JW: Atlas of the Heart. Gower, New York, 1988.

Figs. 6.30, 6.42, 6.49, 6.67, 6.78, 6.81 from Kassner EG: Atlas of Radiologic Imaging. Gower, New York, 1989.

Fig. 6.35 redrawn from Hurst JW: The Heart, 2nd ed. McGraw-Hill, New York, 1970. Courtesy of Robert C. Schlant, MD, Atlanta, GA; from Hurst JW: Atlas of the Heart. Gower, New York, 1988.

Fig. 6.39 redrawn from Hurst JW: The Heart, 4th ed. McGraw-Hill, New York, 1978. Courtesy of Joel M. Felner, MD, Atlanta, GA; from Hurst JW: Atlas of the Heart. Gower, New York, 1988.

Fig. 6.44 redrawn from Perloff JK: The Clinical Recognition of Congenital Heart Disease. WB Saunders, Philadelphia. 1978. Courtesy of James J. Acker, MD, Knoxville, TN; from Hurst JW: Atlas of the Heart. Gower, New York, 1988.

Fig. 6.48 redrawn from Carabello BA, Grossman W: Calculation of stenotic valuve orifice area. In Grossman W (ed): Cardiac Catheterization and Angiography, 3rd ed. Lea & Febiger, Philadelphia, 1986; from Chatterjee K, 1992.

Fig. 6.58 redrawn from Rackley CE: Value of ventriculography in cardiac function and diagnosis. In Fowler NO (ed): Diagnostic Methods in Cardiology. FA Davis, Philadelphia, 1975; from Hurst JW: The Heart, 6th ed. McGraw-Hill, New York, 1986.

Figs. 6.68, 6.74 redrawn from Iskandrian AS: Nuclear Cardiac Imaging: Principles and Applications. FA Davis, Philadelphia, 1987; from Hurst JW: Atlas of the Heart. Gower, New York, 1988.

Fig 6.72 from Lintermans JP: Two-dimensional Echocardiography in Infants and Children. Martinus Nijhoff, Dordrecht, 1986; from Hurst JW: Atlas of the Heart. Gower, New York, 1988.

REFERENCES

1. Abernathy WS, Willis PW III. Thromboembolic complications of rheumatic heart disease. Cardiovasc Clin 5:131, 1973.
2. Baker C, Sommerville J. Clinical features and surgical treatment of fifty patients with severe aortic stenosis. Guys Hosp Rep 108:101, 1959.
3. Baker CG, Finnegan TRL: Epilepsy and mitral stenosis. Br Heart J 19:159, 1957.
4. Baumgartner H, Kratzer H, Helmreich G, et al: Evaluation of aortic regurgitation by color-coded two-dimensional Doppler echocardiography—Usefulness of different jet parameters for quantitation. Am J Noninvas Cardiol 3:185, 1989.

5. Boltwood CM, Tei C, Wong M, et al: Quantitative echocardiography of the mitral complex in dilated cardiomyopathy: The mechanism of functional mitral regurgitation. Circulation 68:498, 1983.

6. Borer JS, Bacharach SL, Greene MV, et al: Exercise-induced left ventricular dysfunction in symptomatic and asymptomatic patients with aortic regurgitation: Assessment with radionuclide cineangiography. Am J Cardiol 42:351, 1978.

7. Braunwald E (1969) Mitral regurgitation: Physiologic, clinical and surgical considerations. N Engl J Med 281:425, 1969.

8. Brouwer CB, Verwers FA, Alpert JS, et al: Isolated aortic stenosis: Analysis of clinical and hemodynamic subsets. J Appl Cardiol 4:555, 1989.

9. Chun PK, Gertz E, Davisa JE, Cheitlin MD: Coronary atherosclerosis in mitral stenosis. Chest 81:36, 1982.

10. Clawson BJ: Rheumatic heart disease. An analysis of 796 cases. Am Heart J 20:454, 1940.

11. Crawley IS, Morris DC, Silverman BD: Valvular heart disease. In Hurst JW (ed): The Heart, 4th ed. McGraw-Hill, New York, 1978.

12. Dalen JE, Alpert JS: Valvular Heart Disease, 2nd ed. Boston, Little, Brown, 1987.

13. David D, Lang RM, Marcus RH, et al: Doppler echocardiographic estimation of transmitral pressure gradients and correlations with micromanometer gradients in mitral stenosis. Am J Cardiol 67:1161, 1991.

14. Dodge HT, Baxley WA: Left ventricular volume and mass and their significance in heart disease. Am J Cardiol 23:528, 1969.

15. Dollar SL, Roberts WC: Morphologic comparison of patients with mitral valve prolapse who died suddenly with patients who died from severe valvular dysfunction or other conditions. J Am Coll Cardiol 17:921, 1991.

16. Edwards JE: On the etiology of acquired valvular disease of the heart. Sem Roentgenol 14:96, 1979.

17. El–Sherif N: Rheumatic tricuspid stenosis: A haemodynamic correlation. Br Heart J 33:16, 1971.

18. Felson B: Chest Roentgenology. WB Saunders, Philadelphia, 1973.

19. Flamm MD, Braiff BA, Kimball R, et al:'Mechanism of effort syncope in aortic stenosis. Circulation 36(suppl 2):II-109, 1967.

20. Frank S, Johnson A, Ross J Jr: Natural history of valvular aortic stenosis. Br Heart J 35:41, 1973.

'21. Gorlin R, Gorlin SG: Hydraulic formula for calculation of the area of the stenotic mitral valve, other cardiac valves and central circulatory shunts. Am Heart J 41:1, 1951.

22. Greves J, Rahimtoola SH, McAnulty JH, et al: Preoperative criteria predictive of late survival following valve replacement for severe aortic regurgitation. Am Heart J 101:300, 1981.

23. Griffith MJ, Carey CM, Byrne JC, et al: Echocardiographic left ventricular wall thickness: A poor predictor of the severity of aortic valve stenosis. Clin Cardiol 14:227, 1991.

24. Hancock EW: The ejection sound in aortic stenosis. Am J Med 40:569, 1966.

25. Hancock EW, Fleming PR: Aortic stenosis. QJ Med 29:209, 1960.

26. Hansing CE, Rowe GG: Tricuspid insufficiency: A study of hemodynamics and pathogenesis. Circulation 45:793, 1972.

27. Harvey WP, Segal JP, Hufnagel CA: Unusual clinical features associated with severe aortic insufficiency. Ann Intern Med 47:27, 1957.

28. Hildner FJ, Javier RP, Cohen LS, et al: Myocardial dysfunction associated with valvular heart disease. Am J Cardiol 30:319, 1972.

29. Holmes AM, Logan WF, Winterbottom T: Transient systolic murmurs in angina pectoris. Am Heart J 76:680, 1968.

30. Holmes JC, Fowler NO, Kaplan S: Pulmonary valvular insufficiency. Am J Med 44:851, 1968.

31. Hood WP Jr, Thompson WJ, Rackley CE, Rolett EL: Comparison of calculations of left ventricular wall stress in man from thin-walled and thick-walled ellipsoidal models. Circ Res 24:575, 1969.

32. Hungenholtz PG, Ryan TJ, Stein SW, et al: The spectrum of pure mitral stenosis: Hemodynamic studies in relation to clinical disability. Am J Cardiol 10:773, 1962.

33. Hunt D, Baxley WA, Kennedy JW, et al: Quantitative evaluation cineaortography in the assessment of aortic regurgitation. Am J Cardiol 31:696, 1973.

34. Hurst JW, Whitworth HB, O'Donoghue S, et al: Heart disease due to ovarian carcinoid: Successful replacement of the pulmonary and tricuspid valves with porcine heterografts and removal of the tumor. In Hurst JW (ed): Clinical Essays on the Heart, vol. 5. New York, McGraw-Hill, 1985.

35. Jeresaty RM: Mitral valve prolapse–click syndrome. Prog Cardiovasc Dis 15:623, 1973

36. Kennedy JW, Twiss RD, Blackmon JR, et al: Quantitative angiocardiography. III. Relationships of left ventricular pressure, volume and mass in aortic valve disease. Circulation 38:838, 1968

37. Kennedy JW, Yarnall SR, Murray JA, et al: Quantitative angiocardiography. IV. Relationships of left atrial and ventricular pressure and volume in mitral valve disease. Circulation 41:817, 1970.

38. Killip T, Lukas DS: Tricuspid stenosis: Physiologic criteria for diagnosis and hemodynamic abnormalities. Circulation 16:3, 1957.

39. Kitchin A, Turner R: Diagnosis and treatment of tricuspid stenosis. Br Heart J 26:354, 1964

40. Klatte EC, Tampas JP, Campbell JA, et al: The roentgenographic manifestations of aortic stenosis and aortic valvular insufficiency. Am J Roentgenol Radium Ther Nucl Med 87:57, 1962.

41. Klein AL, Obarski TP, Stewart WJ, et al: Transesophageal Doppler echocardiography of pulmonary venous flow: A new marker of mitral regurgitation severity. J Am Coll Cardiol 18:518, 1991.

42. Klughaupt M, Flamm MD, Hancock EW, et al: Nonrheumatic mitral insufficiency: Determination of operability and prognosis. Circulation 39:307, 1969.

43. Kostucki W, Vandenbossche JL, Friart A, et al: Pulsed Doppler regurgitant flow patterns of normal valves. Am J Cardiol 58:309, 1986.

44. Lee YC, Scherlis L, Singleton RT: Mitral stenosis: Hemodynamic, electrocardiographic and vector cardiographic studies. Am Heart J 69:559, 1965.

45. Newman GE, Bounous PW, Jones RH, et al: Noninvasive assessment of hemodynamic effects of mitral valve commissurotomy during and exercise in patients with mitral stenosis. J Thorac Cardiovasc Surg 78:750, 1979.

46. Nicks R, Cartmill T, Bernstein L: Hypoplasia of the aortic root: The problem of aortic valve replacement. Thorax 25:339, 1970.

47. Nutter DO, Wickliffe C, Gilbert CA, et al: The pathophysiology of idiopathic mitral valve prolapse. Circulation 52:297, 1975.

48. Osbakken M, Bove AA, Spann JF: Left ventricular function in chronic regurgitation with reference to end-systolic pressure, volume and stress relations. Am J Cardiol 47:193, 1981.

49. Perloff JK, Harvey WP: Clinical recognition of tricuspid stenosis. Circulation 22:346, 1960.

50. Pomerance A: Pathogenesis of aortic stenosis and its relation to age. Br Heart J 34:569, 1972.

51. Pridie RB, Benham MB, Oakley CM: Echocardiography of the mitral valve in aortic valve disease. Br Heart J 33:296, 1971.

52. Rackley CE: Quantitative evaluation of left ventricular function by radiographic techniques. Circulation 54:862, 1976.

53. Rackley CE: Value of ventriculography in cardiac function and diagnosis. Cardiovasc Clin 6:283, 1975.

54. Rackley CE, Dear HD, Baxley WA, et al: Left ventricular chamber volume, mass and function in severe coronary artery disease. Circulation 41:605, 1970.

55. Rackley CE, Hood WP Jr: Aortic valve disease. In Levine HJ (ed): Clinical Cardiovascular Physiology. Grune & Stratton, New York, 1976.

56. Rackley CE, Hood WP Jr: Quantitative angiographic evaluation pathophysiologic mechanisms in valvular heart disease. In Sonnenblick EJ, Lesch M (eds): Valvular Heart Disease. Grune & Stratton, New York, 1976.

57. Rackley CE, Russell RO Jr, Mantle JA, et al: Recognition of acute myocardial infarction. In Rackley CE, Russell RO Jr (eds): Coronary Artery Disease: Recognition and Management. Futura, Mount Kisco, NY, 1979.

58. Radford DJ, Bloom KR, Izukawa T, et al: Echocardiographic assessment of bicuspid aortic valves: Angiographic and pathological correlates. Circulation 53:80, 1976.

59. Rahko PS: Doppler and echocardiographic characteristics of patients having an Austin Flint murmur. Circulation 83:1940, 1991.

60. Rapaport E: Natural history of aortic and mitral valve disease. Am J Cardiol 35:221, 1975.

61. Reigenbaum H: Echocardiography. Lea & Febiger, Philadelphia, 1976.

62. Ronan JA Jr, Steelman RB, de Leon AC Jr, et al: The clinical diagnosis of acute severe mitral insufficiency. Am J Cardiol 27:284, 1971.

63. Rowe JC, Bland EF, Spague HB, et al: The course of mitral stenosis without surgery: Ten and twenty year perspectives. Ann Intern Med 52:741, 1960.

64. Schwartz R, Meyerson RM, Lawrence LT, et al: Mitral stenosis, massive pulmonary hemorrhage and emergency valve replacement. N Engl J Med 272:755, 1966.

65. Selzer A, Cohn KE: Natural history of mitral stenosis: A review. Circulation 45:878, 1972.

66. Selzer A, Katayama F: Mitral regurgitation: Clinical patterns, pathophysiology and natural history. Medicine 51:337, 1972.

67. Selzer A, Naruse DY, York E, et al: Electrocardiographic findings in concentric and eccentric left ventricular hypertrophy. Am Heart J 63:320, 1962.

68. Shelburne JC, Rubenstein D, Gorlin R: A reappraisal of papillary muscle dysfunction. Am J Med 46:862, 1969.

69. Sherrid M, Goyal A, Delia E, et al: Unsuspected mitral stenosis. Am J Med 90:189, 1991.

70. Stott DK, Marpole DG, Bristow JD, et al: The role of left atrial transport in aortic and mitral stenosis. Circulation 41:1031, 1970.

71. Szekely P, Turner R, Snaith L: Pregnancy and the changing pattern of rheumatic heart disease. Br Heart J 35:1293, 1973.

72. Whipple RL, Morris DC, Felner JM, et al: Echocardiographic manifestations of the flail aortic valve leaflet syndrome. J Clin Ultrasound 5:417, 1977.

73. Winkle RA, Lopes MG, Fitzgerald JW, et al: Arrhythmias in patients with mitral valve prolapse. Circulation 52:73, 1975.

74. Wood P: Aortic stenosis. Am J Cardiol 1:553, 1958.

75. Wood P: An appreciation of mitral stenosis. Br Heart J 1:1051, 1954.

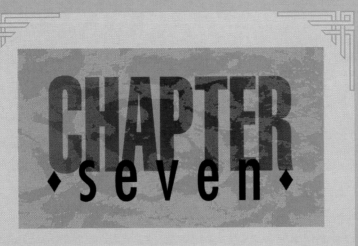

CHAPTER seven

CONGENITAL HEART DISEASE

J. WILLIS HURST, MD

ELIZABETH W. NUGENT, MD

ROBERT H. ANDERSON, MD

JOSEPH S. ALPERT, MD

Congenital cardiac defects are caused by environmental factors and chromosomal abnormalities, such as trisomy, deletion, and mosaicism. The rubella virus may cause patency of the arterial duct and is associated with peripheral pulmonary arterial stenoses.

The overall incidence of congenital heart disease is 8 per 1000 live births; the prevalence of specific lesions is shown in Figure 7.1. The prevalence of congenital heart disease in adults differs from that in children (Fig. 7.2). This is the result of operation and/or mortality in the more complex forms of congenital heart disease.

The complications of congenital heart disease are death, congestive heart failure, arterial oxygen unsaturation with consequent cyanosis and cerebral thrombus, bacterial endocarditis, pulmonary arterial hypertension and pulmonary vascular obstructive disease, retardation of growth and development, and exertional intolerance and restrictions. Many patients with congenital heart disease have no complications for many years.

The following discussion is limited because the list of all types of malformations is virtually unlimited.

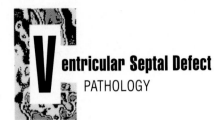

Ventricular Septal Defect
PATHOLOGY

A ventricular septal defect (VSD) is defined as an opening in the ventricular septum that separates the left and the right ventricles. Seventy-five percent of these are perimembranous (Fig. 7.3); they may open into the inlet (Fig. 7.4A) or outlet (Fig. 7.4B) components of the right ventricle, or they may become confluent. Defects in the septum may also be located within the muscular septum; these are termed muscular defects (Figs. 7.5, 7.6). Defects located in the outflow tract roofed by the conjoint leaflets of the aortic and the pulmonary

FIGURE 7.1 PREVALENCE OF SPECIFIC LESIONS OF CONGENITAL HEART DISEASE

	CASES OF CONGENITAL HEART DISEASE (%)				
LESION	KEITH	NADAS	MITCHELL	HOFFMAN	FYLER
Ventricular septal defect	28.3	19.4	29.5	31.3	16.6
Pulmonary stenosis	9.9	7.5	8.6	13.5	3.5
Patent arterial duct	9.8	15.5	8.3	5.5	6.5
Atrial septal defect, secundum	7.0	4.5	7.4	6.1	3.1
Ventricular septal defect with pulmonary stenosis*	9.7	10.5	6.4	3.7	9.4
Aortic stenosis	7.1	5.7	3.8	3.7	2.0
Aortic atresia	1.5	NL	3.1	0.6	7.9
Atrioventricular septal defect†	3.4	2.7	3.6	3.7	5.3
Coarctation of aorta	5.1	8.1	2.6	5.5	8.0
Peripheral pulmonary stenosis	NL	1.0	3.6	NL	NL
Endocardial fibroelastosis	0.9	NL	2.4	NL	NL
Complete transposition	4.9	4.0	2.6	3.7	10.5
Common arterial trunk	0.7	0.8	1.7	2.5	1.5
Total anomalous pulmonary venous connection	1.4	1.3	NL	0.6	2.8
Tricuspid atresia	1.2	1.0	1.2	NL	2.7
Double-outlet right ventricle	0.5	0.2	1.0	0.6	1.6
Pulmonary atresis without ventricular septal defect	0.7	0.3	0.01	0.6	3.3
No. of patients	15,104	10,624	56,109	19,502	2,251

*Includes tetralogy of Fallot.
†Includes partial and complete.
NL = not listed.
(Reproduced with permission; see Figure Credits)

FIGURE 7.2 PREVALENCE OF CONGENITAL HEART DISEASE IN ADULTS

LESION	PETER BENT BRIGHAM*	U MASS†
Atrioventricular septal defect	46%	31%
Ventricular septal defect	23%	18%
Pulmonary stenosis	15%	15%
Patent arterial duct	6%	7%
Coarctation	3%	10%
Tetralogy	2%	5%
Other	5%	15%

*Dexter Lab, Peter Bent Brigham Hospital (1960–1970). 13% of all catheterizations.
†University of Massachusetts Medical Center (1976–1985). 2.5% of all catheterizations.

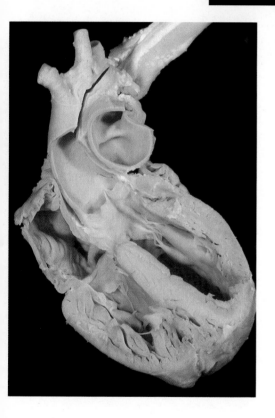

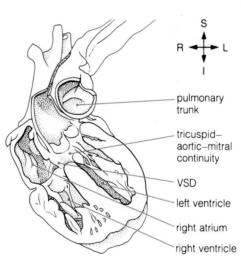

FIGURE 7.3   Simulated four-chamber, long-axis section of a heart with a perimembranous inlet VSD. Characteristic of the defect, its posteroinferior border is made up of an extensive area of fibrous continuity between the mitral, aortic, and tricuspid valves. The aortic valve is located in the roof of the defect. (Reproduced with permission; see Figure Credits)

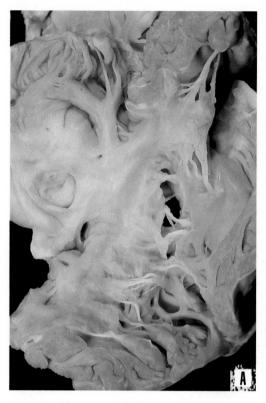

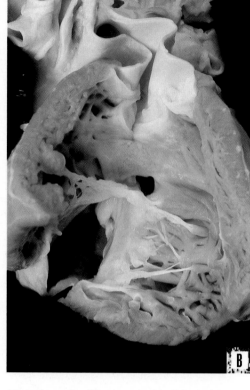

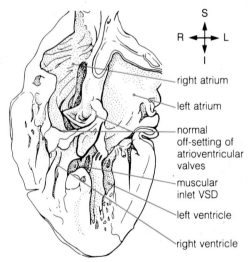

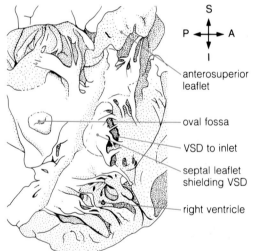

FIGURE 7.4 Perimembranous VSDs photographed from the right ventricular aspect. These VSDs may extend to open primarily into the inlet **(A)** or the outlet **(B)** components of the right ventricle. (Reproduced with permission; see Figure Credits)

S
P ← → A
I

anterosuperior leaflet

oval fossa

VSD to inlet

septal leaflet shielding VSD

right ventricle

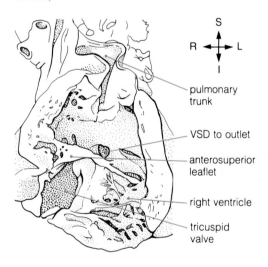

S
R ← → L
I

pulmonary trunk

VSD to outlet

anterosuperior leaflet

right ventricle

tricuspid valve

FIGURE 7.5 Simulated four-chamber, long-axis section of a muscular inlet defect embedded within the musculature of the septum. This VSD can be differentiated from a perimembranous defect opening to the inlet of the right ventricle by a muscle bar that forms the roof of the defect, separating it from the septal attachments of the tricuspid and mitral valves (see Fig. 7.3). (Reproduced with permission; see Figure Credits)

S
R ← → L
I

right atrium

left atrium

normal off-setting of atrioventricular valves

muscular inlet VSD

left ventricle

right ventricle

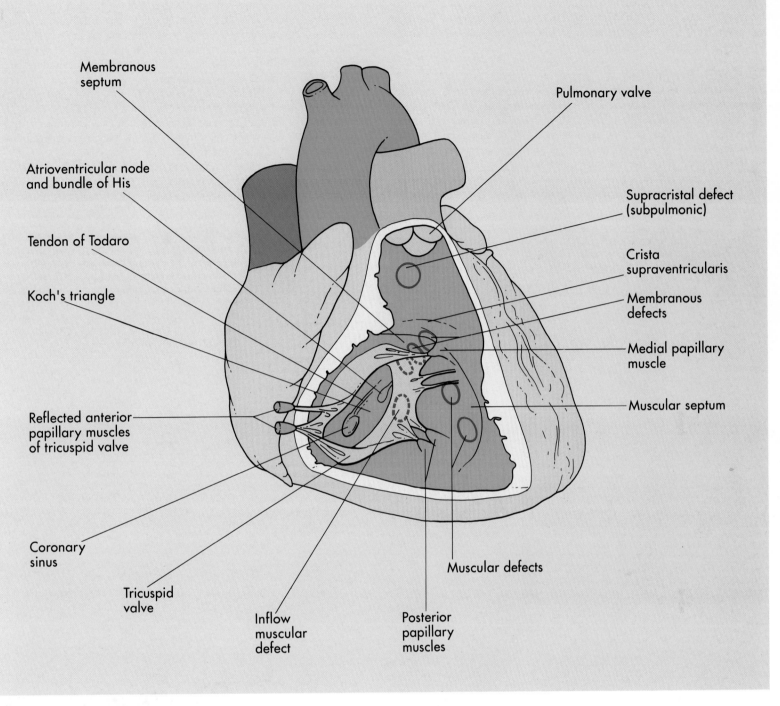

Membranous
septum

Atrioventricular node
and bundle of His

Tendon of Todaro

Koch's triangle

Reflected anterior
papillary muscles
of tricuspid valve

Coronary
sinus

Tricuspid
valve

Inflow
muscular
defect

Posterior
papillary
muscles

Muscular defects

Pulmonary valve

Supracristal defect
(subpulmonic)

Crista
supraventricularis

Membranous
defects

Medial papillary
muscle

Muscular septum

FIGURE 7.6   Location of the common defects in the ventricular septum. The tricuspid valve has been removed to allow visualization of a membranous inflow septal defect. Muscular septal defects can occur in many locations, but the supracristal or subpulmonic defects create special problems. (Reproduced with permission; see Figure Credits)

valves are termed doubly committed juxta-arterial defects (Fig. 7.7). A ventricular septal defect that is located immediately beneath the leaflets of the aortic valve may result in aortic regurgitation because of an associated defect in the structure of the aortic valve annulus.

PATHOPHYSIOLOGY

Patients with VSDs can be divided into three groups according to the associated altered physiology. This depends upon the size of the defect and the reaction of the pulmonary arterioles. The first group is composed of patients with a small defect (less than 0.5 cm²/m²), no elevation of the pulmonary arterial pressure, and a small left-to-right shunt. The patient is at little risk except for endocarditis. In the second group the defect is of medium size (0.5 to 1.0 cm²/m²); the pulmonary arterial and the right ventricular systolic pressures may become elevated to about 80% of the left ventricular systolic pressure (Fig. 7.8). A moderate-sized left-to-right shunt is present, and volume overload of the left atrium and the left ventricle occurs. In the third group, the hole is 1.0 cm²/m² or larger. It is as large as the aortic valve orifice, so that the systolic pressure is equal in the aorta, the left ventricle, the right ventricle, and the pulmonary arteries. The amount of blood delivered to the lungs and the periphery is determined by the pulmonary and peripheral vascular resistance.

There may be very little left-to-right shunting at birth, because the pulmonary vascular resistance is high. After birth the pulmonary vascular resistance decreases and the left-to-right shunt increases, which may lead to left ventricular failure. This is usually detected clinically 3 to 12 weeks after birth; however, in premature infants it may occur earlier.

The large pulmonary blood flow can lead to pulmonary arteriolar disease and a high systolic pressure in the right ventricle and the pulmonary arteries. When the pulmonary arterial resistance exceeds the systemic arterial resistance, a

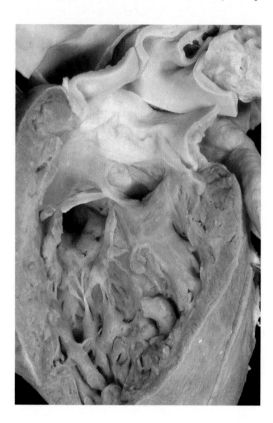

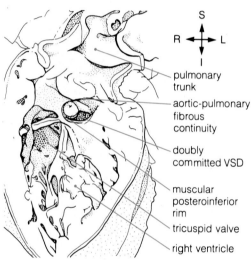

pulmonary trunk

aortic-pulmonary fibrous continuity

doubly committed VSD

muscular posteroinferior rim

tricuspid valve

right ventricle

FIGURE 7.7   Outlet defect with a muscular posteroinferior rim, separating the margin from the area of the membranous septum. A fibrous roof is formed by the continuity between the leaflets of the aortic and pulmonary valves. Such a defect is well described as being doubly committed and juxta-arterial, although some may recognize it as supracristal. (Reproduced with permission; see Figure Credits)

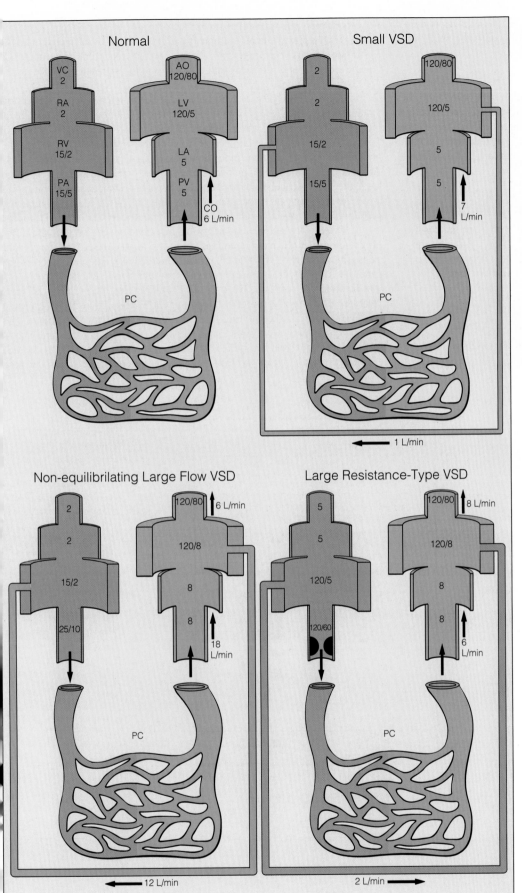

FIGURE. 7.8 Pathophysiology of ventricular septal defect (VSD). The top left panel shows the normal state. The top right panel depicts a small VSD. Pressures are unchanged from that of normal, but there is a small left-to-right shunt from left ventricle (LV) to right ventricle (RV). Oxygenated (red) blood shunts from the RV where it mixes with deoxygenated (blue) blood. The resultant oxygen saturation of the blood in the RV and pulmonary arteries (PA) is therefore considerably higher than normal. The shunt results in a slightly increased pulmonary blood flow (from 6 to 7 L/min). There are no major changes in hemodynamics, and the stimulus for hypertrophy of the LV and RV is minimal. The bottom left panel depicts a large VSD in which considerable amounts of blood (12 L/min) flow from the LV to RV. The hole in the ventricular septum is not so large, however, that RV pressure and LV pressure become equal. Consequently, during ventricular systole, the pressure in the LV is considerably higher than that in the RV, and blood flows from LV to RV. There is a marked increase in pulmonary blood flow (18 L/min), a combination of the systemic venous return (6 L/min), and the left-to-right shunt (12 L/min). The bottom right panel shows a VSD in combination with pulmonary vascular disease. Marked RV systolic hypertension and pulmonary arterial systolic hypertension have developed because of the pulmonary vascular disease. The RV is dilated and hypertrophied. LV and RV systolic pressures are equal, and there is a very small right-to-left shunt. Thus, desaturated blood is found in the LV, and systemic arterial blood is desaturated as compared with normal. This results in clinically detectable cyanosis of the patient. Total cardiac output (CO) represents a combination of pulmonary blood flow (6 L/min) and the right-to-left shunt (2 L/min). This gives a total systemic CO of 8 L/min. (VC = vena cava; RA = right atrium; PC = pulmonary capillaries; PV = pulmonary veins; LA = left atrium; AO = aorta) (Modified and used with permission; see Figure Credits)

right-to-left shunt and arterial oxygen unsaturation are found; this is termed Eisenmenger's syndrome. The pulmonary vasculature is abnormal in such cases.

CLINICAL MANIFESTATIONS

VSD may occur as an isolated defect or in combination with other anomalies. The incidence is the same in males and females. The defect is seen primarily in children and young adults. This observation is accounted for by three factors: (1) VSDs tend to close spontaneously; (2) VSDs are closed surgically in childhood; (3) VSDs lead to pulmonary vascular disease (Eisenmenger's syndrome), which is associated with early demise (see Fig. 7.9).

SYMPTOMS

Infants, children, and adults with small defects have no symptoms. Infants with moderately large defects develop heart failure at 3 to 12 weeks of age; parents notice breathing difficulty and fatigue during feeding. Patients with severe pulmonary hypertension and arterial oxygen unsaturation develop heart failure, hemoptysis, and cerebral thromboses.

PHYSICAL EXAMINATION

When the defect is small, a loud, usually holosystolic murmur is heard with maximal intensity at the mid to lower left sternal border. It may be midsystolic or decrescendo, suggesting that the defect is located in the muscular septum. A thrill may be present. Loud murmurs tend, however, to occur more commonl with large shunts than with small ones (Fig. 7.10). The pulmonary componen of the second sound is normal, and the right and left ventricles produce norma precordial pulsations.

Infants with large defects, who have large left-to-right shunts together witl pulmonary arterial hypertension, exhibit different features. A thrill may be fel to the left of the mid to lower sternum. A loud holosystolic murmur is heard i the same area, with a low-pitched, diastolic rumble at the apex. The latter signi fies a pulmonary-to-systemic blood flow ratio of 2:1 or more. The second sound i normally split, and the pulmonary closure sound is abnormally loud. The righ and the left ventricular precordial pulsations are hyperactive. Respiratory dis tress, liver enlargement, or rales may be detected. With time the shunt ma diminish as the defect becomes smaller, right ventricular outflow tract obstruc tion develops, or pulmonary arteriolar disease increases. When the defec becomes smaller, the murmur and second heart sound are altered in a predictabl way; the murmur becomes less loud with increasing pulmonary hypertension and the intensity of the pulmonary component of the second sound increases.

Eisenmenger's syndrome, seen in older children and adults, also has typica features. Cyanosis is apparent and a prominent a wave is detected in the inter nal jugular veins. A left anterior precordial lift signifies right ventricular hyper trophy. Pulmonary valve closure and pulsation of the pulmonary trunk may be palpable in the second left intercostal space. The murmur generated by the VSE is located in early systole and may be faint. The second sound is loud due to ar

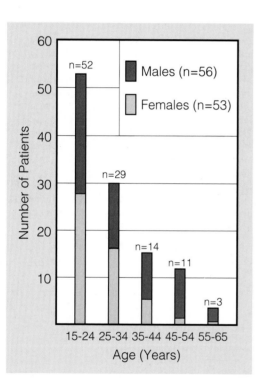

FIGURE. 7.9 Age and sex distribution in 109 adults with a late diagnosis of congenital, isolated VSD. (Reproduced with permission; see Figure Credits) (Reprinted with permission from Physicians World Communicatios Group)

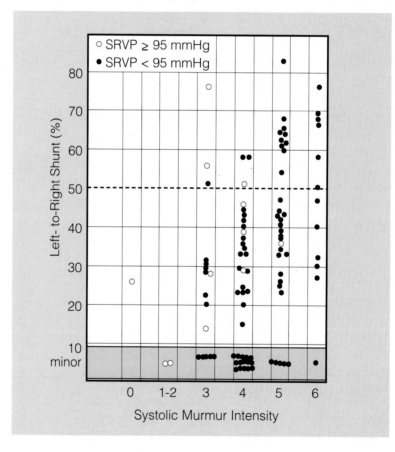

FIGURE. 7.10 Intensity grade of systolic murmur and size of left-to-right shunt expressed as a percentage of pulmonary flow (SRVP = systolic right ventricular pressure; • patients with SRVP <95 mmHg; o = patients wi SRVP >95 mmHg; horizontal line denotes a shunt size of 50%) (Reproduced with permission; see Figure Credits) (Reprinted with permission from Physicians World Communications Grou

increased intensity of closure of the pulmonary valve. The murmur of pulmonary valve regurgitation, called a Graham-Steell murmur, may be heard along the left sternal border. It may be mistaken for a murmur of aortic regurgitation. The systolic murmur of tricuspid regurgitation may also be heard. With time, signs of heart failure may be detected. Any patient with a defect located immediately beneath the aortic valve may have aortic regurgitation due to prolapse of an aortic valve cusp.

LABORATORY STUDIES

Chest Radiography The chest film is normal in patients with a small VSD. The chest radiograph of a patient with a moderate-sized VSD shows a slightly enlarged heart with prominent pulmonary arteries (Figs. 7.11, 7.12). The chest film of a patient with Eisenmenger's syndrome demonstrates an enlarged heart with large pulmonary arteries (Fig. 7.13). The tapering of the right branch of the pulmonary artery suggests pulmonary hypertension.

Electrocardiography The electrocardiogram (ECG) may be normal in patients with a small interventricular septal defect. In the ECG of a patient with a moderate-sided defect the increased QRS voltage suggests left ventricular hypertrophy (Fig. 7.14). The presence of right ventricular hypertrophy is evident in the ECG of a patient with Eisenmenger's syndrome (Fig. 7.15).

Echocardiography Echocardiography is very useful in the diagnosis of congenital heart disease. Color Doppler is extremely useful in detection and localization of the VSD.[6] Perimembranous defects are juxta-aortic, being directly related to the central fibrous skeleton supporting the aortic valve. The muscular defects are surrounded by muscle, while the doubly committed juxta-arterial defects are roofed by aortic and pulmonary valves in fibrous continuity (Fig. 7.16–7.18). A Doppler recording of a patient with an isolated interventricular septal defect is shown in Figure 7.19.

Cardiac Catheterization The amount of left-to-right shunt may be identified by an increase in oxygen saturation in the right ventricle. When the defect is small, the right ventricular and the pulmonary arterial systolic pressures are normal. When the left-to-right shunt is large, the pulmonary arterial systolic pressure may approach systemic levels and the left atrial pressure may be elevated. When there is severe elevation of pulmonary arterial resistance, as in Eisenmenger's syndrome, the shunt becomes right-to-left or bidirectional.

Cardiac angiography and aortography are used to identify aortic regurgitation, patency of the arterial duct, location of the great arteries, and the number of defects (Fig. 7.20).

Other Imaging Modalities Magnetic resonance imaging can also delineate VSDs (Figs. 7.21, 7.22).

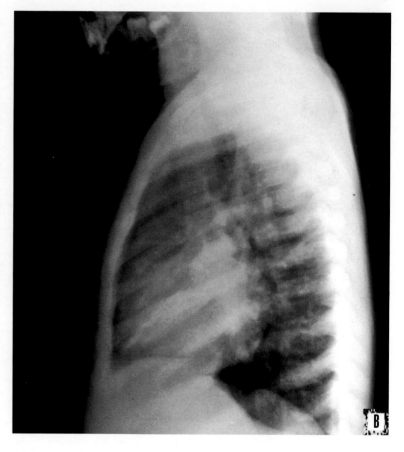

FIGURE 7.11 **(A)** Posteroanterior chest radiograph of a 3-year-old child with a moderate-sized VSD. Moderate generalized cardiac enlargement and increased pulmonary blood flow are seen. The right pulmonary artery is increased in size. **(B)** Lateral view shows generalized cardiac enlargement, particularly of the left atrium. (Reproduced with permission; see Figure Credits)

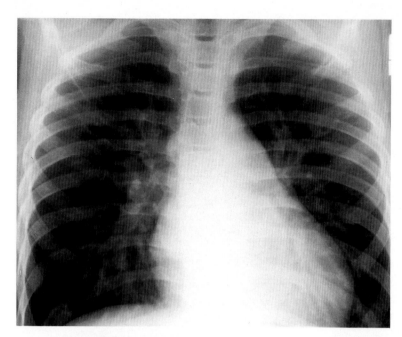

FIGURE 7.12   Moderate-sized VSD with a pulmonary/systemic blood flow ratio of 2.5. There is left ventricular and mild left atrial enlargement and increased pulmonary vascularity. (Reproduced with permission; see Figure Credits)

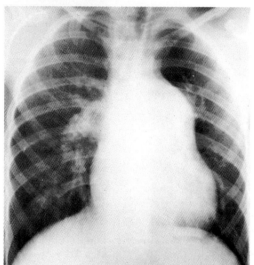

FIGURE 7.13   Posteroanterior chest film of a 12-year-old child with a large VSD and Eisenmenger's syndrome. The main and central pulmonary arteries are markedly dilated, while the peripheral segmental branches appear attenuated. (Reproduced with permission; see Figure Credits)

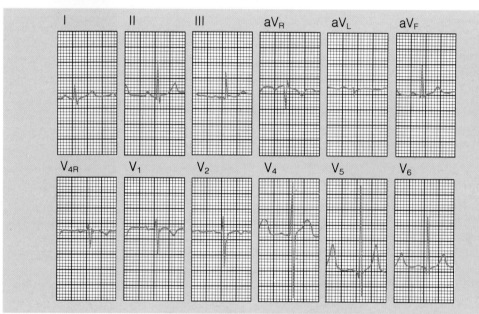

FIGURE 7.14   ECG of a 7-year-old child with a moderate-sized VSD, demonstrating large QRS complexes in leads V_4 and V_5. The mean QRS vector is posteriorly directed at $^+70°$ in the frontal plane. The amplitude is large suggesting left ventricular hypertrophy; the mean T vector is directed at $^+60°$ in the frontal plane and slightly posteriorly. (Reproduced with permission; see Figure Credits)

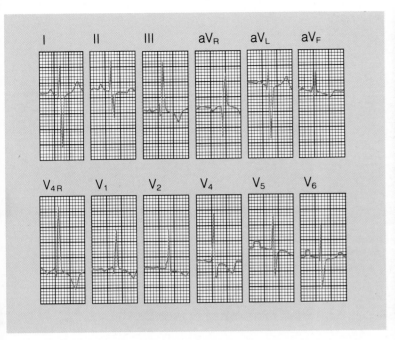

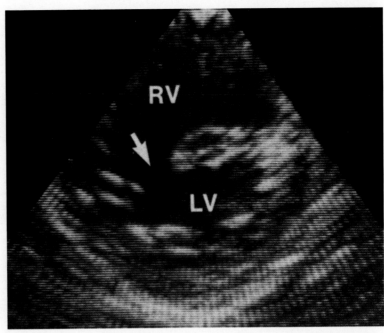

FIGURE 7.15 ECG of a 7-year-old child with an interventricular septal defect and Eisenmenger's syndrome, demonstrating evidence of right ventricular hypertrophy and prolonged QRS complexes. Standardization is normal in leads I, II, III, aV$_R$, aV$_L$, aV$_F$, and V$_{4R}$, one half standardized in V$_1$, and one quarter standardized in leads V$_2$, V$_4$, V$_5$, and V$_6$. (Reproduced with permission; see Figure Credits)

FIGURE 7.16 Cross-sectional echocardiography from a patient with a large muscular VSD. The parasternal short-axis view through the left ventricle (LV) at the level of the papillary muscles shows that the defect (*arrow*) is located in the inferior portion of the septum near the cardiac apex (RV = right ventricle). (Reproduced with permission; see Figure Credits)

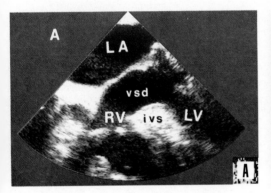

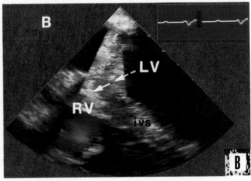

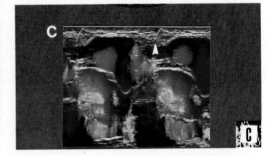

FIGURE 7.17 **(A)** Transesophageal echocardiogram of a VSD. **(B)** Color-flow Doppler demonstrates left-to-right blue jet across the defect during systole (*arrows*). **(C)** Color-flow M-mode and ECG indicate that the blue flow occurs in systole, after the QRS complex (*arrow*). (Reproduced with permission; see Figure Credits)

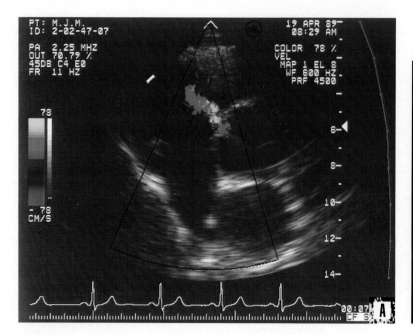

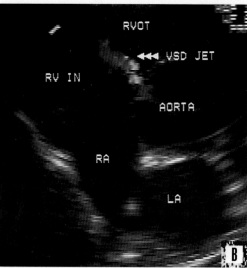

FIGURE 7.18 **(A)** Freeze-frame of a color-coded Doppler echocardiogram from a 26-year-old man with a small membranous defect in the interventricular septum, immediately below the aortic annulus. The echocardiogram is from the left parasternal short-axis view of the aortic valve. The flow is into the right ventricle and produces a red color, indicating that the flow is toward the transducer on the precordium. **(B)** Black-and-white representation. (LA = left atrium; RA = right atrium; RVOT = right ventricular outflow tract; RVIN = right ventricular inflow) (Reproduced with permission; see Figure Credits)

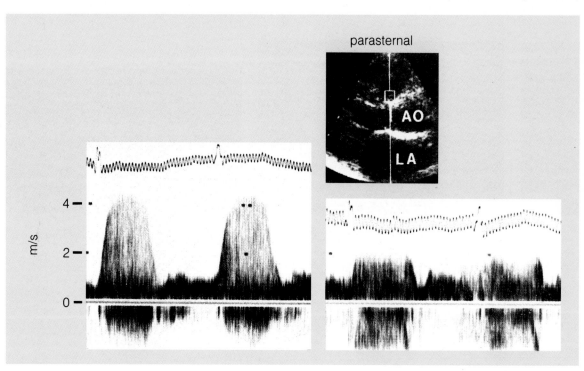

parasternal

FIGURE 7.19 **(A)** High-velocity jet through a VSD toward the transducer recorded with continuous-wave Doppler. **(B)** With pulsed Doppler, the VSD can be localized. The maximal velocity gives a calculated pressure difference of 80 mmHg between the ventricles; the systolic blood pressure of 100 mmHg indicates a right ventricular systolic pressure of around 20 mmHg. (AO = aorta; LA = left atrium) (Reproduced with permission; see Figure Credits)

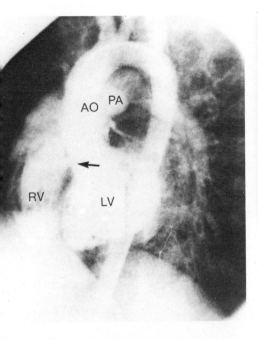

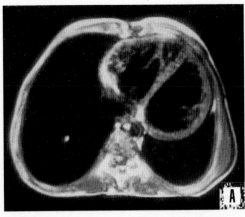

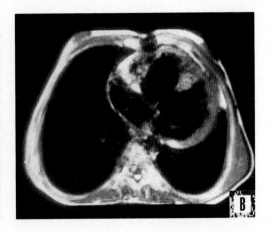

FIGURE 7.21 Transverse sections of ECG-gated spin-echo MR images of perimembranous VSD. **(A)** Section through the posteroinferior part of the ventricular septum shows that the septum is intact at this level. **(B)** A more cephalic section shows a VSD at the level of the central fibrous body. Note that the VSD is in continuity with the septal leaflet of the tricuspid valve. (Reproduced with permission; see Figure Credits)

FIGURE 7.20 Left anterior oblique view of a left ventricular angiogram in a 5-year-old child with a small perimembranous VSD (*arrow*). (RV = right ventricle; LV = left ventricle; AO = ascending aorta; PA = pulmonary artery) (Reproduced with permission; see Figure Credits)

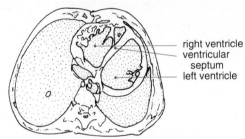

right ventricle
ventricular septum
left ventricle

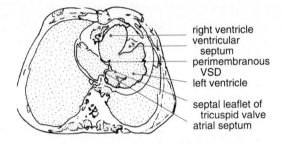

right ventricle
ventricular septum
perimembranous VSD
left ventricle
septal leaflet of tricuspid valve
atrial septum

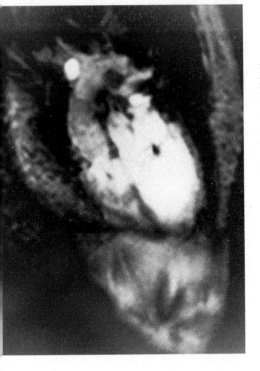

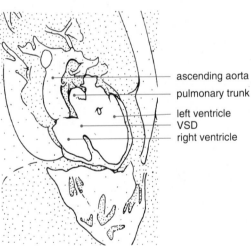

ascending aorta
pulmonary trunk
left ventricle
VSD
right ventricle

FIGURE 7.22 Cine MR image of a muscular VSD associated wlth transposition of the great arteries. The ventricular septum is seen in profile on this oblique craniocaudal section. The VSD is entirely surrounded by the muscular portion of the ventricular septum. The aorta arises from the morphologic right ventricle and the pulmonary trunk arises from the morphologic left ventricle in this patient with transposition of the great arteries. (Reproduced with permission; see Figure Credits)

NATURAL HISTORY

About one fourth of small interventricular defects close spontaneously within 1 1/2 years, one half close in 4 years, and even more are closed at 10 years.[1] With time some large defects become smaller, and a few may close.

Infants with large defects develop congestive heart failure. A small proportion develops subvalvar pulmonary stenosis, which produces a syndrome similar to tetralogy of Fallot.

Eisenmenger's syndrome is more likely to develop in patients beyond 1 year of age whose pulmonary systolic pressure is in excess of half of the systemic arterial pressure.[52]

A small number of patients (less than 1%) develop aortic regurgitation, while about 10% develop endocarditis during the first 30 years of life.[52]

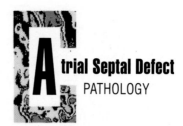

Atrial Septal Defect
PATHOLOGY

In all types of atrial septal defects, or interatrial communications, there is through-and-through opening between the left and the right atria[11] (Fig. 7.23). Only those within the oval fossa, termed *ostium secundum* defects, are true septa

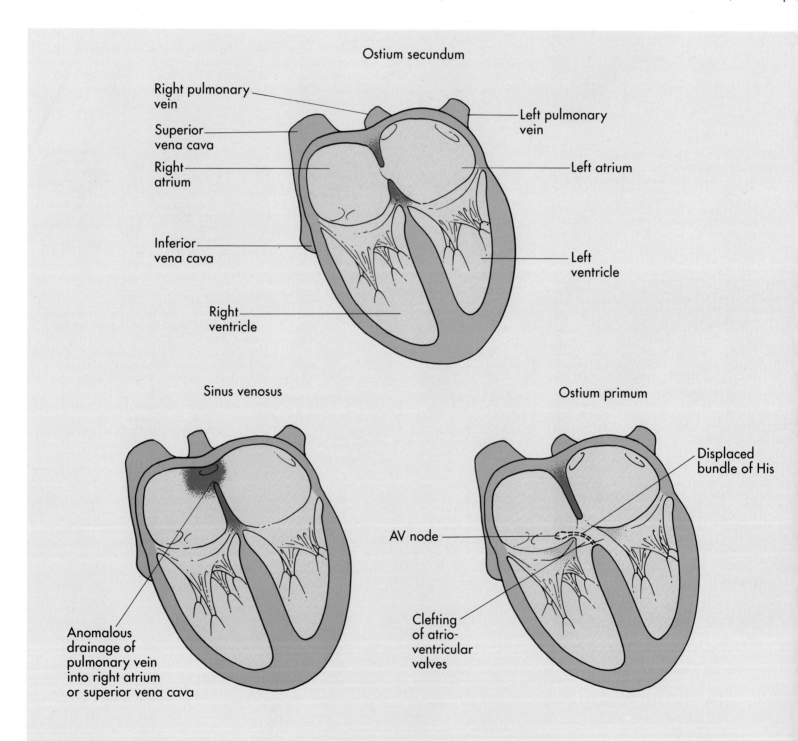

FIGURE 7.23   Interatrial septal defects. (Reproduced with permission; see Figure Credits)

defects (Fig. 7.24). Secundum defects range from patency of the oval foramen, through minimal to major deficiency of the floor of the fossa (Fig. 7.25), to various degrees of perforation of the floor. The *sinus venosus* defect is an interatrial communication in the mouth of the superior or inferior caval veins, existing outside the environs of the oval fossa (Fig. 7.26). Anomalous entrance of one or more pulmonary veins into the right atrium occurs in most patients with this defect. *Coronary sinus defects*, created at the mouth of the sinus because of unroofing of its atrial course, are very rarely found (Fig. 7.27). An atrial septal defect (ASD) within the oval fossa associated with mitral stenosis is termed Lutembacher's syndrome. The *ostium primum* defect is an atrioventricular septal defect (see discussion below).

PATHOPHYSIOLOGY

The ostium secundum defect produces a left-to-right shunt even though left atrial pressure may be the same or only a few millimeters of mercury higher than

the pressure in the right atrium. Left and right atrial pressures are equal when the area of the atrial septal defect exceeds 1.0 cm². The shunt may be large because the right atrium and the right ventricle offer little resistance to filling, and the tricuspid valve is large. Thus, right heart compliance is less than left heart compliance. During diastole when all four cardiac chambers are in communication, flow is directed to the most compliant chambers, producing a net left-to-right shunt (Fig. 7.28). Usually the pulmonary arterial system tolerates a large increase in pulmonary blood flow with little rise in pulmonary arterial pressure. Some patients, however, develop pulmonary hypertension, reversal of the shunt, and arterial oxygen unsaturation; this state is termed *Eisenmenger's physiology*. Mitral valve prolapse may also be present.

The sinus venosus defect produces an abnormal physiologic state similar to that found with ostium secundum. The abnormal physiology associated with Lutembacher's syndrome depends upon the severity of the mitral stenosis and the size of the ASD.

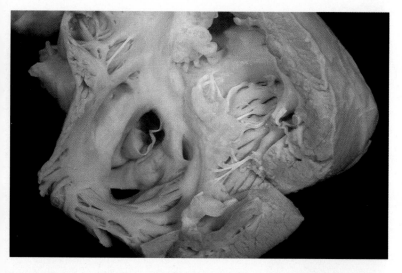

FIGURE 7.24   Interatrial communication within the oval fossa resulting from a deficiency of the floor of the fossa. This septal defect is usually described as

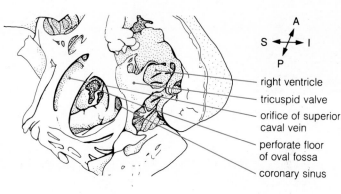

an ostium secundum defect, even though the floor of the fossa is made up of the primary atrial septum. (Reproduced with permission; see Figure Credits)

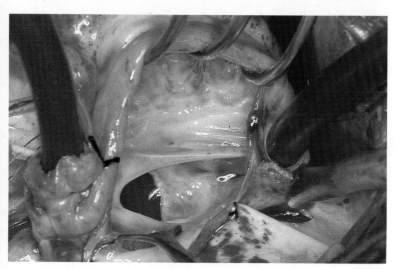

FIGURE 7.25   When the entire floor of the fossa is deficient, a large hole is created. (Reproduced with permission; see Figure Credits)

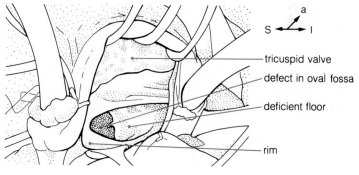

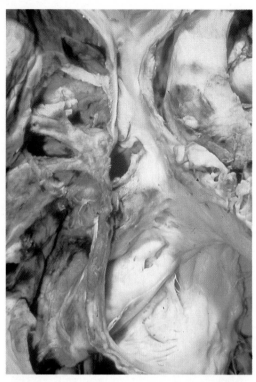

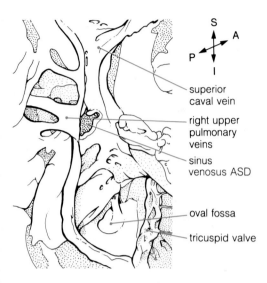

FIGURE 7.26   Sinus venosus defect: an interatrial communication in the mouth of the superior caval vein resulting from the biatrial connection of the superior caval and right upper pulmonary veins. It is outside the confines of the true atrial septum (the environs of the oval fossa), although it unequivocally produces an interatrial defect. (Reproduced with permission; see Figure Credits)

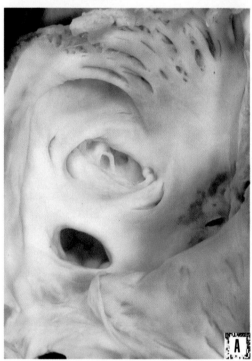

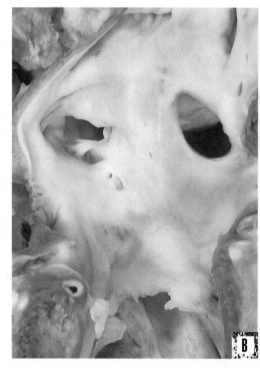

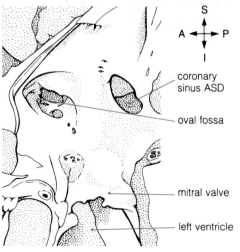

FIGURE 7.27   An interatrial communication through the mouth of the coronary sinus viewed from the right **(A)** and left **(B)** atrial aspects. The defect, which is outside the confines of the oval fossa, results from unroofing of the coronary sinus. There is a total lack of the party wall normally separating the coronary sinus from the left atrium (unroofed coronary sinus). Usually this lesion co-exists with a persistent left superior caval vein connected to the roof of the left atrium, but this anomalous venous connection is lacking in this particular heart. (Reproduced with permission; see Figure Credits)

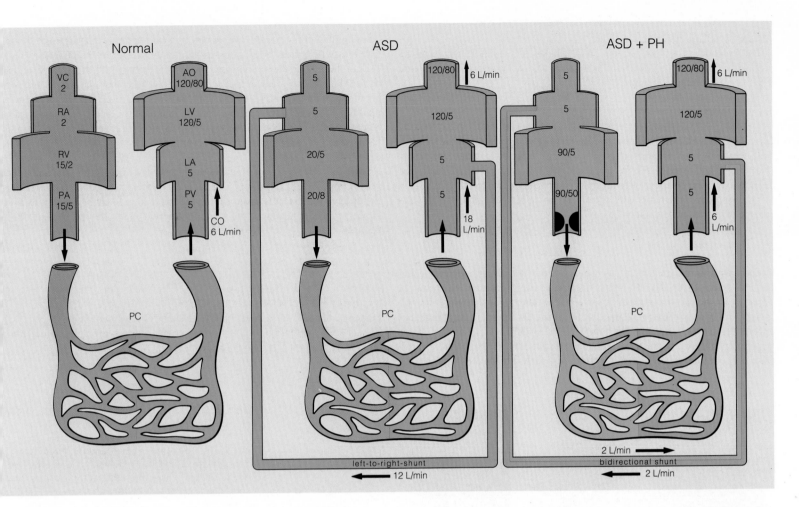

FIGURE 7.28 Pathophysiology of atrial septal defects (ASDs). The left panel depicts normal hemodynamics. The middle panel demonstrates the changes that occur in ASD without pulmonary hypertension (PH). The right ventricle (RV) is dilated and modestly hypertrophied. RV compliance is greater than left ventricular (LV) compliance and, consequently, there is a net flow from the left atrium (LA) to the right atrium (RA) of 12 L/min. There is a pulmonary blood flow of 18 L/min. Left and right heart pressures are within the normal range although right-sided pressures are slightly higher. The right panel demonstrates ASD with pulmonary vascular disease. RV systolic and pulmonary arterial pressures rise considerably, possibly achieving systemic arterial levels. The RV becomes dilated and hypertrophied and RV compliance now equals LV compliance. Consequently, there are small bidirectional shunts at the atrial level (2 L/min each). Forward cardiac output (CO) is maintained at 6 L/min. If the RV or LV fails, systemic CO will fall. (VC = vena cava; PA = pulmonary artery; PC = pulmonary capillaries; PV = pulmonary veins; AO = aorta)(Modified with permission; see Figure Credits)

CLINICAL MANIFESTATIONS

Atrial septal defect is twice as common in females as in males. It may be associated with Holt–Oram syndrome, Ellis–van Creveld syndrome, and thrombocytopenia–absent radius syndrome.[39]

SYMPTOMS

Most patients with ostium secundum defects are asymptomatic until the fourth or fifth decade of life.[19] Patients in their late teens and early twenties may experience fatigue and dyspnea. Atrial fibrillation, heart failure, and pulmonary hypertension may occur during or after the fourth decade of life. Endocarditis is rare.

The symptoms of patients with sinus venosus defects are similar to those of patients with ostium secundum defects.

PHYSICAL EXAMINATION

Patients with secundum defects may appear entirely normal, although some may have a slender build. An abnormal pulsation of the pulmonary trunk may be detected in the second intercostal space to the left of the sternum (the pulmonary artery area). A right ventricular lift of the left anterior precordium may be present. The second sound is almost always widely split; it remains so on inspiration and expiration (the so-called fixed split S_2). The pulmonary component of the second sound is usually normal or slightly increased in intensity. An opening snap of the tricuspid valve may be heard with large left-to-right shunts. There may be a diamond-shaped systolic murmur heard in the pulmonary area. A diastolic rumble due to increased blood flow through the tricuspid valve may be heard at the lower left sternal border. In adults this murmur may be mistaken for the murmur of mitral stenosis. The early systolic click and the late systolic murmur of mitral valve prolapse may be heard at the apex. Pulmonary valve regurgitation due to dilation of the pulmonary artery and pulmonary valve annulus may be detected in older patients even when the pulmonary arterial pressure is only slightly elevated.

The sinus venosus defect produces similar physical signs. When the pulmonary veins from the right upper lobe or middle lobe enter the superior caval vein and the atrial septal defect is small, the second heart sound may be abnormally split. However, fixed splitting of the second sound occurs in only 80 percent of the patients.

LABORATORY STUDIES

Chest Radiography   The chest film of a patient with an atrial septal defect shows a large pulmonary trunk, large pulmonary arterial branches, a small aorta, and right ventricular enlargement (Figs. 7.29, 7.30). Pulmonary hypertension leads to marked enlargement of the right ventricle and pulmonary arteries. The lung fields are clear (Fig. 7.31).

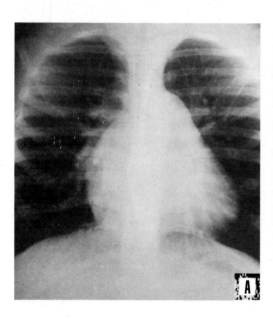 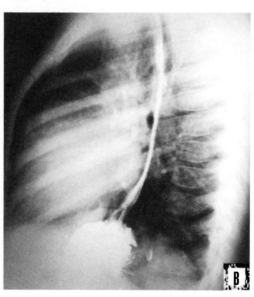

FIGURE 7.29   **(A)** Frontal chest radiograph of a 4-year-old child with a secundum ASD, a large left-to-right shunt, and normal pulmonary arterial pressures. The aorta is small and the main pulmonary artery and its branches are large. **(B)** On the left lateral view, the right ventricle appears to be large. (Reproduced with permission; see Figure Credits)

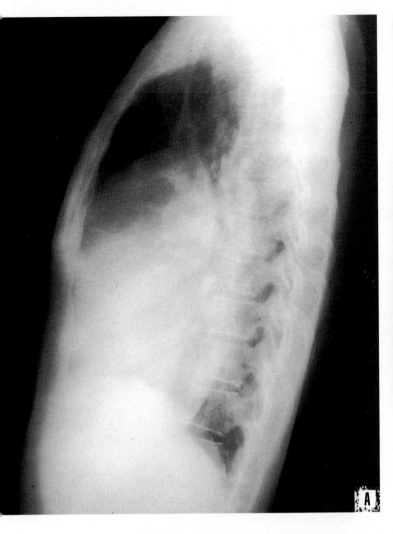

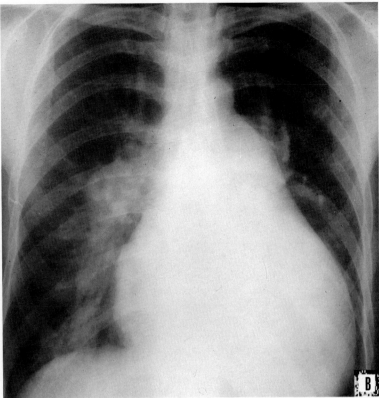

FIGURE 7.30 **(A)** Left lateral projection of a patient with a large secundum ASD and a large left-to-right shunt (pulmonary blood flow three times systemic blood flow). Note massive filling of the retrosternal space by the large right ventricle. Also note the left ventricle pushed posteriorly over the spine. There was no left ventricular enlargement. **(B)** Posteroanterior projection. Note the enlarged cardiac silhouette due to the large right ventricle, markedly enlarged main pulmonary artery segment, and huge pulmonary arterial markings. There is no left ventricular enlargement. The right ventricle forms the apex of the heart. (Reproduced with permission; see Figure Credits)

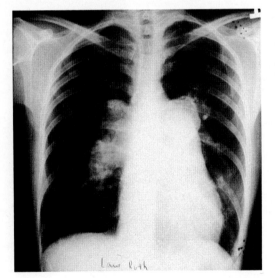

FIGURE 7.31 Posteroanterior projection of a 40-year-old cyanotic woman with a large secundum ASD and with no residual left-to-right shunt and a large right-to-left shunt at the atrial level. Note the massive enlargement of the main pulmonary artery and the primary proximal pulmonary artery branches. This is in contrast to the absence of pulmonary vascular markings in the lateral one third of the lung fields. (Reproduced with permission; see Figure Credits)

Electrocardiography In the typical ECG of a secundum defect there is a right ventricular conduction delay with an rSr' or rSR configuration to the QRS complex in lead V₁ (Fig. 7.32). The PR interval may be long, and Wolff–Parkinson–White (WPW) configuration is occasionally seen, with a short PR interval.

Echocardiography The M-mode echocardiogram reveals evidence of volume overload of the right ventricle. The right atrium and the right ventricle are increased in size, and paradoxical motion of the ventricular septum is evident (Fig. 7.33).

The cross-sectional echocardiogram can identify a secundum ASD with a sensitivity of approximately 90% (Figs. 7.34–7.36), while the sinus venosus defect can be demonstrated in only 50% of patients.[48]

Cardiac Catheterization Patients with ASDs exhibit an increase in the oxygen saturation of the blood in the right atrium, right ventricle, and pulmonary artery; the pulmonary arterial systolic pressure is usually normal. Increase in pulmonary blood flow causes a small pressure gradient across the pulmonary valve. The level of pressure in the left and right atria is usually normal, with the left atrial pressure no more than 3 mmHg higher than the right atrial pressure.

The site of abnormal pulmonary venous connections may be identified by selective injection of contrast material. Aortography is used to identify a patent arterial duct, which may occur in some patients.

Other Imaging Modalities Nuclear magnetic resonance and CT scanning can also clearly delineate atrial septal defects (Fig. 7.37).

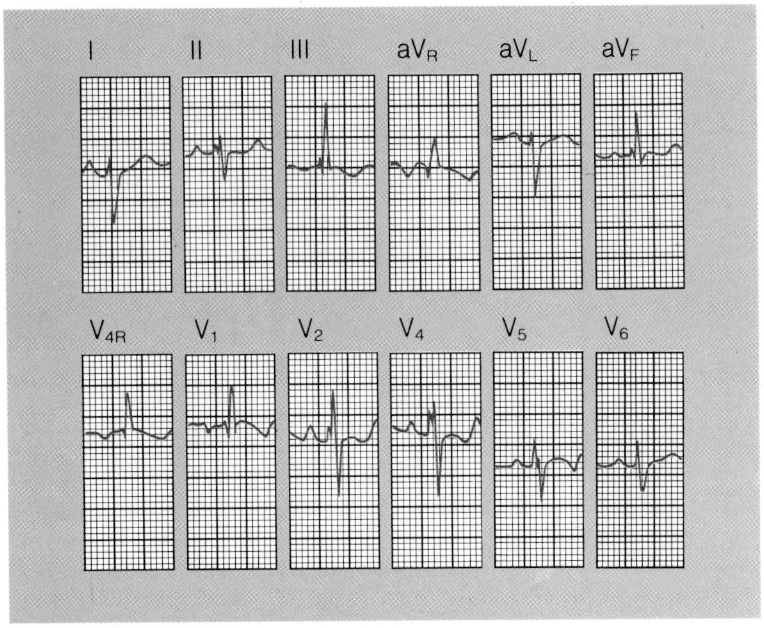

FIGURE 7.32 ECG from a 5-year-old child with ostium secundum ASD. The mean QRS vector is directed to the right and anteriorly; the mean T vector is directed to the left and posteriorly. The configuration of the QRS complex in lead V₁ is rsR'. (Reproduced with permission; see Figure Credits)

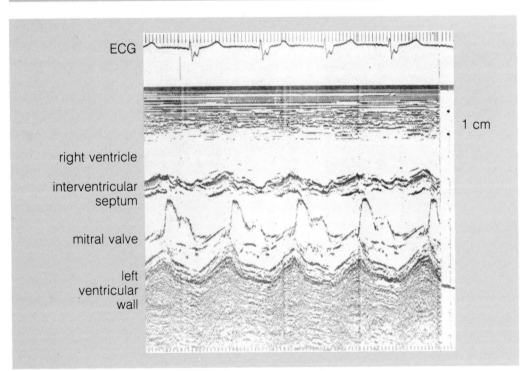

FIGURE 7.33 M-mode echocardiogram from a child with a secundum ASD. There is increased right ventricular cavity dimension (2.4-cm end-diastolic diameter) and anterior systolic motion of the interventricular septum characteristic of right ventricular diastolic overload. (Reproduced with permission; see Figure Credits)

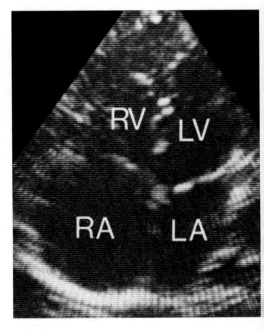

FIGURE 7.34 Cross-sectional echocardiogram from a patient with a large secundum ASD. The apical four-chamber view shows the enlarged right atrium (RA) and right ventricle (RV). The right ventricle forms the apex. An area of echocardiography dropout is present in the mid-portion of the interatrial septum. (LA = left atrium; LV = left ventricle) (Reproduced with permission; see Figure Credits)

NATURAL HISTORY

Spontaneous closure of the secundum defect rarely occurs beyond infancy. A small percentage of these patients develop heart failure as infants, but almost all are asymptomatic and lead normal lives until adulthood. Symptoms begin to appear in the twenties, and by age 40 most patients have dyspnea and fatigue.[19] Severe pulmonary hypertension develops in a few patients in their twenties.[20] However, severe pulmonary vascular disease is usually not seen before the age of 30. It is impossible to predict which patients will develop the disease. Pregnancy may accelerate or exaggerate pulmonary hypertension. On rare occasions, a patient may have a paradoxical embolus and brain abscess. Bacterial endocarditis is rare.

The natural history of a sinus venosus defect is similar to that of the secundum ASD.

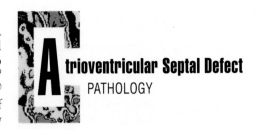

Atrioventricular Septal Defect
PATHOLOGY

A defect in the lower portion of the atrial septum and in the upper portion of the ventricular septum due to complete absence of the normal atrioventricular septal structures is termed an atrioventricular septal defect (AVSD), or sometimes endocardial cushion defect. The absence of atrioventricular septation

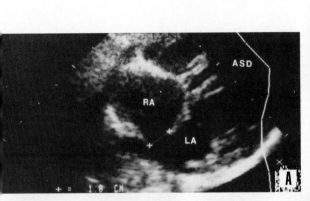

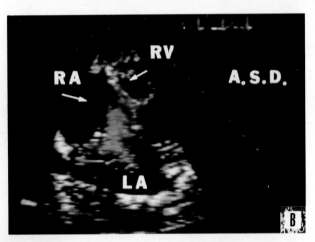

FIGURE 7.35 **(A)** Subcostal two-dimensional image of a secundum ASD 1 cm in diameter. **(B)** Stop-frame image of a two-dimensional flow mapping study. This late-systolic frame shows the direct imaging of left-to-right shunt flow across the secundum defect. (RV = right ventricle; RA = right atrium; LA = left atrium) (Reproduced with permission; see Figure Credits)

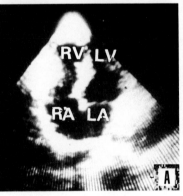
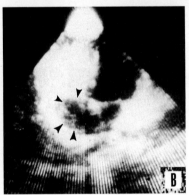
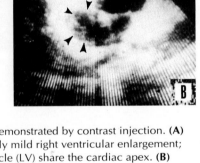

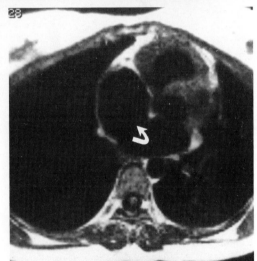
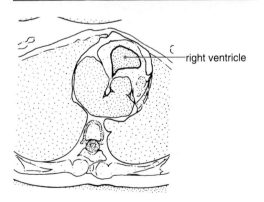

right ventricle

FIGURE 7.37
Transverse image of a patient with a secundum ASD and pulmonary arterial hypertension. Transverse images show the defect in the secundum septum (*curved arrow*). Note the increase in thickness of the walls of the right ventricle (RV). (Reproduced with permission; see Figure Credits)

FIGURE 7.36 Left-to-right shunt demonstrated by contrast injection. **(A)** In the four-chamber view, there is only mild right ventricular enlargement; the right ventricle (RV) and left ventricle (LV) share the cardiac apex. **(B)** Contrast injection reveals that there is a strong jet of unopacified blood passing from left to right (*arrows*). This finding led to the performance of a scintigraphic shunt study, revealing a moderate-sized ASD (>2:1). (Reproduced with permission; see Figure Credits)

results in a common atrioventricular junction guarded by a basically common valve. The left ventricular component of this valve is a three-leaflet structure; the so-called cleft (Fig. 7.38) represents the space between the two leaflets that are tethered in both ventricles, bridging the ventricular septum.[2a]

There are several anatomic types of abnormalities. The *ostium primum* or *partial* type of defect (Fig. 739A) is characterized by a tongue of leaflet tissue that joins the facing surfaces of the bridging leaflets, dividing the basically common orifice into right and left components. The left valve then has a three-leaflet arrangement; the cleft is located between the left ventricular portions of the bridging leaflets. The leaflets themselves, together with the connecting tongue, are bound to the septum as they bridge, so that shunting through the AVSD occurs exclusively at the atrial level.

The *complete* type (often termed common atrioventricular canal or common valve orifice) is characterized by a failure of the common junction to partition into separate atrioventricular orifices. The opening between the atria and the ventricles is thus protected by a common valve (Fig. 7.39B) The complete type is subdivided into three subgroups (Fig. 7.40). In *Type A* the superior bridging leaflet extends only marginally into the right ventricle; the commissure between the superior and anterosuperior leaflets on the right ventricle is attached by short cords to the ventricular septum. An interventricular connection is present between the bridging leaflets. In *Type B* the superior bridging leaflet extends further into the right ventricle. Cords from the leaflet are attached to an anomalous anterior papillary muscle in the right ventricle, but no cords attach to the ventricular septum. In Type C there is extensive bridging of the free-floating

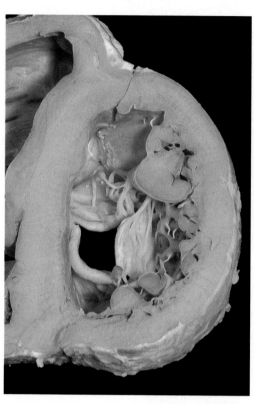

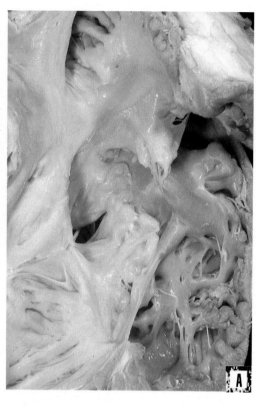

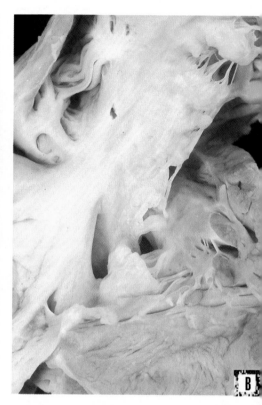

FIGURE 7.38   Short-axis section of an AVSD is viewed from beneath to show the trifoliate nature of the left atrioventricular valve. The abnormality in the mitral valve, frequently described as a cleft, is the space between the left ventricular components of the bridging leaflets. The left valve bears no resemblance to the mitral valve other than its residence within the left ventricle. (Reproduced with permission; see Figure Credits)

FIGURE 7.39   The ostium primum (**A**) and the complete types of AVSD (**B**), which represent absence of the normal atrioventricular septal structures, have directly comparable morphology. The atrial septum is virtually intact in both hearts. In the primum defect the bridging leaflets guard-

ing the common atrioventricular junction are joined by a connecting tongue, but they are separate structures in the heart with a common valve orifice. (Reproduced with permission; see Figure Credits)

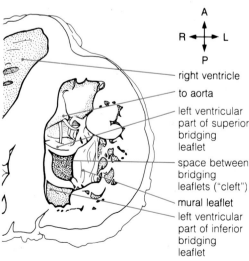

A
R ←→ L
P

- right ventricle
- to aorta
- left ventricular part of superior bridging leaflet
- space between bridging leaflets ("cleft")
- mural leaflet
- left ventricular part of inferior bridging leaflet

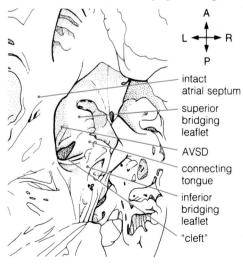

A
L ←→ R
P

- intact atrial septum
- superior bridging leaflet
- AVSD
- connecting tongue
- inferior bridging leaflet
- "cleft"

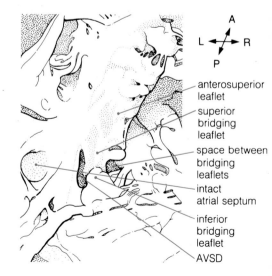

A
L ←→ R
P

- anterosuperior leaflet
- superior bridging leaflet
- space between bridging leaflets
- intact atrial septum
- inferior bridging leaflet
- AVSD

superior leaflet with diminution in size of the anterosuperior leaflet of the right ventricle. The commissure between the two is supported by the anterior papillary muscle of the right ventricle.[44]

The AVSDs discussed above are the varieties most commonly seen in practice; however there are many other defects that are associated with AVSDs. Often a narrowed left ventricular outflow tract with marked disproportion between the inlet and the outlet dimensions of the left ventricle is seen in conjunction with the three-leaflet arrangement of the left atrioventricular valve (Fig. 7.41).

PATHOPHYSIOLOGY

The pulmonary arterial and the right ventricular pressures are normal or slightly elevated in patients with communication between the two atria but no shunt at the ventricular level; the pulmonary blood flow is also increased. These findings simulate those of a large ostium secundum ASD. In contrast the pulmonary arterial and the right ventricular pressures are usually elevated with a large VSD. The arrangement of the leaflets of the valves guarding the abnormal atrioventricular junction may cause severe regurgitation; blood may also be shunted from the left ventricle into the right atrium.

CLINICAL MANIFESTATIONS

About 3% of children with congenital heart disease have some type of AVSD; the female to male ratio is 1.3:1. About 50% or more of patients with the complete type have Down's syndrome.[14]

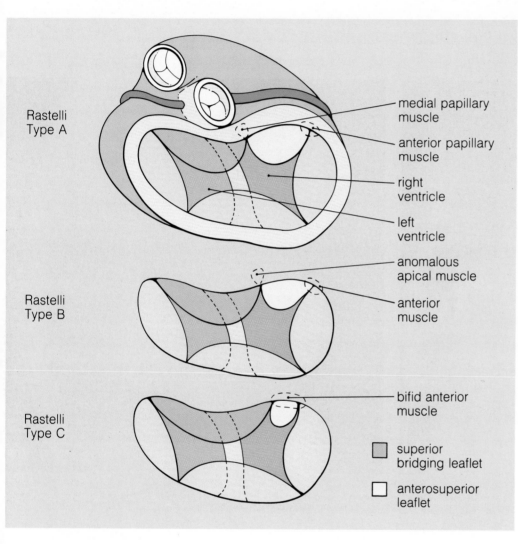

Rastelli Type A

Rastelli Type B

Rastelli Type C

- medial papillary muscle
- anterior papillary muscle
- right ventricle
- left ventricle
- anomalous apical muscle
- anterior muscle
- bifid anterior muscle
- ▨ superior bridging leaflet
- ☐ anterosuperior leaflet

FIGURE 7.40   This schematic drawing illustrates the variable extent of bridging of the superior leaflet in AVSD with common valve orifice. As the superior leaflet extends further into the right ventricle, the anterosuperior leaflet decreases in size. The commissure between the two is supported by a papillary muscle, which occupies a variable location within the right ventricle. (Reproduced with permission; see Figure Credits)

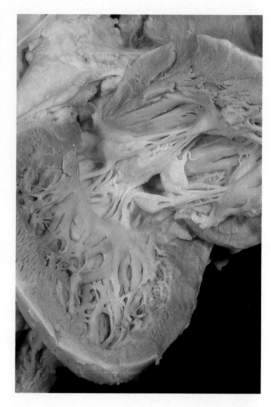

FIGURE 7.41   A view of the outlet component of the left ventricle in a heart with an ASVD shows the marked discrepancy between the inlet and outlet dimensions along with the three-leaflet arrangement of the left atrioventricular valve. (Reproduced with permission; see Figure Credits)

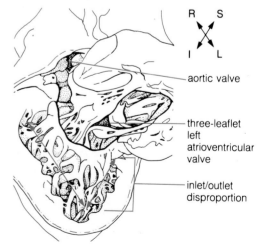

- aortic valve
- three-leaflet left atrioventricular valve
- inlet/outlet disproportion

SYMPTOMS

Children with the partial type of AVSD are usually asymptomatic and simulate patients with secundum ASD, unless there is regurgitation through the left atrioventricular valve. Slight regurgitation may produce no symptoms, while severe regurgitation results in poor weight gain, fatigue, dyspnea, frequent upper respiratory infections, and heart failure.

Patients with the complete type of AVSD are often seriously ill and develop heart failure at an early age. If the defect is not treated surgically, death will occur in about half of patients during the first year of life.

PHYSICAL EXAMINATION

The abnormalities noted on physical examination of patients with partial defects are similar to patients with secundum ASDs, unless the arrangement of the left valve permits regurgitation. Accordingly when regurgitation is present, a systolic murmur is heard at the apex. When the regurgitation is severe, it also results in a diastolic rumble at the apex.

Patients with complete defects exhibit physical abnormalities similar to those found in patients with interventricular septal defects. There may be an anterior precordial lift and a large pulsation at the apex. A murmur of left or right valve regurgitation, which can be separated from the murmur of VSD, may be detected. There is fixed splitting of the second sound. The pulmonary component of the second sound may be louder than normal, because pulmonary hypertension is commonly present.

LABORATORY STUDIES

Chest Radiography   The partial lesion with regurgitation through the left atrioventricular valve is characterized by right and left ventricular hypertrophy, left atrial enlargement, and increased pulmonary blood flow (Fig. 7.42). The complete defect produces a very large heart with evidence of considerable increase in pulmonary blood flow.

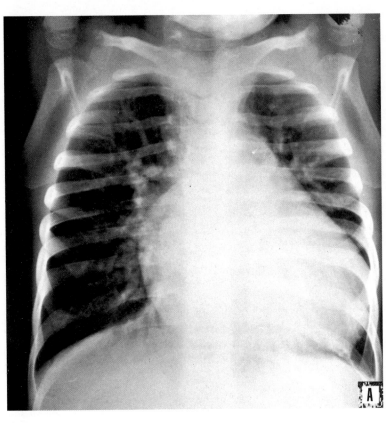

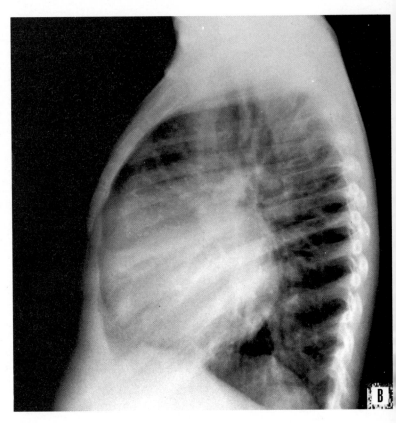

FIGURE 7.42   (A) Posteroanterior chest film of a 4-year-old child with a complete AVSD shows marked cardiac enlargement with increased pulmonary blood flow. (B) On the lateral view left atrial enlargement is evident. (Reproduced with permission; see Figure Credits)

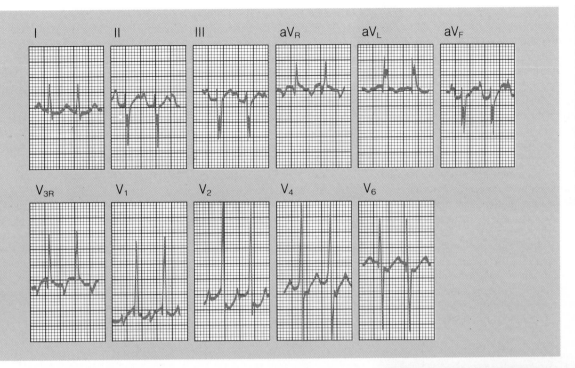

I   II   III   aV_R   aV_L   aV_F

V_3R   V_1   V_2   V_4   V_6

FIGURE 7.43 This ECG was obtained in an infant with a complete AVSD, a large left-to-right shunt, and severe pulmonary arterial hypertension. The mean QRS vector is directed to the left (-70°) and anteriorly. This is caused by left anterior-superior division block plus right ventricular delay or right bundle branch block (QRS duration is 0.09 to 0.10 sec which is prolonged for an infant). Biatrial abnormality and biventricular hypertrophy are present. (Reproduced with permission; see Figure Credits)

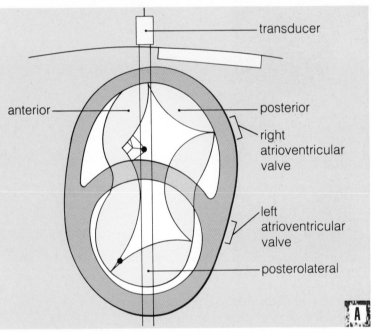

transducer

anterior

posterior

right atrioventricular valve

left atrioventricular valve

posterolateral

A

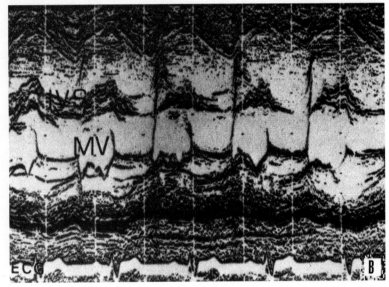

IVS

MV

ECG

B

FIGURE 7.44 (**A**) This diagram represents a transverse cut of a heart with a complete form of AVSD. The orientation of the two bridging leaflets allows a diastolic movement at right angles to the interventricular septum, creating an echocardiographic hole between the anteroposterior leaflet of the right valve and the posterolateral cusp of the left valve. (**B**) In the M-mode echocardiogram an apparent common atrioventricular valve occupies the whole heart. The superimposition of the leaflet, together with the different degrees of atrioventricular valve septal overriding, may explain this picture. No echoes from the anteroseptal leaflet of the left valve are seen (MV, left atrioventricular valve; IVS, interventricular septum). (Partially redrawn; reproduced with permission; see Figure Credits)

Electrocardiography   A partial defect without "mitral" regurgitation may be associated with right ventricular conduction delay. However, the mean QRS vector may be located to the left and superiorly because of displaced atrioventricular conduction tissue. Regurgitation through the left atrioventricular valve, when present, may produce left ventricular hypertrophy. First-degree heart block may be present.

A complete malformation may produce a long P-R interval, a wider than average QRS duration, biatrial abnormality, right bundle branch block plus left anterior-superior division block, with a mean QRS vector rotated to the left and anteriorly, and biventricular hypertrophy (Fig. 7.43).

Echocardiography   An M-mode echocardiogram of a patient with a complete form of AVSD reveals an increase in right ventricular dimensions and anterior systolic movement of the ventricular septum, suggesting right ventricular diastolic overload of the right ventricle (Fig. 7.44).

A cross sectional echocardiogram can detect an ASD and attachment of the bridging leaflets to the ventricular septum, thus demonstrating the AVSD (Fig. 7.45). In patients with the complete type of AVSD, floating of the leaflets differentiates the atrial and ventricular components of the lesion. Echoes taken in the short axis demonstrate the three-leaflet nature of the left valve, showing that the cleft is the space between the left ventricular components of the bridging leaflets. The extent of bridging of the superior leaflet into the right ventricle indicates the presence of subtypes A, B, and C as described by Rastelli and his colleagues[44] (see Fig. 7.43).

Cardiac Catheterization   There is an increase i oxygen saturation between the superior caval vein and the right atrium i patients with partial or complete types of AVSD. Whenever the right ventricu lar and the pulmonary systolic pressures exceed 60 mmHg in such patients, th possibility of a complete lesion must be considered. A complete defect produce nearly identical systolic pressures in the right ventricle, the pulmonary arter and the systemic arterial system.

The left ventriculogram shows a characteristic gooseneck abnormality an shunting of blood from the left ventricle to the right ventricle (Fig. 7.46) Evidence of regurgitation through the left atrioventricular valve and shuntin from the left ventricle to the right atrium may also be evaluated.

NATURAL HISTORY

A patient with an ASD located low in the atrial septum (ostium primum) with no regurgitation through the left atrioventricular valve has the same prognosis as the patient with a secundum defect. Such patients may have a trifo liate left valve that does not permit any regurgitation; they are then more susceptible to endocarditis than patients with secundum defects. When regurgitation is present, the prognosis is determined by its extent; heart failure may occur early in such patients. Infants with complete defects develop congestive heart failure and die unless surgical intervention is successful.

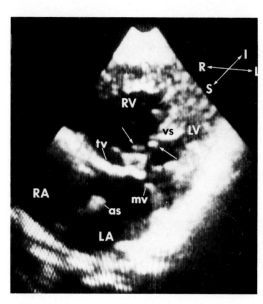

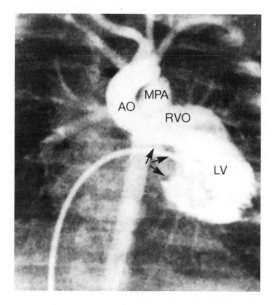

FIGURE 7.45   This cross-sectional echocardiogram in the apex view was obtained in a child with type A complete AVSD. The common anterior leaflet to the right (tv) and the left (mv) valves appears to be attached to the crest of the ventricular septum (vs) by multiple cords (*arrows*). The area of the ostium primum defect lies between the lowermost edge of the atrial septum (as) and the valve (RV, right ventricle; LV, left ventricle; RA, right atrium; LA, left atrium). (Reproduced with permission; see Figure Credits)

FIGURE 7.46   Posteroanterior view of the left ventricular angiogram from a child with complete AVSD demonstrates the characteristic gooseneck deformity (*arrows*) of the outflow tract of the left ventricle (LV). Opacification of the right ventricular outflow tract (RVO) and the pulmonary trunk (MPA) before, or in the absence of, atrial opacification reflects the presence of the interventricular communication (AO, aorta). (Reproduced with permission; see Figure Credits)

Total Anomalous Pulmonary Venous Connections
PATHOLOGY

Total anomalous pulmonary venous connection (TAPVC) is said to be present when all of the pulmonary veins enter the right atrium or a systemic vein rather than the left atrium. In this condition the pulmonary veins leave the lungs and join a common venous structure, which then terminates in a systemic venous location. Occasionally two or more veins terminate in the right atrium or a systemic vein. The sites of termination that are located above the diaphragm are the left innominate vein, the coronary sinus (Fig. 7.47), the right atrium, the superior caval vein (Fig. 7.48), and the azygous veins.[4] The sites of termination that are located below the diaphragm are the portal vein, the venous duct, and the gastric vein (Fig. 7.49). The oval foramen is always present and patent.

Rarely, no major veins leave the common venous structure; in such cases small veins enter the esophageal wall. This condition is called atresia of the common pulmonary vein.

PATHOPHYSIOLOGY

There must be a communication between the left and the right side of the heart in order for life to be sustained, since all of the blood from the pulmonary and systemic circulations eventually returns to the right atrium. The systemic arterial oxygen saturation is low when there is obstruction to the flow in the pulmonary veins.[15]

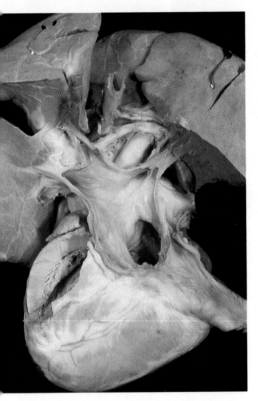

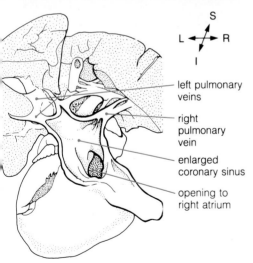

FIGURE 7.47
Total anomalous pulmonary venous connection to the coronary sinus can be seen in this heart dissected from behind. (Reproduced with permission; see Figure Credits)

left pulmonary veins

right pulmonary vein

enlarged coronary sinus

opening to right atrium

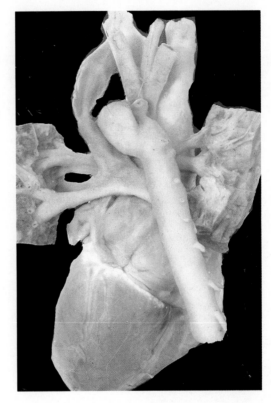

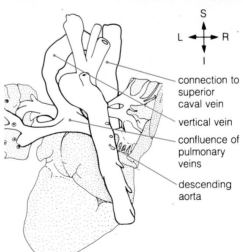

FIGURE 7.48
Total anomalous pulmonary venous connection to the superior caval vein can be seen in this heart viewed from behind. (Reproduced with permission; see Figure Credits)

connection to superior caval vein

vertical vein

confluence of pulmonary veins

descending aorta

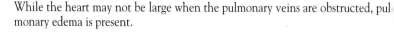

CLINICAL MANIFESTATIONS

SYMPTOMS

Cyanosis in the infant is apparent. The symptoms of heart failure occur in the majority of patients by the age of three months. Most infants are thin and do not gain weight normally.

PHYSICAL EXAMINATION

The infant is usually cyanotic and has an increased respiratory rate. The liver is large, and the jugular venous pulse is elevated. The right ventricular pulsation is hyperdynamic, and the second sound is abnormally split. The split remains during inspiration and expiration; the sound of pulmonary valve closure is usually abnormally loud. There may be a grade 2–3 systolic murmur heard at the left sternal border; a tricuspid diastolic rumble may be heard at the lower sternal border. A continuous murmur may be heard over the common venous structure.

While the heart may not be large when the pulmonary veins are obstructed, pulmonary edema is present.

LABORATORY STUDIES

Chest Radiography   The heart is usually enlarged with an increase in pulmonary blood flow; pulmonary edema may be present. When all of the venous blood enters the innominate vein, a characteristic radiographic contour is seen; it is usually described as the "snowman" or "figure-of-eight" appearance (Fig. 7.50).[26]

Electrocardiography   The ECG shows right atrial abnormality and right ventricular hypertrophy. There may be a qR pattern in the precordial leads.

Echocardiography   The M-mode echocardiogram shows volume overload of the right ventricle when the pulmonary venous system is not obstructed. Signs of pulmonary hypertension may be present when the pul-

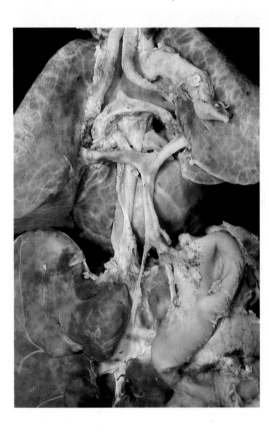

FIGURE 7.49   This heart dissected and viewed from behind shows totally anomalous infradiaphragmatic pulmonary venous connection. The venous channel breaks up and terminates in the gastric veins. (Reproduced with permission; see Figure Credits)

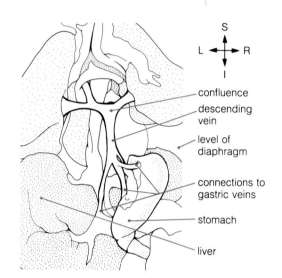

- confluence
- descending vein
- level of diaphragm
- connections to gastric veins
- stomach
- liver

monary veins are obstructed. The common venous structure may be seen behind the right atrium. Cross-sectional echocardiography may outline the site of drainage.[45]

Cardiac Catheterization   The oxygen saturation is increased at the site of abnormal venous connection; similar saturations are found in all chambers of the heart. The right ventricular and the pulmonary arterial pressures are elevated. The pulmonary wedge pressure is elevated in patients who have obstruction of the pulmonary veins.

Pulmonary angiography usually reveals the abnormal venous connection.

Contrast material may be injected into the common venous structure in order to identify the sites of termination and obstruction.

NATURAL HISTORY

Without treatment most patients with pulmonary hypertension and pulmonary venous obstruction die by the age of three months, while patients with pulmonary hypertension alone live longer. The usual clinical picture is heart failure and death within one year.[15]

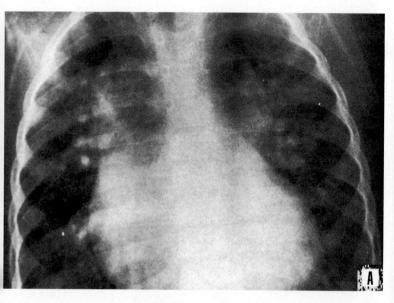

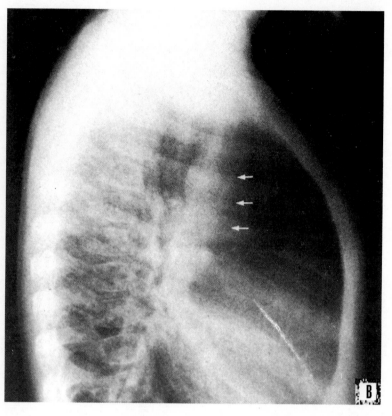

FIGURE 7.50   (**A**) Frontal chest film illustrates the typical "snowman" appearance of total anomalous pulmonary venous return to a left vertical vein. The pulmonary arterial vascularity is increased as the result of left-to-right shunting. (**B**) On the lateral view the density (*arrow*) anterior to the trachea represents the left vertical vein. No thymic tissue is present behind the sternum. (Reproduced with permission; see Figure Credits)

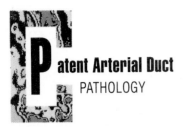

Patent Arterial Duct
PATHOLOGY

In patent arterial duct (also termed *patent ductus arteriosus*, PDA) the arterial duct connects the pulmonary trunk and the aorta, running from the origin of the left pulmonary artery to the aorta just distal to the origin of the left subcla-vian artery[10] (Fig. 7.51). The duct normally closes within 3 weeks of birth, becoming the arterial ligament[53] (Fig. 7.52).

A patent duct may be associated with coarctation of the aorta or ventricular septal defect. Patency of the duct may also be associated with conditions such as pulmonary atresia with intact ventricular septum. In such cases it is advanta-geous if the duct remains open; however, even when needed, it does tend to close.

PATHOPHYSIOLOGY

The blood flows from the aorta through the duct to the pulmonary artery throughout the heart cycle, unless the pulmonary arterial vascular resistance is sufficiently elevated to alter this pattern. As pulmonary vascular resistance rises,

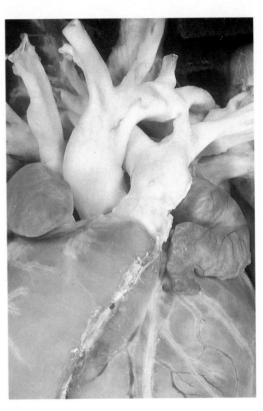

FIGURE 7.52
Normal heart from a 6-week-old infant in which the arterial duct constricts as it is transformed into the arterial ligament. The lumen is completely obliterated by this stage. (Reproduced with permission; see Figure Credits)

FIGURE 7.51   Heart with persistent patency of the arterial duct sectioned to replicate the view obtained by the echocardiographer from the suprasternal window. The duct is seen extending above the left pulmonary artery to the descending aorta. (Reproduced with permission; see Figure Credits)

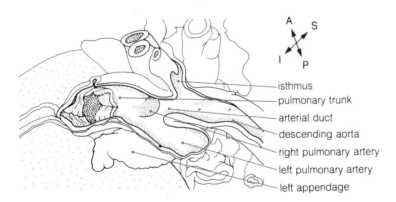

- isthmus
- pulmonary trunk
- arterial duct
- descending aorta
- right pulmonary artery
- left pulmonary artery
- left appendage

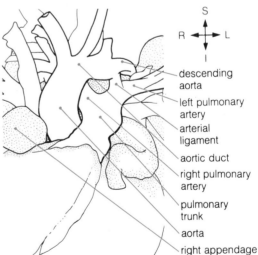

- descending aorta
- left pulmonary artery
- arterial ligament
- aortic duct
- right pulmonary artery
- pulmonary trunk
- aorta
- right appendage

the diastolic component of the left-to-right shunt is first to disappear. The left-to-right shunt may be small or large.

The blood flow through a high-resistance patent duct is small, causing little hemodynamic difficulty. The increased work of the left ventricle created by the increased volume is small; the pulmonary arteriolar resistance and the pulmonary arterial pressure are not elevated.

A large duct offers little resistance to blood flow; the pressure in the pulmonary artery is about the same as it is in the aorta. The volume load on the left ventricle is large, causing dilation and hypertrophy. Pulmonary congestion may develop, because the increased pressure in the left atrium and the pulmonary capillaries and the large pulmonary arterial blood flow develop at a time when the pulmonary arterioles are not fully capable of protecting the lungs. The patient with a moderate-sized or large duct may also have a right ventricle that becomes hypertrophic due to a pressure load created by pulmonary arteriolar vasoconstriction.

When the pulmonary vascular resistance equals or exceeds that of the systemic system, unsaturated blood is shunted from the pulmonary artery to the aorta. When this occurs, the patient's feet may appear more cyanotic than the right hand (Fig. 7.53).

CLINICAL MANIFESTATIONS

Patency of the arterial duct occurs more often in premature infants than in full-term babies, and more often in females than males. It is also common in infants whose mothers contracted rubella during the first trimester of pregnancy;[26] males and females are equally affected in this case.

SYMPTOMS

Patients with small left-to-right shunts through patent ducts have no symptoms, but they are subject to infective endarteritis. Patients with large left-to-right

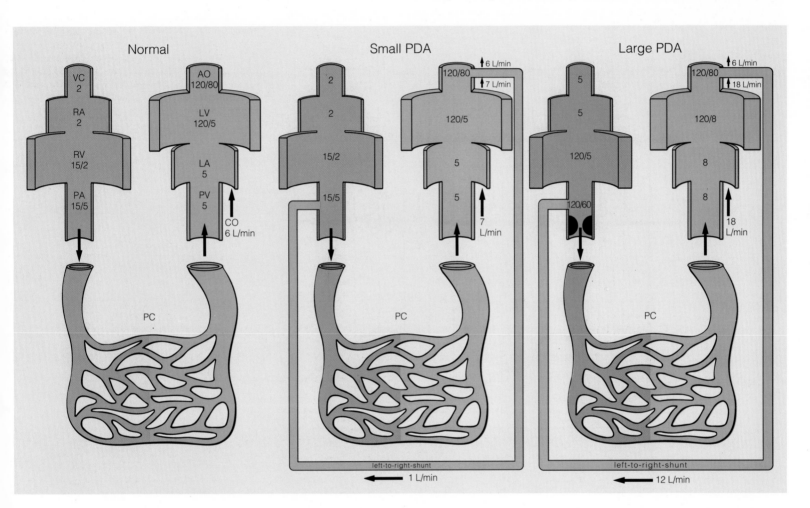

FIGURE 7.53   Pathophysiology of patent ductus arteriosus (PDA). The left panel depicts normal hemodynamics. The middle panel shows the changes occurring with a small PDA. The limited communication between the aorta (AO) and the pulmonary artery (PA) allows a small left-to-right shunt (1 L/min). Pulmonary blood flow and left ventricular cardiac output (CO) are increased by 1 L/min to a total of 7 L/min. The right panel depicts a large PDA and early pulmonary vascular disease. Although pulmonary arterial and aortic systolic pressures are equal, there is still enough difference in systemic arterial (aortic) compliance and pulmonary arterial compliance to maintain a left-to-right shunt of 12 L/min. Pulmonary blood flow is the result of systemic venous return (6 L/min) and the left-to-right shunt (12 L/min). With increasing pulmonary vascular disease, the left-to-right shunt will gradually disappear, leaving either a net right-to-left shunt or balanced shunting. (VC = vena cava; RA = right atrium; PC = pulmonary capillaries; PV = pulmonary veins; LA = left atrium; RV = right ventricle; LV = left ventricle) (Modified with permission; see Figure Credits)

shunts may develop heart failure during the first few weeks of life. If heart failure does not develop at that age, it may not occur until after the third decade. Growth may be retarded. Premature infants may have respiratory distress syndrome followed by heart failure.

PHYSICAL EXAMINATION

The peripheral arterial pulse may be brisk; the pulse pressure may be 45 mmHg or more. When the shunt is large, the apical impulse may be forceful and displaced to the left. A right ventricular lift may be prominent in infants with the respiratory distress syndrome and in children or adults with pulmonary arterial hypertension.

The murmur varies with age, size of the shunt, and magnitude of the pulmonary arterial pressure and resistance. The typical murmur is heard in the sec- ond left intercostal space near the sternum and below the clavicle. The murmur is termed *continuous*, which implies that it builds up in systole, envelops the second sound, and trails off in diastole (Fig. 7.54). The second component of the second sound may be loud; however, the sound may also be masked by the peak intensity of the murmur. The diastolic component of the murmur may be faint or inaudible in newborns, in patients with pulmonary hypertension, and in patients with small shunts. Patients with moderate-sized left-to-right shunts may have a diastolic rumble at the apex, resulting from increased mitral flow. Patients with pulmonary hypertension may have a loud pulmonary valve closure sound followed by the diastolic murmur of pulmonary valve regurgitation.

The continuous murmur of a patent arterial duct must be differentiated from the murmur of the normal venous hum and the murmurs associated with aortopulmonary septal defect, coronary arteriovenous fistula, or rupture of the sinus

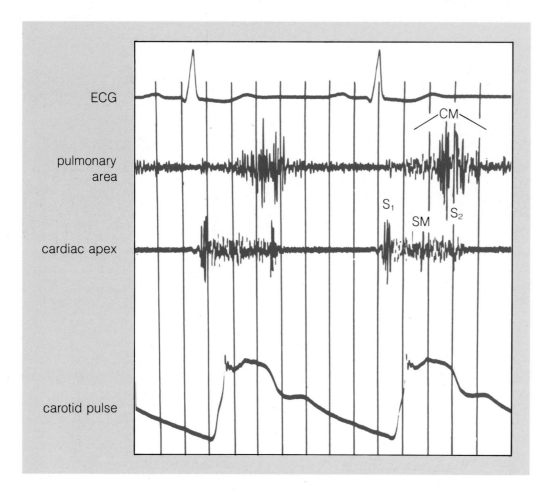

FIGURE 7.54   Phonocardiographic tracings recorded in an 18-year-old female with a patent arterial duct. A continuous murmur (CM) present at the pulmonary area has its peak around the time of the second heart sound (S_2). A pansystolic murmur (SM) is also seen at the apex. It is due to mitral regurgitation associated with dilation of the left ventricle. (Reproduced with permission; see Figure Credits)

of Valsalva. Whenever a continuous murmur is heard in areas other than the second left intercostal space it is prudent to consider an abnormality other than a patent duct.

Cyanosis and clubbing of the toes and fingers of the left hand may be evident in patients in whom the shunt is reversed because of severe pulmonary hypertension.

LABORATORY STUDIES

Chest Radiography The chest film of a patient with a small patent arterial duct may be normal. When the duct permits a moderate-sized left-to-right shunt, slight cardiac enlargement, large pulmonary arteries, and a normal-sized aorta are evident (Fig. 7.55). When severe pulmonary hypertension is present, the pulmonary arteries are usually very large (Fig. 7.56).

Electrocardiography The ECG of a patient with a small patent arterial duct may be normal. In contrast, the patient with a moderate-sized left-to-right shunt may show an increase in QRS voltage, suggesting left ventricular enlargement (Fig. 7.57). The ECG in the presence of pulmonary hypertension often shows right ventricular hypertrophy.

Echocardiography M-mode echocardiography can be used to detect left atrial enlargement. The left ventricular diastolic dimension and the mean velocity of circumferential fiber shortening are increased.

Color Doppler ultrasonography can be used to detect patent arterial duct, while continuous-wave Doppler can be used to measure the flow through it[47] (Figs. 7.58, 7.59).

Cardiac Catheterization The arterial oxygen saturation is increased in the pulmonary artery, and the magnitude of the left-to-

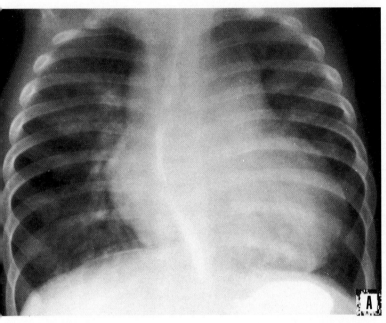

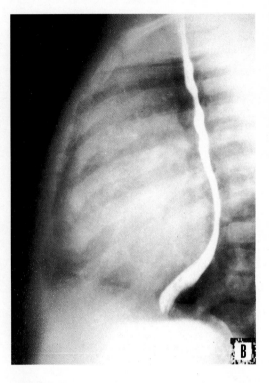

FIGURE 7.55 Chest radiographs of a 1-month-old infant with a large patent arterial duct. **(A)** On the posteroanterior view, moderate cardiac enlargement with increased pulmonary flow is seen. **(B)** Lateral view shows right ventricular hypertrophy and marked left atrial enlargement. (Reproduced with permission; see Figure Credits)

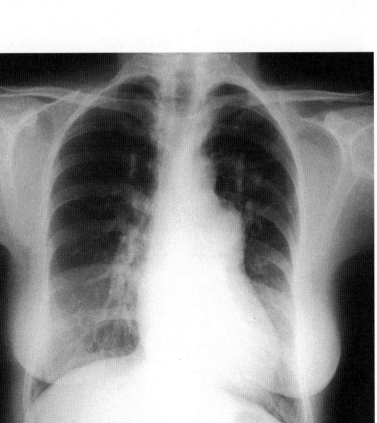

FIGURE 7.56 Posteroanterior projection of a 30-year-old woman with elevated pulmonary vascular resistance due to a patent ductus arteriosus ligated in childhood. Pulmonary hypertension secondary to progressive pulmonary vascular disease has continued. Note the enlarged main pulmonary artery and primary pulmonary branches with clear peripheral lung fields. (Reproduced with permission; see Figure Credits)

right shunt can be calculated. The pulmonary pressure is normal in patients with small or moderate-sized shunts, but it may be increased in patients with large shunts or pulmonary vascular disease. Aortography can be used to visualize the duct and the pulmonary arteries (Fig. 7.60).

NATURAL HISTORY

Patients may live a normal life span. The complications are infective endarteritis, heart failure, and the consequences of pulmonary hypertension. Bacterial endarteritis may occur regardless of the size of the duct. Heart failure related to ductal patency may cause death in premature or young infants. Pulmonary hypertension and reversal of shunt may lead to the complications of erythrocytosis, including cerebral thrombosis.

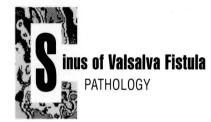

Sinus of Valsalva Fistula
PATHOLOGY

A posterior (noncoronary) sinus of Valsalva aneurysm may rupture into the right atrium, while a right coronary sinus of Valsalva aneurysm may rupture into the right ventricle.[46] Rupture may occur spontaneously or following trauma. Infective endocarditis may produce a fistula that causes a similar clinical picture.

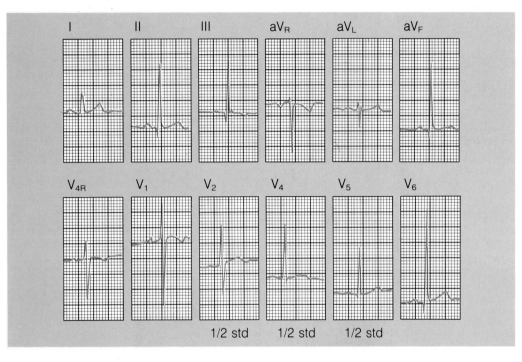

FIGURE 7.57 ECG of a 14-year-old child with a patent arterial duct. The mean QRS vector is large and directed slightly posteriorly and slightly at 65 degrees in the frontal plane and slightly posteriorly, signifying left ventricular hypertrophy. The mean T vector at $^+$25 degrees in the frontal plane to the left and is flush with the frontal plane. Note that leads V_2, V_4, and V_5 are one half standardized. (Reproduced with permission; see Figure Credits)

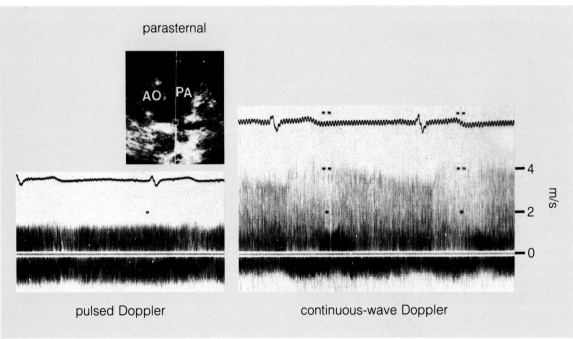

FIGURE 7.58 With a patent arterial duct and normal pulmonary arterial pressure, continuous flow with high velocities into the pulmonary artery can be recorded. The velocity increases in systole and is highest at end systole, when the pressure difference between the aorta (AO) and the pulmonary artery (PA) is greatest. With pulsed Doppler, this flow is shown to originate at the bifurcation, but the recording in the direction of flow may no longer be clear because of aliasing. The flow velocity signal from the patent duct is less evident during systole, when flow into the pulmonary artery is seen as a darker band away from the transducer. (Reproduced with permission; see Figure Credits)

in addition to the characteristic signs of endocarditis.

The rupture may produce chest pain and pulmonary congestion. The murmur is continuous and is heard lower on the chest than is the murmur of a patent arterial duct. The murmur may be to-and-fro. The type of murmur is determined by the location of the fistula. Neck vein pulsation is abnormal when the sinus-ruptures into the right atrium. Aneurysm of the right sinus is commonly associated with a ventricular septal defect. The exact diagnosis is usually confirmed by cardiac catheterization and angiography, although the clinical features are virtually diagnostic.[31]

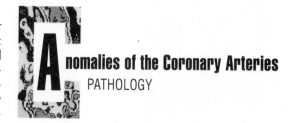

Anomalies of the Coronary Arteries
PATHOLOGY

Many anomalies of the coronary arteries have been identified since the advent

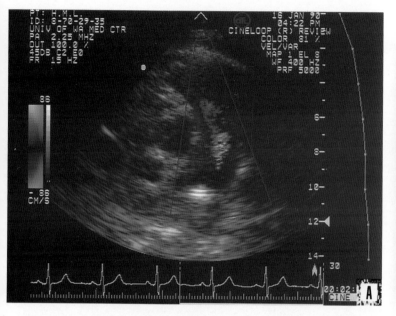

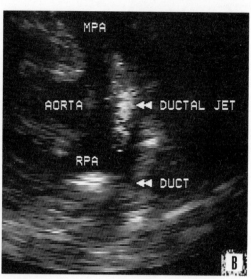

FIGURE 7.59 **(A)** Freeze-frame of color-flow Doppler image from a 24-year-old woman with a patent ductus arteriosus. The red color indicates that the flow is coming toward the transducer, placed in the left parasternal short-axis plane for the aortic valve, i.e., at the left parasternal margin at the third left inter-space. The green and yellow dots indicate turbulent flow. Note that the diastolic flow extends back almost to the pulmonary valve. **(B)** Black-and-white representation. (MPA = main pulmonary artery; RPA = right pulmonary artery) (Reproduced with permission; see Figure Credits)

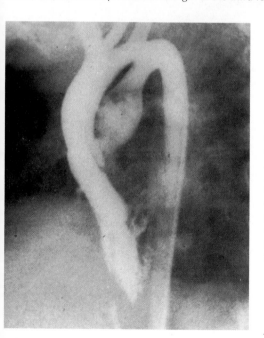

FIGURE 7.60

Left ventriculogram and aortogram obtained in an 11-month-old child with mitral stenosis and a patent arterial duct. The left anterior oblique projection demonstrates the aorta and a large patent duct. Washout of contrast material within the duct results from right-to-left shunting. (Reproduced with permission; see Figure Credits)

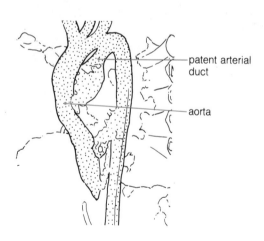

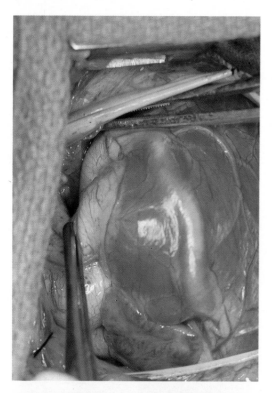

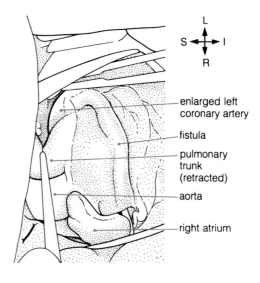

FIGURE 7.61
Operative view shows a large fistula extending between the enlarged left coronary artery and the cavity of the right ventricle. (Reproduced with permission; see Figure Credits)

enlarged left coronary artery

fistula

pulmonary trunk (retracted)

aorta

right atrium

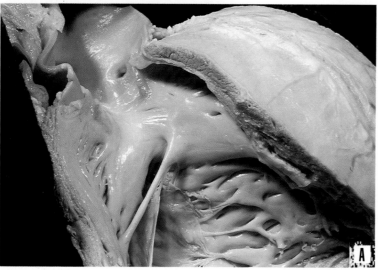

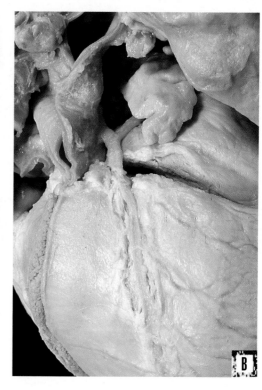

FIGURE 7.62 In this example of anomalous origin of the left coronary artery from the pulmonary trunk the opened pulmonary trunk (**A**) reveals the coronary orifice, and the course of the artery can be seen (**B**). (Reproduced with permission; see Figure Credits)

of coronary arteriography. Only two anomalies are discussed here: coronary arteriovenous fistula (Fig. 7.61) and origin of the left coronary artery from the pulmonary trunk (Figs. 7.62, 7.63).

A coronary arteriovenous fistula is usually recognized by the presence of a continuous murmur over the precordium below the area where the murmur of a patent arterial duct is usually heard. Left ventriculography and coronary arteriography confirm the diagnosis (Fig. 7.64).

When the left coronary artery arises from the pulmonary trunk (see Fig. 7.62), the patient may develop myocardial damage (see Fig. 7.63). The ECG may show myocardial infarction (Fig. 7.65). An infant may appear to be in pain from the effort of sucking a bottle. The ECG may show ST-segment displacement during the episode (see Fig. 7.65). Endocardial fibroelastosis may also be present in such patients. Both these types of coronary anomalies may be corrected by surgery.

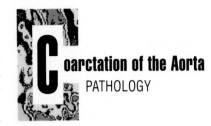

Coarctation of the Aorta
PATHOLOGY

Coarctation of the aorta is a narrowing of the aorta almost always in the region of the arterial duct. The lesion may be an isolated shelf (Fig. 7.66), a waist lesion (Figs. 7.67, 7.68), or a more elongated tubular narrowing of a segment of

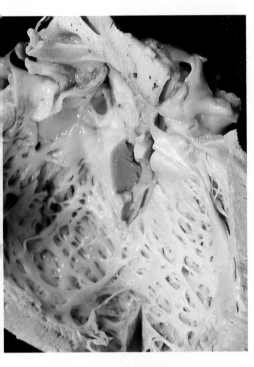

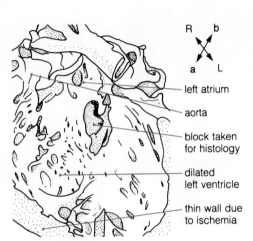

left atrium

aorta

block taken for histology

dilated left ventricle

thin wall due to ischemia

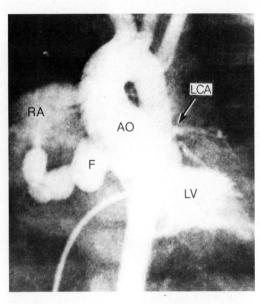

FIGURE 7.64 Posteroanterior view of a left ventricular (LV) angiogram in a child shows a coronary arteriovenous fistula (F) from the left coronary artery (LCA) to the right atrium (RA) (AO, aorta). (Reproduced with permission; see Figure Credits)

FIGURE 7.63 This dilated and ischemic left ventricle is found in the setting of anomalous origin of the left coronary artery from the pulmonary trunk. (Reproduced with permission; see Figure Credits)

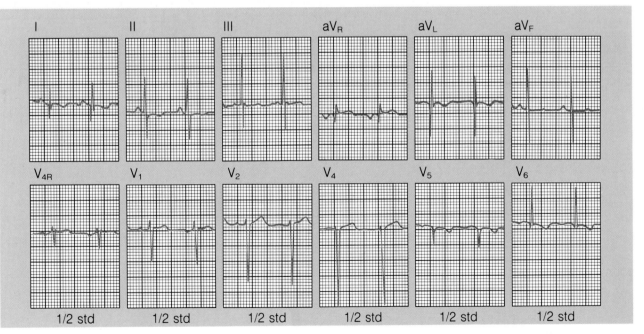

FIGURE 7.65
Twelve lead ECG in an infant whose left coronary artery originates from the pulmonary trunk illustrates the signs of myocardial lateral infarction (chest leads recorded at one half standard voltage). (Reproduced with permission; see Figure Credits)

the aortic arch (Fig. 7.69). Collateral circulation in coarctation usually occurs when the arterial duct is closed.

Coarctation may be associated with left ventricular endocardial fibroelastosis, subendocardial fibrosis (Fig. 7.70), patent arterial duct, ventricular septal defect (VSD) (Fig. 7.71), bicuspid aortic valve (in almost half of cases) (Fig. 7.72), subaortic obstruction, complete transposition, double-outlet right ventricle with subpulmonary VSD (the Taussig–Bing anomaly), aberrant right subclavian artery, or anomalies of the mitral valve, particularly the parachute deformity. Coarctation also accompanies those lesions with univentricular atrioventricular connection to the left ventricle, such as double-inlet or tricuspid atresia, in which there is a discordant ventriculoarterial connection and a restrictive VSD.

PATHOPHYSIOLOGY

The systolic and diastolic blood pressures are elevated above normal levels in the patient's arms. The systolic blood pressure is less in the legs than it is in arms, while the diastolic pressure is near or slightly lower than normal. In so cases the blood pressure is normal in the upper extremities and decreased in lower extremities. The elevated pressure is due to a combination of mechan obstruction and humoral factors.[40]

CLINICAL MANIFESTATIONS

Almost half of patients with Turner's syndrome have coarctation of the ac Approximately half of infants with coarctation experience heart failure dur the first few months of life. About 20% of patients with severe heart failure a coarctation have isolated coarctation, about 20% have a patent arterial du and about one half have a VSD.[14] Almost half of the patients have a bicus aortic valve. The male to female ratio is 3:1 in patients with isolated coarctat and 1:1 when other lesions are present.

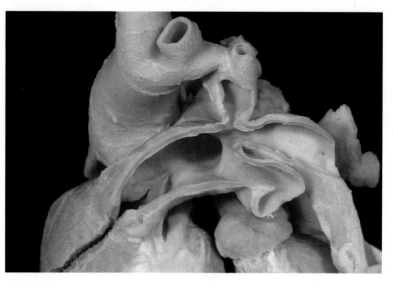

FIGURE 7.66 Heart specimen with preductal coarctation sectioned to replicate the view obtained by the echocardiographer from the suprasternal window. The coarctation shelf is continuous with the wall of the arterial duct, and it is composed of ductal tissue. (Reproduced with permission; see Figure Credits)

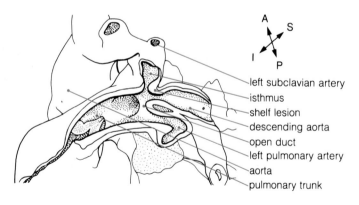

left subclavian artery
isthmus
shelf lesion
descending aorta
open duct
left pulmonary artery
aorta
pulmonary trunk

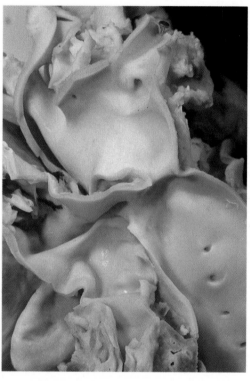

FIGURE 7.67
Coarctation with an open arterial duct du to a waist lesion in t immediate preductal position. The narrow ing is an infolding of the aortic wall rather than a discrete intra minal shelf.
(Reproduced with pe mission; see Figure Credits)

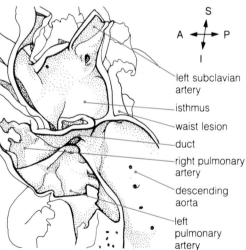

left subclavian artery
isthmus
waist lesion
duct
right pulmonary artery
descending aorta
left pulmonary artery

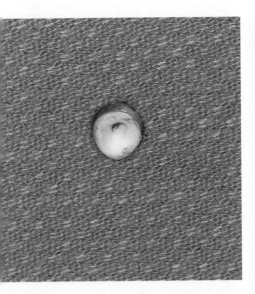

IGURE 7.68 Short, coarcted segment emoved from a patient. The extreme narrowness f the lumen is caused by the shelf-like projection f the coarctation tissue. (Reproduced with per- nission; see Figure Credits)

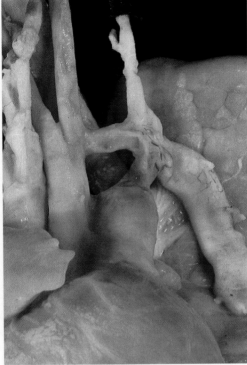

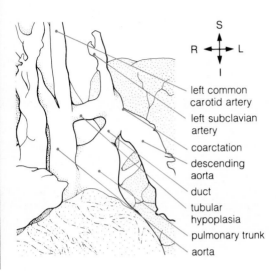

FIGURE 7.69 Severe tubular hypoplasia of the segment of aortic arch between the left common carotid and the left subclavian arteries. This heart also has discrete coarctation in the preductal location (not shown). (Reproduced with permission; see Figure Credits)

left common carotid artery

left subclavian artery

coarctation

descending aorta

duct

tubular hypoplasia

pulmonary trunk

aorta

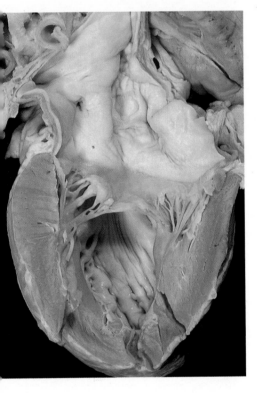

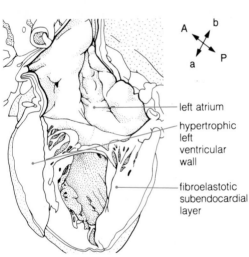

left atrium

hypertrophic left ventricular wall

fibroelastotic subendocardial layer

FIGURE 7.70 Heart from a 5-year-old child who died with severe, unoperated aortic coarctation with a closed arterial duct. There is extensive hypertrophy of the left ventricle with marked subendocardial fibrosis. (Reproduced with permission; see Figure Credits)

Symptoms

The symptomatic infant may have heart failure with dyspnea, difficulty in feeding, and poor weight gain. Older patients are usually asymptomatic, although a child may complain of intermittent claudication of the legs. The symptoms of heart failure may occur after age 40. Endarteritis or endocarditis may occur at any age.

Physical Examination

The infant may exhibit signs of heart failure. The murmur of coarctation (see below) may not be audible until heart failure is improved. There may be murmurs related to associated defects.

Older children and adults may exhibit more characteristic signs of coarctation of the aorta. The trunk may reveal more muscular development than the lower extremities. There may be signs of Turner's syndrome (ovarian agenesis) in female patients. The blood pressure may be normal or only slightly elevated in the arms. A lower pressure in one arm compared with the other suggests that the corresponding subclavian artery arises below the coarctation. The blood pressure is less in the legs than it is in the arms in patients with coarctation, whereas normally it is higher in the legs than in the arms; the latter is true because the size of the muscles in the legs of the normal person produces a cushion around the arteries. One third of patients have no hypertension, and two thirds have slight to moderate elevation of blood pressure. It is important to record the blood pressure in the arms after exercise because this may produce an abnormal elevation of pressure when compared with normal patients.

There is a prominent arterial pulsation noted in the neck. Palpation of the apex impulse of the left ventricle may suggest left ventricular hypertrophy. The femoral arterial pulsations may be diminished or absent, and collateral arterial vessels may be seen and palpated in the intercostal spaces in the back.

The aortic component of the second sound may be increased in intensity; an early systolic click at the apex suggests the presence of a bicuspid aortic valve.

The systolic murmur of coarctation is best heard in the interscapular region; it may be faint or inaudible anteriorly. Continuous murmurs are usually heard over the collateral vessels on the back in older children and adults. A bicuspid aortic valve may cause a systolic murmur, a systolic click, and the murmur of aortic regurgitation. The murmurs due to associated conditions, such as VSD or a patent arterial duct, may also be heard.

Laboratory Studies

Chest Radiography   The chest film of the infant with heart failure shows cardiac enlargement and, when there is an associated duct or VSD, an increase in pulmonary blood flow. The aortic arch gives the appearance of the figure 3 and the barium-filled esophagus resembles the letter E. Rib notching is seen after 8 years of age (Figs. 7.73, 7.74). The proximal portion of the aorta is enlarged, especially when there is aortic stenosis due to a bicuspid aortic valve.

Electrocardiography   The ECG in an infant with heart failure may show a right atrial abnormality, right ventricular hypertrophy, biventricular hypertrophy; the T waves may be inverted in the left precordial leads. The ECGs of older children and adults may be normal (Fig. 7.75) or they may show left atrial abnormality, left ventricular hypertrophy, and left anterior hemiblock.

Echocardiography   Left ventricular function can be assessed using M-mode echocardiography. The coarctation itself can be viewed with cross-sectional echocardiography; associated defects may also be visualized (Figs. 7.76, 7.77).

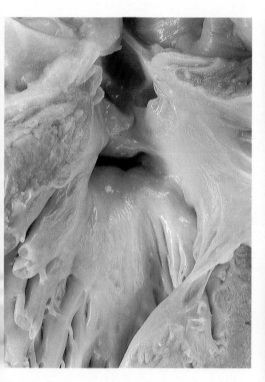

FIGURE 7.71 Heart sectioned to show the left ventricular aspect of a malaligned VSD. The outlet septum is deviated into the left ventricle, thus producing subaortic obstruction. Severe preductal coarctation is also exhibited. (Reproduced with permission; see Figure Credits)

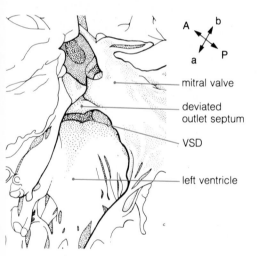

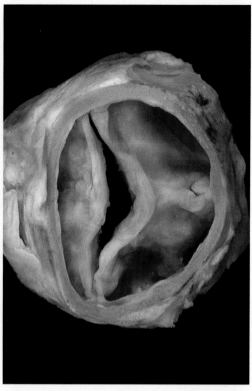

FIGURE 7.72 Bifoliate (bicuspid) aortic valve viewed from above. The raphe is seen clearly, suggesting fusion of the right and left coronary leaflets. The valve is also thickened and stenotic. (Reproduced with permission; see Figure Credits)

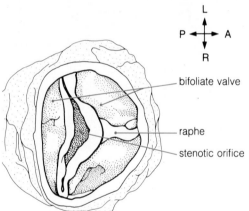

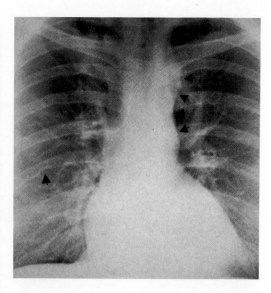

FIGURE 7.73 Large notch in the seventh posterior rib (right lung, *arrow*) in the chest film of this adult with coarctation of the aorta. The vascularity is normal with a normal-sized left ventricular contour (left lung, *arrows*). The transverse aortic arch and the upper descending thoracic aorta are distorted. The findings regarding the thoracic aorta in this case cannot be differentiated from those of an aortic dissection. The notched rib is the premier radiographic finding in the differential. Note what is probably the precoarctation aortic dilation (*right upper arrow*), as well as what is probably a postcoarctation dilation of the aorta (*right lower arrow*). (Reproduced with permission; see Figure Credits)

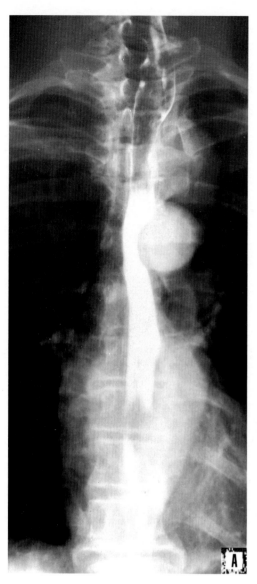

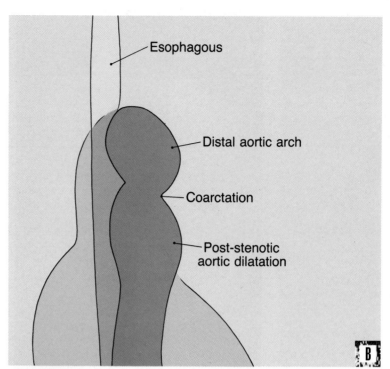

Esophagous

Distal aortic arch

Coarctation

Post-stenotic
aortic dilatation

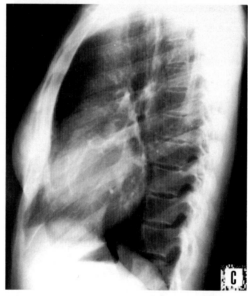

FIGURE 7.74　(A) Frontal chest view with barium
in the esophagus demonstrating the E, or inverted 3,
of coarctation of the aorta. There are two discrete
impressions on the esophagus: a proximal indentation caused by the aortic arch and dilated subclavian artery and a distal indentation caused by the
dilated poststenotic segment of the descending
aorta. (B) Appearance of the coarctation (note the
inverted 3). (C) In another patient, the image of the
aortic arch cannot be identified on the lateral chest
x-ray. Apparent absence of the aortic arch on the lateral projection suggests the diagnosis of coarctation
of the aorta. (Reproduced with permission; see
Figure Credits)

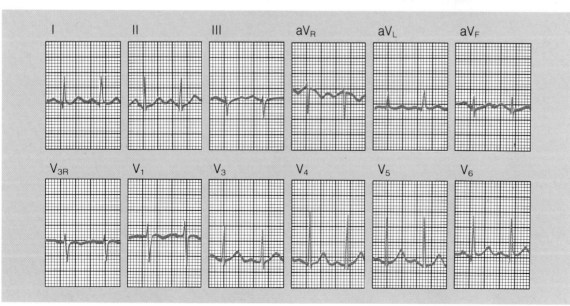

FIGURE 7.75　ECG of an 8-year-
old girl with coarctation of the aorta.
The findings are normal, as is often
the case with this anomaly. Blood
pressure in the arms was 170/110
mmHg. Early in life the ECG may
show right ventricular hypertrophy;
later in life, with sufficient hypertension and aortic valve stenosis, the
ECG may show left ventricular
hypertrophy. (Reproduced with permission; see Figure Credits)

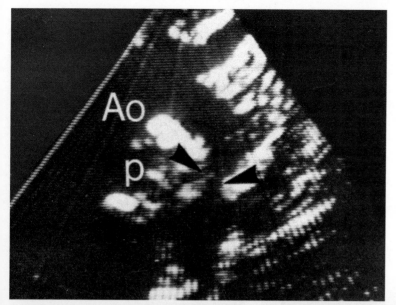

FIGURE 7.76   Cross-sectional echocardiography performed on a patient with coarctation of the aorta. On the suprasternal notch long-axis view an area of narrowing is seen just beyond the origin of the left subclavian artery (*arrows*). Poststenotic dilation of the descending aorta is apparent. (Ao = aorta; p = right pulmonary artery). (Reproduced with permission; see Figure Credits)

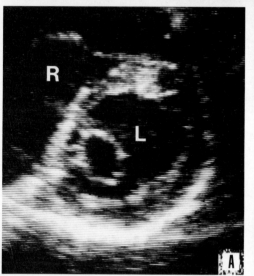

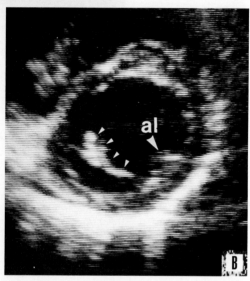

FIGURE 7.77   Two-dimensional echocardiograms of parachute mitral valve and bicuspid aortic valve in a patient with coarctation of the aorta. **(A)** Parasternal short-axis view in diastole. **(B)** In systole, the line of coaptation of the mitral leaflet tissue is noted (*small arrows*). The anterolateral (al) papillary muscle is hypoplastic and none of the chordae attach to it. **(C)** A short-axis cut somewhat closer to the apex shows the posteromedial (pm) papillary muscle to be slightly larger than usual and all of the mitral chordae attaching to it. **(D)** In the high parasternal short-axis view, the line of coaptation of the aortic leaflets (*arrowheads*) shows that this is a bicuspid valve. (R = right ventricle; L = left ventricle; la = left atrium; rvot = right ventricular outflow tract) (Reproduced with permission; see Figure Credits)

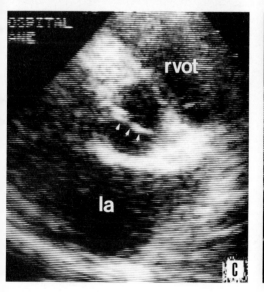

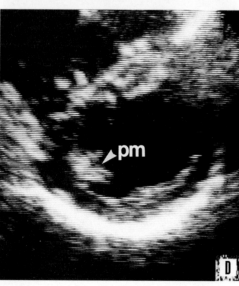

Cardiac Catheterization   A systolic pressure difference may be detected between the left ventricle and the femoral artery, although this difference may not be present when there is a large VSD or arterial duct. Other defects, such as aortic valve stenosis or regurgitation, VSD, or arterial duct, may be detected. Aortography reveals the exact site and length of the coarctation (Figs. 7.78).

Other Imaging Modalities   CT scanning and nuclear magnetic resonance imaging may clearly delineate the coarctation as well as associated anatomic abnormalities (Fig. 7.79).

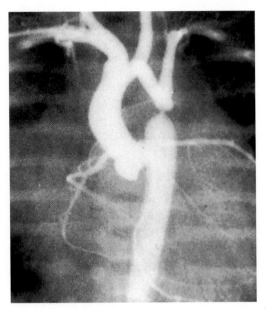

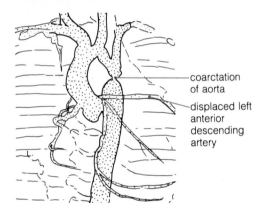

FIGURE 7.78
Contrast material injected into a patient through a catheter inserted from the right subclavian artery. On the frontal view, tight coarctation of the aorta is present distal to the left subclavian artery. The segment of the arch as far proximally as the innominate artery is mildly hypoplastic. Mild post-stenotic dilation is present beyond the coarctation. The left anterior descending coronary artery branch is displaced by an enlarged left ventricle. (Reproduced with permission; see Figure Credits)

— coarctation of aorta

— displaced left anterior descending artery

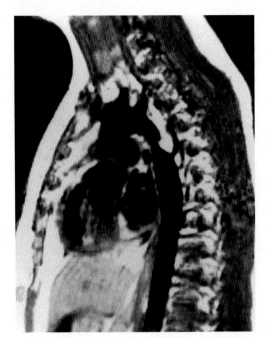

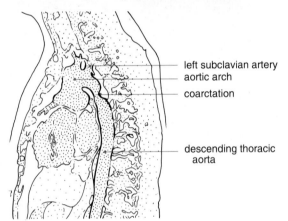

FIGURE 7.79   Left anterior oblique section of a spin-echo MR image of the entire thoracic aorta. The coarcted segment appears as a narrowing at the junction between the aortic arch and the descending thoracic aorta. The left subclavian artery is dilated. The descending thoracic aorta is normal. (Reproduced with permission; see Figure Credits)

left subclavian artery
aortic arch
coarctation

descending thoracic aorta

NATURAL HISTORY

About 20% of infants with heart failure have coarctation of the aorta. Most of these babies respond to medical treatment, including digitalis; as collateral circulation develops, the signs of heart failure gradually decrease. Some patients, particularly those with associated defects, require surgery in infancy. Restenosis occurs in some patients operated on at this age, irrespective of the type of surgery employed.

Older patients with hypertension may have rupture of the aorta, rupture of a berry aneurysm in the brain, endocarditis, or heart failure. Because of this, surgery is indicated early during childhood. The blood pressure returns to normal in most patients following surgery, but it may remain elevated without renal disease or restenosis of the coarctation site. This postoperative hypertension seems to occur less frequently in patients who are operated on early in childhood.[30]

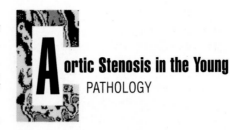

Aortic Stenosis in the Young
PATHOLOGY

Congenital heart disease is the usual cause of aortic valve stenosis in infants and children and it may be the cause in adults. Certain features of this condition in children justify a separate discussion on the subject (See Chapter 6 for a discussion of aortic valve stenosis in adults.)

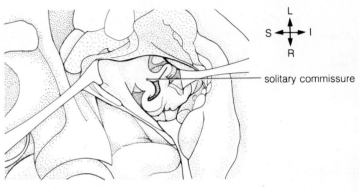

FIGURE 7.80   Operative view shows a unicuspid, unicommissural, and stenotic aortic valve. (Reproduced with permission; see Figure Credits)

solitary commissure

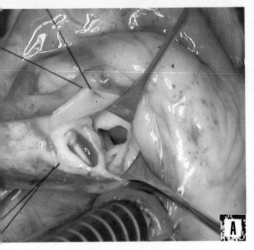

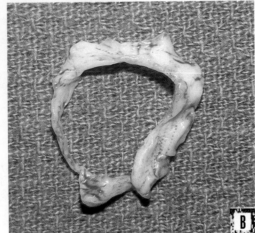

FIGURE 7.81   (**A**) Operative view through the aortic valve shows subvalvular aortic stenosis produced by a fibrous shelf. (**B**) The resected shelf encircled the outflow tract. (Reproduced with permission; see Figure Credits)

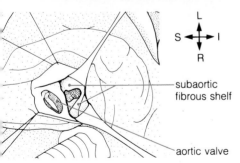

subaortic fibrous shelf

aortic valve

PATHOPHYSIOLOGY

Aortic stenosis, or left ventricular outflow tract obstruction can be divided into three types: valvular, including bicuspid (see Chapter 6) and unicuspid (see Fig. 7.80) variants; subvalvular, including shelf-like (Fig. 7.81) or muscular (Fig. 7.82)variants; or supravalvular, including hourglass, (Fig. 7.83), hypoplastic, and membranous variants. Valvular congenital stenosis is common, whereas the other types of obstruction are rare. Left ventricular hypertrophy and endocardial fibroelastosis may be present, and a bicuspid aortic valve is common. Coarctation of the aorta is the most commonly associated defect.

The reader is referred to the discussion of abnormal physiology of aortic valve stenosis in adults in Chapter 4.

CLINICAL MANIFESTATIONS
SYMPTOMS

The majority of children are asymptomatic even when the stenosis is severe, but dyspnea, fatigue, syncope, angina, and sudden death may occur.

Infants with severe stenosis develop heart failure within the first few weeks of life; this is considered a medical emergency. Those with less severe stenosis may develop heart failure during the first six months of life.

Children with subvalvular stenosis are usually asymptomatic. The syndrome is recognized because of a systolic murmur, often thought to be due to a ventricular septal defect. Although subvalvular stenosis may be due to development of a fibrous shelf, obstuction may also be caused by muscular hypertrophy. This con-

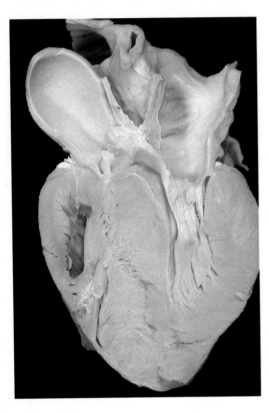

FIGURE 7.82 This simulated parasternal long-axis section shows how hypertrophic cardiomyopathy produces severe asymmetric thickening of the ventricular septum, which results in subaortic obstruction. (Reproduced with permission; see Figure Credits)

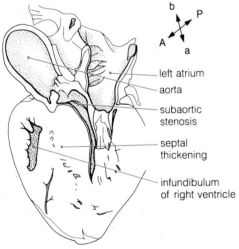

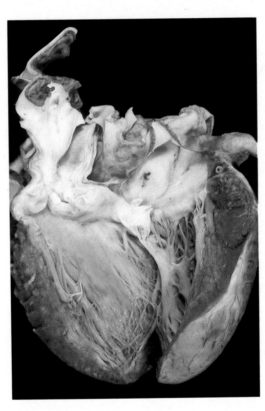

FIGURE 7.83 This heart photographed from the left ventricular aspect shows severe narrowing of the aortic outflow at the level of the commissural ridge, an example of the hourglass variant of supravalvular aortic stenosis. (Reproduced with permission; see Figure Credits)

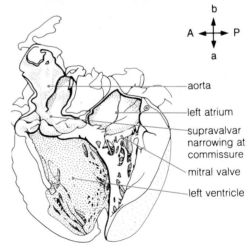

ition is known as asymmetric septal hypertrophy, or when more extensive, as idiopathic hypertrophic subaortic stenosis. This condition is usually part of the hypertrophic cardiomyopathy. This occurs more commonly in males; older children and adults with this condition have syncope, angina, and heart failure.

Patients with supravalvular aortic stenosis have symptoms that are similar to those with valvular or subvalvular aortic stenosis except that heart failure in the newborn is rare.

PHYSICAL EXAMINATION

Peripheral arterial pulses may be diminished in infants with severe aortic valve stenosis. When severe heart failure is present, a murmur may not be detected. Older children and adults may have a systolic thrill in the aortic area, a sustained apex impulse during systole, an aortic ejection click at the apex, an atrial gallop, a diminished aortic valve closure sound, paradoxical splitting of the second sound, and a diamond-shaped, systolic murmur in the aortic area. A murmur of aortic regurgitation may be detected.

The systolic murmur of subvalvular aortic stenosis is often mistaken for that of a ventricular septal defect. The discrete, shelf-like type of obstuction causes aortic regurgitation in one half of cases. An aortic ejection click is not heard, and when aortic regurgitation is present, a two-peaked pulse is palpated in the carotid artery. (The muscular type of subvalvular stenosis–hypertrophic cardiomyopathy–is discussed in Chapter 8.)

One type of supravalvular aortic stenosis may be familial, transmitted as an autosomal-dominant trait. Another type, usually called Williams syndrome, occurs sporadically; it is characterized by supravalvular aortic stenosis, characteristic facies (high forehead, epicanthic folds, and underdevploped bridge of the nose and mandible), hypercalcemia, and mental retardation. Peripheral pulmonary artery stenoses may be found in both types of supravalvular aortic stenoses.

Chest Radiography The heart of a patient with valvular aortic stenosis is usually of normal size, although there may be post-stenotic dilation of the aorta.

The chest film of a patient with subvalvular aortic stenosis is usually normal. The left ventricle may become prominent, but post-stenotic dilation of the aorta does not occur.

The chest x-ray film of a patient with supravalvular aortic stenosis is usually normal, and post-stenotic dilation of the aorta does not occur.

Electrocardiography Symptomatic infants with valvular aortic stenosis may show biventricular hypertrophy. The ECG may be normal in older children and adults with mild stenosis, but it usually shows various stages of left ventricular hypertrophy when the stenosis is severe.

The ECG of a patient with the shelf-like type of subvalvular aortic stenosis may be similar to the ECG seen in patients with valvular stenosis.

The ECG of the muscular variety of aortic stenosis associated with idiopathic cardiac hypertrophy usually reveals left ventricular hypertrophy; the ST-T waves may be bizarre. The QRS complex may be typical of the WPW phenomenon.

The ECG of supravalvular aortic stenosis may reveal left ventricular hypertrophy. Right ventricular hypertrophy may also be present in patients with peripheral stenoses of the pulmonary arteries.

Echocardiography M-mode and cross-sectional echocardiographic studies reveal the obstructive lesions in patients with valvular, subvalvular, and supravalvular aortic stenosis (Fig. 7.84).

Doppler studies permit an assessment of the systolic pressure gradient across discrete forms of left ventricular outflow tract obstruction.

Cardiac Catheterization Complete right and left heart catheterization should be performed on symptomatic infants with left ventricular outflow tract obstruction in order to determine the cardiac output and to

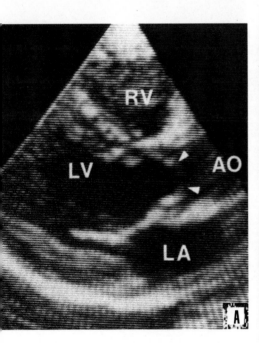

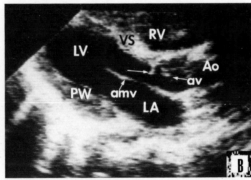

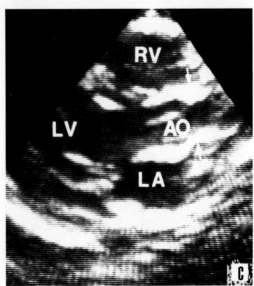

FIGURE 7.84 Cross-sectional echocardiograms in the parasternal long-axis view in three patients with aortic stenosis. (**A**) In aortic valve stenosis the aortic valve cusps (*arrows*) are thickened and domed with diminished cusp separation (AO, aorta; LA, left atrium; LV, left ventricle; RV, right ventricle). (**B**) In discrete, fibrous subvalvular aortic stenosis a thin, discrete shelf (unlabeled arrow) is seen attached to the interventricular septum (VS) in the left ventricular (LV) outflow tract immediately below the aortic valve (av) (PW, posterior left ventricular wall; amv, anterior leaflet of the mitral valve). (**C**) In supravalvular aortic stenosis an hourglass-type constriction is seen on the external aspects of the aorta (*arrows*) with a corresponding narrowing of the aortic lumen. (Reproduced with permission; see Figure Credits)

identify the systolic pressure gradient across the obstruction. Associated lesions may also be discovered at cardiac catheterization. Older children and adults who exhibit only a murmur and have no symptoms may be studied initially with noninvasive means. The visualization of the left ventricular anatomy by left ventriculography and aortography may be useful and coronary arteriography is essential in adult patients to identify the presence or absence of coronary disease.

NATURAL HISTORY

Most infants with severe valvular aortic stenosis develop heart failure within the first year of life.[34] One third of patients with less severe stenosis gradually develop a greater left ventricular-aortic pressure gradient; the ECG may reveal more left ventricular hypertrophy, and heart failure may develop. Syncope or sudden death may occur as complications of valvular aortic stenosis. Infective endocarditis is always a threat even with slight valve stenosis.

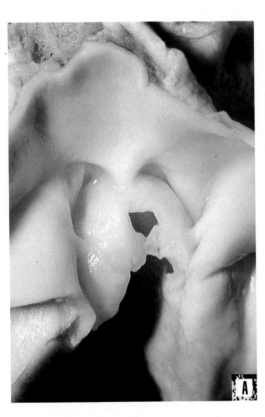
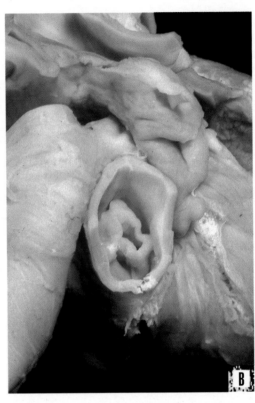
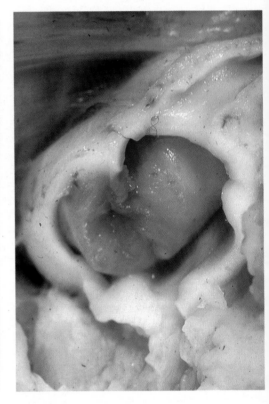

FIGURE 7.85 **(A)** Heart specimen showing a dome-shaped stenosis of an initially three-leaflet pulmonary valve from a neonate. **(B)** Domed stenosis of the pulmonary valve from an older child. The poststenotic dilated pulmonary trunk is cut away to show the rubbery valve leaflets. (Reproduced with permission; see Figure Credits)

FIGURE 7.86 Severely dysplastic leaflets of the pulmonary valve. Stenosis is produced as a consequence of the leaflet's sheer bulk. (Reproduced with permission; see Figure Credits)

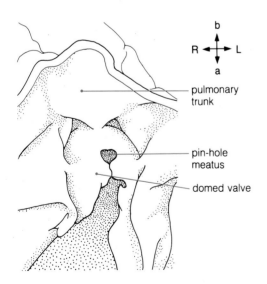
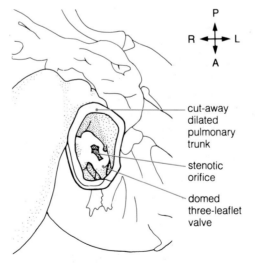
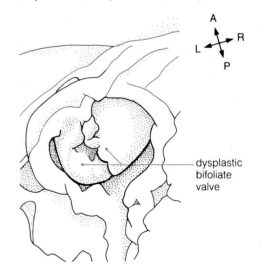

The infant with subvalvular aortic stenosis rarely develops heart failure;[56] Older children and adults may have syncope, arrhythmias, and sudden death. Endocarditis is not uncommon.

The complications of supravalvular aortic stenosis are similar to those of valvular aortic stenosis.

Pulmonary Stenosis With Intact Ventricular Septum

PATHOLOGY

Isolated congenital *pulmonary valve stenosis*, when seen in infancy, is usually due to a small opening at the top of a dome-shaped structure[55] (Fig. 7.85), and less often is due to valvular dysplasia[10] (Fig. 7.86). *Supravalvular stenosis* may also occur; it may be localized, segmental, diffuse, or due to multiple peripheral pulmonary artery stenoses. *Subvalvular stenosis* commonly occurs at the infundibular level of the right ventricle, but it may also occur in hypertrophic cardiomyopathy (Fig. 7.87). (See Chapters 6 and 8 for further discussion.)

PATHOPHYSIOLOGY

While the area of the normal pulmonary orifice at birth is about 0.5 cm^2, it increases with age until it reaches about 2 cm^2/m^2. The valve orifice area must be decreased 60% to produce a significant obstruction in blood flow.

With pulmonary stenoses, the right ventricular systolic pressure is greater than the pulmonary arterial systolic pressure. The pressure in the right ventricle may be 240 mmHg or higher.

The significance of a right ventricle–pulmonary artery gradient must always be assessed in the light of the pulmonary blood flow. When the pulmonary arterial blood flow is normal, a right ventricle–pulmonary artery gradient of less than 50 mmHg is considered to present mild stenosis. A gradient greater than 100 mmHg indicates severe stenosis.

When the right ventricle fails, right ventricular end-diastolic and right atrial mean pressures are increased. The oval foramen may open, and a right-to-left shunt may develop, producing arterial oxygen unsaturation and cyanosis.

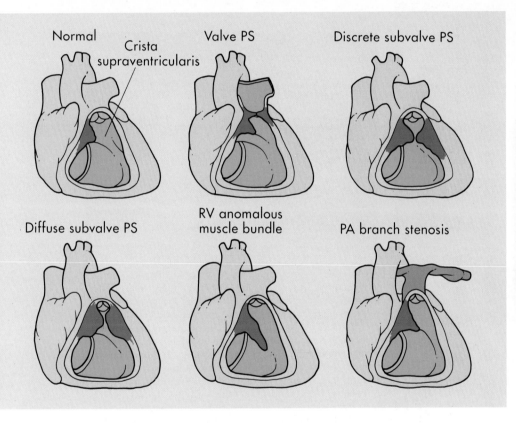

FIGURE 7.87   Anatomic sites at which obstruction to right ventricular outflow may occur. (PS = pulmonary stenosis; RV = right ventricular; PA = pulmonary artery) (Reproduced with permission; see Figure Credits)

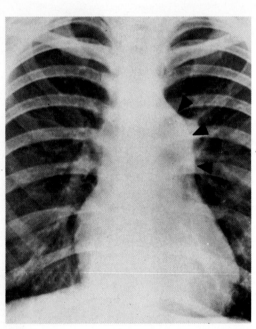

FIGURE 7.88   Chest radiograph of a patient with pulmonary valve stenosis. The pulmonary trunk is enlarged (*arrows*) with normal pulmonary vascularity. (Reproduced with permission; see Figure Credits)

Stagnant cyanosis may occur in patients with poor cardiac output without right-to-left shunts because of the increased extraction of oxygen from the blood in the capillaries of the skin.

CLINICAL MANIFESTATIONS
SYMPTOMS

Many patients with right ventricular outflow tract obstruction may be asymptomatic, but some have dyspnea and fatigue. Young infants may have symptoms of heart failure.

PHYSICAL EXAMINATION

Patients with dysplastic pulmonary valves may be short with low-set ears and mental retardation; this is termed Noonan's syndrome.[38] Cyanosis is uncommon except in patients with an interatrial communication and severe pulmonary valve obstruction.

A prominent a wave may be seen in the jugular venous pulse of patients with pulmonary valve stenosis. Right ventricular hypertrophy may be detected as an anterior lift located to the left of the midsternal area; systolic thrill may be felt in the pulmonary area. An early systolic click may be heard in patients with dome-shaped valves, but it may not be heard with severe stenosis or dysplastic valves. An atrial gallop may be present. The pulmonary closure sound is delayed; it may be inaudible when there is severe stenosis. A diamond-shaped, systolic murmur is heard in the pulmonary area. The more severe the stenosis, the later the murmur peaks in systole. With severe stenosis the murmur may mask aortic valve closure.

Subvalvular stenosis may occur as a part of idiopathic cardiac hypertrophy. The systolic murmur may be heard in such patients, but an ejection click is not audible. An atrial gallop may be heard.

Supravalvular pulmonary stenosis may be found in patients with Noonan's syndrome, the congenital rubella syndrome, and Williams' syndrome (hypercalcemia, typical facies, mental retardation, and dental abnormalities). The symptoms and the physical findings are similar to those of valvular stenosis, except there is no ejection click and the second sound may be normal. Systolic murmurs may be heard over the back when there are peripheral pulmonary arterial stenoses. A continuous murmur may be heard over the back when a diastolic gradient accompanies the pulmonary branch stenosis.

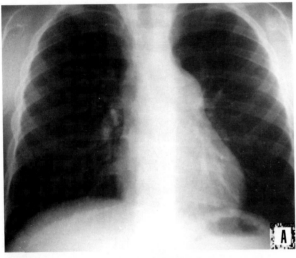

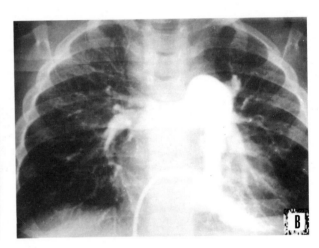

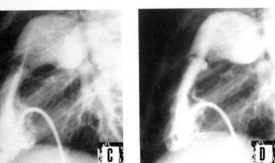

FIGURE 7.89   Pulmonary valve stenosis with patent foramen ovale. **(A)** X-ray shows average-sized heart with prominent, convex main pulmonary artery. Pulmonary arteries are visible in the hilar regions but are sparse in the middle and outer thirds of the lung fields. **(B)** Selective right ventricular angiocardiogram opacifies the right ventricle with hypertrophied walls and the main pulmonary artery and branches. The poststenotic dilatation of the main pulmonary artery accounts for the convex prominence of the left heart border on the x-ray **(A)**. (C,D) Lateral films show the narrow jet through the central small orifice of the radiolucent, thickened, stenotic pulmonary valve **(C)**. **(D)** The column of blood traversing the narrow opening has widened. Poststenotic dilatation is evident on lateral views, as well as frontal. There is very little evidence in early systole **(C)** or late systole **(D)** of accompanying infundibular hypertrophy. (Reproduced with permission; see Figure Credits)

Chest Radiography

Since the heart size is usually normal, a huge heart indicates a critical state. The right ventricle may appear large in the left lateral view. Usually the pulmonary trunk and its left branch are dilated, and the right pulmonary artery is normal in size (Figs. 7.88, 7.89). Pulmonary blood flow may be decreased when there is a right-to-left shunt at the atrial level. The pulmonary trunk is not dilated in patients with subvalvular or supravalvular stenosis.

Electrocardiography

Right ventricular hypertrophy and right atrial abnormality are seen in the ECG of a patient with moderate or severe pulmonary valve stenosis (Fig. 7.90). Patients with dysplasia of the pulmonary valve may have a superiorly located mean QRS vector.[27]

Echocardiography

2D imaging outlines the level of stenosis while Doppler is very useful at predicting the pressure gradient.[54]

Abnormalities associated with valvular (Fig. 7.91), and infundibular (Fig. 7.92) pulmonary stenoses can be differentiated by cross-sectional echocardiography.

Cardiac Catheterization

In patients with valvular stenosis the right ventricular systolic pressure is elevated, and there is a pressure gradient across the pulmonary valve. When the stenosis is severe, it may be unwise to pass the cardiac catheter into the pulmonary trunk. The arterial oxygen saturation is normal, unless there is a right-to-left shunt at the atrial level.

Subpulmonary stenosis may be detected by analyzing the right ventricular pressure curves in pull-back pressure tracings, since the gradient occurs within the right ventricle. It is important to exclude associated congenital heart defects.

Suprapulmonary stenoses produce systolic pressure differences across obstructions throughout the pulmonary arteries. The pulse pressure may be wide in the pulmonary trunk, and the right ventricular systolic pressure is elevated.

Valvular, subvalvular, and supravalvular pulmonary stenoses, including stenosis of branches of the pulmonary artery, produce characteristic abnormalities

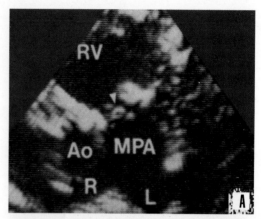

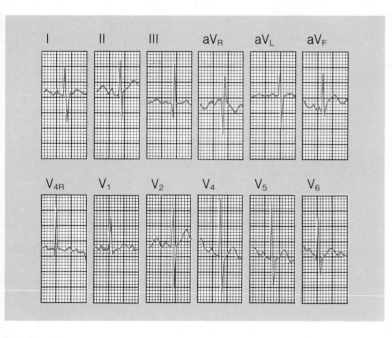

FIGURE 7.90   ECG of a 7-month-old infant with pulmonary valve stenosis. The P waves are pointed, and the mean QRS vector is directed slightly to the right (+95 degrees) and anteriorly. The mean T vector is directed at +50 degrees in the frontal plane and slightly anteriorly. These abnormalities signify right ventricular hypertrophy. (Reproduced with permission; see Figure Credits)

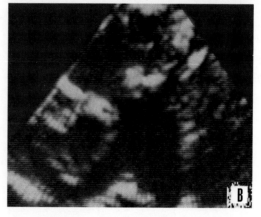

FIGURE 7.91
Cross-sectional echocardiograms in the parasternal short-axis view obtained through the base of the heart in diastole **(A)** and systole **(B)** from a patient with severe pulmonary valve stenosis. The pulmonary valve (*arrow*) is thickened, and the annulus is severely narrowed. There is poststenotic dilation of the pulmonary trunk (MPA). (Ao = aorta; L = left pulmonary artery; R = right pulmonary artery; RV = right ventricle) (Reproduced with permission; see Figure Credits)

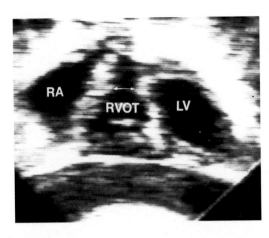

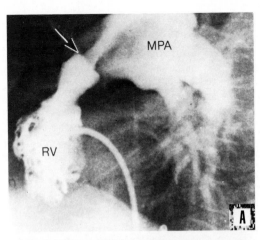

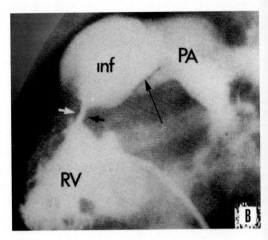

FIGURE 7.92   Cross-sectional echocardiogram in the subxiphoid coronal view (L-4) of the right ventricular outflow tract (RVOT). A narrowed infundibular area (*arrows*) that is associated with pulmonary stenosis can be seen. The RVOT is small compared with the left ventricle (LV), only a portion of which is seen from this view. (RA = right atrium) (Reproduced with permission; see Figure Credits)

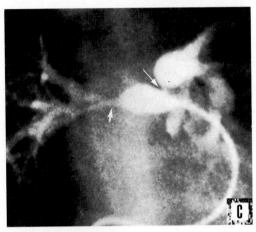

FIGURE 7.93   **(A)** Lateral view of a right ventricular (RV) angiogram of typical valvular pulmonary stenosis. The pulmonary valve (*arrow*) is domed, and a narrow jet of contrast enters the dilated pulmonary trunk (MPA). **(B)** Lateral right ventriculogram demonstrates very severe stenosis (*white and black arrows*) at the level of the ostium of the infundibulum (inf) in patient with congenital isolated infundibular pulmonary stenosis. The subarterial infundibular chamber and the pulmonary trunk (PA) are dilated. The pulmonary valve (*long black arrow*) is slightly thickened. **(C)** Injection of contrast medium into a pulmonary artery shows a focal stenosis at the origin of the left pulmonary artery (*long arrow*) and a more diffuse stenosis of the right pulmonary artery (*short arrow*). (Reproduced with permission; see Figure Credits)

FIGURE 7.94   Severe obstruction to the left upper pulmonary vein demonstrated with a jet of contrast entering the left atrium (*arrow*) at the narrowed junction of the pulmonary vein to the left atrium. The transseptal catheter used for injected has been pulled back into the left atrium. (Reproduced with permission; see Figure Credits)

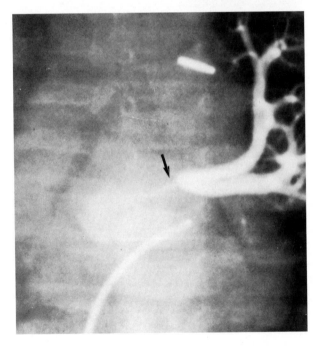

that can be identified by right ventricular and pulmonary arterial angiography (Figs. 7.93, 7.94). Doming of the pulmonary valve is not seen in patients with dysplasia of the valve.

NATURAL HISTORY

Patients with mild-to-moderate pulmonary valve stenosis have good prognoses; only a few progress to severe obstruction,[35] which may produce heart failure and early death in young infants and adults;[33] patients are subject to infective endocarditis. Paradoxical emboli may occur through a patent oval foramen, and brain abscess is possible.

Patients with subvalvular stenosis may have good survival curves although severity is usually progressive. Patients with supravalvular stenosis usually have a stable course; however, the artery distal to the obstruction may rupture or thrombose, and infective arteritis is possible.

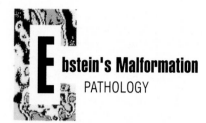

Ebstein's Malformation
PATHOLOGY

The basic pathologic defect in Ebstein's malformation is downward displacement of the dysplastic tricuspid valve leaflets into the right ventricle. The right atrium is large, and the functional component of the right ventricle is smaller than normal.[29] The annular attachment of the anterosuperior leaflet of the valve is normally positioned, while the mural (inferior) and septal leaflets are attached

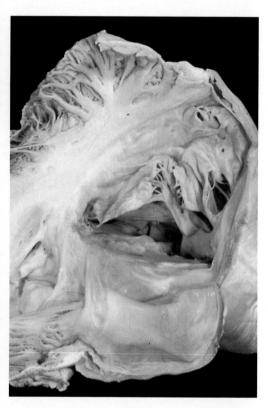

FIGURE 7.95 The right atrial aspect of the right atrioventricular junction in this example of Ebstein's malformation shows a normal focal attachment of the anterosuperior leaflet of the tricuspid valve with marked downward displacement of the septal and the mural leaflets. (Reproduced with permission; see Figure Credits)

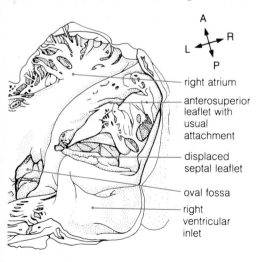

A
L — R
P

- right atrium
- anterosuperior leaflet with usual attachment
- displaced septal leaflet
- oval fossa
- right ventricular inlet

FIGURE 7.96 The atrial aspect of the abnormal right atrioventricular junction in this example of Ebstein's malformation shows linear attachment of the grossly abnormal anterosuperio leaflet of the tricuspid valve. The valve is consequently much more deformed than that shown in Figure 7.95. (Reproduced with permission; see Figure Credits)

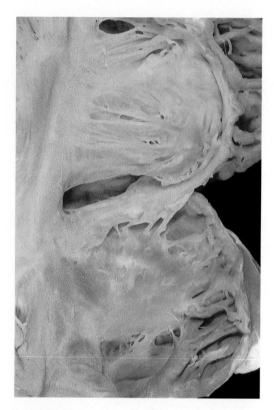

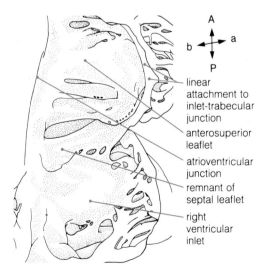

A
b — a
P

- linear attachment to inlet-trabecular junction
- anterosuperior leaflet
- atrioventricular junction
- remnant of septal leaflet
- right ventricular inlet

to the right ventricle below the atrioventricular junction. The papillary muscle and cords are abnormally formed, but the major variant in morphology depends on whether the diseased edges of the leaflets are attached in focal (Fig. 7.95) or linear (Fig. 7.96) fashion. Linear attachment produces much more severe anatomic derangement. There is almost always an additional septal defect.

PATHOPHYSIOLOGY

The compliance of the right ventricle is decreased, and tricuspid regurgitation is usually present. These abnormalities may lead to a right-to-left shunt at the atrial level.[28]

CLINICAL MANIFESTATIONS
SYMPTOMS

Infants develop symptoms of heart failure and cyanosis, while older children and adults may be asymptomatic or may have dyspnea on effort.[51] Patients with Ebstein's malformation have palpitation due to supraventricular tachycardia; syncope and sudden death may occur.

PHYSICAL EXAMINATION

Infants are usually cyanotic; older children and adults may exhibit clubbing of the fingers and toes. A small percentage of patients have no left-to-right shunt, and therefore have no cyanosis.

Palpation of the precordium may not reveal abnormal pulsations, but the liver may be enlarged. The jugular venous pulse reflects the presence of tricuspid regurgitation. The first sound is loud and abnormally split. The second sound is also abnormally split. Atrial and ventricular gallop sounds are heard. Murmurs of tricuspid regurgitation or stenosis may be detected.

LABORATORY STUDIES

Chest Radiography   The chest film may be normal in mild cases, but it usually shows a large heart. The right atrium is large, and pulmonary blood flow is diminished. The radiograph often resembles that of pericardial effusion (Fig. 7.97).

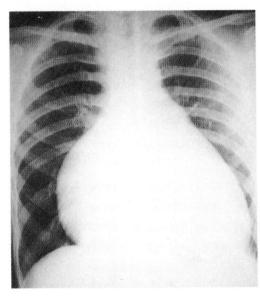

FIGURE 7.97   This chest radiograph of a 12-year-old boy with Ebstein's malformation shows marked cardiomegaly and diminished pulmonary flow (Reproduced with permission; see Figure Credits)

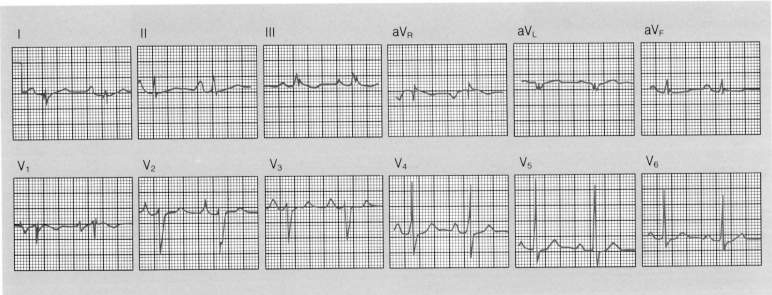

FIGURE 7.98   In this ECG of a 20-year-old male with Ebstein's malformation extremely large P waves and intraventricular conduction delay are evident. The P-R interval is 0.20 second. The P wave abnormality is due to a right atrial abnormality. The last portion of the P wave is negative in lead V₁ suggesting a left atrial abnormality. The prominent negative P wave in lead V₁ is, however, caused by a very large right atrium which directs the terminal portion of the P wave posteriorly.

Electrocardiography Large P waves are commonly present. The P-R interval may be long, and right bundle branch block is common (Fig. 7.98). The Wolff-Parkinson-White syndrome is present in 10% of patients.[51]

Echocardiography The echocardiographic abnormalities are specific for Ebstein's malformation (Fig. 7.99). The tricuspid valve is large, and its closure is delayed when compared to mitral valve closure.[17]

Cardiac Catheterization Because patients with Ebstein's malformation are prone to arrhythmias, they are at greater risk of having an arrhythmia during cardiac catheterization. Death can occur during cardiac catheterization. Tricuspid regurgitation and right-to-left shunts may be rec-

ognized. A right ventricular pressure curve is not recorded at the usual location but at the apex and right ventricular outflow tract.

An angiogram of the right ventricle shows abnormal valve morphology and tricuspid regurgitation (Fig. 7.100).

NATURAL HISTORY

Ebstein's malformation is a serious abnormality; half of patients who are recognized as having the disease die early in infancy.[17] Those who survive and are identified later in life often die in early adult life. Mild cases probably go unrecognized.

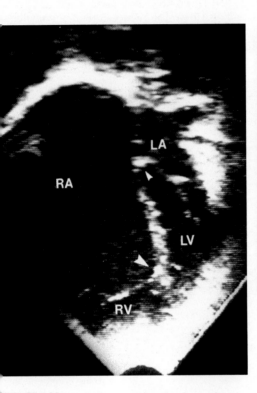

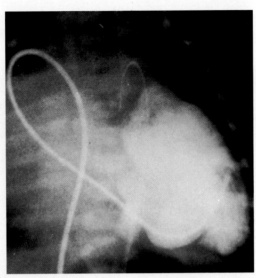

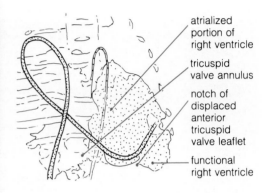

atrialized portion of right ventricle

tricuspid valve annulus

notch of displaced anterior tricuspid valve leaflet

functional right ventricle

FIGURE 7.100 Frontal projection of a right ventriculogram, obtained by injecting contrast material into the functional right ventricle, shows the position of the tricuspid valve annulus overlying the left spinal margin. The notch formed by the displaced anterior tricuspid valve leaflet is demonstrated, Note the dilated and smooth-walled atrialized portion of the right ventricle. (Reproduced with permission; see Figure Credits)

FIGURE 7.99 Cross-sectional echocardiogram in the apical four-chamber view of Ebstein's malformation shows marked displacement of septal tricuspid attachment to the interventricular septum (*large arrow*) relative to the attachment of the mitral leaflet (*small arrow*). The right atrium (RA) is very large and includes the atrialized portion of the right ventricle (RV) (LA, left atrium; LV, left ventricle). (Reproduced with permission; see Figure Credits)

Tetralogy of Fallot

PATHOLOGY

The four abnormalities that comprise the tetralogy of Fallot (Fig7.101) are a large ventricular septal defect (VSD), origination of the aorta from both ventricles above the septal deficiency, infundibular right ventricular outflow tract obstruction, and right ventricular hypertrophy.[10] Frequently there may be valvular and supravalvular stenosis.

PATHOPHYSIOLOGY

The VSD is usually about the size of the aortic valve, and both are larger than the right ventricular outflow tract. Accordingly, the systolic pressure is the same in the right and left ventricles and the aorta, but it is lower than normal in the pulmonary trunk. When the resistance to pulmonary blood flow is great, there is a right-to-left shunt and cyanosis (Fig. 7.102). When the resistance to pulmonary blood flow is not high, the pulmonary blood flow may be normal or increased, and the arterial oxygen saturation may be normal; this clinical picture is termed *acyanotic tetralogy of Fallot*. When the right ventricular outflow tract obstruction is very severe, pulmonary blood flow may also occur through collateral arteries or a patent arterial duct, which may close, producing a further reduction of the pulmonary blood flow. The right ventricular infundibular stenosis may gradually increase; it also transiently increases with physical maneuvers or with drugs that increase contractility.

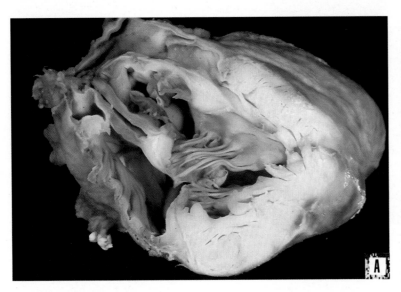

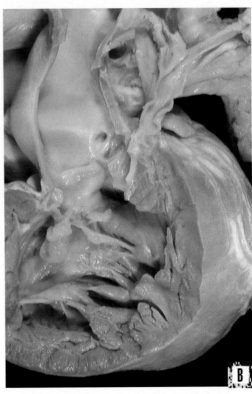

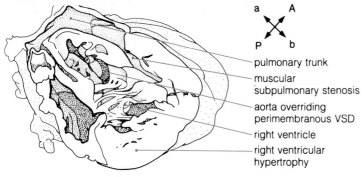

pulmonary trunk
muscular subpulmonary stenosis
aorta overriding perimembranous VSD
right ventricle
right ventricular hypertrophy

FIGURE 7.101

(A) Simulated paracoronal subcostal section of a heart with tetralogy of Fallot. A perimembranous VSD, muscular subpulmonary obstruction as a consequence of anterocephalad deviation of the outlet septum, overriding of the aortic valve, and marked right ventricular hypertrophy are apparent. (B) The right ventricular aspect of this heart shows muscular pulmonary atresia in the setting of tetralogy of Fallot. There is a perimembranous VSD, and the confluent pulmonary arteries are fed through an arterial duct. (Reproduced with permission; see Figure Credits)

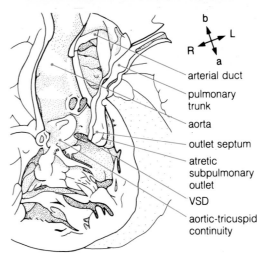

arterial duct
pulmonary trunk
aorta
outlet septum
atretic subpulmonary outlet
VSD
aortic-tricuspid continuity

Children with tetralogy of Fallot may develop dyspnea and faintness after exercise. These symptoms are relieved by assuming the squatting position, which increases peripheral arterial resistance, decreases the right-to-left shunt, and increases pulmonary blood flow.

Hypoxic episodes may be caused by a decrease in peripheral arterial resistance, which decreases pulmonary blood flow. These spells may also be due to any stimulus causing a dynamic increase in the infundibular muscular obstruction.

CLINICAL MANIFESTATIONS
SYMPTOMS

Infants with tetralogy of Fallot are usually discovered because of cyanosis, although all patients with the condition are not cyanotic. Patients may become more cyanotic as the arterial duct closes and as they grow older. A few patients have a left-to-right shunt at birth, but with increasing infundibular stenosis they develop a right-to-left shunt. Tetralogy of Fallot is the cause of cyanosis in 75% of children who are older than 2 years.[26]

Infants have hypoxic spells that can result in syncope and death. Children have dyspnea on effort, which is relieved by squatting.

PHYSICAL EXAMINATION

Cyanosis is usually present except in patients with acyanotic tetralogy of Fallot (see above). Clubbing occurs after 3 or 4 months of age, but heart failure rarely occurs.

There is an anterior lift of the precordium, suggesting right ventricular hyper-trophy. A systolic murmur is usually heard to the left of the midsternal area. The murmur ends before the second sound, which is usually single because the pulmonary closure sound is not heard. The murmur of an arterial duct may be heard until the duct closes.

LABORATORY STUDIES

Chest Radiography   The heart size is not increased, but the configuration is abnormal because of the small pulmonary trunk. The right ventricle appears large on the lateral radiograph. The aortic arch is on the right side in one quarter of patients. Blood flow to the lungs is diminished (Figs. 7.103, 7.104).

Electrocardiography   The ECG shows right ventricular hypertrophy and a right atrial abnormality (Fig. 7.105). When the mean QRS vector is directed far to the right or superiorly, it is likely that an additional defect is present.

Echocardiography   The echocardiogram shows abrupt ending of the septum below the overriding aorta. Right ventricular hypertrophy, a narrow outflow tract, and a dilated aorta are evident (Fig. 7.106).

Cardiac Catheterization   The right and left ventricular pressures are equal, and the right atrial pressure is normal. The pulmonary arterial pressure is usually low, but it may be normal. A hypoxic spell may be precipitated when the cardiac catheter occludes a small right ventricular outflow tract. Pull-back pressure recordings identify the level of right ventricular outflow tract obstructions. There is right-to-left shunt at the ventricular level, and the peripheral arterial blood oxygen saturation is diminished.

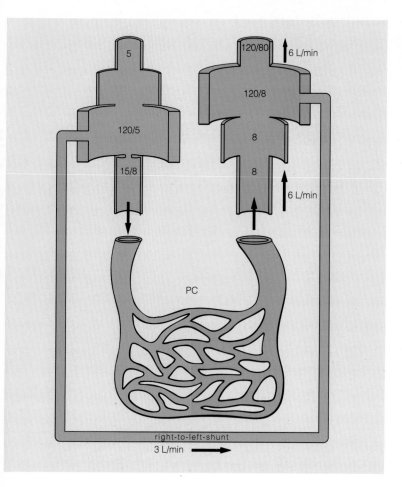

FIGURE 7.102   Pathophysiology of tetralogy of Fallot. Note the high systolic pressures in the right ventricle and the normal pulmonary arterial pressures. There is a right-to-left shunt through the ventricular septal defect. (Modified with permission; see Figure Credits)

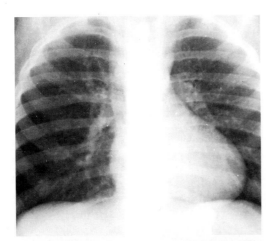

FIGURE 7.103 Chest film of a 3-year-old boy with tetralogy of Fallot. A boot-shaped heart with a right aortic arch and mildly diminished pulmonary flow are seen. (Reproduced with permission; see Figure Credits)

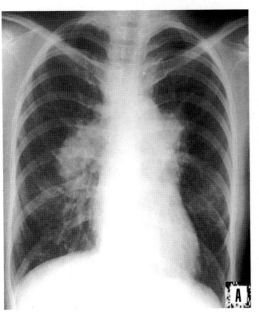

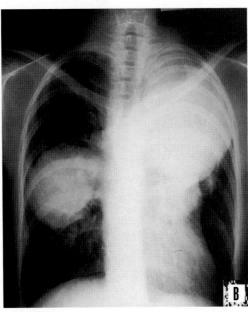

FIGURE 7.104 Posteroanterior projections of the chest of a 30-year-old woman with tetralogy of Fallot who had bilateral Blalock–Taussig shunts in 1948. The x-rays were taken in 1965 **(A)** and again in 1971 **(B)**. There are aneurysms of both right and left pulmonary arteries with severe pulmonary hypertension and pulmonary vascular disease. In 1972, the patient died of rupture of the left pulmonary aneurysm. (Reproduced with permission; see Figure Credits)

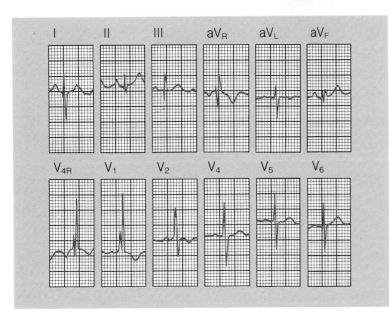

FIGURE 7.105 ECG recorded from a 3-year-old boy with tetralogy of Fallot. The P waves are prominent, and right ventricular hypertrophy is apparent. (Reproduced with permission; see Figure Credits)

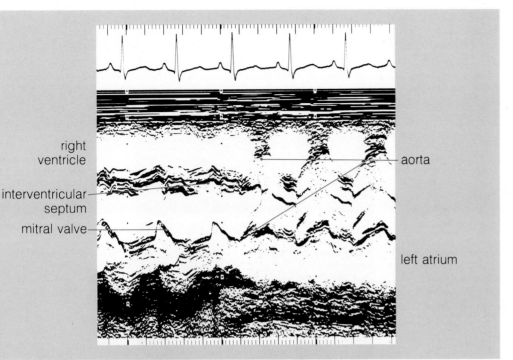

FIGURE 7.106 M-mode echocardiogram in a child with tetralogy of Fallot. There is aortic override of the interventricular septum and aortic–mitral valve continuity. (Reproduced with permission; see Figure Credits)

right ventricle

interventricular septum

mitral valve

aorta

left atrium

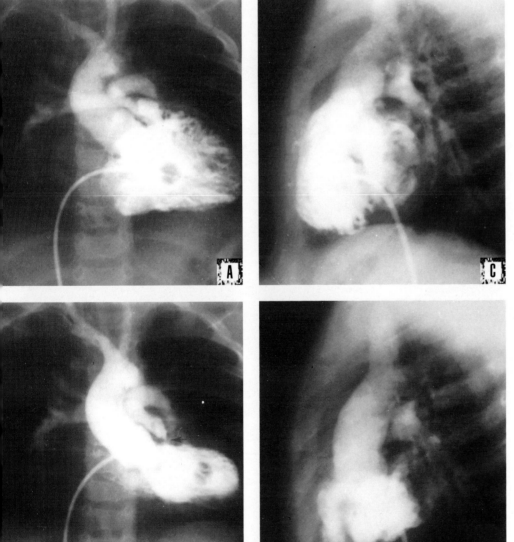

infundibular pulmonic stenosis

FIGURE 7.107 Angiocardiograms of tetralogy of Fallot. Selective right ventricular angiocardiogram in simultaneous frontal (**A**) and lateral (**B**) projections shows equal opacification of the large, overriding aorta that arches to the left and of the infundibular narrowing (*arrow*), infundibular chamber, small pulmonary annulus, and hypoplastic main pulmonary artery and more nearly normal-sized, confluent right and left pulmonary arteries. In lateral view, (**B**), the high VSD is opacified as systemic venous blood shunts right to left into the left ventricle posteriorly. Selective left ventricular injection (**C,D**) demonstrates dense opacification of the large aorta and the small pulmonary artery. Extreme infundibular pulmonic stenosis (*arrow*) is seen even better than on right ventricular injection (**A,B**). In the lateral projection (**D**), the VSD is opacified by blood shunting into the right ventricle. (Reproduced with permission; see Figure Credits)

Right and left ventriculography and coronary arteriography are valuable tools used to identify anomalies of the coronary arteries (Fig. 7.107).

Other Imaging Modalities All of the key features of tetralogy of Fallot are clearly demonstrated by MRI (Figs. 7.108–7.110).

NATURAL HISTORY

Severe cyanosis and hypoxic spells indicate a poor prognosis.[5] Patients develop polycythemia and cerebral thromboses; thrombi in the pulmonary arteries, brain abscess, and infective endocarditis may also occur.[13] Without surgical treatment about 25% of infants die during the first year, 50% die by the age of 3, and 75% die by the age of 10. Only a small percentage live beyond age 30; a few case reports describe patients beyond this age.[3] The natural history and deaths at an early age are profoundly improved by surgical intervention.

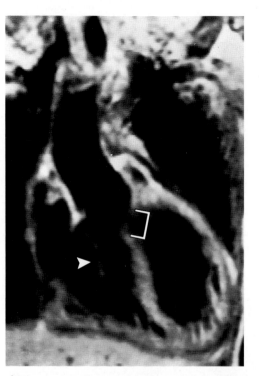

FIGURE 7.108 Gated spin-echo MR image of tetralogy of Fallot. The coronal section shows the right ventricle connecting with the aorta via a perimembranous VSD (*bracket*). The septal leaflet of the tricuspid valve (*arrow*) is adjacent to the VSD.
(Reproduced with permission; see Figure Credits)

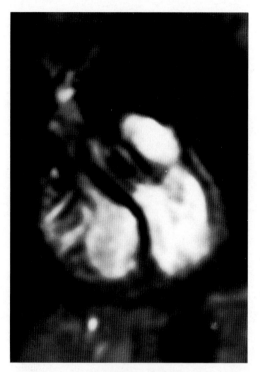

FIGURE 7.109 Cine MR image of tetralogy of Fallot. The left anterior oblique projection shows the aorta overriding the ventricular septum. The connections between the left and right ventricles and the aorta are approximately the same size. The VSD is located beneath the aortic valve.
(Reproduced with permission; see Figure Credits)

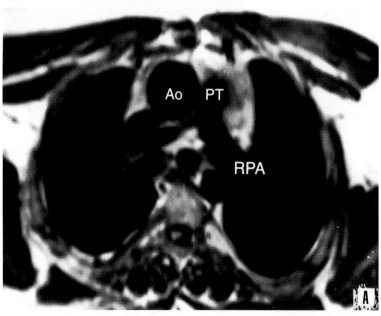

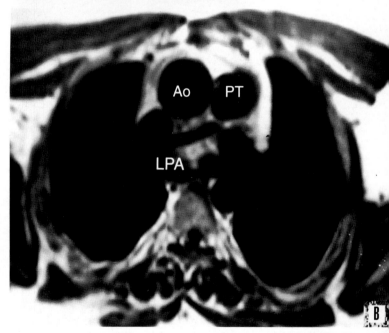

FIGURE 7.110 Gated spin-echo MR images of tetralogy of Fallot. **(A)** Axial section at the level of the right pulmonary artery shows a small pulmonary trunk and a normal-sized right pulmonary artery. **(B)** A more caudal section shows a hypoplastic left pulmonary artery. (Reproduced with permission; see Figure Credits)

Tricuspid Atresia

PATHOLOGY

The right atrioventricular connection is completely absent in most patients with tricuspid atresia (Fig. 7.111). A few patients have imperforate valves, usually in the setting of Ebstein's malformation (Fig. 7.112). A right-to-left shunt must be present for the patient to survive. An atrial septal defect or a patent oval foramen is present, and a ventricular septal defect (VSD) (Fig. 7.113) usually permits blood to enter a rudimentary right ventricle. The blood flow from the ventricular mass is then determined by its ventriculoarterial connection, which is usually concordant. When the ventriculoarterial connection is discordant, as in transposition, coarctation is usually present and a restrictive VSD produces subaortic obstruction.[42,49]

PATHOPHYSIOLOGY

The right atrial pressure is higher than the left atrial pressure, producing a prominent a wave in the right atrium. Blood in the left ventricle is always desaturated. With concordant ventriculoarterial connections pulmonary blood flow is decreased, because the right ventricle, the pulmonary artery, or the VSD is small. In such cases an arterial duct may be present to deliver desaturated

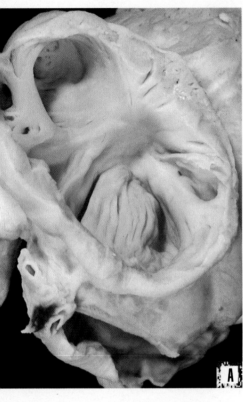

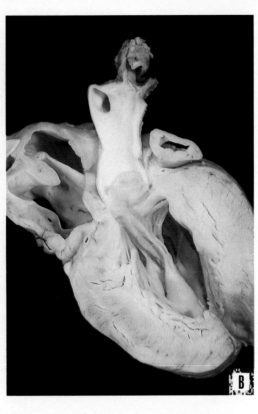

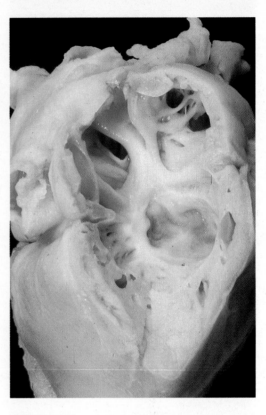

IGURE 7.111   Classic tricuspid atresia is lmost always due to complete absence of the ight atrioventricular connection. As viewed from he right atrium (**A**), the atrial chamber is blind-nding with a muscular floor. The so-called dim-le points to the left ventricular outflow tract, as hown in the simulated four-chamber section (**B**).

This view also shows the atrioventricular groove tissue interposing between the atrial floor and the ventricular mass. The rudimentary right ventricle is anterosuperiorly located and is not seen in this section. (Reproduced with permission; see Figure Credits)

FIGURE 7.112   This view of the posterior aspect of the right atrioventricular junction shows the much rarer variant of tricuspid atresia produced by an imperforate tricuspid valve in the setting of Ebstein's malformation. (Reproduced with permission; see Figure Credits)

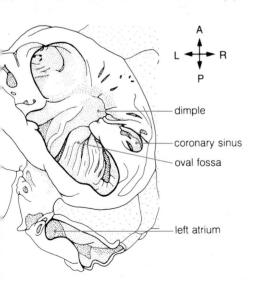

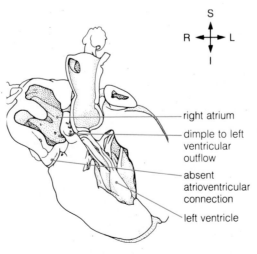

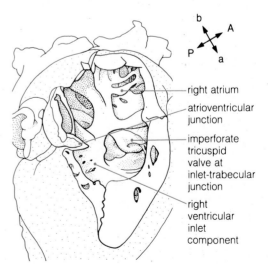

blood to the lungs. When the great arteries are discordantly connected (transposed), blood flow to the lungs may be increased.

CLINICAL MANIFESTATIONS
SYMPTOMS

Two different clinical pictures may occur. When the great arteries are concordantly connected, cyanosis is present from birth. Paroxysmal hypoxic spells may occur; squatting is evident at a later age. When the VSD is large and the right ventricle and the pulmonary trunk are also large, pulmonary blood flow is increased. An increase in pulmonary blood flow also occurs when the great

arteries are discordantly connected. This leads to symptoms of heart failure with slight cyanosis.

PHYSICAL EXAMINATION

Severe or slight cyanosis may be present; clubbing of the fingers appears later in the first year of life. A prominent a wave is seen in the internal jugular veins, and the liver may be enlarged. When there is a VSD and decreased pulmonary blood flow, the second sound is single. A systolic murmur may be heard to the left of the midsternal region, or there may be no murmur. When there is an increase in pulmonary blood flow, the apex impulse is forceful and the second

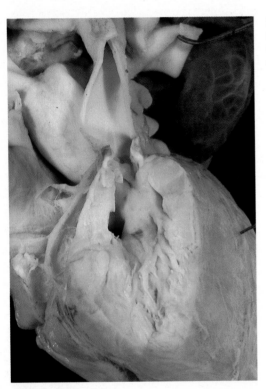

FIGURE 7.113
Discordant ventriculoarterial connection (transposition) and a restrictive VSD are seen in the rudimentarry right ventricle from a case of tricuspid atresia. The heart also exhibits severe isthmic hypoplasia and coarctation. (Reproduced with permission; see Figure Credits)

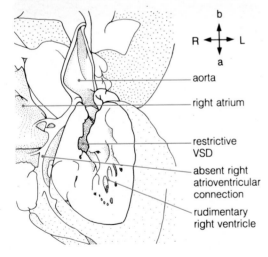

aorta

right atrium

restrictive VSD

absent right atrioventricular connection

rudimentary right ventricle

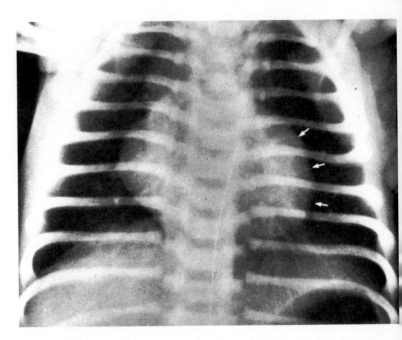

FIGURE 7.114   Chest radiograph of an infant with tricuspid atresia shows decreased pulmonary arterial vascularity and cardiomegaly. The prominent right lower cardiac border results from the enlarged right atrium. The very round prominent left cardiac border results from enlargement of left ventricle (*arrows*). When the ventricular septal defect is large or there is associated discordant ventriculoarterial connection, blood flow to the lungs is increased. However, the pulmonary blood flow is diminished in most patients with tricuspid atresia. (Reproduced with permission; see Figure Credits)

sound is split. A loud systolic murmur and a thrill may be best heard in the left midsternal area; a diastolic rumble may be heard at the apex. Signs of heart failure may be present.

LABORATORY STUDIES

Chest Radiography   The heart is usually normal in size; however, it may be enlarged in patients with an increase in pulmonary arterial blood flow. The right heart border is straight because of the small right ventricle. The blood flow to the lungs is usually diminished. However, when the VSD and the right ventricle are large or when the great arteries are transposed, the blood flow to the lungs is increased (Fig. 7.114).

Electrocardiography   The ECG usually shows left ventricular hypertrophy (mean QRS vector located between 0° and -90°) and right atrial abnormality (Fig. 7.115). When the great arteries are transposed, the mean QRS axis is located between 0° and +90°.[9]

Echocardiography   M-mode echocardiography usually reveals a rudimentary right ventricle; the tricuspid valve is not seen[?]. Cross-sectional echocardiography reveals absence of the right atrioventricular connection and many of the associated defects (Fig. 7.116).[24]

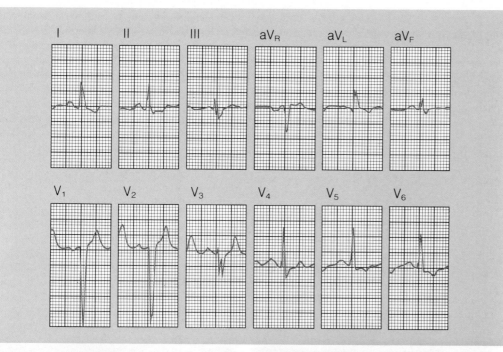

FIGURE 7.115   Left ventricular hypertrophy is evident in this ECG from a 31-year old woman with congenital tricuspid atresia, who survived because of atrial and ventricular septal defects. The P waves are large. Left bundle branch block is present (QRS duration 0.12 sec). The mean QRS vector is directed at 0° and posteriorly. The mean T vector is directed +180° to the right and anteriorly. These electrocardiographic abnormalities are caused by a dilated left ventricle. (Reproduced with permission; see Figure Credits).

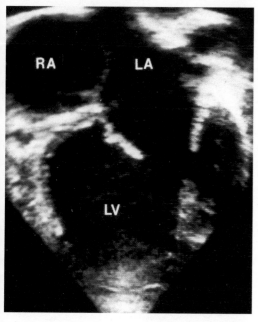

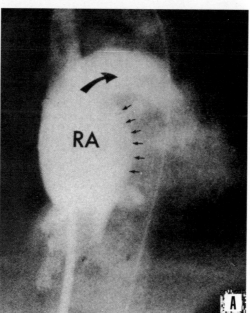

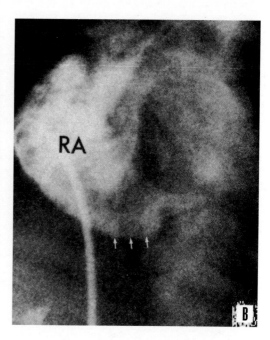

FIGURE 7.116   Cross-sectional echocardiogram in the apical four-chamber view of a patient with tricuspid atresia shows that a single atrioventricular valve–the mitral valve–is present (LA, left atrium; LV, left ventricle; RA, right atrium). (Reproduced with permission; see Figure Credits).

FIGURE 7.117   (**A**) This selective right atriogram in the frontal projection is from a patient with tricuspid atresia and right-to-left atrial shunting through a sinous venosus-type atrial septal defect (*curvilinear arrow*). The remainder of the atrial septum is intact (*small black arrows*). (**B**) In the hepatoclavicular projection the right atriogram demonstrates the smooth floor of the right atrium (RA, *white arrows*). (Reproduced with permission; see Figure Credits).

Cardiac Catheterization   The right atrial pressure is abnormally elevated, and it is higher than the left atrial pressure. The catheter passes from the right atrium into the left atrium; the right ventricle cannot be entered through the tricuspid valve. With normally related great arteries the pulmonary pressure and flow depend on the size of the VSD, the right ventricle, the pulmonary artery, and the pulmonary valve. Accordingly the pulmonary blood flow may be diminished or increased. When there is no VSD, pulmonary blood flows via an arterial duct or, rarely, aortopulmonary collateral arteries. When the great arteries are transposed, the catheter may enter the pulmonary trunk from the left ventricle. Angiocardiography usually reveals the entire anatomy (Fig. 7.117).

NATURAL HISTORY

Cyanosis is evident in most of the infants at birth. It usually progresses with closure of the arterial duct or as the VSD becomes smaller.[43] About one half of patients die by six months of age, about two thirds die by one year of age, and 90% die by ten years of age. Life expectancy is longer when there is moderate blood flow to the lungs. Hypoxia and its complications are the most common cause of death, but heart failure may occur. When pulmonary atresia is present, the life expectancy is three months.

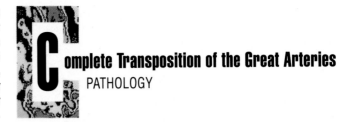

Complete Transposition of the Great Arteries
PATHOLOGY

The pulmonary trunk arises from the left ventricle and the aorta arises from the right ventricle in the setting of a concordant atrioventricular connection (Figs. 7.118, 7.119). Other abnormalities must be present for the patient to survive, including the VSD (Fig. 7.120), found in one third of patients, an atrial septal defect, or patency of the arterial duct.[41] Other associated abnormalities include pulmonary valve stenosis, subpulmonary stenosis (Fig. 7.121), aneurysm of the ventricular septum, and adherence of the anterior (pulmonary) leaflet of the mitral valve to the ventricular septum.

PATHOPHYSIOLOGY

Patients with complete transposition are able to survive because of the patent

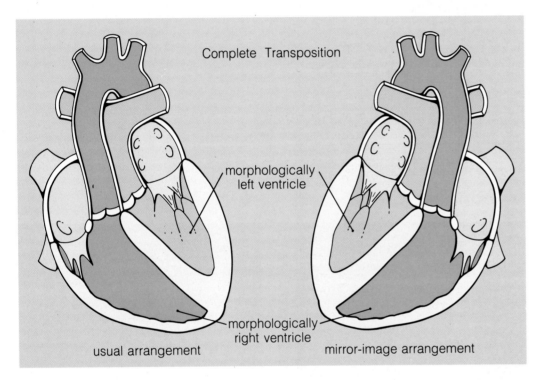

FIGURE 7.118   This diagram shows the chamber connections that create the combination best described as complete transposition. This condition may be found with usually arranged (solitus) and mirror-image (inversus) atrial chambers, but not with atrial isomerism. (Reproduced with permission; see Figure Credits)

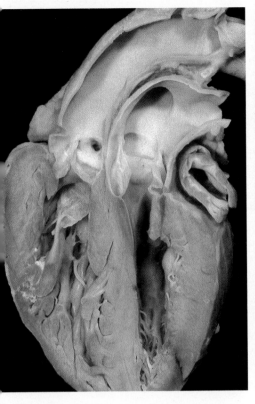

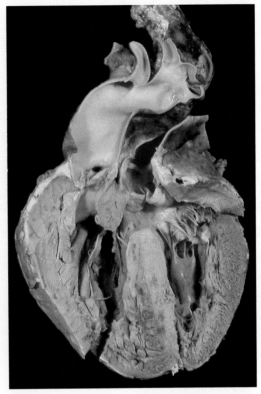

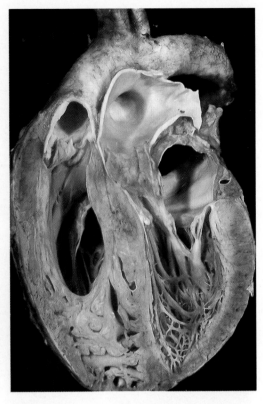

FIGURE 7.119 A simulated four-chamber long-axis section through the ventricular outlets shows the discordant ventriculoarterial connection that, combined with a concordant atrioventricular connection, is the hallmark of complete transposition of the great arteries. (Reproduced with permission; see Figure Credits)

FIGURE 7.120 A subpulmonary VSD in the setting of complete transposition has a completely muscular right ventricular margin. The overriding pulmonary valve and the narrowed subaortic outflow tract arise as the consequence of malalignment of the outlet septum. This lesion can be considered as one variant of the Taussig–Bing malformation. (Reproduced with permission; see Figure Credits)

FIGURE 7.121 A simulated four-chamber section through the ventricular outlets shows severe subpulmonary obstruction in the setting of complete transposition of the great arteries. A discrete subpulmonary fibrous shelf that coexists with an anomalous attachment of the anterolateral papillary muscle of the mitral valve is the cause of the obstruction. A similar shelf produces subaortic obstruction if found in the setting of concordant ventriculoarterial connection. (Reproduced with permission; see Figure Credits)

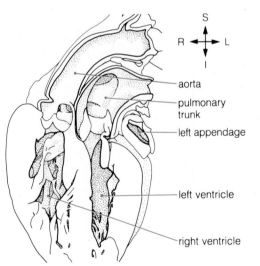

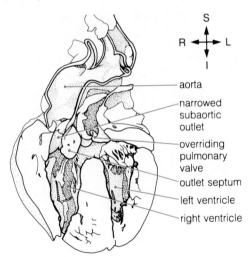

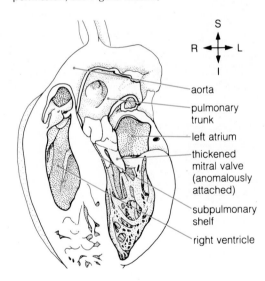

oval foramen, VSD, or patent arterial duct. The physiologic derangement depends on the type and severity of these associated defects.

CLINICAL MANIFESTATIONS

The condition is two to three times more common in males than in females. Complete transposition occurs in slightly less than 10% of children who are recognized as having congenital heart disease; about one third of the untreated patients die within the first week of life.[41]

SYMPTOMS

The physician and parents note the infant's discomfort due to hypoxia and heart failure.

The infant with an intact ventricular septum or a small VSD has intense cyanosis; breathing difficulty is apparent. An anterior precordial lift may be present. The first sound is loud and the second sound is split, signifying the presence of aortic and pulmonary valves. Murmurs may not be heard.

Cyanosis may be slight when a large VSD is present; these patients may have signs of heart failure and difficulty in breathing. The right and left ventricular pulsations are prominent. The sound of closure of the pulmonary valve is audible. A systolic murmur is usually present to the left at the lower end of the sternum; a diastolic rumble may be heard at the apex.

FIGURE 7.122   On this chest film of a three-week-old infant with complete transposition a VSD is probably absent or very small, and the main pulmonary artery segment is not seen. There is slight cardiac enlargement with a narrow mediastinum. (Reproduced with permission; see Figure Credits)

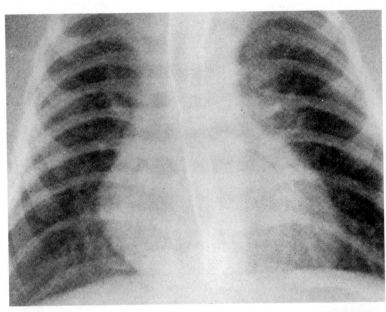

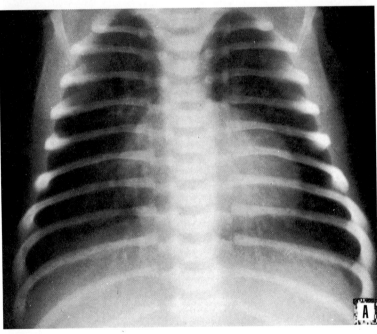

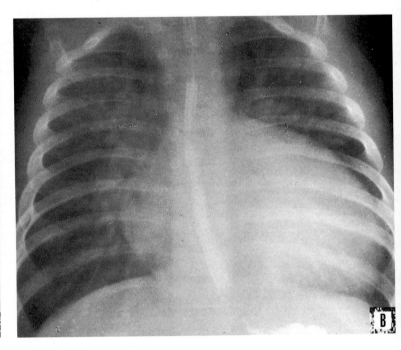

FIGURE 7.123   Chest radiographs of an infant with complete transposition and a large VSD were obtained at age one month (**A**) and at age five months (**B**). Marked cardiac enlargement and pulmonary plethora developed during the four-month interval, as pulmonary vascular resistance decreased and pulmonary arterial blood flow increased. The egg-on-side contour of the heart and the narrow cardiac base characteristic of complete transposition are evident in both films (Reproduced with permission; see Figure Credits).

Chest Radiography   The chest film of a patient with complete transposition an intact ventricular septum is shown in Fig. 7.122. The pulmonary flow may appear normal, but is usually increased. The shadow of the great arteries may appear narrow due to the displaced pulmonary trunk. The heart is large, giving an egg-on-side appearance. On the chest film of a patient with a large interventricular septal defect the pulmonary blood flow is increased, the shadow of the great arteries is narrow, and the heart is large (egg-on-side appearance) (Fig. 7.123).

Electrocardiography   The abnormalities in the ECG vary with the age of the patient and the existence of interventricular septal defect. When the infant with transposed great arteries has an intact ventricular septum, the P waves may be tall. Abnormal right ventricular forces develop toward the end of the first week of life. Upright T waves in leads V_1 and V_{3R} signify that right ventricular hypertension is present. Older infants have right ventricular hypertrophy (Fig. 7.124). When the patient has a large VSD, ECG shows biatrial abnormalities and biventricular hypertrophy.

Echocardiography   Cross-sectional echocardiography reveals the origination of pulmonary trunk from the left ventricle and the aorta

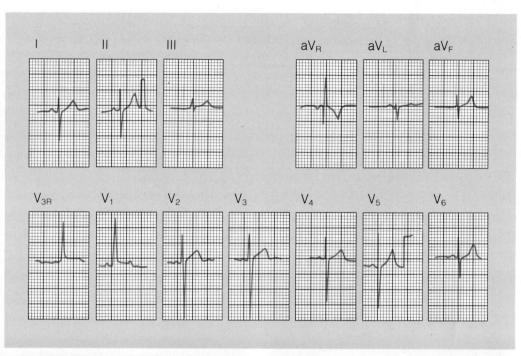

FIGURE 7.124   Electrocardiogram of an infant with complete transposition of the great arteries. The mean QRS vector is directed to the right and anteriorly and the T vector is directed at +50 degrees in the frontal plane and anterior; indicating right ventricular hypertrophy. (Reproduced with permission; see Figure Credits)

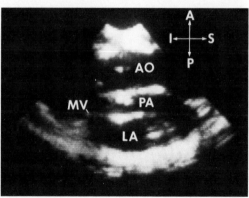

FIGURE 7.125   Both great arteries are visualized in the cross-sectional echocardiogram in the para sternal long-axis view from a patient with complete transposition and intact ventricular septum. The pulmonary trunk (PA) is identified posterior to the aorta (AO) by its sharp posterior angulation around the superior aspect of the left atrium (LA) (MV, mitral valve) (Reproduced with permission; see Figure Credits)

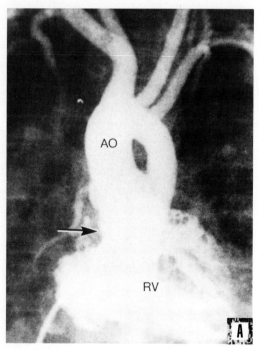

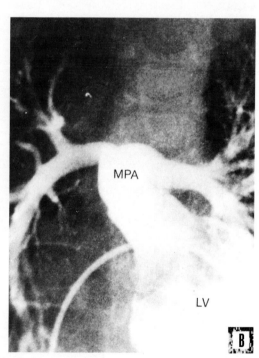

FIGURE 7.126   (**A**) Posteranterior view of the right ventricular angiogram from a patient with complete transposition and intact ventricular septum demonstrates that the aorta (AO) arises from the heavily trabeculated right ventricle (RV) above a subaortic infundibulum (arrow). (**B**) On the left ventricular angiogram the pulmonary trunk (MPA) can be seen arising from the smooth-walled left ventricle (LV). (Reproduced with permission; see Figure Credits)

from the right ventricle (Fig. 7.125). Associated lesions can also be identified.

Cardiac Catheterization   Systemic arterial oxygen saturation may be extremely low in patients without a VSD, but only slightly low in patients with a large VSD. The oxygen saturation in the pulmonary artery is always higher than in a systemic artery. The right ventricular systolic pressure is at systemic levels, as is the left ventricular pressure if a large VSD, patent arterial duct, or pulmonary valve stenosis is present. Angiography outlines the associated abnormalities (Fig. 7.126).

Cardiac catheterization should be performed on a patient suspected of having complete transposition. Atrial septostomy should be performed if the atrial septum is intact.

NATURAL HISTORY

Without treatment 50% of patients with complete transposition die during the first month of life, and 90% die within the first year. Patients with intact ventricular septum die of hypoxia and its complications; patients with a large VSD die of heart failure and pulmonary vascular disease.[18,37] Patients with a VSD and pulmonary valve stenosis have the best prognosis.

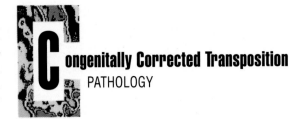

Congenitally Corrected Transposition
PATHOLOGY

The great arteries are transposed in the setting of a discordant atrioventricular connection. The pulmonary trunk arises from the morphologically left ventricle, which in turn is connected to the right atrium. The aorta arises from the morphologically right ventricle, which is connected to the left atrium (Fig. 7.127). The mitral valve is usually located on the right side along with the left ventricle (Fig. 7.128A), and the tricuspid valve is located on the left side with the right ventricle (Fig. 7.128B). The course of the coronary arteries is arranged in mirror-image fashion.

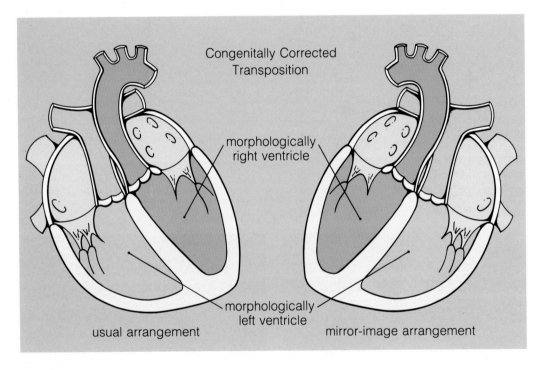

FIGURE 7.127   This diagram shows the chamber connections producing the combination best described as congenitally corrected transposition. Like complete transposition, this lesion may exist with usually arranged or mirror-image atrial chambers, but not with atrialisomerism. (Reproduced with permission; see Figure Credits)

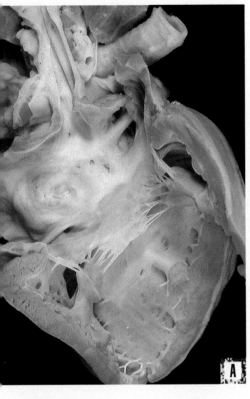
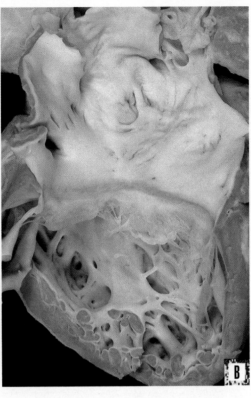

FIGURE 7.128   The discordant atrioventricular connection that is the hallmark of congenitally corrected transposition is shown here in the setting of a heart with the usual atrial arrangement. (**A**) The right atrium is connected to the right-sided, morphologically left ventricle, while the left atrium is connected to the left-sided morphologically right ventricle (**B**). (Reproduced with permission; see Figure Credits)

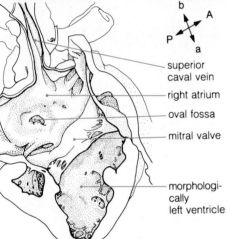

superior
caval vein

right atrium

oval fossa

mitral valve

morphologi-
cally
left ventricle

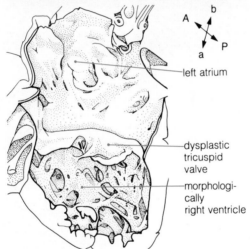

left atrium

dysplastic
tricuspid
valve

morphologi-
cally
right ventricle

FIGURE 7.129   A simulated paracoronal subcostal section of a heart shows a perimembranous inlet VSD along with subpulmonary obstruction due to fibrous tissue tags in a heart with congenitally corrected transposition. (Reproduced with permission; see Figure Credits)

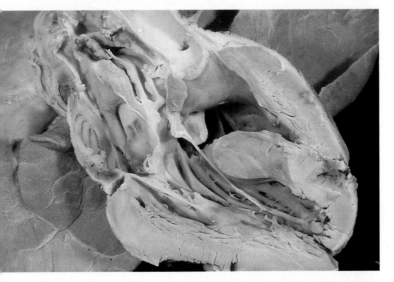

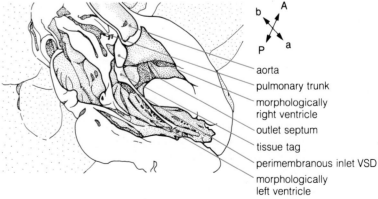

aorta

pulmonary trunk

morphologically
right ventricle

outlet septum

tissue tag

perimembranous inlet VSD

morphologically
left ventricle

PATHOPHYSIOLOGY

A VSD is usually present (Fig. 7.129). An Ebstein-like malformation may be seen in the left-sided, morphologically right ventricle where the tricuspid valve is located. Pulmonary stenosis or atresia is also commonly present (see Fig. 7.129)[44a]. When pulmonary stenosis and an interventricular septal defect are present, the condition hemodynamically resembles tetralogy of Fallot. Oth[e] serious anomalies are common. Atrioventricular conduction abnormalities ma[y] be present and evidence of the existence of the condition may be detecte[d] before delivery.

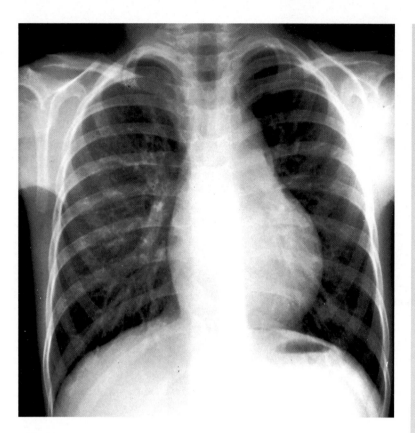

FIGURE 7.130 On the posteroanterior chest radiograph of a patient with congenitally corrected transposition of the great vessels note the straight upper-left heart border. This is produced by the aorta originating from the systemic ventricle, which in corrected transposition, is the anatomic right ventricle. (Reproduced with permission; see Figure Credits)

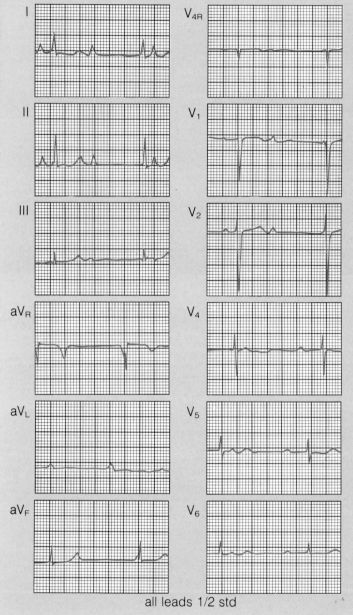

all leads 1/2 std

FIGURE 7.131 On the ECG of a six-year-old patient with congenitally corrected transposition of the great arteries, Q waves are evident at V_{4R} and the R waves are small at V_1. Complete atrioventricular block is present, the ventricular rate is about 50 per minute, and the atrial rate is 85 per minute. (Reproduced with permission; see Figure Credits)

CLINICAL MANIFESTATIONS

SYMPTOMS

Symptoms depend on the associated abnormalities. They include dyspnea and rhythm disturbance.

PHYSICAL EXAMINATION

The second sound may be louder than usual, because the aortic valve is located nearer the chest wall than it is normally. Murmurs depend on the associated defects that are present. Therefore when a patient appears to have tetralogy of Fallot but the second component of the second sound is loud, congenitally corrected transposition should be considered.

LABORATORY STUDIES

Chest Radiography   A straight upper-left heart border representing the contour of the transposed aorta is a characteristic finding on the chest film (Fig. 7.130).

Electrocardiography   The ECG often shows atrioventricular block including complete heart block, with Q waves in the right precordial leads (Fig. 7.131).

Echocardiography   Cross-sectional echocardiography enables identification of the morphology of the abnormally connected right and left ventricles, the pulmonary trunk and the aorta, and the nature and number of associated defects (Fig. 7.132).

Cardiac Catheterization   Cardiac catheterization may also identify many of the associated abnormalities, and ventricular angiograms are characteristic (Fig. 7.133).

NATURAL HISTORY

The natural history depends on the associated defects. Many of the defects can be corrected by surgery, but there is a question as to the capability of the morphologically right ventricle to maintain a normal cardiac output throughout a complete and normal lifespan.

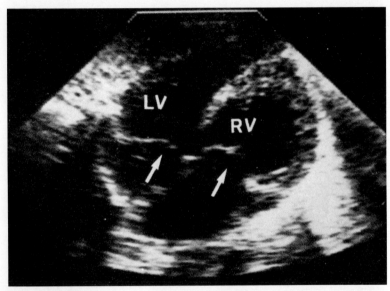

FIGURE 7.132   This cross-sectional echocardiogram in the apical four-chamber view from an infant shows congenitally corrected transposition (ventricular inversion with L-transposition of the great arteries). In a normal heart the right-sided atrioventricular valve is closer to the apex than the left-sided atrioventricular valve, but in ventricular inversion the opposite is true (*arrows*) (LV, morphologically left ventricle; RV, morphologically right ventricle). (Reproduced with permission; see Figure Credits)

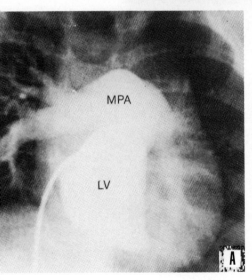
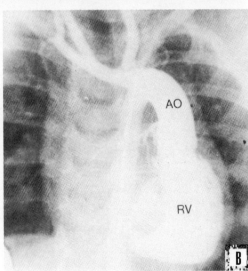

FIGURE 7.133   (**A**) As seen on the posteroanterior view of the left ventricular (LV) angiogram in a child with corrected transposition of the great arteries, the pulmonary trunk (MPA) arises from the smooth-walled left ventricle, which receives systemic venous blood. (**B**) On the posteroanterior view of the right ventricular (RV) angiogram the ascending aorta (AO) arises to the left of the pulmonary trunk from the more heavily trabeculated right ventricle, which receives the pulmonary venous blood. The ventricular septum, seen here perpendicular to the frontal plane, is intact. (Reproduced with permission; see Figure Credits)

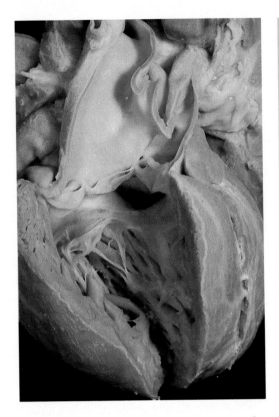

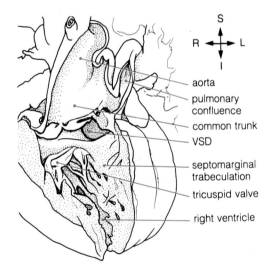

FIGURE 7.134 The right ventricular aspect of this heart exposes a common arterial trunk. The common truncal valve overrides a subarterial VSD with a muscular posterointerior rim. The pulmonary arteries arise from a short confluent channel that originates from the common trunk (type 1). (Reproduced with permission; see Figure Credits)

aorta
pulmonary confluence
common trunk
VSD
septomarginal trabeculation
tricuspid valve
right ventricle

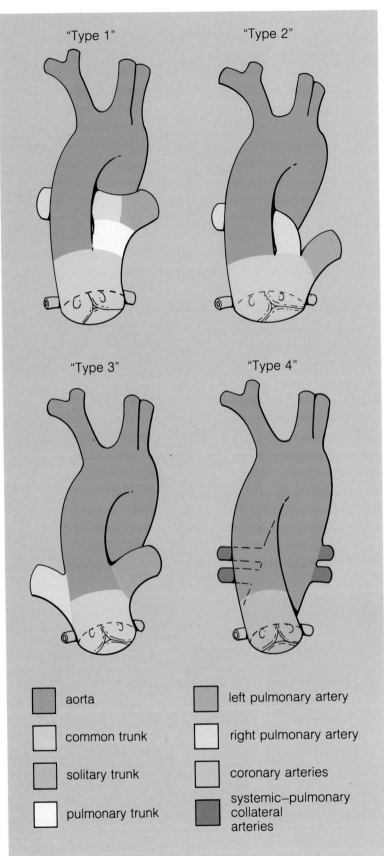

"Type 1" "Type 2"

"Type 3" "Type 4"

aorta

common trunk

solitary trunk

pulmonary trunk

left pulmonary artery

right pulmonary artery

coronary arteries

systemic–pulmonary collateral arteries

FIGURE 7.135 This diagram demonstrates the variability in the origin of the pulmonary arteries from a common arterial trunk; four types are conventionally described. The so-called type 4 is not strictly a common trunk, since the intrapericardial pulmonary arteries are completely absent, and blood supply to the lungs is derived from systemic–pulmonary collateral arteries and supplied directly to intraparenchymal branches. While it can be argued embryologically that the trunk in this circumstance is common, it could also be an aorta. It is preferable to describe it as a solitary arterial trunk. (Reproduced with permission; see Figure Credits)

Common Arterial Trunk
PATHOLOGY

When a single artery leaves the heart through a common valve above a VSD to supply the systemic, pulmonary, and coronary arteries, it is labeled a common arterial trunk or truncus arteriosus (Fig. 7.134). There are four types of arterial trunks (Fig. 7.135). The first type (see Fig. 7.134) is characterized by partial sep-

aration of the common trunk, so that a vestige of the pulmonary trunk is present; the pulmonary arteries pass to the lungs from this vestige. In the second variant the right and left pulmonary arteries arise separately from the posterior portion of the common trunk. The third type is rare; characteristically the right and left pulmonary arteries arise from the lateral aspects of the common trunk.[7] The fourth type, also the most controversial, is characterized by a solitary trunk with total absence of the intrapericardial pulmonary arteries. The argument centers on whether the solitary trunk in this setting is an aorta or a common trunk. It is probably best described simply as a solitary arterial trunk; clinically it is considered an example of pulmonary atresia with VSD (see above).

A common trunk can be identified when it can be shown that the coronary arteries, the aorta, and the pulmonary arteries arise directly from it. Other abnormalities are associated with this defect. Obstructive lesions, in particular

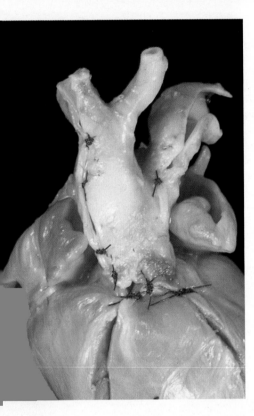

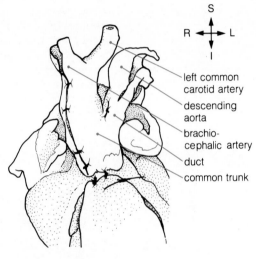

FIGURE 7.136 In this heart with a common arterial trunk the descending aorta is supplied from the common trunk via an arterial duct. The interruption of the aortic arch is between the left common carotid and the left subclavian arteries. (Reproduced with permission; see Figure Credits)

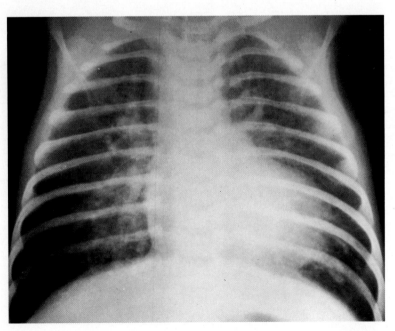

FIGURE 7.137
Posteroanterior chest radiograph of an infant with common arterial trunk shows mild cardiomegaly, increased pulmonary vascular markings, and a right aortic arch. (Reproduced with permission; see Figure Credits)

interruption of the arch (Fig. 7.136), may occur in the aortic pathway from the trunk. The descending aorta is then supplied through the arterial duct. A right aortic arch occurs in about 20% of patients, and a single coronary artery occurs in 5%. Branches of the right coronary artery may traverse the anterior wall of the right ventricle.[2] One of the pulmonary arteries may be absent. The truncal valve may be abnormal with two to five leaflets.[16]

PATHOPHYSIOLOGY

Patients with common arterial trunks (types 1, 2, 3) have an increase in pulmonary blood flow, because the contents of the right and the left ventricles are expelled into the common conduit from which the pulmonary arteries arise. There is a slight decrease in Po_2. Truncal regurgitation of variable severity is common.

Type 4 presents more usually as pulmonary atresia with a VSD. The condition of patients with duct-dependent blood supply is more precarious than that of patients in whom the blood supply is through the bronchial arteries. The collateral arteries give surprisingly good blood supply during the neonatal period. Fortunately this congenital anomaly is rare.

CLINICAL MANIFESTATIONS

SYMPTOMS

The symptoms and signs of a common arterial trunk depend on the amount of pulmonary blood flow. Most patients have an increase in pulmonary blood flow. Heart failure may be severe, and poor growth is evident during the first few weeks of life. Patients with solitary trunks are severely hypoxic and die early in life.

PHYSICAL EXAMINATION

Cyanosis may be noted in patients with type 1, 2, or 3 common arterial trunk; it is more severe when the pulmonary arteries are small. The systemic arterial pulsation may be prominent. An abnormal parasternal lift may be noted, and the apex impulse may be large. The second heart sound is single, and a systolic click may be detected. A systolic murmur may be heard in the third and fourth intercostal spaces near the left sternal border. Truncal regurgitation is commonly heard. A continuous murmur may be heard over the lung fields due to the torrential increase in pulmonary arterial blood flow.

LABORATORY STUDIES

Chest Radiography   The chest film reveals a large heart, a large arterial trunk, and increased pulmonary blood flow. A right aortic arch is common (Fig. 7.137). In rare cases the pulmonary arteries are small, the heart may be only slightly enlarged, and the pulmonary blood flow may be normal or decreased.

Electrocardiography   The ECG shows increased QRS voltage and biventricular hypertrophy (Fig. 7.138).

Echocardiography   Two separate arterial valves cannot be recorded, and the left atrium may be enlarged. Otherwise the M-mode echocardiogram is similar to that of tetralogy of Fallot. Cross-sectional echocardiography can distinguish between these diagnoses when the pulmonary arterial origin is visualized (Fig. 7.139).

Cardiac Catheterization   Bidirectional shunting and systemic arterial oxygen desaturation are observed. When the pulmonary arteries are small, the oxygen desaturation may be severe. An effort must be made to advance the catheter into both pulmonary arteries. Pulmonary hypertension is usually present, and the pulmonary vascular resistance must be determined.

Right ventricular angiography is used to identify the VSD and to visualize the arterial trunk and the pulmonary arteries. Angiographic study of a solitary arterial trunk reveals no central pulmonary arteries; the lungs are supplied through large systemic-to-pulmonary collateral arteries.

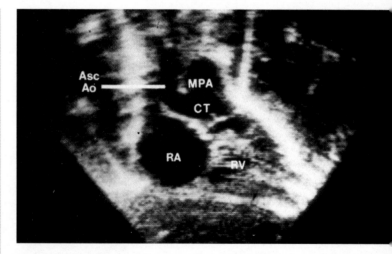

FIGURE 7.139   Cross-sectional echocardiogram in the subxiphoid long-axis view (L-3) from a patient with common arterial trunk and an interrupted aortic arch shows that the pulmonary artery segment is large and the ascending aorta (Asc Ao) is small. No transverse aortic arch can be seen from any view, since the ascending aorta ends at the left carotid branch (CT, common trunk; MPA, pulmonary trunk; RA, right atrium; RV, right ventricle) (Reproduced with permission; see Figure Credits)

FIGURE 7.138   In this ECG of a three-year-old child with common arterial trunk the P waves are prominent and peaked in lead V_2, suggesting right atrial abnormality. The mean QRS vector is directed at +90° and anteriorly. The QRS complex is large. The mean T vector is directed at +120° and posteriorly. (Reproduced with permission; see Figure Credits)

NATURAL HISTORY

The majority of children with common arterial trunk, if untreated surgically, die before the age of one year of heart failure and severe pulmonary vascular disease. A few have complications of erythrocytosis and endocarditis. Patients with small pulmonary arteries live longer.

Eisenmenger's Complex and Reaction

PATHOLOGY

Pulmonary vascular disease in patients with congenital heart disease may eliminate the possibility of corrective surgery and lead to shortened life expectancy. As pulmonary vascular disease develops in patients with congenital cardiac lesions and a left-to-right shunt, pulmonary arterial pressure gradually increases with increasing pulmonary vascular resistance. As pulmonary vascular resistance and pressure rise, the magnitude of the left-to-right shunt decreases, eventually disappearing (a phenomenon known as *balanced shunting*). Progression of pulmonary vascular disease leads to a net right-to-left shunt with resultant systemic arterial hypoxemia and clinical cyanosis, the so-called Eisenmenger's reaction. The term *Eisenmenger's syndrome*, strictly speaking, refers to the combination of lesions decribed by Eisenmenger, i.e., a VSD, an over-riding aorta, severe pulmonary vascular disease, and a right-to-left shunt.[8,12]

PATHOPHYSIOLOGY

across the pulmonary vascular bed is normally quite low, with the normal mean pulmonary arterial pressure being only 12 ± 2 mmHg. The low resistance of the pulmonary vascular bed is the result of the thin media of the precapillary pulmonary arterioles as compared with the thicker media of systemic arterioles.

As pulmonary vascular disease commonly develops, pulmonary arterioles undergo a variety of changes that lead to thicker walls and, hence, higher vascular resistance. Ultimately, pulmonary vascular resistance equals or exceeds systemic vascular resistance. Patients with Eisenmenger's reaction have pulmonary vascular resistance that equals or exceeds systemic vascular resistance.

Pulmonary vascular disease involves three alterations in the normal microscopic architecture of the pulmonary vascular bed: (1) increased muscularity of small pulmonary arteries; (2) intimal hyperplasia, scarring, and, at times, vessel thrombosis; (3) a reduced number of intra-acinar arteries. Increased muscularity of small pulmonary arteries is apparently a response of vascular smooth muscle to increased wall tension secondary to increased intraluminal pressure, i.e., pulmonary hypertension. Furthermore, pulmonary arterial smooth muscle is found in the distal vascular bed of pulmonary hypertensive individuals; this is not the case with normotensive subjects. The increase in pulmonary arterial muscle mass is due to hyperplasia rather than to hypertrophy, with new smooth muscle cells formed locally from mesenchymal cells.

Intimal hyperplasia, fibrosis, and vessel thrombosis are prominent histologic features of advanced pulmonary vascular disease. As intimal thickening progresses, intimal cells are replaced by hyalinized, collagenous tissue leading to so-called onion-skin lesions. Thrombosis of small pulmonary arteries may be followed by recanalization. Thus, individuals with severe pulmonary vascular disease have decreased numbers of intra-acinar pulmonary arteries accompanied by

FIGURE 7.140 MODIFIED HEATH–EDWARDS HISTOLOGIC CLASSIFICATION OF PULMONARY VASCULAR DISEASE

GRADE	CHANGE	GRADE	CHANGE
I	Vascular smooth muscle hypertrophy in small pulmonary arteries	IV	Plexiform lesions—dilated segments of artery with intraluminal capillary-like channels
II	Vascular smooth muscle hypertrophy and intimal hyperplasia in small pulmonary arteries	V	Grade IV changes, plus extensive fibrosis of the media and intima of small pulmonary arteries
III	Intimal hyperplastic cells replaced by collagen, producing an "onion-skin" appearance of small pulmonary arteries	VI	Acute arteritis with fibrinoid necrosis

(Reproduced with permission; see Figure Credits)

increased pulmonary arterial smooth muscle.[21,23,25,50]

In 1958, Heath and Edwards introduced a comprehensive histologic classification of pulmonary vascular disease, which has subsequently been modified. Six grades of worsening pathologic change have been identified,[21] as shown in Figure 7.140. Grade I consists of vascular smooth muscular hypertrophy in small pulmonary arteries. In grade II changes, smooth muscle hypertrophy and mild-to-severe intimal hyperplasia occur. Grade III changes consist of replacement of intimal cells by hyalinized, collagenous tissue leading to onion-skinning of the small pulmonary arteries. In grade IV patients, so-called plexiform lesions are observed. These consist of locally dilated segments of small pulmonary arteries with thin, damaged walls and with large numbers of intraluminal cellular septae, giving the arterial lumen the appearance of being filled with capillary-like channels. Grade V changes include all of grade IV changes and extensive fibrosis of the media and intima of small pulmonary arteries.[50] Thin-walled vessels often rupture producing small foci of hemosiderosis. Grade VI changes involve an acute arteritis with fibrinoid necrosis. The higher histologic grades of pulmonary vascular disease severity correlate with increasingly severe hemodynamic and angiographic evidence of pulmonary vascular disease[50] and pulmonary hypertension (Fig. 7.141).

Virmani and Roberts have categorized the anatomic changes of pulmonary vascular disease into three grades: grade 1 changes consist of medial thickening; grade 2 changes are defined as medial thickening and intimal thickening; grade 3 changes consist of medial and intimal thickening plus plexiform lesions.

Increased flow, increased pressure, embolism, thrombosis, hypoxia, acidosis, and a number of vasoactive substances produce pulmonary hypertension by a

FIGURE 7.141 COMPARISON OF ANGIOGRAPHIC, HEMODYNAMIC, AND HISTOLOGIC FEATURES OF PULMONARY VASCULAR DISEASE

ANGIOGRAPHIC FEATURES	GROUP A: NORMAL HEMODYNAMICS	GROUP B: ≠ FLOW NORMAL PRESSURE	GROUP C: ≠ FLOW ≠ PRESSURE	GROUP D: ≠ PVR	GROUP E: PULMONARY VENOUS HYPERTENSION
Resistance to hand injection	Low	Low	Low to moderate	Increased	Variable
Reflux of contrast	Rare	Rare	Frequent (27%)	Usual (63%)	Occasional (10%)
Proximal muscular arteries (1–2 mm)	Straight	Dilated	Dilated ± tortuous	Dilated, tortuous	Dilated or constricted
Tapering of muscle arteries	Even, gradual	Even, rapid	Uneven, rapid	Uneven, rapid; beading	Even, rapid (lower lobes)
Supernumerary vessels (monopedial branching)	Numerous from elastic and muscular arteries	Numerous, dilated	Reduced, especially from elastic arteries	Reduced to sparse or absent	Reduced, constricted
Capillary blush	Full, granular blush around each artery	Full, granular	Full reticular–granular (18%)	Sparse, patchy (94%)	Sparse-full, coarse, recticular (18%)
Small veins (1–2 mm)	Narrow, orderly arborization	Dilated	Dilated	Normal	Dilated
V/A diameter ratio; mean ± SD	V/A = 1.04 ± 0.28	V/A = 0.99 ± 0.23	V/A = 0.87 ± 0.18	V/A = 0.93 ± 0.22	V/A = 1/43 ± 0.33 (P <0.001)
Heath–Edwards histology grade	Normal to I	Normal to II	Normal to early III	Early III, late III, IV, and V	II to eary III

↑ = increased; PUR = pulmonary vascular resistance; V = vein; A = artery. (Reproduced with permission; see Figure Credits)

variety of mechanisms. Common to all etiologies is pulmonary vasoconstriction. Moreover, pulmonary hypertension begets more pulmonary hypertension. Initially, pulmonary hypertension leads to endothelial cell injury, secondary to increased intraluminal hydrostatic shear forces applied to the endothelium. Endothelial proliferation results. At the same time, increased wall tension within the pulmonary arteries leads to vascular smooth muscle hyperplasia. Both of these processes progressively restrict the lumen of small pulmonary arteries, leading to increased vascular resistance and further elevation of pulmonary arterial pressure. A vicious spiral is engendered with sustained pulmonary hypertension leading to continuing endothelial injury and vascular smooth muscle hyperplasia, which inturn lead to worsening pulmonary hypertension. Eventually, arteries that lack smooth muscle layers dilate, thrombose, or rupture with resultant cellular repair and proliferation, leading to dilatation or plexiform lesions.

Early in the course of pulmonary vascular disease, pulmonary vasoconstriction plays an important role. Late in the natural history of pulmonary vascular disease, fixed, nonreactive, anatomic obstruction predominates.

Patients with increased pulmonary arterial pressure *and* flow develop pulmonary vascular disease at an earlier age and of greater severity than patients with increased pulmonary flow only. In addition, patients with left-to-right shunts who live at higher elevations will have moderate arterial hypoxemia; they develop pulmonary vascular disease at an earlier age than patients with similar defects living at sea level. The rate of development of pulmonary vascular disease differs markedly from person to person despite similar congenital defects and similar magnitudes of left-to-right shunting (Fig. 7.142).

CLINICAL MANIFESTATIONS

SYMPTOMS

Patients with severe pulmonary vascular disease usually complain of effort intolerance, with dyspnea on exertion and undue fatigue. Syncope also occurs, but chest pain is less frequent.

PHYSICAL EXAMINATION

The physical examination is strikingly abnormal in these patients: central cyanosis, digital clubbing, a prominent right ventricular left and pulmonary arterial impulse, and a loud P_2 are almost always present. Jugular venous filling is normal with a prominent a wave in patients without right heart failure. Individuals with right ventricular failure may demonstrate jugular venous distension with CV waves secondary to tricuspid regurgitation. A normal or slightly reduced arterial pulse contour is observed in most patients with Eisenmenger's reaction. A right ventricular S_3 is commonly present.

LABORATORY STUDIES

Chest Radiography   The chest roentgenogram confirms the presence of an enlarged right ventricle and central pulmonary arteries. The peripheral lung fields are oligemic. Enlargement of other cardiac chambers is

FIGURE 7.142 CAUSES OF EISENMENGER'S REACTION*

DEFECT	NO. OF CASES	AGE AT DIAGNOSIS (MEAN RANGE)	
Ventricular septal defect	51	9.2 yr	(2 mo–35 yr)
Patent atrial duct	17	11.6 yr	(2 mo–37 yr)
Secundum ASD	9	20.8 yr	(6 yr–36 yr)
Endocardial cushion defect	5	5.2 yr	(19 mo–10 yr)
Combined lesions	9	5.6 yr	
Total	91		

Colorado General Hospital (1950–1965) (Reproduced with permission; see Figure Credits)

common and depends on the underlying form of congenital heart disease (Fig. 7.143; see also Figs. 7.13, 7.31, 7.56).

Electrocardiography   The ECG invariably demonstrates one of the patterns of right ventricular hypertrophy. Depending on the underlying congenital cardiac defect, associated left ventricular hypertrophy may also be observed.

Echocardiography   Echocardiographic examination confirms the presence of right ventricular and pulmonary arterial enlargement. Tricuspid or pulmonic valve regurgitation is often disclosed by Doppler. The pulmonic valve tracing demonstrates the loss of the right atrial kick.

Cardiac Catheterization   Common hemodynamic features of Eisenmenger's reaction, regardless of etiology, include arterial hypoxemia, markedly elevated pulmonary arterial pressure and pulmonary vascular resistance. Right atrial hypertension results from right ventricular failure. Erythrocytosis is common. Balanced shunting or net right-to-left shunting of blood is observed.

NATURAL HISTORY

Although it was once felt that patients with Eisenmenger's reaction had a grave prognosis, more recent observations have demonstrated that despite functional limitations, most of these patients lead active lives with little risk of death or other complications, such as stroke, before the third decade of life. However, survival beyond 50 years of age is uncommon. Once balanced shunting or net right-to-left shunting develops, operative mortality for closure of the congenital defect is high and postoperative functional results are poor. Pulmonary vascular disease usually fails to regress postoperatively and right ventricular failure supervenes, leading to further deterioration in exercise tolerance.[57]

Complications of Eisenmenger's reaction include right ventricular failure with or without syncope, arrhythmias, pulmonary infarction with or without hemorrhage, paradoxical embolism, brain abscess, bacterial endocarditis, spontaneous abortions, and gout. Terminal events include fatal arrhythmias, heart failure, pulmonary infarction and hemorrhage, brain abscess, and infectious endocarditis.

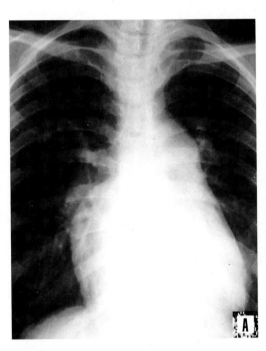
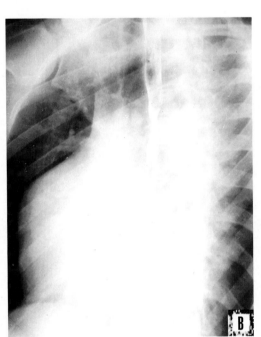
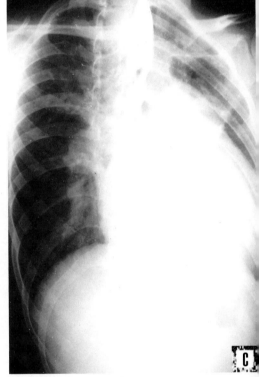

FIGURE 7.143   Eisenmenger's syndrome in a woman with ASD and high pulmonary vascular resistance. **(A)** Chest x-ray shows cardiomegaly with marked enlargement of the right atrium and of the main pulmonary artery. Pulmonary arterial markings are evident in the hilar regions but are pruned in the mid-lung field. Right ventricular hypertrophy is present on the ECG. Enlargement of the right ventricle is not shown in this frontal view although it was evident in the left **(B)** and right **(C)** anterior oblique views. Barium swallow shows left aortic arch and no evidence of left atrial enlargement. **(B)** Marked anterior enlargement of the heart due to increased size of the right atrium and ventricle. The esophagram is normal. **(C)** Enlargement of the anterior (right) ventricle. Normal esophagram shows no evidence of left atrial enlargement. (Reproduced with permission; see Figure Credits)

ACKNOWLEDGEMENT

This chapter is based in part on Nugent EW, Plauth WH Jr, Edwards JE, et al: Congenital heart disease. In Hurst JW (ed): The Heart, 6th ed. McGraw-Hill, New York, 1986. The majority of the illustrations of cardiac morphology shown in this chapter are of hearts in the Cardiopathological Museum of Children's Hospital of Pittsburgh. The photographs were taken with the permission and extensive collaboration of J.R. Zuberbuhler, MD. His considerable help is gratefully acknowledged.

FIGURE CREDITS

Figs. 7.3–7.5, 7.7, 7.14, 7.24, 7.25, 7.27, 7.32, 7.38, 7.39, 7.41, 7.46, 7.47, 7.49, 7.51, 7.52, 7.57, 7.61, 7.66–7.72, 7.80–7.83, 7.85, 7.86, 7.93(B) 7.95, 7.96, 7.101, 7.113, 7.118–7.121, 7.127–7.129, 7.134–7.136 from Hurst JW (ed): Atlas of the Heart. Gower, New York, 1988.

Figs. 7.1, 7.13, 7.29, 7.46, 7.65, 7.93A, 7.97, 7.103, 7.131 from Hurst JW: The Heart, 6th ed. McGraw-Hill, New York, 1986.

Fig. 7.6 redrawn and modified from Dillard DH, Miller DW Jr: Atlas of Cardiac Surgery. Macmillan, New York, 1983.

Fig. 7.8, 7.9, 7.28, 7.53, 7.102 modified from Selzer A: Principles of Clinical Cardiology: An Analytic Approach. WB Saunders, Philadelphia 1975.

Figs. 7.9, 7.10 redrawn from Otterstad JE: Ventricular septal defect in adults. Prim Cardiol 165, Apr 1986.

Figs. 7.11, 7.13, 7.29, 7.42, 7.55, 7.97, 7.103, 7.130 courtesy of the X-ray Department, Henrietta Egleston Hospital for Children, Atlanta, GA.

Figs. 7.12, 7.17, 7.18, 7.23, 7.30, 7.31, 7.35–7.37, 7.56, 7.59, 7.77, 7.87, 7.89, 7.94, 7.104, 7.107, 7.140–7.143 from Chatterjee K, et al: Cardiology : An Illustrated Text–Reference. Gower, New York, 1992.

Figs. 7.14, 7.15, 7.32, 7.42, 7.43, 7.55, 7.57, 7.90, 7.105, 7.106, 7.115, 7.131, 7.138 redrawn and courtesy of the Electrocardiography Laboratory, Henrietta Egleston Hospital for Children, Atlanta, GA.

Figs. 7.16, 7.34, 7.76, 7.84(A,C), 7.91 from Silverman NH, Snider AR: Two-Dimensional Echocardiography in Congenital Heart Disease. Appleton & Lang, Norwalk, CT, 1982 .

Figs. 7.19, 7.58 from Hatle L, Angelsen B: Doppler Ultrasound in Cardiology. Lea & Febiger, Philadelphia, 1985.

Figs. 7.20, 7.93, 7.126, 7.133 courtesy of the Cardiac Catheterization Laboratory, Henrietta Egleston Hospital for Children, Atlanta, GA.

Figs. 7.21, 7.22,, 7.79, 7.108–7.110 from Soto B, Kassner EG, Baxley WA: Imaging of Cardiac Disorders. Gower, New York, 1992.

Fig. 7.26, 7.111, 7.112 from Becker AE, Anderson RH: Cardiac Pathology. Raven, New York, 1983.

Fig. 7.33, 7.84(B), 7.93(A), 7.126, 7.161 from Nugent EW, Plauth WH, Jr, Edwards JE, et al: in Hurst JW: The Heart, 6th Ed. McGraw–Hill, New York, 1988.

Fig 7.40 from Wilcox BR, Anderson RH: Surgical Anatomy of the Heart. Raven Press, New York, 1985.

Fig. 7.44 partially redrawn from Lundstrom N-R: Pediatric Echocardiography–Cross-sectional, M-mode, and Doppler. Elsevier, Amsterdam, 1980.

Fig. 7.45 from Hagler DJ, Tajik AJ, Seward JB, Mair DD, Ritter DG: Real-time wide angle sector echocardiography:Atrioventricular canal defects. Circulation 59:140, 1980; with permission of the American Heart Association, Inc.

Fig. 7.48 courtesy of Leon Gerlis, MD, Leeds, UK; and from Hurst JW (ed): Atlas of the Heart.

Figs. 7.50, 7.60, 7.78, 7.93(B,C), 7.100, 7.117 from Freedom RM, Culham JAG, Moes CAF: Angiocardiography of Congenital Heart Disease. Macmillan, New York, 1984.

Fig. 7.54 redrawn from Tavel ME: Clinical Phonocardiography and External Pulse Recording. Year Book, Chicago, 1972.

Figs. 7.62 and 7.63 courtesy of A Smith, MD, Liverpool, UK; and from Hurst JW (ed): Atlas of the Heart.

Figs. 7.64, 7.137 from Hurst JW (ed): The Heart, 5th ed. McGraw-Hill, New York, 1982.

Figs. 7.73, 7.78, 7.88, 7.122 from Elliott LP, Schiebler GL: The X-Ray Diagnosis of Congenital Heart Disease in Infants, Children, and Adults. Charles C Thomas, Springfield, IL, 1979.

Fig. 7.74 from Kassner EG: Atlas of Radiologic Imaging. Gower, New York, 1989.

Fig. 7.75 redrawn from Gooch AS, Maranhao V, Goldberg H: Congenital Heart Disease. FA Davis, Philadelphia, 1969.

Figs. 7.92, 7.99, 7.116, 7.139 from Williams RG, Bierman FZ, Sanders SP: Echocardiographic Diagnosis of Cardiac Malformations. Little, Brown, Boston, 1986.

Fig. 7.98 redrawn from Goldfarb MS, Lutz JF, Hurst JW, in Hurst JW (ed): Clinical Essays on the Heart, vol 4. McGraw-Hill, New York, 1984.

Fig. 7.114 from Gedgaudas E, Moller JH, Castaneda-Zuniga WR, Amplatz K: Cardiovascular Radiology. WB Saunders, Philadelphia, 1985.

Fig. 7.115 redrawn courtesy of the Electrocardiography Laboratory, Emory Hospital and Emory Clinic, Atlanta, Georgia.

Fig. 7.123A, from Brinsfield et al in Hurst JW (ed):The Heart, 4th ed. McGraw-Hill, New York.

Fig. 7.124 redrawn from Fink BW: Congenital Heart Disease: A Deductive Approach to its Diagnosis. Year Book Medical Publishers, Chicago, 1985.

Fig. 7.125 from Hagler DJ, Tajik AJ, Seward JB, Mair DD, Ritter DG: Wide angle two-dimensional echocardiographic profiles of conotruncal abnormalities. Mayo Clin Proc 55:73, 1980.

Fig. 7.132 from Lintermans JP: Two-Dimensional Echocardiographyc in Infants and Children. Dordrecht, Martinus Nijhoff, 1986.

Fig. 7.141 modified from Nihill MR, McNamara DG: Magnification pulmonary wedge angiography in the evaluation of children with congenital heart disease and pulmonary hypertension. Circulation 58:1094, 1978.

Fig. 7.143 from Brammel HL, et al: The Eisenmenger syndrome: A clinical and physiologic reappraisal. Am J Cardiol 28:679, 1971.

REFERENCES

1. Alpert BS, Cook DH, Varghese PJ, et al: Spontaneous closure of small ventricular septal defects: 10-year follow-up. Pediatrics 63:204, 1979.
2. Anderson KR, McGoon DC, Lie JT: Surgical significance of the coronary arterial anatomy in truncus arteriosus communis. Am J Cardiol 41:76, 1978.
2a.Becker AE, Anderson RH: Atrioventricular septal defects: What's in a name? J Thoracic Cardiovasc Surg 83: 461, 1982.
3. Bertranaou EG, Blackstone EH, Hazelrig JB, et al: Life expectancy without surgery in tetralogy of Fallot. Am J Cardiol 42:458, 1978.
4. Blake HAR, Hall J, Manion WC,: Anomalous pulmonary venous return. Circulation 32:406, 1965.
5. Bonchek LI, Starr A, Sunderland CO, et al: Natural history of tetralogy of Fallot in infancy: Clinical classification and therapeutic implications. Circulation 48:386, 1973.
6. Capelli H, Andrade JL, Somerville J: Classification of the site of ventricular septal defect by 2-dimensional echocardiography. Am J Cardiol 51:1474, 1983.
7. Collett RW, Edwards JE,: Persistent truncus arteriosus: A classification according to anatomic types. Surg Clin North Am 29:1245, 1949.
8. Dexter L: Pulmonary vascular disease in acquired and congenital heart disease. Arch Int Med 139:922, 1979.
9. Dick M, Fyler DC, Nadas AS: Tricuspid atresia: Clinical course in 101 patients. Am J Cardiol 36:327, 1979.
10. Edwards JE: Classification of congenital heart disease in the adult. In Roberts WC (ed): Congenital Heart Disease in Adults, Cardiovasc Clin series 10/1. FA Davis, Philadelphia, 1979.
11. Edwards JE: The pathology of atrial septal defect. Semin Roentgenol 1:24, 1966.
12. Eisenmenger V: Die angeborenun Defecte der Kammerscheidwand der Herzens. Z Klin Med 32:1, 1897.
13. Ferencz C: The pulmonary vascular bed in tetralogy of Fallot: I. Changes associated with pulmonary stenosis. Bull Johns Hopkins Hosp 106:81, 1960.
14. Fyler DC: Report of the New England regional infant cardiac program. Pediatrics 65(suppl 2):375, 1980.
15. Gatham GE, Nadas AS: Total anomalous pulmonary venous connection. Clinical and physiologic observations of 75 pediatric patients. Circulation 42:143, 1970.
16. Gelband H, Van Meter S, Gersony WM: Truncal valve abnormalities in infants with persistent truncus arteriosus. A Clinicopathologic study. Circulation 45:397, 1972.
17. Giuliani ER, Fuster V, Brandenburg RO, Mair DD: Ebstein's anomaly: The clinical features and natural history of Ebstein's anomaly of the tricuspid valve. Mayo Clin Proc 54:163, 1979.
18. Gutgesell HP, Garson A, McNamara DG: Prognosis for the newborn with transposition of the great arteries. Am J Cardiol 44:96, 1979.
19. Hamilton WT, Haffajee CE, Dalen JE, et al: Atrial septal defect secundum: Clinical profile with physiologic correlates in children and adults. In Roberts WC (ed): Congenital Heart Disease in Adults. FA Davis, Philadelphia, 1979.
20. Haworth SG: Pulmonary vascular disease in secundum atrial septal defect in childhood. Am J Cardiol 51:265, 1983.

21. Heath D, Edwards JE: The pathology of hypertensive pulmonary vascular disease. A description of six grades of structural changes in the pulmonary arteries with special reference to congenital cardiac defects. Circulation 18:533, 1958.

22. Hoffman JIE, Christianson R: Congenital heart disease in a cohort of 19,502 births with long-term follow up. Am J Cardiol 42:641, 1978.

23. Hoffman JIE, Rudolph AM, Heymann MA: Pulmonary vascular disease with congenital heart lesions: Pathologic features and causes. Circulation 64:873, 1981.

24. Houston AB, Gregory NL, Coleman EN: Two-dimensional sector scanner echocardiography in cyanotic congenital heart disease. Br Heart J 39:1076, 1977.

25. Hutchins GM, Ostrow PT: The pathogenesis of two forms of hypertensive pulmonary vascular disease. Am Heart J 92:797, 1976.

26. Keith JD, Rowe RD, Vlad P: Heart Disease in Infancy and Childhood, 3rd ed. Macmillan, New York, 1978.

27. Koretzky ED, Moller JH, Korns ME, et al: Congenital pulmonary stenosis resulting from dysplasia of valve. Circulation 40:43, 1969.

28. Kumar AE, Fyler DC, Miettinen OS,Nadas AS: Ebstein's anomaly. Clinical profile and natural history. Am J Cardiol 28:84, 1971.

29. Lev M, Liberthson RR, Joseph RH, et al: The pathologic anatomy of Ebstein's disease. Arch Pathol 90:334, 1970.

30. Maron BJ: Coarctation of the aorta in the adult. In Roberts WC (ed): Congenital Heart Disease In Adults. FA Davis, Philadelphia, 1979.

31. Meyer J, Wukasch DC, Hallman GL, Cooley DA: Aneurysm and fistula of the sinus of Valsalva: Clinical considerations and surgical treatment in 45 patients. Ann Thorac Surg 19:170, 1975.

32. Mitchell SC, Korones SB, Berendes HW: Congenital heart disease in 56,109 births: Incidence and natural history. Circulation 43:323, 1971.

33. Mody MR: The natural history of uncomplicated valvular pulmonic stenosis. Am Heart J 90:317, 1975.

34. Moss AJ, Adams FH, Emmanouilides GC: Heart Disease In Infants, Children, and Adolescents, 2nd ed., Williams & Wilkins, Baltimore, 1977.

35. Nadas AS (ed): Pulmonary stenosis, aortic stenosis, ventricular septal defect: Clinical course and indirect assessment (Report from the Joint Study on the Natural History of Congenital Heart Defects). Circulation 56 (suppl 1):1, 1977.

36. Nadas AS, Fyler DC: Pediatric Cardiology, 3rd ed. WB Saunders, Philadelphia, 1972.

37. Newfeld EA, Paul MH, Muster AJ, Idriss FS: Pulmonary vascular disease in transposition of the great vessels and intact ventricular septum. Circulation 59:525, 1979.

38. Noonan JA: Hypertelorism with Turner phenotype: A new syndrome with associated congenital heart disease. Am J Dis Child 116:373, 1968.

39. Noonan JA: Syndromes associated with cardiac defects, In Engle MA, Brest AN (eds): Pediatric Cardiovascular Disease. FA Davis Company, Philadelphia, 1981.

40. Parker FB Jr, Streeten DHP, Farrell B, et al: Preoperative and postoperative renin levels in coarctation of the aorta. Circulation 66:513, 1982.

41. Paul MH: Transposition of the great arteries. In Moss AJ, Adams FH, Emmanouilides GC: Moss' Heart Disease In Infants, Children, and Adolescents, Williams & Wilkins, Baltimore, 1983.

42. Rao PS: A unified classification for tricuspid atresia. Am Heart J 99:799, 1980.

43. Rao PS: Natural history of the ventricular septal defect in tricuspid atresia and its surgical implications. BR Heart J 39:276, 1977.

44. Rastelli GC, Kirklin JW, Titus JL: Anatomic observations on complete form of persistent atrioventricular canal with septal reference to atrioventricular valves. Mayo Clin Proc 41:296, 1968.

44a.Ruttenburg HD: Corrected transposition (L-transposition) of the great arteries and splenic syndromes. In Adams FH, Emmanouilides GC (eds) Moss' Heart Disease in Infants, Children, and Adolescents. Williams & Wilkens, Baltimore, 1983.

45. Sahn DJ, Allen HD, Lange LW, Goldberg SJ: Cross-sectional echocardiographic diagnosis of the sites of total anomalous pulmonary venous drainage. Circulation 60:1317, 1979.

46. Sakakibara S, Konno S: Congenital aneurysm of the sinus of Valsalva. Anatomy and classification. Am Heart J 63:405, 1962.

47. Serwer GA, Armstrong BE, Anderson PAW: Continuous wave Doppler ultrasonographic quantitation of patent ductus arteriosus flow. J Pediatr 100:297, 1982. 28.

48. Shub C, Dimopoulos IN, Seward JB, et al: Sensitivity of two-dimensional echocardiography in the direct visualization of atrial septal defect utilizing the subcostal approach: Experience with 154 patients. J Am Coll Cardiol 3:127, 1983.

49. Tandon R, Edwards JE: Tricuspid atresia. A reevaluation and classification. J Thorac Cardiovasc Surg 67:530, 1974.

50. Virmani R, Roberts WC: Pulmonary arteries in congenital heart disease: A structure–function analysis. In Roberts WC (ed): Congenital Heart Disease in Adults. FA Davis, Philadelphia, 1979.

51. Watson H: Natural history of Ebstein's anomaly of the tricuspid valve in childhood and adolescence. An international cooperative study of 505 cases. Br Heart J 36:417, 1974.

52. Weidman WH, Blount SG Jr, Dushane JW, et al: Clinical course in ventricular septal defect. Circulation 56 (suppl 1):56, 1977.

53. Wells HG: Persistent patency of the ductus arteriosus. Am J Med Sci 136:381, 1908.

54. Weyman AE, Dillon JC, Fiegenbaum H, et al: Echocardiographic differentiation of infundibular from valvar pulmonary stenosis. Am J Cardiol 36:21, 1975.

55. White PD, Hurst JW, Fennell RH: Survival to the age of 75 years with congenital pulmonary stenosis and patent foramen ovale. Circulation 2(4):558, 1950.

56. Wright GB, Keane JF, Nadas AS, Berard, WF, Castaneda AR: Fixed subaortic stenosis in the young: Medical and surgical course in 83 patients. Am J Cardiol 52:830, 1983.

57. Young D, Mark H: Fate of the patient with Eisenmenger Syndrome. Am J Cardiol 28:658, 1971.

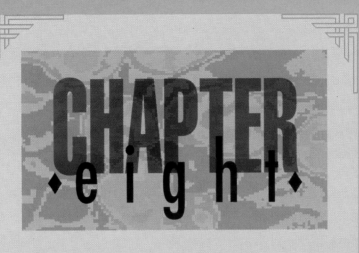

CHAPTER ·eight·

MYOCARDIAL DISEASE: MYOCARDITIS

J. WILLIS HURST, MD

NANETTE K. WENGER, MD

WALTER H. ABELMANN, MD

ANTON E. BECKER, MD

JOSEPH S. ALPERT, MD

CARDIOMYOPATHY

J. WILLIS HURST, MD

NANETTE K. WENGER, MD

JOHN F. GOODWIN, MD

ANTON E. BECKER, MD

JOSEPH S. ALPERT, MD

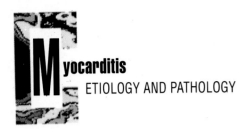

Myocarditis

ETIOLOGY AND PATHOLOGY

Myocarditis is an inflammatory response within the myocardium due to a variety of causes. Among the most common are infectious diseases caused by viral, bacterial, mycotic, rickettsial, or parasitic organisms.[17,21,36] Infectious myocarditis is a common complication in patients who are immunocompromised due to disease or immunosuppressive drugs.

In the United States and Europe virus infections, such as coxsackievirus type B (especially strains Bl to B5 and A4), are responsible of most cases of myocarditis (Fig. 8.1).[1] In South America the most common cause of myocarditis is *Trypanosoma cruzi;* which is responsible for Chagas' disease.[29] In New Zealand, Australia, and Uruguay, where sheep are raised in abundance, echinococcosis is often seen.[24] Trichinosis caused by eating uncooked pork is a serious but rare cause of myocarditis.

Bacterial myocarditis is most often due to staphylococci, streptococci, pneumococci, or meningococci. A suppurative response prevails, and microabscesses are common (Fig. 8.2). Tuberculosis in some parts of the world is still a common cause of myocarditis (Fig. 8.3), often complicated further by hemorrhagic pericarditis. Other causes of bacterial myocarditis, such as syphilis, are rare (Fig. 8.4).

Drug-induced myocarditis may result from direct toxic effect on the myocardium or from an immune reaction, termed allergic or hypersensitivity myocarditis (Fig. 8.5). Drug-induced toxic myocarditis is usually dose-dependent and cumulative. Drugs that cause myocarditis are manifold; well-known examples are emetine, barbiturates, the ophylline, the herbicide paraquat, amphetamines, and a number of immunosuppressive agents. Allergic or hypersensitivity myocarditis is not dose-dependent; it usually regresses when administration of the drug is stopped.

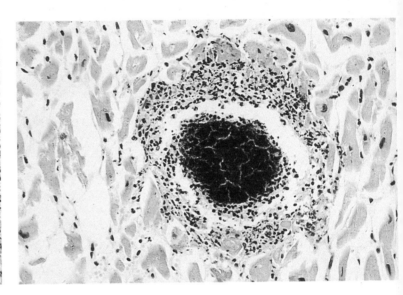

FIGURE 8.2   Histologic section of myocardium with a microabscess containing a colony of staphylococci due to sepsis. (Reproduced with permission; see Figure Credits)

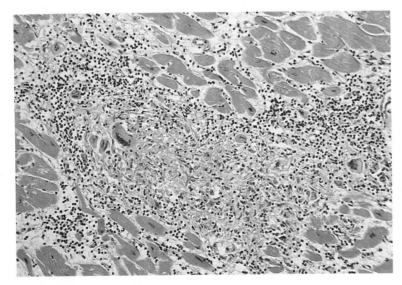

FIGURE 8.1   Histologic section of myocardium from a patient with viral myocarditis. Extensive loss of myocytes is accompanied by massive infiltration of inflammatory cells, mainly lymphocytes. (Reproduced with permission; see Figure Credits)

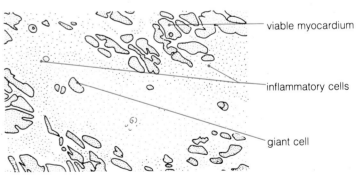

FIGURE 8.3   Histologic section of myocardium showing a granulomatous inflammation with multinucleated giant cells in a case of tuberculous myocarditis. (Reproduced with permission; see Figure Credits)

FIGURE 8.4 RARER FORMS OF MYOCARDITIS

ETIOLOGY	DISTINCTIVE FEATURES			REFERENCE
	PHYSICAL EXAMINATION	LABORATORY	MORPHOLOGIC MANIFESTATIONS	
BACTERIAL				
Diphtheria	—	Complete heart block	—	See Hurst, The Heart, 6th ed.
Tuberculosis	Arrhythmias	Arrhythmias	Tubercles with caseation	Claiborne: Am J Cardiol 33:920, 1974
Typhoid fever (*Salmonella*)	Early: peripheral circulatory collapse; ? endotoxin effect Late: congestive heart failure	—	Coronary arteritis Abscesses	Diem: Am J Trop Med Hyg 23:218, 1974
Scarlet fever Rheumatic fever	—		Valve lesions Aschoff bodies	Ewy: Am Heart J 78:238, 1969
Meningococcemia	Circulatory collapse	Disseminated intravascular coagulation	Petechiae	Denmark: Arch Intern Med 127:238, 1971
Infective endocarditis	—	—	Valve vegetations Microabscesses	Roberts: Cardiovasc Med 3:699, 1978
Staphylococcal Pheumococcal Gonococcal infection	—	—	Abscesses Valve vegetations	—
Clostridial infection	—	—	Air cysts with organisms in wall	Roberts: Am Heart J 74:482, 1967
Psittacosis (*Chlamydia psittaci*)	—	—	Psittacosis inclusion bodies in plasma cells	Sutton: Am Heart J 81:597, 1971
Chlamydia trachomatis	Heart failure	—	—	Grayston: JAMA 246:2823, 1981
Brucellosis	—		—	Buczynska-Hencner: Pol Tyg Lek 20:761, 1966
Actinomycosis	—	—	Abscesses with actinomycotic granules	Edwards: Am J Dis Child 41:419, 1931
Tetanus	—	—	Nerve cell degeneration	Murphy: Med J Aust 2:542, 1970
Tularemia	—	—		
Melioidosis	Mimic AMI	Mimic AMI	Abscesses	Baumann: Ann Intern Med 67:836, 1967
Legionnaires' disease	Heart failure	—		Gross: Chest 79:232, 1981
SPIROCHETAL				
Syphilis	Arrhythmias, heart block Conduction abnormalities	Arrhythmias, heart block Conduction abnormalities	Gumma	Boss: Ann Intern Med 55:824, 1961
Leptospirosis	Valve "pseudostenosis" Arrhythmias	Arrhythmias	Focal hemorrhage Edema Necrosis	Nusynowitz: Haw Med J 23:41, 1963
Relapsing fever	Vasoconstriction Hypotension Heart failure Conduction abnormalities, arrhythmias	Conduction abnormalities, arrhythmias	—	Judge: Arch Pathol 97:136, 1974
Lyme disease	—	Conduction abnormalities Complete heart block	—	Steere: Ann Intern Med 93:8, 1980

(Reproduced with permission; see Figure Credits)

FIGURE 8.4 RARER FORMS OF MYOCARDITIS

ETIOLOGY	DISTINCTIVE FEATURES			REFERENCE
	PHYSICAL EXAMINATION	LABORATORY	MORPHOLOGIC MANIFESTATIONS	
RICKETTSIAL				
Typhus	—	—	Vasculitis	Woodward: Ann Intern Med 53:1130, 1960
Rocky Mountain spotted fever	Hypovolemia, hypotension Peripheral vascular collapse	—	Vasculitis	Walker: Arch Pathol Lab Med 104:171, 1980
Q fever	—	—	—	Barraclough: Br Med J 2:423, 1975
VIRAL				
Coxsackie B	Congestive heart failure, arrhythmias	Arrhythmias —	—	Bell: Am Heart J 82:133, 1971
Echovirus	—	—	—	Bell: Am Heart J 82:133, 1971
Poliomyelitis	Pulmonary edema Vascular collapse		—	Trimbos: Folia Med Neerl 1963, p. 49
Influenza	Peripheral circulatory failure Arrhythmias, complete heart block	Arrhythmias, complete heart block	Myofiber necrosis	Verel: Am Heart J 92:290, 1976
Mumps	—	complete heart block	—	Arita: Br Heart J 46:342, 1981
Infectious mononucleosis (virus Epstein-Barr)	—	—	Abnormal perivascular lymphocytes	Hudgins: JAMA 235:2626, 1976
Viral hepatitis	—	—	—	Bell: JAMA 218:387, 1971
Rubella	Congestive heart failure	ECG: mimic AMI	Extensive myocardial vacuolation necrosis	Ainger: Cardiol Dig 2:21, 1967
Rubeola	Pericarditis Arrhythmias	—	—	Guistra: AMA J Dis Child 79:487, 1950
Rabies	—	—	—	Roux: Coeur Med Intern 15:37, 1976
Varicella	—	Bundle branch block Arrhythmia	Eosinophilic intranuclear inclusion bodies	Fiddler: Br Heart J 39:1150, 1977
Mycoplasma pneumoniae	Myalgia	ECG: mimic AMI Arrhythmias	—	Ponka: Acta Med Scand 206:77, 1979
Lymphocytic choriomeningitis	—	—	—	Thiede: Arch Intern Med 109:104, 1962
Viral encephalitis	—	—	—	Ungar: Am J Clin Pathol 18:48, 1948
Herpes simplex	—	—	—	Bell: Am Heart J 74:309, 1967
Cytomegalovirus	—	—	Intranuclear inclusion bodies	Wilson: Br Heart J 34:865, 1972
Variola	—	—	—	—
Herpes zoster	—	—	—	—
Adenovirus infection	—	—	—	Henson: Am J Dis Child 121:334, 1971
Arbovirus infection	Arrhythmias Heart failure	Arrhythmias	—	Obeyesekere: Am Heart J 85:186, 1973
Respiratory syncytial virus	—	—	—	Giles: JAMA 236:1128, 1976
Viral hemorrhagic fever	Shock	—	Myocardial hemorrhage	Milei: Am Heart J 104:1385, 1982

(Reproduced with permission; see Figure Credits)

FIGURE 8.4 RARER FORMS OF MYOCARDITIS

ETIOLOGY	DISTINCTIVE FEATURES			REFERENCE
	PHYSICAL EXAMINATION	LABORATORY	MORPHOLOGIC MANIFESTATIONS	
MYCOTIC				
Blastomycosis	—	—	Tubercle with caseation and giant cells	Baker: Am J Pathol 13:139, 1937
Candidiasis	Debilitated or immunosuppressed host	ECG: Bundle branch block, AV block, mimic AMI	Multiple abscesses with pseudohyphae, yeast forms	Franklin: Am J Cardiol 38:924, 1976
Aspergillosis	Debilitated or immunosuppressed host	—	Granulomas or microabscesses; mycelial and filamentous forms	Williams: Am J Clin Pathol 61:247, 1974
Histoplasmosis	—	—	Granulomas H. capsulatum in phagocytes	Owen: Am J Med 32:552, 1962
Sporotrichosis	—	—		Collins: Arch Dermatol 56:523, 1947
Coccidioidomycosis	—	—	Miliary granulomas with C. immitis spherules	Reingold: Am J Clin Pathol 20:1044, 1950
Cryptococcosis	—	—	C. neoformans in granulomas	Jones: Br Heart J 27:462, 1965
Mucormycosis	Debilitated or immunosuppressed host	—	Septic thromboses	Virmani: Am J Clin Path 78:42, 1982
PROTOZOAL				
Chagas' disease	Congestive heart failure	BBB; CHB	—	Acquatella: Circulation 62:787, 1980
Sleeping sickness (trypanosomiasis)	Arrhythmias, conduction abnormalities	Frequent ECG abnormalities and arrhythmias	—	Poltera: Br Heart J 38:827, 1976
Toxoplasmosis	—	Arrhythmias	Parasitized myofiber→rupture	Leak: Am J Cardiol 43:841, 1979
Malaria	Peripheral circulatory collapse	—	Parasitized RBC Myocardial vascular occlusion	Herrera: Arch Inst Cardiol Mex 30:26, 1960
Leishmaniasis	Angina	—	Clasmatocytes with Leishman-Donovan bodies	Benhamou: Arch Mal Coeur 31:81, 1938
Balantidiasis	—	—	—	Sidorov: Ann Anat Pathol 12:711, 1935
Sarcosporidiosis	—	—	Sarcocysts in myofiber with basophilic bodies	Aral: J Mt Sinai Hosp 15:367, 1949
Amebiasis	—	—	Microabscesses	Markowitz: Am J Clin Pathol 62:619, 1974

(Reproduced with permission; see Figure Credits)

FIGURE 8.4 RARER FORMS OF MYOCARDITIS

| ETIOLOGY | DISTINCTIVE FEATURES | | | REFERENCE |
	PHYSICAL EXAMINATION	LABORATORY	MORPHOLOGIC MANIFESTATIONS	
HELMINTHIC				
Trichinosis			—	
Echinococcosis				Murphy: J Thorac Cardiovasc Surg 61:443, 1971
Schistosomiasis	Cor pulmonale	—	Microscopic pseudo-tubercle or granuloma	Lima: Rev Inst Med Trop São Paulo, 11:290, 1969
Ascariasis	—	—	—	Ferreira: Rev Med Aeroaut 15:35, 1963
Heterophydiasis	—	—	—	Africa: Acta Med Philippina, Mono. Series, no. 1, 118, 1940
Filariasis	Congestive heart failure	Eosinophilia	Pericardial effusion Restrictive endocarditis	Tatibouet: Semaine Hop Paris 37:3418, 1961
Paragonimiasis	—	—	—	Kean: Parasites of the Human Heart. New York, Grune & Stratton, 1964, p.104
Strongyloidiasis	—	—	—	Kyle: Ann Intern Med 29:1014, 1948
Cysticercosis	—	—	Myocardial scolex-containing cysts	Ibarra-Perez: South Med J 65:484, 1972
Visceral larva migrans	—	—	Allergic granulomatosis	Becroft: NZ Med J 63:729, 1964

Note (—) indicates no distinctive physical findings, laboratory data, or morphologic manifestations other than heart failure and nonspecific cardiac enlargement. (Reproduced with permission; see Figure Credits)

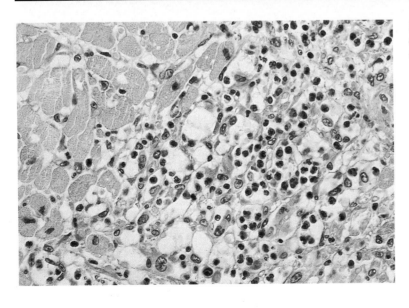

FIGURE 8.5 Histologic section of myocardium with a dense infiltration of inflammatory cells, predominately eosinophilic cells, suggesting hypersensitivity myocarditis. (Reproduced with permission; see Figure Credits)

sulfonamides are the best-known drugs in this category, but others, such as penicillin, streptomycin, tetracycline, and phenylbutazone, have been reported to cause myocarditis.

Autoimmune myocarditis is also reported in patients with rheumatic fever, systemic lupus erythematosus, and rheumatoid arthritis. Active myocarditis under these circumstances is usually of a temporary nature, but occasionally it may have a profound effect on the clinical profile of the autoimmune disease. In years past it was not uncommon for children to die as a result of rheumatic myocarditis. Necrotizing arteritis of coronary arteries in infancy, known as Kawasaki's disease (mucocutaneous lymph node syndrome), may belong to this category; in the acute stage of the disease it is often accompanied by myocarditis (Fig. 8.6).

Finally, particular types of myocarditis occur that cannot be related to a known etiology. These include idiopathic myocarditis granulomatous myocarditis, giant cell myocarditis (Fig. 8.7), and Fiedler's myocarditis. Myocarditis often coexists with pericarditis.[1] Considerable discussion has developed concerning the etiology, classification, prognosis, and management of patients with idiopathic myocarditis. Universal agreement has not been reached. Figure 8.8 outlines the diagnostic categories for idiopathic myocarditis based on myocardial biopsy (Fig. 8.9).

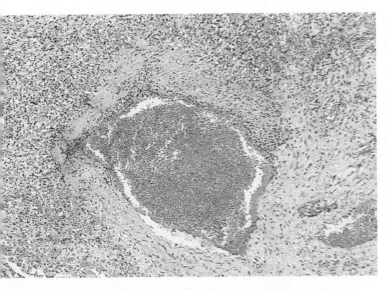

IGURE 8.6   Histologic section of a coronary artery from a patient with Kawasaki's disease. Note an extensive inflammatory cellular infiltrate affecting the arterial wall and spreading onto adjacent tissues. (Reproduced with permission; see Figure Credits)

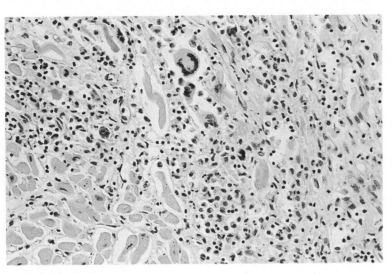

FIGURE 8.7   Histologic section of myocardium from a patient with idiopathic giant cell myocarditis. Note inflammatory foci containing giant cells. (Reproduced with permission; see Figure Credits)

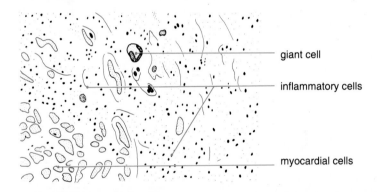

giant cell

inflammatory cells

myocardial cells

FIGURE 8.8 DIAGNOSTIC CATEGORIES OF IDIOPATHIC MYOCARDITIS*

FIRST BIOPSY	SUBSEQUENT BIOPSIES
Active myocarditis with myocytic necrosis (with or without fibrosis)	Ongoing (persistent myocarditis)
	Resolving (healing myocarditis)
Borderline myocarditis (biopsy results not diagnostic; suggest rebiopsy)	Resolved (healed myocarditis; this group may have some of the features of dilated cardiomyopathy)
No evidence of myocarditis	

*Suggested by the Dallas Myocarditis Panel. (Reproduced with permission; see Figure Credits)

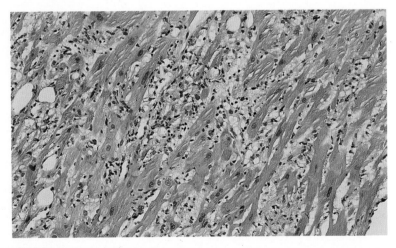

FIGURE 8.9   Endomyocardial biopsy from a 50-year-old man demonstrates the features of idiopathic myocarditis. There is a marked, predominantly lymphocytic, interstitial inflammatory cell infiltrate with evidence of myocyte damage. (Reproduced with permission; see Figure Credits)

PATHOPHYSIOLOGY

Myocardial cells are damaged by the invading organisms. In addition evidence suggests that certain organisms activate the autoimmune system; this in turn damages the heart muscle. Myocarditis due to rheumatic fever is an example of this type of myocardial damage. Infections such as diphtheria have a special affinity for the conduction system.[3,22]

Both ventricles are usually involved. The right and the left ventricular diastolic volumes and pressures may increase; myocardial contractility may diminish. Atrial and ventricular tachycardia may occur, further compromising cardiac function. Complete heart block and shock may occur with diphtheria; right bundle branch block is common in patients with Chagas' disease.

CLINICAL MANIFESTATIONS

No effort is made here to characterize the unique features of all causes of myocarditis. As indicated earlier, specific causes are common to certain geographic areas. In addition, myocarditis due to rheumatic fever and myocarditis due to diphtheria have different clinical manifestations. These examples indicate that the clinical setting and the systemic manifestations of a large number of clinical conditions due to infectious agents vary considerably. The purpose of this discussion is to emphasize the damage that is done to the heart muscle rather than to describe the entire clinical picture related to specific etiologies. The clinical clues used to recognize myocarditis are similar regardless of the etiology.

SYMPTOMS

The individual may have no complaints relative to the heart if there is minimal cardiac involvement in the overall process of infection. Severe involvement of the heart may produce cardiac failure, which in turn may lead to fatigue, dyspnea, and palpitations. The chest pain of pericarditis may be associated with myocarditis. Syncope and sudden death may occur secondary to arrhythmia or heart block.[37]

PHYSICAL EXAMINATION

Fever and tachycardia are often present; the latter is often out of proportion to the fever. Bradycardia may be present, usually due to an atrioventricular conduction disturbance.

The heart may be enlarged, and hypotension may be present. Neck vein abnormalities and pulsus alternans are often detected. The apex impulse may be diffuse; atrial and ventricular gallop sounds are commonly heard. The first heart sound may be faint, and new murmurs of mitral and tricuspid regurgitation are sometimes present.[38] A pericardial rub may be heard, and the liver may be enlarged.

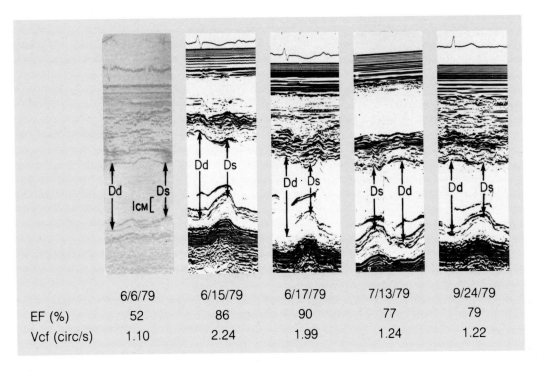

	6/6/79	6/15/79	6/17/79	7/13/79	9/24/79
EF (%)	52	86	90	77	79
Vcf (circ/s)	1.10	2.24	1.99	1.24	1.22

FIGURE 8.10 Serial M-mode echocardiograms from a 34-year-old male with acute viral myocarditis who presented with cardiogenic, shock. The first study shows hypokinesis of the posterior wall of the left ventricle. Nine days later movement of the posterior wall is normal. (Dd = left ventricular end-diastolic diameter; Ds = left ventricular end-systolic diameter; EF ([%]) = ejection fraction percentage ([normal = 55 %]); Vcf = mean velocity of circumferential fiber shortening ([normal = 1.29 ± 0.23 circ/sec]). (Reproduced with permission; see Figure Credits)

Atrial and ventricular arrhythmias and conduction abnormalities may account for the abnormal rhythm found in patients on physical examination.

LABORATORY STUDIES

Chest Radiography   The chest film may show enlargement of the left and right ventricles and evidence of heart failure.

Electrocardiography   The electrocardiogram (ECG) may show nonspecific low voltage of the QRS complexes, nonspecific ST–T wave abnormalities, sinus and atrial tachycardia, conduction defects including right or left bundle branch block, atrioventricular block of varying degrees, and, on rare occasion, signs of acute infarction.

Echocardiography   This technique identifies increased ventricular chamber size, wall-motion abnormalities, and pericardial effusion. It is especially useful in following the progress of patients with myocarditis (Fig. 8.10) [25]

Cardiac Catheterization   Cardiac catheterization is not performed in patients who have diagnostic evidence of myocarditis. On rare occasion it may be needed to exclude certain other diseases, such as coronary artery disease or valvular heart disease.

Radionuclide Studies   Ventricular function and wall-motion abnormalities can be identified with radionuclide ventriculography. Patients with myocarditis may show global myocardial dysfunction or regional wall-motion abnormalities. A gallium scan showing considerable uptake in the myocardium is believed to indicate an active inflammatory process; in certain cases it suggests that therapy with corticosteroids may be helpful.[26]

Endomyocardial Biopsy   Endomyocardial biopsy of the right or left ventricle can be performed safely (Fig. 8.11); at times a specific etiology may be discovered. In the past it was believed that when the biopsy revealed considerable inflammation, the condition might respond more readily to corticosteroid medication.[9,18] Recent studies have indicated that a myocardial biopsy did not usually reverse information that could be used to guide the therapy that is currently available.[18a]

Routine and Special Laboratory Test   Routine laboratory tests may reveal eosinophilia, elevated sedimentation rates, and elevated creatine kinase levels. Test for specific infectious agents, such as acute and convalescent antibody titers, are useful, but the results are often negative.

NATURAL HISTORY

Most patients with mild myocarditis recover completely. However, severe myocarditis is a serious condition, and, depending on its etiology, the recovery rate is variable. Many patients either die from heart failure or cardiac arrhythmia, or develop chronic dilated cardiomyopathy. A few patients with severe myocarditis recover and exhibit no cardiac dysfunction. One problem in establishing the natural history of myocarditis is the inability to determine the cause of dilated cardiomyopathy.[6]

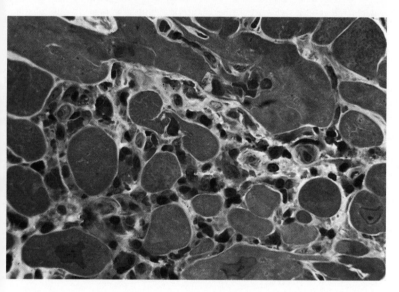
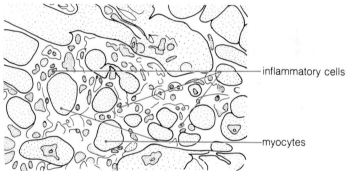

FIGURE 8.11   Endomyocardial biopsy containing a lymphocytic inflammatory infiltrate indicative of active myocarditis. (Reproduced with permission; see Figure Credits)

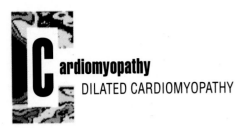

Cardiomyopathy
DILATED CARDIOMYOPATHY

ETIOLOGY AND PATHOLOGY

Dilated cardiomyopathy (DCM), formerly known as congestive cardiomyopathy is the most common form of myocardial disease. By definition the term *cardiomyopathy* indicates that the term is not known.[29a] Most forms of specific heart muscle disease[29a] such as alcoholic disease, infiltrations, granulomatous, collagen vascular diseases, infections, deficiency diseases, and drugs produce a dilated form of heart muscle disease (see p.285). In no more than 50% of cases of DCM the cause may be a previous viral infection. In the remainder the cause is not yet known. The cause of dilated cardiomyopathy is usually difficult or impossible to establish in an individual patient. It is likely that many different causes are responsible, eventually leading to irreversible myocardial damage and, as a final common pathway, becoming clinically manifest as *idiopathic* (or more accurately identified as *cryptogenic*) *dilated cardiomyopathy*. It can, on occasion, be distinguished from specific heart muscle disease resulting from a specific etiology (e.g., Chagas' cardiomyopathy; Fig. 8.12).

Ischemic cardiomyopathy due to atherosclerotic coronary artery disease may simulate other types of cardiomyopathy. Some physicians object to this term since the primary problem is coronary disease, because all types of dilated cardiomyopathy may display angina and electrocardiographic abnormalities simulating infarction of the myocardium and because ischemic heart muscle disease due to coronary atherosclerosis may not be associated with angina or other signs of infarction.

The pathology of dilated cardiomyopathy is characterized by gross dilation of the chambers of the heart, accompanied by marked hypertrophy (Fig. 8.13). Interstitial myocardial fibrosis is usually present (Figs. 8.14–8.16). In a number of cases the endocardium is thickened and often shows hyperplasia of smooth muscle cells; lymphocytes may be recognized. This finding is often interpreted as an indication that the disease is initiated by myocarditis, which in its end stage results in dilated cardiomyopathy.[32]

PATHOPHYSIOLOGY

During the early stages of the condition, stroke volume is reduced. Cardiac output is maintained at a normal level by an increase in heart rate. While this type of compensation is adequate at rest, it may not be adequate during exercise, when there may be an increase in left ventricular end-diastolic and left atrial pressures.

Later in the course of the disease the stroke output and the cardiac output become decreased. Eventually, as dictated by Laplace's law (see Fig. 2.7), dilation becomes increasingly harmful. Myocardial wall tension and pressure increase, as do the oxygen demand and the metabolic needs of the myocardium. There is also a decreased rate of myocardial fiber shortening and a decrease in the maximal rate of rise of pressure (max dP/dT) and in the velocity of ejection. The systolic and the diastolic volumes of the ventricles are increased and the ejection fraction is decreased, while the left ventricular end-diastolic pressure is increased.[20]

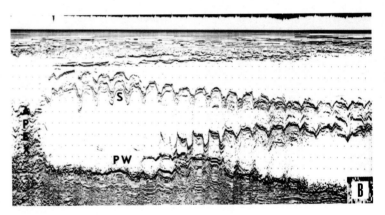

FIGURE 8.12   (A) Comparison of Chagas' cardiomyopathy with non-Chagas' cardiomyopathy and the normal cardiac condition. The values next to each figure refer to the ratio of septal-to-posterior wall thickening at the ventricular level. In normal hearts and non-Chagas' myopathies, the posterior wall thickening is greater than septal at all levels. In Chagas' patients with arrhythmias (AR) and with congestive cardiomyopathy (CHF) a reversal of thickening ratios is seen in the more apical segments. In other words, relative to the septum the posteroapical segments are more scarred and less contractile. This pattern of septal scarring appears unique to Chagas' heart disease. **(B)** M-mode sweep of Chagas' cardiomyopathy. Note that the posterior wall shows very little sign of thickening while the septum is exaggerated. (Reproduced with permission; see Figure Credits)

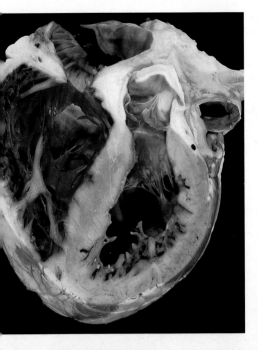

FIGURE 8.13 Cross section of a heart showing biventricular chamber dilation with wall hypertrophy in dilated congestive cardiomyopathy. (Reproduced with permission; see Figure Credits)

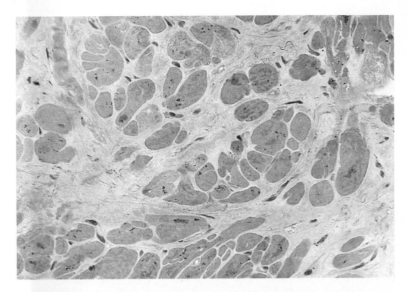

FIGURE 8.14 Histologic section in dilated congestive cardiomyopathy showing hypertrophied myocytes amid dense fibrosis. There is no evidence of inflammatory infiltrate. (Reproduced with permission; see Figure Credits)

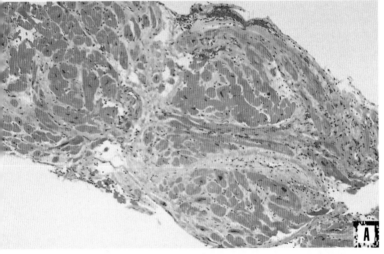

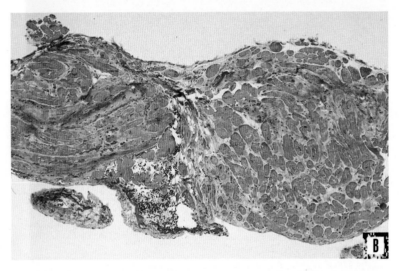

FIGURE 8.15 Endomyocardial biopsy from an 18-year-old, demonstrating characteristic features of idiopathic dilated cardiomyopathy. **(A)** There is moderate myocyte hypertrophy associated with interstitial fibrosis. This is highlighted on the trichrome stain **(B)**, where the collagen stains blue. Note the characteristic pericellular pattern of interstitial fibrosis. (A, hematoxylin & eosin; B, Masson's trichrome) (Reproduced with permission; see Figure Credits)

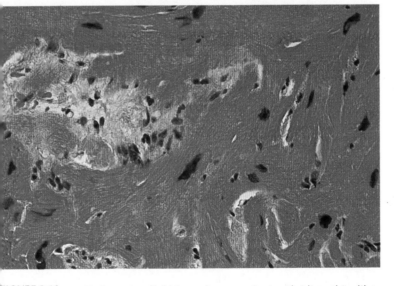

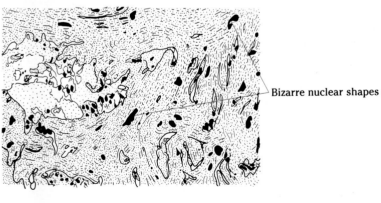

Bizarre nuclear shapes

FIGURE 8.16 Endomyocardial biopsy from a patient with idiopathic dilated cardiomyopathy. Note the bizarre nuclear shapes characteristic of this entity. (Hematoxylin & eosin; magnification x200.) (Reproduced with permission; see Figure Credits)

The pulmonary venous pressure rises, producing dyspnea. The pulmonary arterial pressure and the pulmonary vascular resistance are often slightly increased. The decrease in cardiac output sets in motion the compensatory mechanisms that, in an effort to correct the fault, produce congestive heart failure (Fig. 8.17). Angina pectoris due to myocardial ischemia may occur; it is thought to be due to an increase in coronary arterial resistance together with the exercise-precipitated elevation in left ventricular end diastolic volume and pressure.[27]

CLINICAL MANIFESTATIONS

Symptoms   The condition is most commonly seen in adult males. The patient may be asymptomatic when first seen. Eventually dyspnea on effort becomes apparent, and the symptoms of advanced heart failure with paroxysmal nocturnal dyspnea and pulmonary edema may develop. The patient may have arrhythmias and chest pain consistent with angina pectoris. Serious arrhythmias

are commonly linked to the severity of hemodynamic disturbance.[19]
Physical Examination   There may be signs of heart failure, but the systemic blood pressure is usually normal or elevated. Pulsus alternans may be present, and the jugular venous pressure is raised. A systolic jugular pulsation may be detected in the internal jugular veins, signifying tricuspid regurgitation. The cardiac impulse indicates left ventricular enlargement. Atrial and ventricular diastolic gallop sounds are usually heard; the systolic murmurs of mitral and tricuspid regurgitation may be detected. There may be reversed splitting of the second sound when left bundle branch block is present. Atrial fibrillation occurs in around 20% of cases.

LABORATORY STUDIES

Chest Radiography   The chest film reveals cardiacenlargement due to dilation of the ventricles and the atria. Signs of heart failure

FIGURE 8.17 FUNCTIONAL ABNORMALITIES IN DILATED CARDIOMYOPATHY

PARAMETER	DILATED CARDIOMYOPATHY
Left ventricular volume	
End-diastolic	Increased
End-systolic	Increased
Left ventricular mass	Increased
Volume/mass ratio	Increased
Systolic function	
Ejection fraction	Decreased
Normalized ejection rate	Decreased
Myocardial fiber shortening	Decreased
Wall stress	Increased
End-diastolic function	
Pressure/volume	Decreased
Wall stress/volume	Decreased
Diastolic function	
Chamber stiffness	Decreased or normal
Myocardial stiffness	Increased or normal
Negative dp/dt	Decreased
Tau	Prolonged

(Reproduced with permission; see Figure Credits)

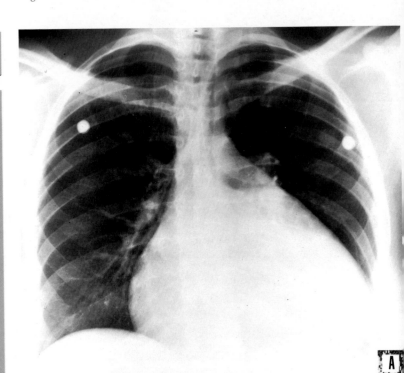

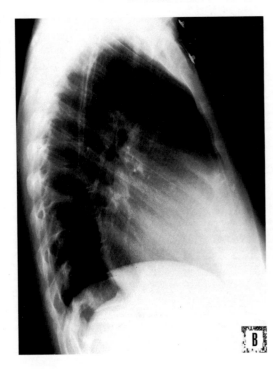

FIGURE 8.18   Chest radiographs of dilated cardiomyopathy. Posteroanterior **(A)** and lateral **(B)** x-rays in a patient with postpartum cardiomyopathy demonstrate cardiomegaly with biventricular enlargement and pulmonary venous hypertension.(Reproduced with permission, see Figure Credits)

re frequently present (Fig. 8.18).

lectocardiography The ECG may show nonspecific T–T wave changes, left ventricular hypertrophy, low voltage, left bundle ranch block (common), atrial abnormalities, atrial arrhythmias, ventricular rrhythmias, atrioventricular conduction defects, and abnormal Q waves suggesting myocardial infarction.[11]

Ambulatory Electrocardiography. Patients with rhythm disturbances should be udied with ambulatory electrocardiography (Holter monitoring) to detect serius ventricular arrhythmias.

chocardiography The echocardiogram reveals dilation of

both ventricles and decreased contractility of the myocardium, especially the posterior free wall of the left ventricle, with paradoxical movement of the septum (Figs. 8.19, 8.20). The free wall and septal thickness are usually normal. Left ventricular thrombi may be seen in the cross-sectional echocardiogram.[7] Echocardiography cannot be used reliably to separate nonischemic from ischemic cardiomyopathy.

Cardiac Catheterization Cardiac catheterization reveals an elevated left ventricular diastolic pressure. Angiography shows dilation of the left and right ventricles, decreased myocardial contractility, decreased ejection fraction, slight mitral regurgitation, and either normal

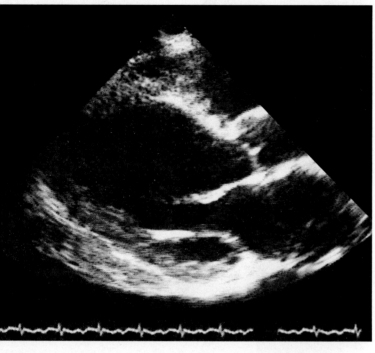

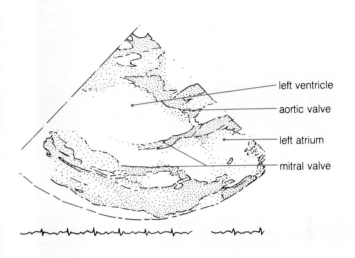

IGURE 8.19 Cross-sectional echocardiogram in the long-axis view ecorded during systole in a 35-year-old male with dilated cardiomyopathy.

The systolic dimension of the left ventricle was 7.4 cm, and the diastolic dimension was 8.6 cm. (Reproduced with permission; see Figure Credits)

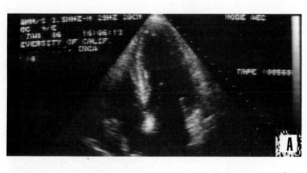

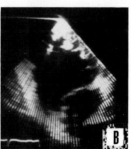

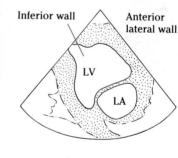

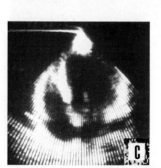

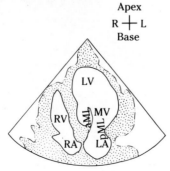

FIGURE 8.20 Cardiomyopathy compared to the normal cardiac condition. (**A**) A four-chamber view from a normal heart. A heart from a patient with cardiomyopathy in two- and four-chamber views (**B** and **C**, respectively). Note that the heart with cardiomyopathy is more spherical than its normal counterpart. The development of a spherical configuration is fairly typical of dilated cardiomyopathy. (Reproduced with permission; see Figure Credits)

coronary arteries, nonobstructive coronary artery disease, or severe obstructive coronary disease (Fig. 8.21). The latter finding usually signifies the presence of ischemic cardiomyopathy, although dilated cardiomyopathy may be accompanied by unrelated coronary atherosclerosis. Echocardiography has largely replaced the use of cardiac catheterization and angiography in such patients.

Radionuclide Studies   Nuclear ventriculography reveals enlargement of both ventricles and global hypokinesis. The ejection fraction may be as low as 10% to 15%. This test may be useful in following the progress of a patient with cardiomyopathy.[13] However, this procedure cannot reliably separate coronary disease from cardiomyopathy.[8]

Thallium scanning may reveal areas of poor perfusion. This test does not always separate nonischemic from ischemic cardiomyopathy.

Endomyocardial Biopsy   Whereas endomyocardial biopsy was formerly used only for research purposes, it is now commonly used in patients who may be candidates for transplantation. Myocarditis may be found, which may dictate certain treatment, or the biopsy may give evidence of a systemic disease that would make cardiac transplantation inadvisable. The procedure is also used to detect the early signs of cardiac rejection in patients who have had a heart transplant.

Other Imaging Modalities   Cardiac MRI clearly delineates the uniformly dilated ventricles of patients with dilated cardiomyopathy (Fig. 8.22). This information can, however, be obtained using simpler and cheaper methods.

HYPERTROPHIC CARDIOMYOPATHY
ETIOLOGY AND PATHOLOGY

Hypertrophic cardiomyopathy is a disease of unknown origin characterized b massive myocardial hypertrophy, and, in some instances, it is inherited as a autosomal dominant trait.[16] It usually involves the mid-and upper parts of th ventricular septum and the adjacent anterior wall of the left ventricle, producir asymmetric hypertrophy (Figs. 8.23, 8.24). However, concentric hypertroph affecting all of the left ventricle or predominately the apex also occurs. The le ventricular cavity is usually small, and the mitral valve may be thickened. Th corresponding septal surface on the left ventricle may show fibroelastosis as secondary effect of mitral valve impact during systole. Hypertrophic cardiomy opathy restricted to the right ventricle may also occur (Figs. 8.25, 8.26).

Microscopically, the disease is characterized by extensive myocardial fiber di array throughout the grossly affected areas (Fig. 8.27). The myocardial cells a markedly hypertrophic, often with a perinuclear halo. The texture is distorted i the sense that bundles may cross each other in different directions, ofte exhibiting whorls or cartwheel configurations. Perpendicular branchings a intercellular junctions are often seen.

The abnormal architecture of the myocardium is generally considered t underlie the abnormal decrease in compliance of the ventricles, which leads t the restricted inflow of blood during diastole.

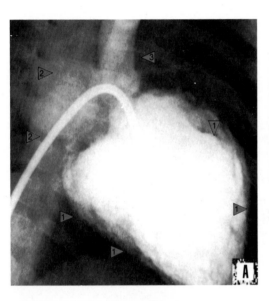
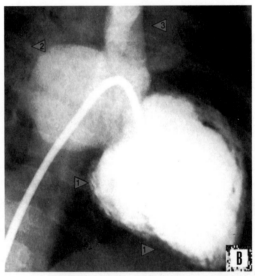

FIGURE 8.21   Left ventriculogram of dilated cardiomyopathy in the right anterior oblique projection in diastole (**A**) and systole (**B**). There is marked left ventricular enlargement (arrows 1) with minimal change in ventricular size between diastole and systole, indicating a very low ejection fraction. Note the dense opacification of the left atrium (arrows 2), which is due to severe mitral insufficiency. (arrow 3 = ascending aorta) (Reproduced with permission; see Figure Credits)

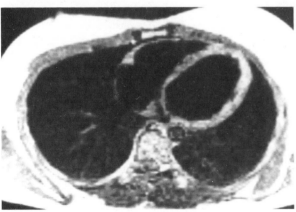
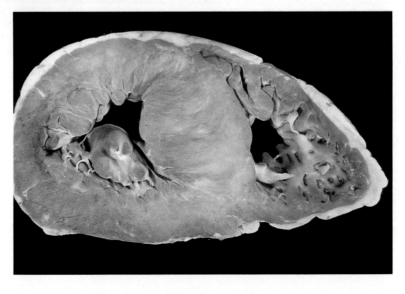

FIGURE 8.22   Transverse MR image of a patient with congestive cardiomyopathy. Note the dilation of the right and left ventricular chambers. (Reproduced with permission; see Figure Credits)

FIGURE 8.23
Cross section through a heart with hypertrophic cardiomyopathy and asymmetry c the affected interventricu lar septum. (Reproduced with permission; see Figure Credits)

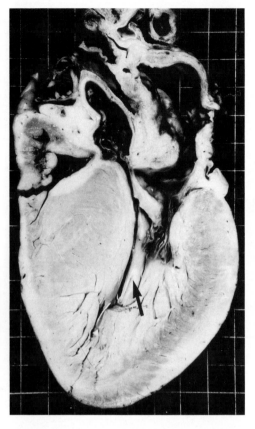

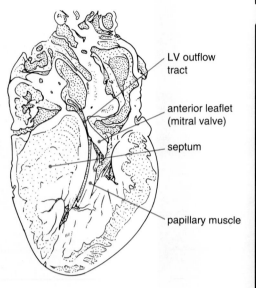

LV outflow
tract

anterior leaflet
(mitral valve)

septum

papillary muscle

FIGURE 8.25 VARIATIONS OF
HYPERTROPHIC CARDIOMYOPATHY

	APPROXIMATE INCIDENCE* (%)
Left Ventricular Involvement	
Asymmetrical hypertrophy	
Ventricular septal hypertrophy	90
Midventricular hypertrophy	1
Apical hypertrophy	3
Posteroseptal and/or lateral wall hypertrophy	1
Symmetrical (concentric) hypertrophy	5

*At the Toronto General Hospital. The incidence of the different types of hypertrophic cardiomyopathy varies considerably among different centers. (Reproduced with permission; see Figure Credits)

FIGURE 8.24 Longitudinal section of the heart of a 32-year-old woman with hypertrophic obstructive cardiomyopathy. Hemodynamic investigation confirmed the presence of hypertrophic cardiomyopathy as well as mitral regurgitation that was partially due to an abnormal mitral valve (insertion of anomalous papillary muscle onto the ventricular surface of a fibrotic anterior mitral leaflet). Note that there is asymmetric hypertrophy with grossly thickened ventricular septum and a narrowed outflow between the upper septum and anterior mitral leaflet. (Reproduced with permission; see Figure Credits)

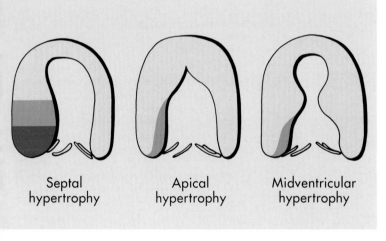

Septal
hypertrophy

Apical
hypertrophy

Midventricular
hypertrophy

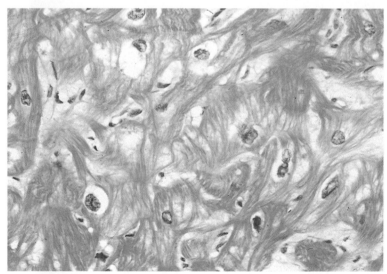

FIGURE 8.26 Three common varieties of asymmetric left ventricular hypertrophy as would be seen in the apical four-chamber view of a two-dimensional echocardiogram. Septal hypertrophy may involve only the basal one third of the septum (subaortic area) or the basal two thirds of the septum (down to the papillary muscles) or it may extend from base to apex, involving the whole septum. In apical hypertrophy, the principal involvement is in the apical one third of the ventricle and there may be considerable asymmetry in this area. The apical hypertrophy may extend up the septum toward the base, in which case obstruction to outflow may occur. In midventricular hypertrophy, the maximal thickening occurs at the level of the papillary muscles. Basal septal hypertrophy may also occur in this variety of hypertrophic cardiomyopathy and thus give rise to midventricular obstruction. (Reproduced with permission; see Figure Credits)

FIGURE 8.27 Histologic section of myocardium in a patient with hypertrophic cardiomyopathy. There are marked hypertrophy of individual myocytes and an abnormal texture known as myocardial disarray. Note the large, hyperchromatic nuclei and the extensive amount of loose intercellular connective tissue. (Reproduced with permission; see Figure Credits)

PATHOPHYSIOLOGY

Over emptying of the left ventricle with an ejection fraction of 80%–90% or more is an important feature of hypertrophic cardiomyopathy. Authorities have argued about the importance of *obstruction* versus *elimination* of the left ventricular cavity (Fig. 8.28). Hypertrophic cardiomyopathy produces a decrease in ventricular compliance, impedance to diastolic filling of the ventricle, and abnormal ventricular contraction. The filling of the ventricle takes a longer time than normal, and there is a greatly prolonged isovolumic relaxation period.[31]

While these diastolic abnormalities are well documented, further study is needed to understand fully the entire diastolic abnormality associated with this disorder.

The obstructive type of the disease is characterized by a peak systolic pressure gradient between the body of the left ventricle and the aorta. The magnitude of the gradient varies from time to time; it is increased by an ectopic beat, increased myocardial contractility, hypovolemia, or decreased systemic blood pressure. The outflow tract of such patients becomes muscle-bound; the anterior leaflet of the mitral valve is entrapped in the obstructing process (Fig. 8.29). The early phase of ventricular contraction is rapid; the subsequent ventricular contraction pattern produces a pulsus bisferiens-type contour in the carotid artery pulsation. Whereas the gradient does not directly correlate with symptoms or prognosis in all patients, it is important in some patients. In most patients the gradient does not indicate true mechanical obstruction because there is no reduction in blood flow.[5a] In a minority of cases, true obstruction does occur.[15a]

Myocardial ischemia occurs because the thickened myocardium needs more blood than normal. Additional causes of myocardial ischemia in such patients are myocardial bridging of the coronary arteries, abnormal diastolic function of the ventricles, and associated but unrelated atherosclerotic coronary disease.

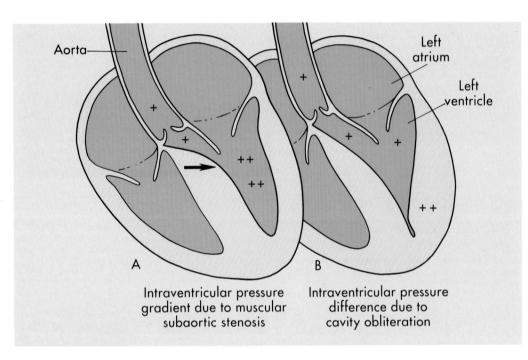

Intraventricular pressure gradient due to muscular subaortic stenosis

Intraventricular pressure difference due to cavity obliteration

FIGURE 8.28 Left ventricular inflow tract pressure. **(A)** In muscular subaortic stenosis, the intraventricular pressure distal to the stenosis is low (+), whereas all ventricular pressures proximal to the stenosis, including the one just inside the mitral valve (the inflow tract pressure) are elevated (++) **(B)** When an intraventricular pressure difference is recorded, it is elevated only in the area of cavity obliteration (++). The intraventricular systolic pressure in all other areas of the left ventricular cavity, including that in the inflow tract just inside the mitral valve, is low (+) and equal to the aortic systolic pressure. Note that in cavity elimination, there is an intraventricular pressure difference between the apex and the inflow tract and also the outflow tract. In muscular subaortic stenosis, there is no intraventricular pressure difference between the apex and the inflow tract pressure. The three areas of the left ventricle represented by the +'s are (from top to bottom) the outflow tract just below the aortic valve, the inflow tract just inside the mitral valve, and the left ventricular apex. (Reproduced with permission; see Figure Credits)

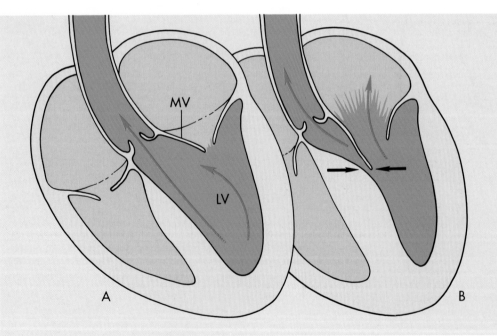

FIGURE 8.29 Proposed mechanism of systolic anterior motion of the anterior mitral leaflet in muscular subaortic stenosis. **(A)** In normal hearts, blood is ejected from the left ventricle in a relatively direct path into the aorta through a wide open outflow tract. **(B)** In muscular subaortic stenosis, the ventricular septum is thickened (left horizontal arrow), resulting in a narrowed outflow tract. Because of this narrowing, the ejection of blood from the ventricle occurs at a high velocity and the ejection path is closer to the anterior mitral leaflet than is normal. As a result, the anterior leaflet is drawn into the outflow tract toward the septum by Venturi effect (right horizontal arrow). Mitral leaflet–septal contact results in obstruction to left ventricular outflow. Mitral regurgitation (upper right oblique arrow) results from the anterior mitral leaflet being out of its normal systolic position. (LV = left ventricle; MV = mitral valve) (Reproduced with permission; see Figure Credits)

CLINICAL MANIFESTATIONS

Symptoms   The patient, who is usually male, may be asymptomatic or may complain of angina or syncope. Late in the course of the condition the patient may complain of dyspnea and palpitation. Death is sudden in 50% of those who die from the disease.

Physical Examination   The general appearance of the patient is usually normal, although the skeletal muscles may be prominent.

Patients with a left ventricular outflow tract pressure gradient may have a diamond-shaped, systolic murmur of late onset that is heard to the left of the midsternal area, at the apex, and less well in the aortic area. The murmur becomes louder when the patient stands or performs a Valsalva maneuver, but it becomes fainter with squatting and handgrip. The murmur may not become louder during the systole that follows an ectopic beat, as it does with aortic valve stenosis. The murmur of mitral regurgitation may be heard. On rare occasion a low-pitched, diastolic rumble may be heard at the apex. Slight aortic regurgitation has also been noted.

The arterial pulse is sharp and ill-sustained, and may be detected easily in the carotid artery. An atrial gallop may be heard and felt at the cardiac apex. During systole the apex impulse may be bifid (Fig. 8.30).

A prominent a wave may be seen in the jugular venous pulse when there is involvement of the right ventricle with obstruction of its outflow tract.[14]

LABORATORY STUDIES

Chest Radiography   The heart may appear normal on the chest radiograph. Alternately, there may be slight-to-moderate cardiac enlargement. The left atrium may be large and, late in the course of the disease, pulmonary congestion may be evident. Valvular calcification is not seen.

Electrocardiography   The ECG usually shows left ventricular hypertrophy with increased amplitude of the QRS complexes. The ST–T wave abnormality may simulate myocardial infarction with elevated ST segments and inverted T waves in some leads. Abnormal Q waves may also suggest myocardial infarction (Fig. 8.31). The T waves may be deeply inverted and large in apical hypertrophic cardiomyopathy. The P–R interval may be short and a delta wave may be noted in the QRS complex, signifying that an atrioventricular bypass tract is present (Wolff–Parkinson–White syndrome).[35] Left atrial enlargement shown by a bifid P wave and ST segment deficiencies is common. Ventricular arrhythmias may be seen on the routine ECG, but they are more often detected by ambulatory monitoring.[10]

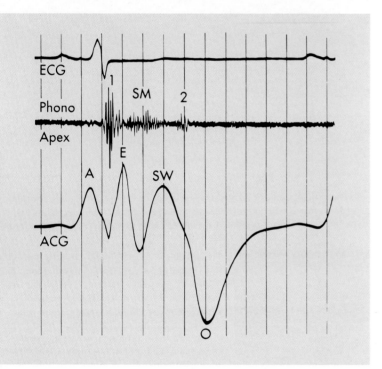

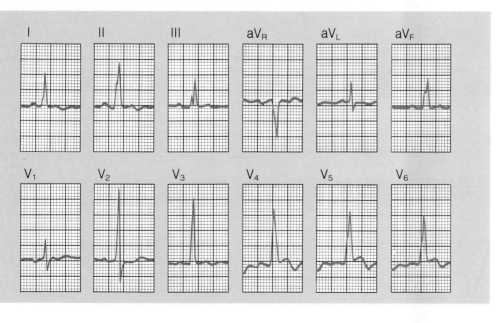

FIGURE 8.30   Apex cardiogram along with phonocardiogram from a patient with obstructive hypertrophic cardiomyopathy. A midsystolic outward motion (SW) after the E point, along with a prominent a wave (**A**), give a triple-humped appearance. The peak of the ejection systolic murmur (SM) coincides with the midsystolic dip. (1 = first heart sound; 2 = second heart sound; 4 = fourth heart sound; ACG = apex cardiogram) (Reproduced with permission; see Figure Credits)

FIGURE 8.31   ECG of a 77-year-old woman with apical hypertrophic cardiomyopathy. There is a normal sinus rhythm, a tall R wave in lead V_1, and very unusual ST and T waves. The ST and T wave abnormalities persisted for years; they simulate the ST and T wave abnormalities of myocardial infarction. (Reproduced with permission; see Figure Credits)

Echocardiography   The M-mode echocardiogram delineates on increased thickness of the ventricular wall (Figs. 8.32–8.34). The septum is often thicker than the posterior left ventricular wall, and it may contract less than the free wall of the left ventricle. The left ventricular cavity size may be decreased. There is abnormal anterior motion of the mitral valve during systole, and its rate of closure is slowed.[12] The aortic valve tends to close in mid-systole. The left atrial size may be increased.

Cross-sectional echocardiography is superior to the M-mode technique in detecting hypertrophy of the septum and studying the mitral apparatus (Fig. 8.35).[7] Doppler echocardiography reveals characteristic LV inflow and outflow-tract tracings (Fig. 8.36).

Cardiac Catheterization   A systolic pressure gradient between the left ventricle and the aorta may be identified when the patient is at rest (Fig. 8.37). The gradient may be provoked with amyl nitrate, a Valsalva maneuver, or isoproterenol; it may also be detected following a ventricular ectopic beat. Catheter entrapment must

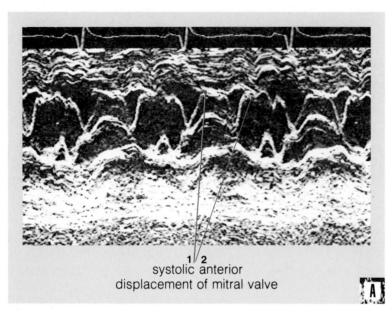

1 2
systolic anterior
displacement of mitral valve

A

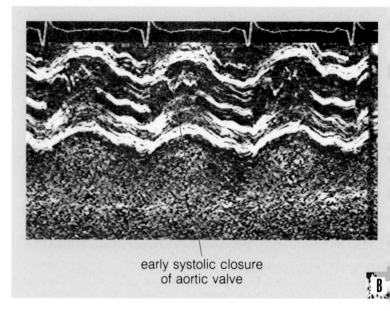

early systolic closure
of aortic valve

B

FIGURE 8.32   M-mode echocardiogram of a middle-aged female with hypertrophic cardiomyopathy and left ventricular outflow tract obstruction demonstrating **(A)** Abnormal systolic anterior displacement of the mitral valve (*arrow 1*) and the position of the anterior mitral valve leaflet during diastole (*arrow 2*); **(B)** Early systolic closure of the aortic valve, suggesting that dynamic obstruction is present. (Reproduced with permission; see Figure Credits)

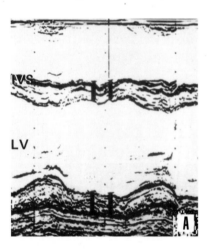

IVS

LV

A

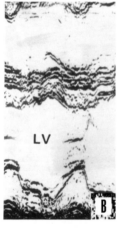

LV

B

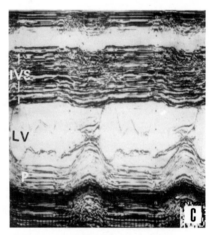

IVS

LV

C

FIGURE 8.33   Symmetric and asymmetric left ventricular hypertrophy. Normal left ventricle **(A)** is contrasted to mild symmetric left ventricular hypertrophy **(B)** and marked asymmetric hypertrophy **(C)**. Note that the a wave or presystolic ventricular filling is more exaggerated in the mild left ventricular hypertrophy. Exaggerated filling during the atrial phase of diastole can be a clue to decreased compliance, which may be more marked for the degree of hypertrophy. (Reproduced with permission; see Figure Credits)

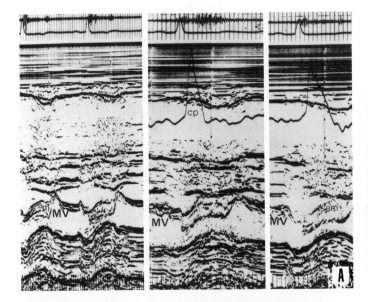

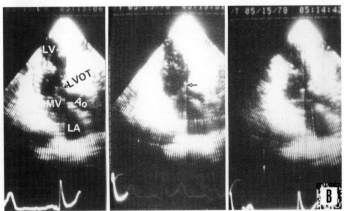

FIGURE 8.34 Provocable outflow tract obstruction. **(A)** Simultaneous M-mode, phonocardiogram, and carotid pulse tracing (cp) during rest (left panel), peak amyl nitrate effect (center), and recovery (right). Note that the systolic anterior motion (sam) of the mitral valve (MV) increases markedly and lies in close apposition to the interventricular septum during the provocation. Note also that the murmur becomes more intense and the carotid pulse loses its dicrotic wave. During recovery, the systolic anterior motion of the mitral valve is much less marked and only barely makes contact with sep-

tum. **(B)** Two-chamber views of the mitral valve and left ventricular outflow tract (LVOT) to demonstrate the site and appearance of systolic anterior motion of the MV. In the left panel, the patient is at rest and the LVOT is open. In the middle panel, the patient has been given amyl nitrate and the recording was made at its fullest effect. Note that the coapted mitral valve chordae tip has moved into the LVOT and now abuts the septum (arrow). In the right panel, the effect has passed and the valve has returned toward its resting position. (Reproduced with permission; see Figure Credits)

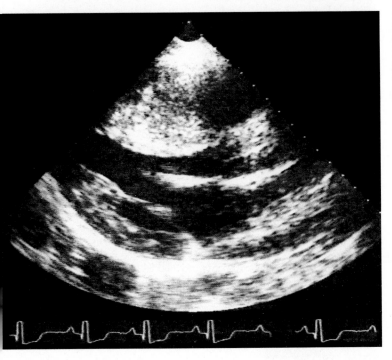

FIGURE 8.35 Diastolic frame of a cross-sectional echocardiogram of a young man who has hypertrophic cardiomyopathy with obstruction showing severe hypertrophy of the septum. (Reproduced with permission; see Figure Credits)

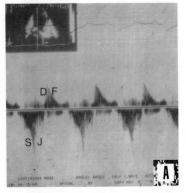

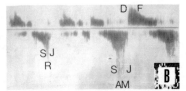

FIGURE 8.36 Doppler of dynamic subvalvular obstruction. **(A)** Continuous-wave Doppler recording from the apical four-chamber view records inflow across the mitral valve during diastole (DF) and outflow tract systolic jet (SJ) typical of dynamic subaortic outflow obstruction. Features of the systolic jet include transient duration, giving the velocity profile the appearance of a horse's tail. **(B)** The systolic jet during rest (R) has a velocity of 2.5 m/sec, suggesting a 25 mmHg subaortic gradient. During amyl nitrate (AM) provocation, the jet increases in velocity to over 4 m/sec, consistent with a gradient of at least 65 mmHg. (Reproduced with permission; see Figure Credits)

be avoided to prevent the spurious recording of an elevated left ventricular pressure.[2]

Left ventriculography, performed at the time of cardiac catheterization, may reveal the thick ventricular muscle in the region of the apex, mid-left ventricle, or subaortic area. A subvalvular membrane is present in the LV outflow tract in a small number of individuals (Fig. 8.38). Coronary arteriography is useful to identify coronary atherosclerosis, which may occasionally coexist with hypertrophic cardiomyopathy.

Other Imaging Modalities Magnetic resonance imaging (MRI) may reveal the thick myocardium of hypertrophic cardiomyopathy (Fig. 8.39).

NATURAL HISTORY

The survival period for patients with hypertrophic cardiomyopathy varies from a short period to a long life. About 50% of patients die suddenly due to an arrhyth-

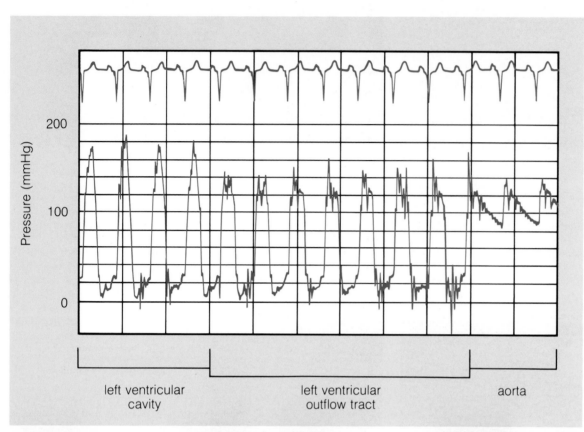

FIGURE 8.37 Obstruction in the outflow tract of the left ventricle in idiopathic hypertrophic subaortic stenosis. To demonstrate the obstruction, the catheter is pulled from the left ventricular cavity through the outflow tract into the aorta. Pressure recordings are shown from the left ventricular cavity, the outflow tract of the left ventricle, and the aorta. (Reproduced with permission; see Figure Credits)

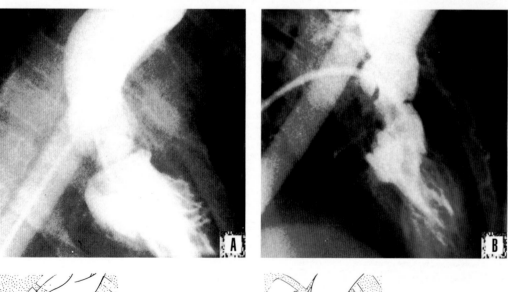

FIGURE 8.38 Left ventriculograms in two patients with subvalvular aortic stenosis (ring type). **(A)** A linear defect is seen beneath the aortic valve during diastole. This proved to be a complete ring of fibrous tissue (diaphragmatic type of subvalvular aortic stenosis). **(B)** A shelf-like deformity of the anterolateral aspect of the left ventricular outflow tract is seen during systole. This proved to be an incomplete subvalvular ring. (Reproduced with permission; see Figure Credits)

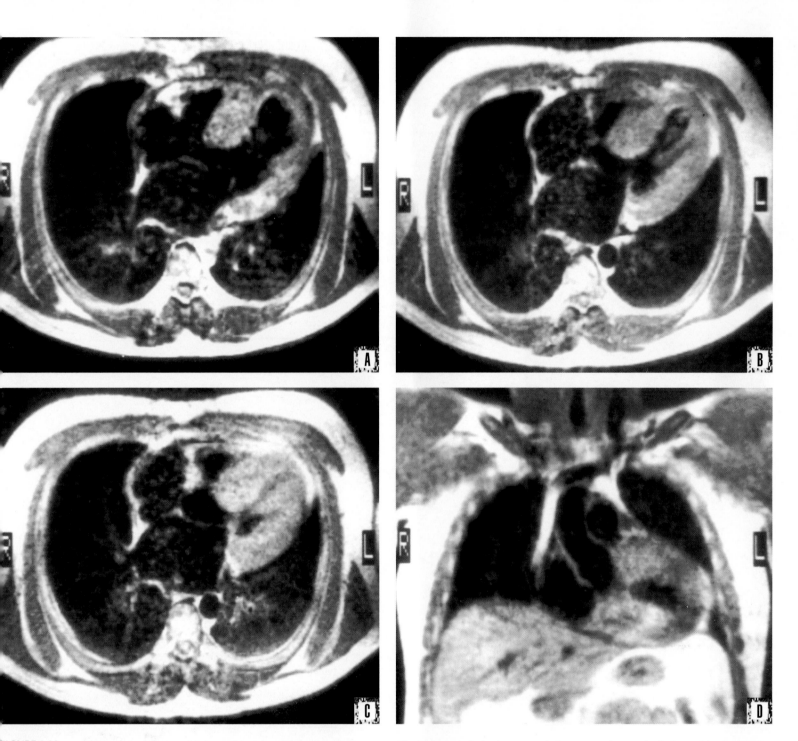

FIGURE 8.39   MRI sections from a 31-year-old male with hypertrophic cardiomyopathy and two episodes of syncope. The transverse sections were made during end-diastole (**A**), mid-diastole (**B**), and end-systole (**C**). The image made in the coronal plane was also made during mid-systole (**D**). Left ventricular hypertrophy is evident, with systolic anterior motion of the mitral valve in all systolic images. (Reproduced with permission; see Figure Credits)

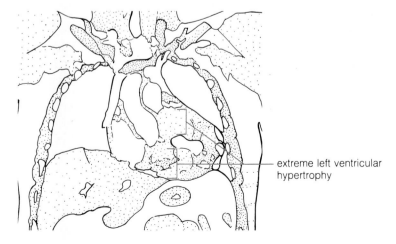

extreme left ventricular hypertrophy

mia or severe left ventricular outflow tract obstruction.[33] Syncope may occur, and it is considered to be a serious and dangerous event. Both supraventricular and ventricular arrhythmias are common. Some patients have pre-excitation due to atrioventricular bypass tracts. When atrial fibrillation develops in this setting, the ventricular rate is very rapid. Congestive heart failure occurs late in the natural course of the condition, often precipitated by atrial fibrillation.[23,34]

Episodes of myocardial ischemia produce angina pectoris in many patients. A few patients experience prolonged chest pain due to myocardial ischemia. This, in addition to the electrocardiographic abnormalities that may simulate myocardial infarction, may lead the physician to erroneously diagnose atherosclerotic coronary artery disease.[28] Systemic hypertension is associated with HCM in some patients.

Infective endocarditis may occur in any patient. Peripheral emboli, which are usually related to atrial fibrillation, occur in about 10% of patients. Severe mitral regurgitation with calcification of the mitral valve may develop, and this contributes to the development of heart failure.

RESTRICTIVE CARDIOMYOPATHY
ETIOLOGY AND PATHOLOGY

Restrictive cardiomyopathy, the least common type of cardiomyopathy, is caused by conditions such as endomyocardial fibrosis (with or without eosinophilia), amyloid disease (Figs. 8.40, 8.41), and hemochromatosis (Table 5.2, Fig. 8.47).[3] The decreased diastolic volume and the diminished ability of the ventricle to

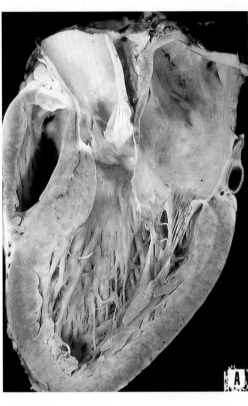
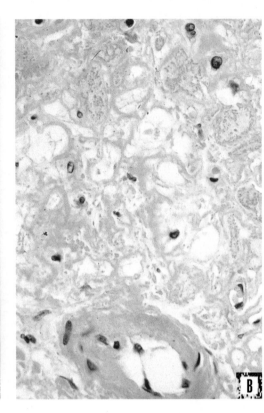
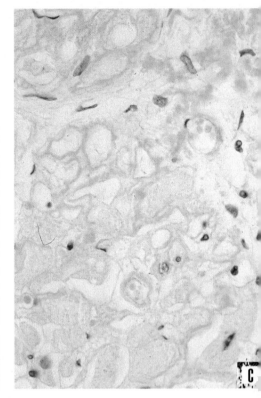

FIGURE 8.40 (A) Long-axis section through a heart with amyloid disease. Note the sandy appearance of the left atrial endocardium. (B) Histologic section shows myocardial cell degeneration and extensive extracellular deposition of amorphous eosinophilic material enclosing the cells. (C) The amyloid stains positive with a Congo red stain. (Reproduced with permission; see Figure Credits)

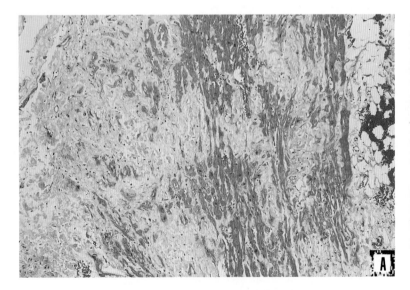
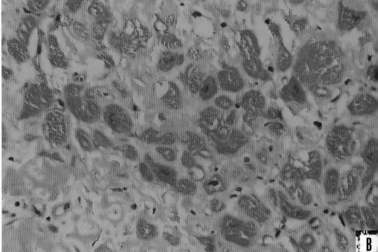

FIGURE 8.41 (A) Endomyocardial biopsy showing replacement of much of the myocardium by amyloid in a patient with multiple myeloma. (B) The higher-power photomicrograph with the myocytes cut in cross section demonstrates the characteristic perimyocytic pattern frequently found in cardiac amyloidosis. (Reproduced with permission; see Figure Credits)

retch in response to a volume load may cause a decrease in cardiac output. Myocardial contraction is usually normal until late in the course of the disease.[5] The ventricular cavity may become small during the late phase of the disease, at which time the condition has been described as *obliterative cardiomyopathy*.[15]

PATHOPHYSIOLOGY

During the early phase of endomyocardial fibrosis restricted ventricular filling is caused by endomyocardial fibrosis; later there may be progressive obliteration of the ventricular cavity with thrombus and fibrous tissue. This process can involve the papillary muscles and the tendinous cords, producing mitral and tricuspid regurgitation.

Early diastolic filling of the ventricles may be normal, but the condition limits diastolic filling during the later part of diastole. Systolic function is preserved until late in the course of the disease. The physiologic picture is similar to that found in constrictive pericarditis. Accordingly the pressure curve in the right ventricle shows a *dip-and-plateau* wave form during diastole; diastolic pressure in the right atrium and the right ventricle may be the same. A small paradoxical pulse may be present. The stroke output is decreased, and tachycardia may be present. Pulmonary hypertension may be present when the left ventricle is severely damaged and mitral regurgitation is present. The right atrium may become enlarged.

The physiologic derangement of Loeffler's endomyocardial fibrosis with eosinophilia and tropical endomyocardial fibrosis without eosinophilia is similar.

Amyloid heart disease differs from other forms of RCM in that ventricular filling is slow throughout diastole in patients with amyloid infiltration of the heart. Early in the course of the disease the contractility is normal, but it decreases later. Ventricular distortion does not occur as it does in endomyocardial fibrosis.

Hemochromatosis also decreases the compliance of the ventricles, thereby limiting diastolic filling.

CLINICAL MANIFESTATIONS

Symptoms The patient with acute eosinophilic endomyocardial disease (Loeffler's disease) may experience fever, dyspnea, and edema. These abnormalities may disappear for a while or continue as fatigue and fever. Gradually the patient develops a syndrome not unlike constrictive pericarditis, with dyspnea, cough, ascites, and edema.

Tropical endomyocardial fibrosis may involve the left, the right or both ventricles. Dyspnea and cough dominate the clinical picture when the left ventricle is predominantly involved. Ascites and edema dominate the clinical picture when the right ventricle is primarily involved. However, usually the clinical picture is a mixture of left and right ventricular forms of the disease. Both ventricles are usually involved in the pathologic process. Arterial fibrillation and embolism are common.

Primary amyloid involvement of the heart produces a similar clinical picture. Angina pectoris may be present when the coronary arteries themselves are involved.

Hemochromatosis of the heart also gives a similar clinical picture. The patient's skin may be bronze in color, and diabetes may be present.

Physical Examination The physical findings may suggest constrictive pericarditis. The cardiac rhythm is usually normal, but atrial fibrillation may be present. The neck veins are distended, and the deep jugular venous pulsation may show a prominent a wave and rapid descent of the x and y waves. Inspiration produces a marked increase in the abnormalities of neck veins.

Amyloid disease may be characterized by isolated heart disease, but systemic features in the primary forms of amyloid may include the presence of a large tongue, petechiae, purpura, peripheral neuropathy, and downward displacement of the submaxillary glands due to involvement of the base of tongue. Postural hypotension may be present, and sick sinus node syndrome may occur.

LABORATORY STUDIES

Chest Radiography The chest film shows moderate cardiomegaly, an enlarged left atrium, and prominent pulmonary veins. Calcium may be seen as a linear streak in the endocardial area of the left ventricular apex in patients with endomyocardial fibrosis.

Electrocardiography The ECG of patients with endomyocardiall fibrosis of the left ventricle may show left ventricular hypertrophy and a left atrial abnormality. Patients with endomyocardial fibrosis of the right ventricle may exhibit low voltage of the QRS complexes and large P waves due to a right atrial abnormality. The ECG associated with amyloid heart disease may show low voltage of the QRS complexes and evidence of a sick sinus node and atrioventricular condition block. Abnormal Q waves suggesting infarction may be present (Fig. 8.42).[4]

Echocardiography The M-mode echocardiogram of patients with endomyocardial fibrosis may not be helpful. The cross-sectional echocardiogram may show obliteration of the ventricular cavities, an increase in left ventricular mass, thrombi in the ventricular cavity, normal ventricular contractility, and a large left atrium.

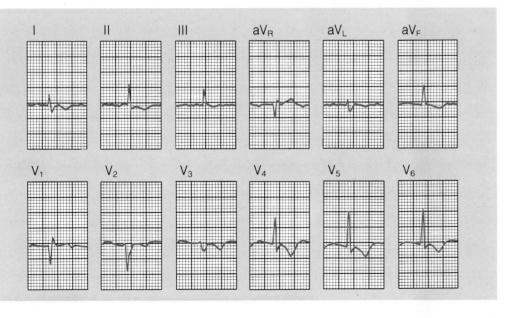

FIGURE 8.42 ECG of a 65-year-old woman with amyloid of the heart and normal sinus rhythm. The P waves are just barely visible in lead aV_R, and the P–R interval is 0.24 sec. Large abnormal Q waves are seen in leads V_1 to V_3. The T waves are deeply inverted in leads I, II, aV_F; and V_2 to V_6. Initially the condition was diagnosed as myocardial infarction with normal coronary arteries. (Reproduced with permission; see Figure Credits)

The cross-sectional echocardiogram in patients with amyloid heart disease may show brilliant echoes involving the myocardium. Bright echoes in amyloid are not diagnostic. The interactive septum is thickened (Fig. 8.43).[7]

Cardiac Catheterization   The pressure curves may simulate those found in constrictive pericarditis with the dip-and-plateau wave form recorded during diastole in the right ventricle (see Fig. 9.26). There may be evidence of tricuspid and mitral valve regurgitation.

Angiography reveals obliterated areas in the apices of the ventricles. The ventricular cavity size may be decreased, and the myocardial wall may be thicker than normal. Contractility is usually normal during the early stages of the disease, while relaxation of the myocardial wall is abnormal.

Radionuclide Studies   Radionuclide ventriculography reveals a normal or a decreased ventricular cavity size; this assists in the differentiation from dilated cardiomyopathy. The relaxation abnormality of the myocardial wall may be identified. Cardiac amyloidosis is less likely to show a distorted ventricular cavity. ^{99m}Tc pyrophosphate scans show abnormal areas of increased myocardial uptake in patients with amyloidosis (Fig. 8.44).

Computed Tomography and Magnetic Resonance Imaging   These modalities may help differentiate several conditions that produce somewhat similar clinical pictures. They may show the thick ventricular muscle and distorted cavity in patients with endomyocardial fibrosis or may reveal a thick pericardium and normal cardiac muscle thickness in patients with constrictive pericarditis.

Endomyocardial Biopsy   Endomyocardial biopsy may be diagnostic of endomyocardial fibrosis, amyloid involvement of the heart, or hemochromatosis.

Other Studies   The hypereosinophilic syndrome is associated with eosinophilic infiltration of tissues, including the heart. The eosinophils may constitute 75% of the total white blood cell count, which may be as high as 100,000/mm³. There may be no recognizable cause of the eosinophilia, but the abnormality may be an immunologic response of some sort. The response may be associated with parasitic infections, or it may be of unknown origin, as in Loeffler's disasease.

Biopsy of the rectal mucosa, gums, skin lesions, and other sites may be performed if one suspects amyloid heart disease, but endomyocardial biopsy is more diagnostic.

NATURAL HISTORY

Patients with restrictive myocardial disease may survive only a few months or a few years.

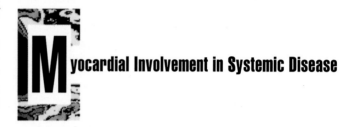

Myocardial Involvement in Systemic Disease

There are several causes of myocardial disease, some of which are limited to the heart, while others represent the heart's participation in systemic disease, as in Pompe's disease (Fig. 8.45) or tumor metastases to the heart (Fig. 8.46). For systemic diseases involving the heart, see Figure 8.46 and Chapters 15 through 27.

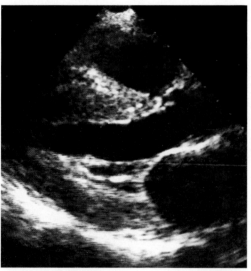

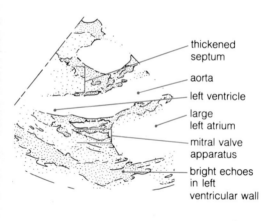

thickened septum
aorta
left ventricle
large left atrium
mitral valve apparatus
bright echoes in left ventricular wall

FIGURE 8.43   Cross-sectional echocardiogram in the long axis view was obtained during systole in a 66-year-old male with amyloid involving the heart. Sparkling echoes involving the myocardium are evident. Both the interventricular septum and the posterior wall are thickened. (Reproduced with permission; see Figure Credits)

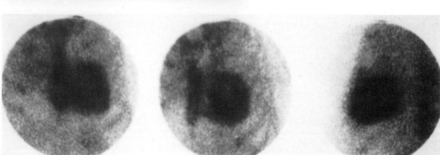

FIGURE 8.44   Markedly abnormal ^{99m}Tc pyrophosphate images in anterior (left), left anterior oblique (center), and left lateral (right) projections taken in a patient with primary amyloidosis. (Reproduced with permission; see Figure Credits)

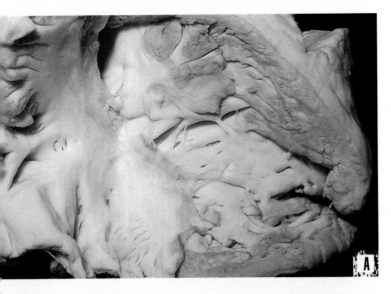

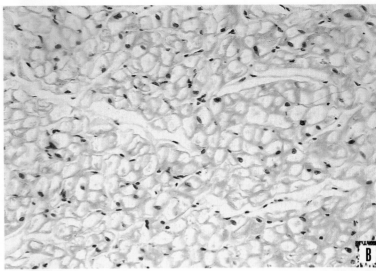

FIGURE 8.45 **(A)** Right ventricular view of the heart in a case of Pompe's disease. Note the pale-staining myocardial wall. **(B)** Histologic section shows vacuolated cells where the glycogen has been washed out. (Reproduced with permission; see Figure Credits)

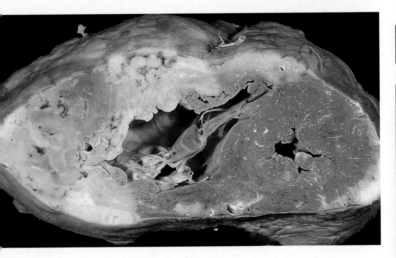

FIGURE 8.46 Extensive tumor involvement of the heart consequent to spread from a primary bronchial carcinoma. (Reproduced with permission; see Figure Credits)

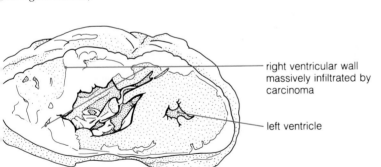

right ventricular wall massively infiltrated by carcinoma

left ventricle

FIGURE 8.47 EXAMPLES OF MYOCARDIAL INVOLVEMENT IN SYSTEMIC DISEASE

Infectious disease
Sarcoidosis
Nutritional disorders
Metabolic disorders
Endocrine disorders
Hematologic diseases
Neurologic and neuromuscular diseases
Collagen vascular diseases
Neoplastic diseases
Chemical and drug effects
Physical causes
Miscellaneous systemic syndromes

(Reproduced with permission; see Figure Credits)

ACKNOWLEDGMENTS

This chapter is based in part on Wenger NK, Abelmann WH, Roberts WC: Myocarditis; and Wenger NK, Goodwin JF, Roberts WC: Cardiomyopathy and myocardial involvement in systemic disease. In Hurst JW (ed): The Heart, 6th ed. McGraw-Hill, New York, 1986.

FIGURE CREDITS

Figs. 8.1–8.3, 8.5, 8.23, 8.40 from Becker AE, Anderson RH: Cardiac Pathology. Raven, New York, 1983.

Figs. 8.4, 8.10, from Hurst JW (ed): The Heart, 6th ed., McGraw-Hill, New York, 1986.

Figs. 8.6, 8.7, 8.11, 8.13, 8.14, 8.19, 8.27, 8.31, 8.35, 8.37, 8.42, 8.45–8.47 from Hurst JW (ed): Atlas of the Heart, Gower, New York, 1988.

Figs. 8.8, 8.9, 8.12, 8.15–8.17, 8.20, 8.22, 8.24–8.26, 8.28–8.30, 8.33, 8.34 8.36, 8.41, 8.44 from Chatterjee K, et al: Cardiology: An Illustrated Text–Reference, Gower, New York, 1992. Fig. 8.44 courtesy of R Lull, MD, San Francisco, CA.

Figs. 8.12, from Acquatella H, et al: M-mode and two-dimensional echocardiography in chronic Chagas' heart disease. Circulation 62:787, 1980. Fig. 8.12A redrawn and modified.

Figs. 8.18, 8.21 from Kassner EG: Atlas of Radiologic Imaging, Gower, New York, 1989.

Figs. 8.19, 8.32, 8.35, 8.43 courtesy of Stephen D. Clements, Jr., MD, Atlanta, GA.

Fig. 8.24 redrawn from Silver MD: Cardiovascular Pathology, Churchill Livingstone, New York, 1983. Courtesy of L. Horlick, MD, Saskatoon, Saskatchewan, Canada.

Figs. 8.26, 8.28, 8.29 modified and redrawn from Wigle ED, et al: Hypertrophic cardiomyopathy: The importance of the site and extent of hypertrophy. A review. Prog Cardiovasc Dis 28:1, 1985.

Fig. 8.30 redrawn from Tavel ME: Clinical Phonocardiography and External Pulse Recording. Year Book, Chicago, 1967.

Fig. 8.37 courtesy of Jerre F. Lutz, MD, Atlanta, GA.

Fig. 8.38 from Soto B, et al: Imaging of Cardiac Disorders, Gower, New York, 1992.

Fig. 8.39 courtesy of Roderic I. Pettigrew, MD, PhD, Atlanta, GA.

REFERENCES

1. Bell GJ, Grist NR: Echoviruses, carditis, and acute pleurodynia. Am Heart J 82:133, 1971.
2. Braunwald E, Morrow AG, Cornell WP, et al: Idiopathic hypertrophic subaortic stenosis: Clinical, hemodynamic and angiographic manifestations. Am J Med 29:24, 1960.
3. Burch GE, Giles TD: The role of viruses in the production of heart disease. Am J Cardiol 29:231, 1972.
4. Carroll JD, Gaasch WH, McAdam KPWJ: Amyloid cardiomyopathy: Characterization by a distinctive voltage/mass relation. Am J Cardiol 49:9, 1982.
5. Chew CYC, Ziady GM, Raphael JM, et al: Primary restrictive cardiomyopathy: Nontropical endomyocardial fibrosis and hypereosinophilic heart disease. Br Heart J 39:399, 1977.
5a. Criley JM, Siegal RJ: A non-obstructive view of hypertrophic cardiomyopathies. In Goodwin JF (ed): Heart Muscle Disease. MTP Press, 1985.
6. Davidoff R, Palacios I, Southern J, et al: Giant cell versus lymphocytic myocarditis: A comparison of their clinical features and long-term outcomes. Circulation 83:953, 1991.
7. DeMaria AN, Bommer W, Lee G, et al: Value and limitations of two-dimensional echocardiography in assessment of cardiomyopathy. Am J Cardiol 46:1224, 1980.
8. Dunn RF, Uren RF, Sadick N, et al: Comparison of thallium-201 scanning in idiopathic dilated cardiomyopathy and severe coronary artery disease. Circulation 66:804, 1982.
9. Edwards WD, Holmes DR Jr, Reeder GS: Diagnosis of active lymphocytic myocarditis by endomyocardial biopsy: Quantitative criteria for light microscopy. Mayo Clin Proc 57:419, 1982.
10. Frank MJ, Watkins LO, Prisant M, et al: Potentially lethal arrhythmias and their management in hypertrophic cardiomyopathy. Am J Cardiol 53:1608, 1984.
11. Gau GT, Goodwin JF, Oakley CM, et al: Q waves and coronary arteriography in cardiomyopathy. Br Heart J 34:1034, 1972.
12. Gilbert BW, Pollick C, Adelman AG, et al: Hypertrophic cardiomyopathy: Subclassification by M-mode echocardiography. Am J Cardiol 45:861, 1980.
13. Goldman MR, Boucher CA: Value of radionuclide imaging techniques in assessing cardiomyopathy. Am J Cardiol 46:1232, 1980.

14. Goodwin JF: The frontiers of cardiomyopathy. Br Heart J 48:1, 1982.
15. Goodwin JF: Cardiomyopathy: An interface between fundamental and clinical cardiology. In Hayase S, Murao S (eds): Cardiology (Proceedings VIII World Congress of Cardiology, Tokyo, 1978). Excerpta Medica, Amsterdam, 1979.
15a. Goodwin JF. Thirty years of cardiomyopathy. In Boraldi G, Camerine F, Goodwin JF (eds): Advances in Cardiomyopathies. Springer-Verleig, Berlin, 1990.
16. Hejtmancik JF, Brink PA, Towbin J, et al: Localization of gene for familial hypertrophic cardiomyopathy to chromosome 14q1 in a diverse US population. Circulation 83:1592, 1991.
17. Kean BH, Breslau RC: Parasites of the Human Heart. Grune & Stratton, New York, 1964.
18. Kereiakes DJ, Parmley WW: Myocarditis and cardiomyopathy. Am Heart J 108:1318, 1984.
18a. Mason J: Personal communication, December 1992.
19. Keren A, Gottlieb S, Tzivoni D, et al: Mildly dilated congestive cardiomyopathy—Use of prospective diagnostic criteria and description of the clinical course without heart transplantation. Circulation 81:506, 1990.
20. Kristinsson A: Diagnosis, natural history and treatment of congestive cardiomyopathy. PhD thesis, University of London, Royal Postgraduate Medical School of London, 1969.
21. Lansdown ABG: Viral infections and diseases of the heart. Prog Med Virol 24:70, 1978.
22. Lerner AM, Wilson FM, Reyes MP: Enteroviruses and the heart (with special emphasis on the probable role of coxsackie viruses, group B, types 1–5). I. Epidemiological and experimental studies. II. Observations in humans. Mod Concepts Cardiovasc Dis 44:7, 11, 1975.
23. Maron BJ, Bonow RO, Cannon RO, et al: Hypertrophic cardiomyopathy—Interrelations of clinical manifestations, pathophysiology, and therapy. N Engl J Med 316:780, 844, 1987.
24. Murphy TE, Kean BH, Venturini A, et al: Echinococcus cyst of the left ventricle: Report of a case with review of the pertinent literature. J Thorac Cardiovasc Surg 61:443, 1971.
25. Nieminen MS, Heikkila J, Karjalainene J: Echocardiography in acute infectious myocarditis: Relation to clinical and electrocardiographic findings. Am J Cardiol 53:1331, 1984.
26. O'Connell JB, Henkin RE, Robinson JA, et al: Gallium-67 imaging in patients with dilated cardiomyopathy and biopsy proven myocarditis. Circulation 70:58, 1984.
27. Opherk D, Schwarz F, Mall G, et al: Coronary dilatory capacity in idiopathic dilated cardiomyopathy: Analysis of 16 patients. Am J Cardiol 51:1657, 1983.
28. Ouzts HG, Turner JL, Douglas JS Jr, et al: Prolonged chest pain suggesting myocardial infarction in patients with hypertrophic cardiomyopathy. In Hurst JW (ed): Update III: The Heart. McGraw-Hill, New York, 1980.
29. Puigbo JJ, Rhode JRN, Barrios HG, et al: Clinical and epidemiological study of chronic heart involvement in Chagas' disease. Bull WHO 34:655, 1966.
29a. Report of the WHO/IFSC Task Force on the definition and classification of cardiomyopathies. Brit Heart J 48: 672, 1980.
30. Roberts WC, Bjua LM, Ferrans VJ: Loeffler's fibroplastic parietal endocarditis, eosinophilic leukemia, and Davies' endomyocardial fibrosis: The same disease at different stages? Pathol Microbiol 35:90, 1970.
31. Sanderson JE, Gibson DG, Brown DJ, et al: Left ventricular filling in hypertrophic cardiomyopathy: An angiographic study. Br Heart J 39:661, 1977.
32. Schaper J, Froede R, Hein S, et al: Localization of the myocardial ultrastructure and changes of the cytoskeleton in dilated cardiomyopathy. Circulation 83:504, 1991.
33. Shah PM, Adelman AG, Wigle ED, et al: The natural (and unnatural) course of hypertrophic obstructive cardiomyopathy—A multicenter study. Circulation 47/48(suppl 4):IV-S, 1973.
34. Spirito P, Chiarella F, Carratino L, et al: Clinical course and prognosis of hypertrophic cardiomyopathy in an outpatient population. N Engl J Med 320:749, 1989.
35. Vacek JL, Davis WR, Bellinger RL: Apical hypertrophic cardiomyopathy in American patients. Am Heart J 108:1501, 1984.
36. Walsh TJ, Hutchins GM, Bulkley BH, et al: Fungal infections of the heart: Analysis of 51 autopsy cases. Am J Cardiol 45:357, 1980.
37. Wentworth P, Jentz LA, Croal EA: Analysis of sudden unexpected death in southern Ontario, with emphasis on myocarditis. Can Med Assoc J 120:676, 1979.
38. Woodward TE, Togo Y, Lee Y–C, et al: Special microbial infections of the myocardium and pericardium. A study of 82 patients. Arch Intern Med 120:270, 1967

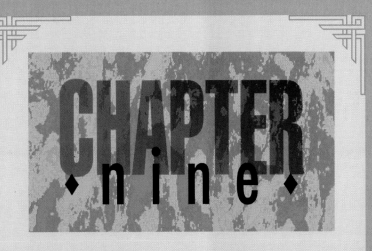

CHAPTER ·nine·

PERICARDIAL DISEASE

J. WILLIS HURST, MD

RALPH SHABETAI, MD

ANTON E. BECKER, MD

JOSEPH S. ALPERT, MD

While there are many causes of pericardial disease, (Fig. 9.1), three clinical syndromes may be defined: acute pericarditis with or without recurrence, pericardial effusion with or without cardiac tamponade, and constrictive pericarditis.

Acute Pericarditis
ETIOLOGY AND PATHOLOGY

Acute pericarditis is usually due to a viral infection, commonly by echovirus or coxsackievirus. The term *idiopathic pericarditis* is used when clinical features are similar to those of a viral infection, but a viral etiology is not demonstrated (see Fig. 9.1).

The pathology of acute pericarditis is determined by the exudative response as it relates to the underlying cause. The pericardial layers are often coated with fibrinous deposits (Fig. 9.2). Cultures of the fibrin deposits and fluid may reveal the etiology. Purulent pericarditis indicates a bacterial cause, often due to direct spread of the infection from other sites in the heart (Figs. 9.3, 9.4) or surrounding structures, such as the lung. A hemorrhagic exudate often indicates a neoplasm's underlying cause; it may also occur in patients with tuberculosis or in those receiving anticoagulant therapy for chronic renal disease. Pericarditis may occur after myocardial infarction or following cardiac surgery. Lupus erythematosus may be the cause, especially in young women. Occasionally cytology of the exudate may indicate the proper diagnosis, such as lymphoma or infectious mononucleosis. In rare cases the histology identifies the underlying cause as fungi or caseous granulomata suggesting tuberculosis (Fig. 9.5).

FIGURE 9.1   ETIOLOGY OF PERICARDITIS*

I. TRAUMA
- A. *Pericardiotomy*
- B. *Indirect trauma to chest*
- C. *Transeptal catheterization*
- D. *Pressure injection of contrast medium*
- E. *Perforation of right ventricle by indwelling catheter*
- F. *Implantation of epicardial pacemaker*
- G. *Blow to chest*
- H. *Perforation of right ventricle with catheter for parenteral nutrition*

II. VIRAL INFECTIONS
- A. *Coxsackieviruses B5, B6*
- B. *Echovirus*
- C. *Adenovirus*
- D. *Infectious mononucleosis*
- E. *Influenza*
- F. *Lymphogranuloma venereum*
- G. *Chickenpox*
- H. *Mycoplasma pneumoniae*
- I. *AIDS*

III. BACTERIAL INFECTIONS
- A. *Staphylococcus*
- B. *Pneumococcus*
- C. *Meningococcus*
- D. *Streptococcus*
- E. *Haemophilus influenza*
- F. *Psittacosis*
- G. *Salmonella*
- H. *Tuberculosis*

IV. AMEBIASIS

V. ECHINOCOCCUS CYSTS

VI. FUNGUS INFECTIONS—HISTOPLAS-MOSIS, ASPERGILLOSIS, BLASTOMYCOSIS, COCCIDIOIDOMYCOSIS

VII. RICKETTSIA

VIII. RADIATION

IX. AMYLOIDOSIS

X. TUMORS
- A. *Primary*
  1. Mesothelioma
  2. Rhabdomyosarcoma
  3. Teratoma
  4. Fibroma
  5. Leiomyofibroma
  6. Lipoma
  7. Angioma
- B. *Metastatic*
  1. Bronchogenic carcinoma
  2. Carcinoma of breast
  3. Lymphoma
  4. Leukemia
  5. Melanoma

XI. SARCOID

XII. COLLAGEN DISEASE
- A. *Rheumatic fever*
- B. *Lupus erythematosus*
- C. *Rheumatoid arthritis*
- D. *Vasculitis*
- E. *Polyarteritis nodosa*
- F. *Scleroderma*
- G. *Dermatomyositis*

XIII. ANTICOAGULANTS
- A. *Heparin*
- B. *Warfarin*

XIV. MYOCARDIAL INFARCTION
- A. *Acute myocardial infarction*
- B. *Postmyocardial infarction (Dressler's syndrome)*

XV. IDIOPATHIC THROMBOCYTOPENIC PURPURA

XVI. DRUGS
- A. *Procainamide*
- B. *Cromolyn sodium*
- C. *Hydralazine*
- D. *Dantrolene*
- E. *Methysergide*

XVII. DISSECTING ANEURYSM

XVIII. INFECTIVE ENDOCARDITIS WITH VALVE RING ABSCESS

XIX. THYMIC CYST

Principal causes of pericardial disease and pericardial heart disease. Many of these conditions can cause pericardial effusion, cardiac tamponade, and/or constrictive pericarditis. The more common causes of these syndromes are mentioned under the syndromes and under specific disorders. (Reproduced with permission; see Figure Credits)

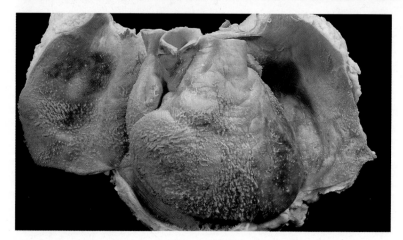

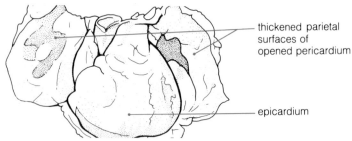

FIGURE 9.2   Heart with pericardium opened to show fibrinous pericarditis, which is most likely of viral origin. (Reproduced with permission; see Figure Credits)

thickened parietal surfaces of opened pericardium

epicardium

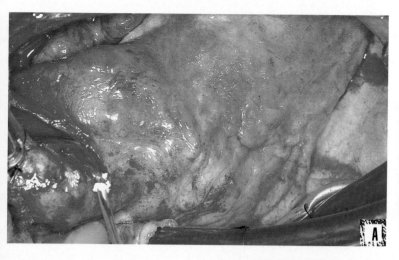
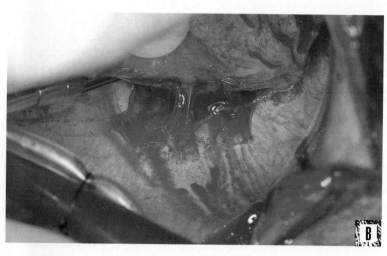

FIGURE 9.3 **(A)** Operative view of the heart showing epicardial surface with fine granular appearance. Bacterial endocarditis extends into the peri- cardium. **(B)** Adhesions extend to the diaphragmatic surface of the heart. (Reproduced with permission; see Figure Credits)

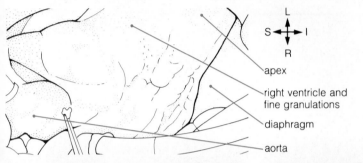
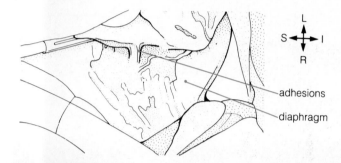

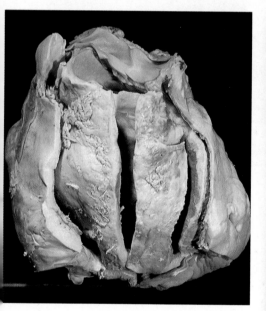

FIGURE 9.4 Chronic purulent pericarditis caused by bacterial infection. (Reproduced with permission; see Figure Credits)

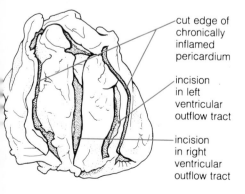

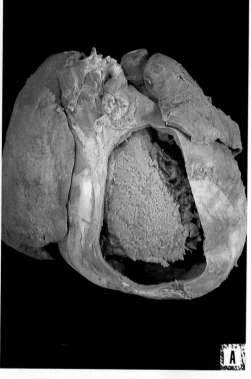

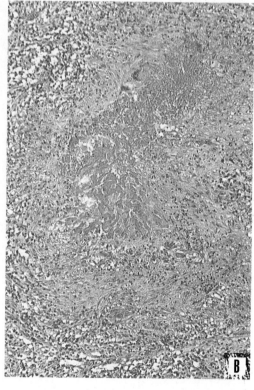

FIGURE 9.5 **(A)** Window cut into the peri- cardium of this grossly enlarged heart exposing fibrinous pericarditis due to tuberculosis.

(B) Histologic section of the pericardium shows caseous necrosis indicative of tuberculosis. (Reproduced with permission; see Figure Credits)

PATHOPHYSIOLOGY

The amount of pericardial fluid is often slightly increased with acute pericarditis, but patients who have considerable fluid are excluded from this discussion (Fig. 9.6). By definition, therefore, hemodynamic alterations do not occur in patients with uncomplicated acute pericarditis. The chest pain produced by pericarditis is caused by stimulation of cardiac branches of the phrenic and intercostal nerves.

CLINICAL MANIFESTATIONS

SYMPTOMS

Patients may develop myalgia and fever a few days before the onset of chest pain. While the pain is usually located in the anterior portion of the chest or precordium, it may radiate to the top of the shoulders. It may be either sharp or crushing, and may be aggravated by inspiration, turning, or swallowing. The pain lessens when the patient leans forward. Patients may have pericarditis without chest pain.

PHYSICAL EXAMINATION

While the physical examination may be normal, it is possible to detect that the patient is trying to avoid deep inspirations that produce pain. A pericardial friction rub is sometimes detected. It is best heard with the patient in a sitting position; the stethoscope is placed on the precordium between the left sternal border and the apex. The rub may be louder during inspiration. It is often triphasic; the components occur with atrial systole, ventricular systole, and ventricular diastole.[17] However, the rub may consist of only one or two of these components. Atrial arrhythmias may occur, possibly due to inflammation of the sinus node, but arrythmia more likely is evidence of accompanying myocarditis.[19]

LABORATORY STUDIES

Chest Radiography   The chest film is usually normal in patients with acute pericarditis with little pericardial fluid and no myocarditis.

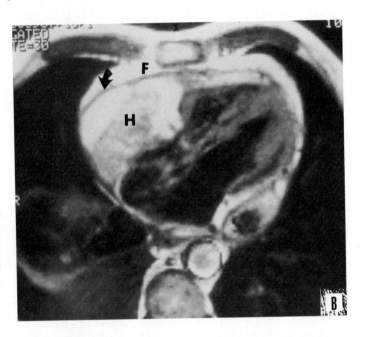

FIGURE 9.6   ECG-gated spin-echo images of two patients with inflammatory effusion and pericardial hematoma. **(A)** The thickened parietal *(arrows)* and visceral pericardium have high-signal intensity, consistent with inflammatory pericardial thickening caused by uremic pericarditis. The nonhemorrhagic effusion (E) causes low intensity. **(B)** The pericardial hematoma (H) produces high-signal intensity on this T1-weighted image. The hematoma has a signal intensity equivalent to the fat (F) on the surface of the parietal pericardium *(curved arrow)*. (Reproduced with permission; see Figure Credits)

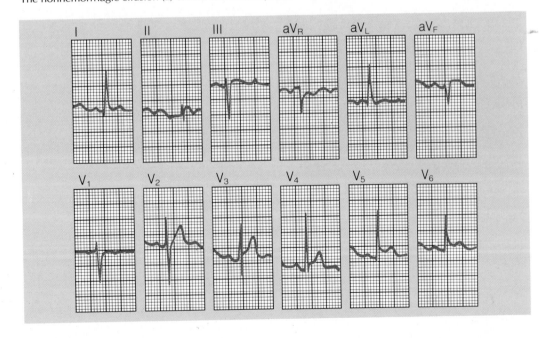

FIGURE 9.7   ECG from a patient with acute pericarditis showing PR-segment depression and ST-segment elevation. (Reproduced with permission; see Figure Credits)

he film may show the disease process etiologically related to the pericarditis, uch as pneumonia or neoplastic disease.

lectrocardiography The electrocardiogram (ECG) of cute pericarditis is characterized by PR-segment depression, normal QRS complexes, and a mean ST-segment vector that is directed toward the cardiac apex Fig. 9.7). Later in the disease course the ST-segment vector becomes smaller, nd as it does, the T-wave vector is abnormally directed away from the cardiac pex (Fig. 9.8).[18] These changes are due to inflammation of the epicardium of he heart. Myocarditis should be considered when atrioventricular block or bundle branch block occurs. Electrocardiographic changes may not appear in uremic pericarditis.

chocardiography The echocardiogram is normal unless ericardial fluid or myocarditis is present.

OTHER LABORATORY ABNORMALITIES

The erythrocyte sedimentation rate is usually elevated. Leukocytosis or ymphocytosis may be present. Cardiac enzyme levels are usually normal. Skin ests for tuberculosis and fungi are often positive in those diseases.

NATURAL HISTORY

The natural history of acute pericarditis often depends on the etiology. The prog- osis of pericarditis follows that of the causative disease itself in the following: remia, collagen disease, acute myocardial infarction, and dissection of the aorta. The natural history of bacterial pericarditis is very different from that of viral ericarditis. Bacterial causes may be fatal unless recognized with subsequent rainage of the pericardium. The natural history of viral or idiopathic pericardi- tis is usually predictable due to the self-limiting nature of viral infections. Fever and pericardial rub usually subside within 2 weeks; however, the disease may recur. When the illness lasts longer than 2 weeks, it is wise to consider a more serious etiology. Regardless of the etiology, acute pericarditis may recur after varying intervals,[4] possibly due to immunologic causes.

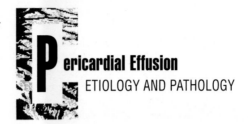

Pericardial Effusion
ETIOLOGY AND PATHOLOGY

Pericardial effusion may be clinically associated with acute or recurrent pericarditis. It may be discovered on routine examination or during the workup of an ill patient. The effusion may be asymptomatic, or it may produce cardiac tamponade.

The common causes of pericarditis with effusion are acute viral or idiopathic pericarditis, collagen disease (especially lupus and rheumatoid arthritis), neoplastic disease (especially breast cancer, bronchogenic carcinoma, and lymphoma), and postpericardiotomy or Dressler's (postmyocardial infarction) syndrome (see Fig. 9.1). Transmural myocardial infarction commonly results in effusion (Fig. 9.9), but in this situation the pathology of the epicardium and pericardium is not specific. Hemorrhagic pericardial effusion may be caused by rupture of the heart due to myocardial infarction or dissecting aortic aneurysm. Pyogenic effusion must not be overlooked, since specific therapy is necessary for cure.

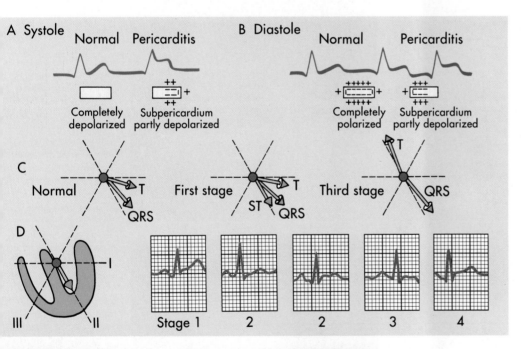

FIGURE 9.8 Electrical basis of ECG changes in acute pericarditis. **(A)** Systolic J–ST displacement. **(B)** Diastolic J–ST "displacement" due to depression of TP interval. **(C)** Spatial representation of QRS, ST, and T vectors. **(D)** Net ST vector, usual orientation: inferiorly, anteriorly, and leftward. Bottom tracing shows representative complexes from stages I, II, III, and IV of ECG evolution of acute pericarditis. (Reproduced with permission; see Figure Credits)

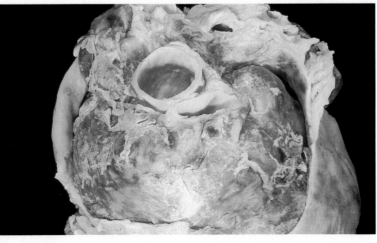

FIGURE 9.9 Fibrinous pericarditis resulting from acute myocardial infarction. (Reproduced with permission; see Figure Credits)

PATHOPHYSIOLOGY

The normal amount of pericardial fluid is approximately 50 mL. The characteristics of the pericardial pressure–volume curve are shown in Figure 9.10.[12] These characteristics are determined by the elastic properties of the pericardium and the speed at which pericardial fluid accumulates. The initial flat portion of the curve indicates fluid accumulation; during this phase the pericardium stretches and adapts to the increasing volume. The intrapericardial pressure is lower than the atrial or ventricular diastolic pressure.

As more fluid accumulates, stretching of the pericardium reaches its limit; at that point the intrapericardial pressure may rise to dangerous levels. The normal filling pressures of the heart are then exceeded and must increase to allow continued cardiac output.[16] When fluid accumulates slowly, the cardiac silhouette may become quite large with no signs of tamponade. When fluid accumulates abruptly, the cardiac silhouette may increase only slightly in size, yet serious tamponade may be present.

CLINICAL MANIFESTATIONS
Pericardial Effusion Without Cardiac Tamponade

Pericardial effusion should be considered when a patient has a disease that may involve the pericardium. Effusion should be suspected, especially when there is any evidence of pericarditis.

SYMPTOMS

There may be no symptoms resulting from pericardial effusion unless acute pericarditis or tamponade is present.

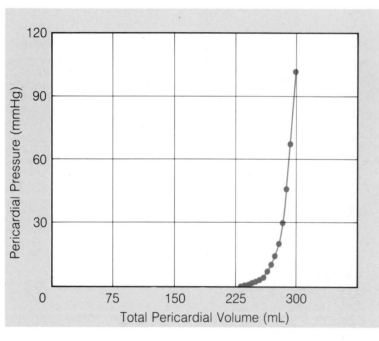

FIGURE 9.10 Pericardial pressure–volume curve of canines. (Reproduced with permission; see Figure Credits)

PHYSICAL EXAMINATION

The physical examination does not usually reveal any evidence of fluid. The neck veins do not show abnormal distention or pulsation. Heart sounds are not usually diminished in intensity by the presence of pericardial fluid; a friction rub may be heard even when there is considerable effusion.

LABORATORY STUDIES

Chest Radiography   Pericardial fluid may be suspected when the chest film is reviewed. An epicardial fat stripe may occasionally be seen in patients with pericardial effusion (Fig. 9.11). However, the typical appearance is an enlarged cardiac shadow with smooth borders and no evidence of pulmonary congestion (Fig. 9.12). The problem, however, is to differentiate among pericardial fluid alone, cardiac enlargement alone, and the presence of both pericardial effusion and cardiac enlargement. Computed tomography (CT) may be used to identify pericardial disease and pericardial effusion (Figs 9.13, 9.14).

Electrocardiography   The ECG may reveal low voltage. Electrical alternans is occasionally present when the heart swings to and fro within an effusion that is large (Fig. 9.15).

Echocardiography   The cross-sectional echocardiogram is both sensitive and specific in identifying pericardial effusion (Figs 9.16–9.18).[9,21] In addition, it may be used to identify chamber enlargement when present.

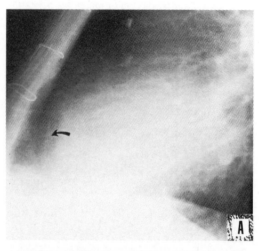

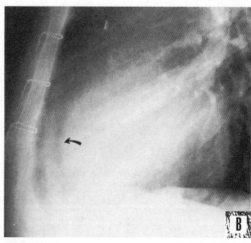

FIGURE 9.11
(A) Lateral radiograph of a patient 3 weeks after a coronary bypass procedure. Normal pericardium is seen as a hairline density *(arrow)* sandwiched between the subepicardial fat stripe interiorly and the mediastinal fat exteriorly. Metallic sutures are evident in the sternum, and a surgical clip marks the origin of a venous graft in the ascending aorta.
(B) The same patient developed postpericardiotomy syndrome 5 weeks postoperatively. In this lateral radiograph the subepicardial fat stripe *(arrow)* is more distinct because of pericardial effusion, and is displaced interiorly by the widened pericardium. (Reproduced with permission; see Figure Credits)

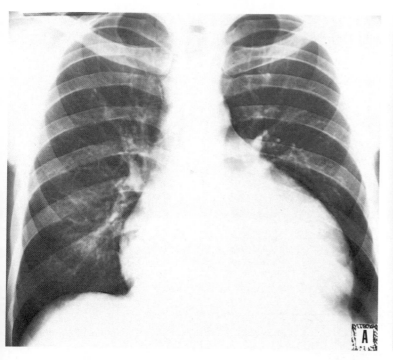

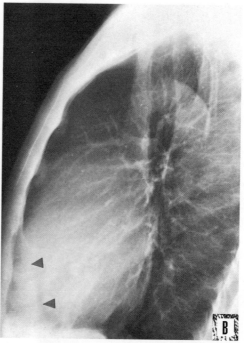

FIGURE 9.12 Chest radiographs demonstrating pericardial effusion. **(A)** Posteroanterior projection shows a large cardiovascular silhouette with prominence of the right and left contours. The cardiac margins are smooth, and structures that normally form the left upper heart border (e.g., left atrial appendage and pulmonary outflow tract) cannot be identified. The contour returns to normal at the level of the vascular pedicle: the aortic arch can be identified on the left, and the middle and upper segments of the superior vena cava on the right. **(B)** The lateral projection shows posterior displacement of the anterior epicardial fat *(arrows)*. The space between the epicardial fat and the anterior chest wall is occupied by pericardial fluid. (Reproduced with permission; see Figure Credits)

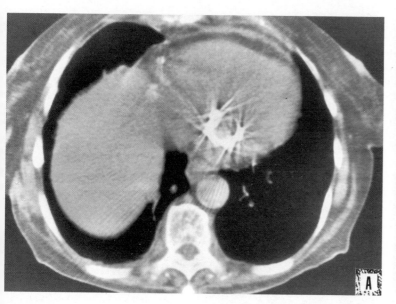

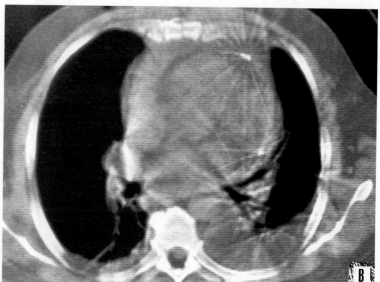

FIGURE 9.13 **(A)** CT scan at the level of a mitral heterograft in a 77-year-old female after mitral valve replacement. Note the anterior pericardial thickening between the more lucent epicardial fat and retrosternal fat. **(B)** Scan of a 53-year-old male, examined because of suspected mediastinitis 2 weeks following coronary bypass surgery, reveals loculated pericardial effusion in the right side of the pericardial space, outlined by the air-containing lung laterally and the epicardial fat medially. Bilateral pleural effusions are also present. The two densities with streak artifacts are surgical clips. (Reproduced with permission; see Figure Credits)

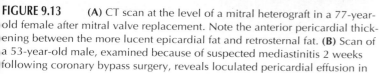

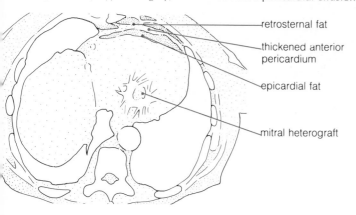

retrosternal fat

thickened anterior pericardium

epicardial fat

mitral heterograft

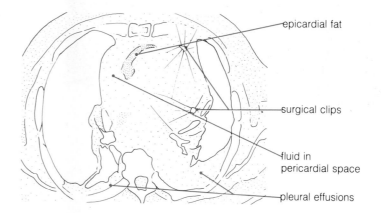

epicardial fat

surgical clips

fluid in pericardial space

pleural effusions

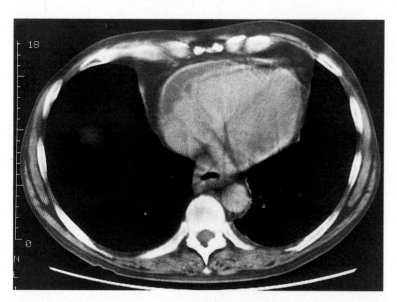

FIGURE 9.14 Axial CT at the level of the ventricles showing an accumulation of pericardial fluid between the visceral pericardium and perietal pericardium. (Reproduced with permission; see Figure Credits)

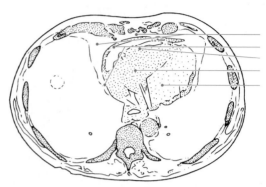

mediastinal fat
parietal pericardium
visceral pericardium
right ventricle
left ventricle

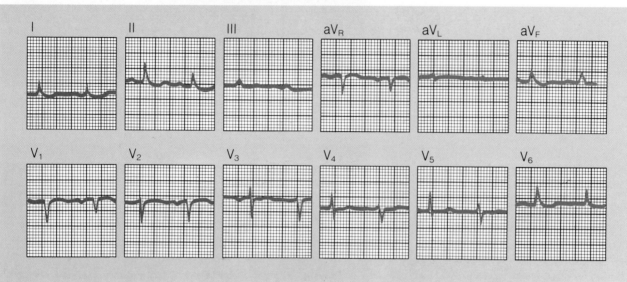

FIGURE 9.15 Electrical alternans of the QRS complex occurring with pericardial effusion. This particular patient also had cardiac tamponade. (Reproduced with permission; see Figure Credits)

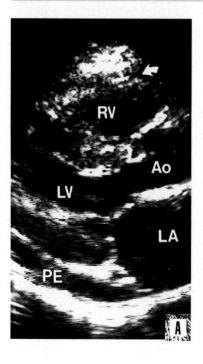

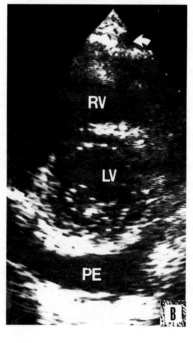

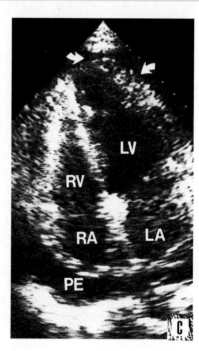

FIGURE 9.16 Parasternal long-axis (**A**) and short-axis (**B**) cross-sectional echocardiograms demonstrating moderate-sized posterior (PE) and small anterior pericardial effusions (arrows). Apical four-chamber view (**C**) shows fluid completely surrounding the heart. (RV = right ventricle; LV = left ventricle; Ao = aorta; LA = left atrium; RA = right atrium) (Reproduced with permission; see Figure Credits)

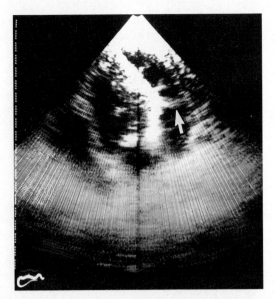

FIGURE 9.17   Two-dimensional apical four-chamber view from a patient with chronic pericardial effusion. The transducer has been angled sharply toward the left, permitting examination of the pericardial space. Within are multiple strand-like structures (arrow) connecting visceral and parietal pericardium. These structures exhibited a great deal of mobility during the cardiac cycle. Such stranding is a sign of chronicity. (Reproduced with permission; see Figure Credits)

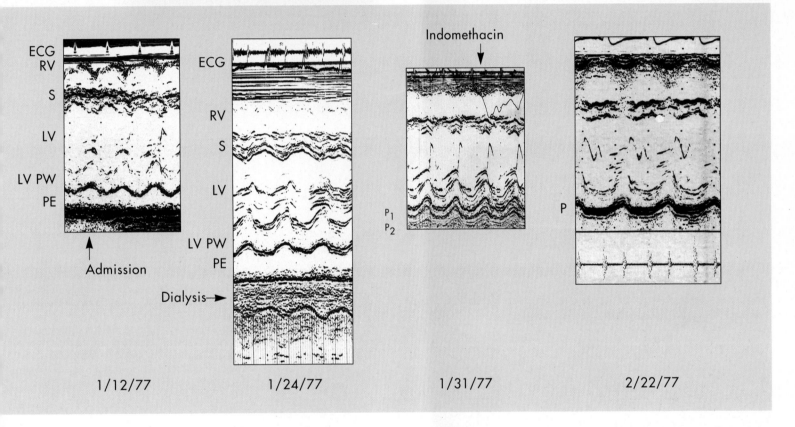

FIGURE 9.18   Serial echograms from a patient with end-stage renal disease and the onset of pericarditis. Moderate effusion was shown (left) and assumed secondary to uremia. The frequency of dialysis was increased, but after 12 days the effusion was larger (left center). Pericarditis was assumed to be inflammatory/infectious and indomethacin was administered. Seven days later (right center) there was resolution of effusion with evidence of pericardial thickening pattern (i.e., parallel motion of pericardial layers P_1 and P_2). Three weeks following detection of this pattern, there was no sign of pericardial space and only mild residual pericardial thickening (right). (Reproduced with permission; see Figure Credits)

Cardiac Catheterization   Pericardial effusion without tamponade is occasionally detected when cardiac catheterization and angiography are performed (Fig. 9.19).

Other Imaging Modalities   Both magnetic resonance imaging and CT scanning are capable of demonstrating pericardial effusion (see Figs. 9.13, 9.14).

Pericardial Aspiration   Pericardial aspiration (Fig. 9.20) is not usually indicated in patients who have either viral or self-limited pericarditis with effusion. This technique should be performed when the clinical course runs longer than 2 weeks despite medical therapy, and bacterial or nonviral infection is considered a possible cause. It is used, for example, to distinguish

between neoplastic effusion and radiation pericarditis in patients with cancer of the breast or lung. Aspiration is also indicated when tamponade from any cause is suspected.

Pericardial Effusion With Cardiac Tamponade

Any disease affecting the pericardium may cause pericardial effusion, which in turn may potentially produce cardiac tamponade. The common causes of tamponade are trauma (including surgical procedures on the heart), cardiac rupture from infarction, dissecting aneurysm, viral or idiopathic pericarditis, neoplastic pericarditis, collagen disease, dialysis-related pericardial disease, and, rarely Dressler's syndrome.[11]

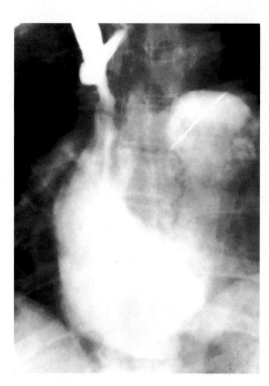

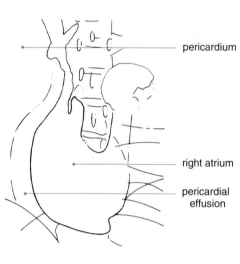

peuricardium

right atrium

pericardial
effusion

FIGURE 9.19   Pericardial effusion demonstrated by contrast medium injected into the right side of the heart. Note the distance between contrast medium located in the right atrium and the right border of the pericardium. (Reproduced with permission; see Figure Credits)

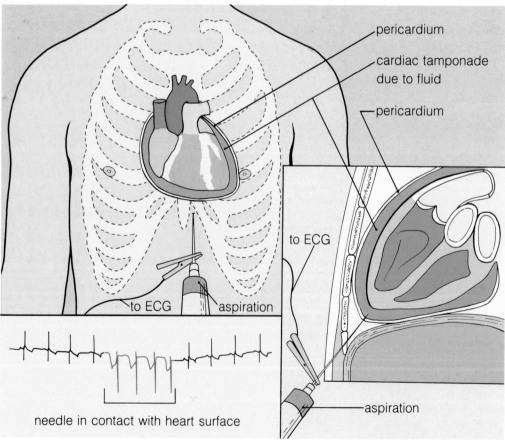

pericardium

cardiac tamponade
due to fluid

pericardium

to ECG

to ECG   aspiration

aspiration

needle in contact with heart surface

FIGURE 9.20   The subxyphoid pericardiocentesis technique: the needle is inserted to the left of the xiphoid and directed toward the midscapular area. The ECG lead is attached to the needle. Negative deflection of the QRS complex represents contact with the heart surface. As the needle is slowly withdrawn, and loses contact with the myocardium, the ECG reverts to normal. (Reproduced with permission; see Figure Credits)

Severe symptoms or death may result from sudden and acute cardiac tamponade, as in cardiac rupture. In less dramatic examples the patient may complain of dyspnea, chest tightness, or pericardial pain.

PHYSICAL EXAMINATION

The external jugular veins are distended, and the systemic arterial pressure may be abnormally low. When the tamponade does not occur rapidly, abnormal pulsations of the internal jugular veins may be identified. The **x** descent becomes prominent and coincides with the carotid pulse. A paradoxical pulse may be detected with the blood pressure cuff unless hypotension is severe.[3] The apex impulse of the heart is decreased in size, but heart sounds may not be diminished in intensity.[6]

LABORATORY STUDIES

Electrocardiography   No signs of cardiac tamponade are detected in the ECG. Electrical alternans may occur with pericardial effusion, but it does not necessarily imply that tamponade is present.

Echocardiography   Cross-sectional echocardiography is extremely useful in identifying pericardial effusion with cardiac tamponade (Fig. 9.21). It reveals evidence of compression of the right atrium and diastolic collapse of the right ventricle.[5,7,13,14]

Cardiac Catheterization   Cardiac catheterization reveals equal diastolic pressure in the two sides of the heart and decreased ventricular volumes. This procedure is usually not necessary, but it is occasionally useful to measure the right atrial and pulmonary wedge pressures. However, echocardiographic studies may be adequate to supply this information.

Pericardial Aspiration   See "Pericardial Effusion Without Cardiac Tamponade" (above).

Skin Tests and Other Laboratory Tests   Skin tests for tuberculosis and fungi aid in defining the etiology of pericarditis with effusion. Blood may also be tested for evidence of collagen disease or prior viral infections.

NATURAL HISTORY

The natural history of pericardial effusion with or without tamponade is determined by the promptness of the diagnosis, the etiology of the disease, and the therapy employed. Viral or idiopathic pericarditis with effusion is usually self-limiting and benign; however, it may recur or lead to constriction. Pericarditis due to bacteria, including the tubercle bacillus, is always serious, but it may be successfully treated when recognized. Effusion due to neoplasm is obviously serious and may contribute to the death of the patient. Effusion due to collagen disease can usually be managed on a long-term basis, although cardiac tamponade may ensue. In general, however, the patient's clinical course is related to the collagen disease. Acute hemorrhagic effusion with tamponade is often lethal when caused by rupture of the heart or aorta.

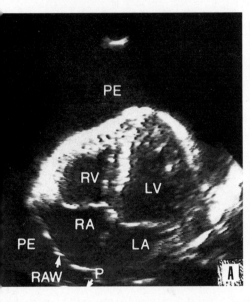
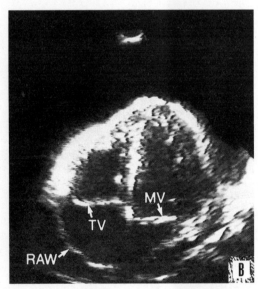
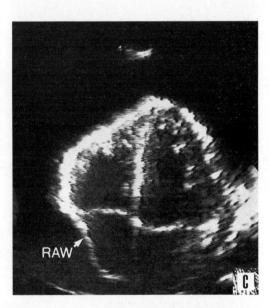

FIGURE 9.21   **(A–C)** Apical four-chamber echocardiograms from a patient with cardiac tamponade demonstrating a large pericardial effusion (PE) surrounding the entire heart. The right atrial wall (RAW) is seen to collapse inwardly on each view, suggesting early tamponade. (RV = right ventricle; RA = right atrium; LV = left ventricle; LA = left atrium; TV = tricuspid valve; MV = mitral value) (Reproduced with permission; see Figure Credits)

Constrictive Pericarditis

ETIOLOGY AND PATHOLOGY

Constrictive pericarditis may develop following pericarditis due to any cause. The majority of cases are idiopathic or postviral, post-traumatic (including surgery on the heart), neoplastic, postradiation treatment to the mediastinum, due to collagen disease (i.e., rheumatoid arthritis), or due to bacterial infections including tuberculosis. Constrictive pericarditis due to bacterial causes is becoming less common.[2]

Constrictive pericarditis is characterized by fibrous tissue encapsulating the heart either locally or diffusely (Fig. 9.22). The cause of injury cannot usually be determined from the current pathological state; an exception is constriction due to massive growth of a tumor. The creamy pericardial fluid found in some examples of constrictive pericarditis may contain calcium (Fig. 9.23); in these cases one may overestimate the amount of calcification of the epicardium when viewing the chest film.

PATHOPHYSIOLOGY

The inflammation of pericarditis produces a fibrous tissue response in the pericardium and epicardium, eventually leading to a fibrosed, tight pericardium and poor diastolic compliance. The fibrous tissue gradually limits diastolic filling of the heart; when a critical point is reached, the hemodynamics of the heart are altered.

The altered physiology of cardiac tamponade and constrictive pericarditis is similar, but there are some distinct differences, as illustrated in Figure 9.24. Cardiac catheterization reveals the abnormalities associated with cardiac tamponade (Fig. 9.25) or with constrictive pericarditis (Fig. 9.26).

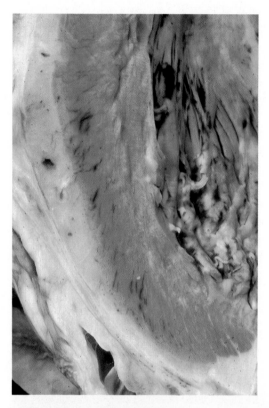

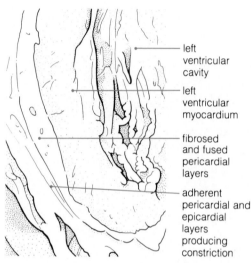

FIGURE 9.22 Constrictive pericarditis with fibrosed pericardial layers encapsulating the heart. (Reproduced with permission; see Figure Credits)

left ventricular cavity

left ventricular myocardium

fibrosed and fused pericardial layers

adherent pericardial and epicardial layers producing constriction

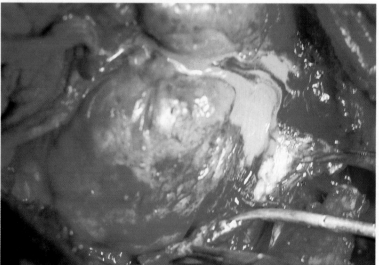

FIGURE 9.23 Creamy fluid with calcium crystals, seen in this operative view of chronic calcific constrictive pericarditis. The radiographic appearance of this heart suggested more extensive calcification than was actually found. (Reproduced with permission; see Figure Credits)

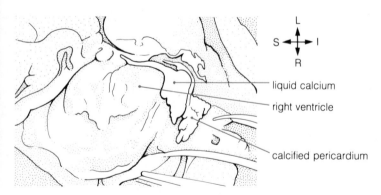

liquid calcium

right ventricle

calcified pericardium

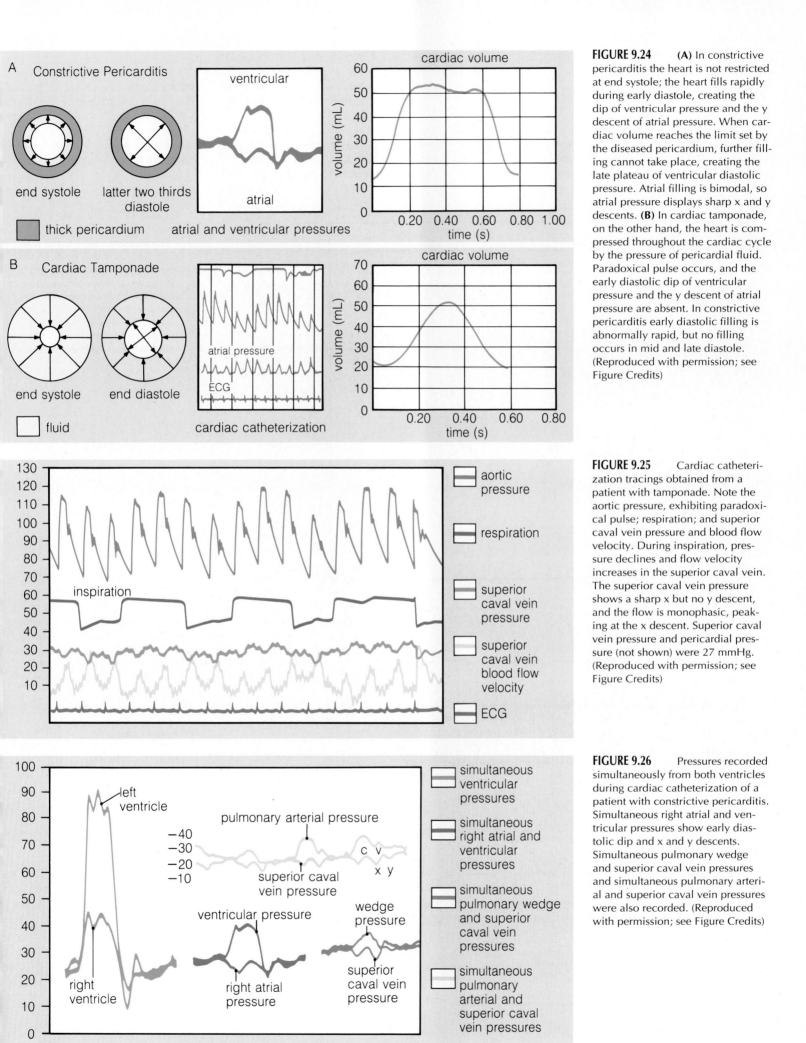

FIGURE 9.24 **(A)** In constrictive pericarditis the heart is not restricted at end systole; the heart fills rapidly during early diastole, creating the dip of ventricular pressure and the y descent of atrial pressure. When cardiac volume reaches the limit set by the diseased pericardium, further filling cannot take place, creating the late plateau of ventricular diastolic pressure. Atrial filling is bimodal, so atrial pressure displays sharp x and y descents. **(B)** In cardiac tamponade, on the other hand, the heart is compressed throughout the cardiac cycle by the pressure of pericardial fluid. Paradoxical pulse occurs, and the early diastolic dip of ventricular pressure and the y descent of atrial pressure are absent. In constrictive pericarditis early diastolic filling is abnormally rapid, but no filling occurs in mid and late diastole. (Reproduced with permission; see Figure Credits)

FIGURE 9.25 Cardiac catheterization tracings obtained from a patient with tamponade. Note the aortic pressure, exhibiting paradoxical pulse; respiration; and superior caval vein pressure and blood flow velocity. During inspiration, pressure declines and flow velocity increases in the superior caval vein. The superior caval vein pressure shows a sharp x but no y descent, and the flow is monophasic, peaking at the x descent. Superior caval vein pressure and pericardial pressure (not shown) were 27 mmHg. (Reproduced with permission; see Figure Credits)

FIGURE 9.26 Pressures recorded simultaneously from both ventricles during cardiac catheterization of a patient with constrictive pericarditis. Simultaneous right atrial and ventricular pressures show early diastolic dip and x and y descents. Simultaneous pulmonary wedge and superior caval vein pressures and simultaneous pulmonary arterial and superior caval vein pressures were also recorded. (Reproduced with permission; see Figure Credits)

Effusive constrictive pericarditis occurs when pericardial fluid is present while the pericardium constricts (Fig. 9.27).[10]

CLINICAL MANIFESTATIONS
SYMPTOMS

Early in the disease process, patients are asymptomatic. There may be a history of prior pericarditis. Later, patients complain of modest dyspnea, peripheral edema, and abdominal swelling due to ascites.

A paradoxical pulse is occasionally found in patients with constrictive pericarditis. The neck veins are distended, and the x and y descents may be prominent in the internal jugular venous pulse (Fig. 9.28). The apex impulse is not prominent, and a protodiastolic pericardial knock may be heard. An enlarged liver, ascites, and severe peripheral edema may be encountered. Many patients with constrictive pericarditis are initially thought to have a malignancy because of weight loss, fatigue, and ascites.

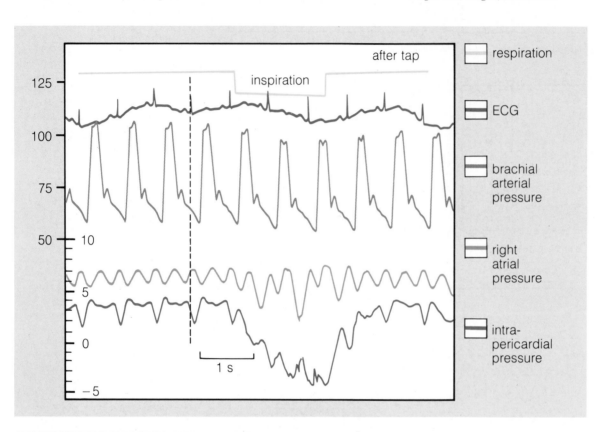

FIGURE 9.27 Cardiac catheterization tracings of a patient with effusive constrictive pericarditis due to bronchogenic carcinoma. The tracings were obtained during pericardiocentesis, which lowered pericardial pressure. However, right atrial pressure elevation persists, and the tracing shows prominent x and y descents and absent respiratory variation. (Reproduced with permission; see Figure Credits)

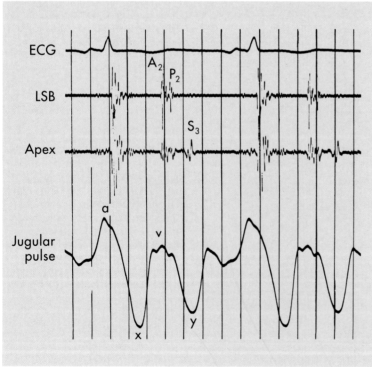

FIGURE 9.28 Jugular venous pulse tracing, phonocardiograms, and electrocardiogram in a patient with constrictive pericarditis. Both x and y descents were deep. A pericardial knock (S_3) and P_2 of lower intensity than A_2 favor the diagnosis of constrictive pericarditis. (LBS = left sternal border; apex = over the apex; a = a wave; v = v wave) (Reproduced with permission; see Figure Credits)

Chest Radiography   The size of the heart may be normal, or it may be slightly enlarged when the pericardium is thick. Pericardial calcification may be seen on the lateral view (Fig. 9.29).

Electrocardiography   Atrial fibrillation may be detected on ECG. The voltage is often diminished, and nonspecific ST–T waves may be present. Less commonly, scars and calcium may involve the myocardium, producing bundle branch block and atrioventricular conduction defects.

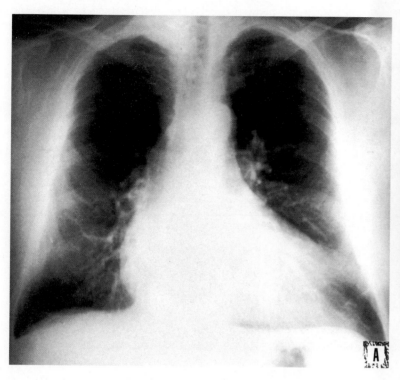
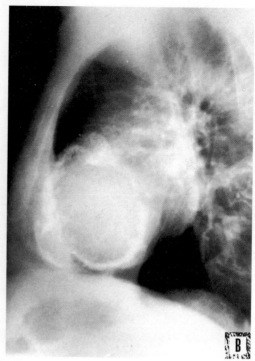
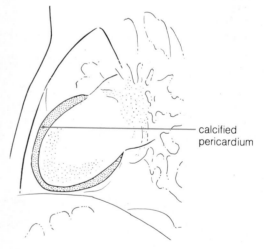

FIGURE 9.29   (**A**) Postero-anterior chest radiograph of a patient with calcific pericarditis. The calcified pericardium is not clearly shown. (**B**) Lateral view demonstrates the calcified pericardium surrounding the heart. The etiology was never established; however, tuberculous pericarditis was suspected. (Reproduced with permission; see Figure Credits)

calcified pericardium

Echocardiography   The echocardiogram may reveal evidence of pericardial calcification and clues to the presence of constrictive pericarditis (Fig. 9.30).

Cardiac Catheterization   Cardiac catheterization reveals equalization of the pulmonary arterial wedge pressure, diastolic pulmonary arterial pressure, diastolic right ventricular pressure, and right atrial mean pressure. The right ventricular pressure curve shows an early diastolic dip and late diastolic plateau (see Fig. 9.26).

Other Imaging Modalities   The thickened, constricting pericardium can be clearly visualized by magnetic resonance imaging (Fig. 9.31).

DIFFERENTIAL DIAGNOSIS

Constrictive pericarditis must be differentiated from cirrhosis of the liver, chronic cor pulmonale, chronic right ventricular failure, and restrictive cardiomyopathy by the techniques described above. It may not be possible, however, to differentiate restrictive cardiomyopathy from constrictive peri-

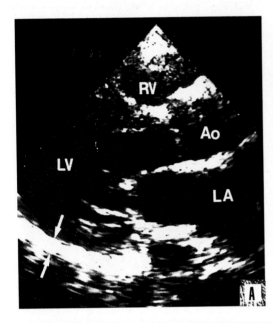
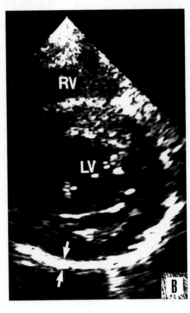
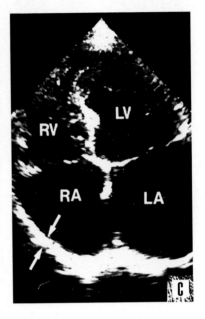

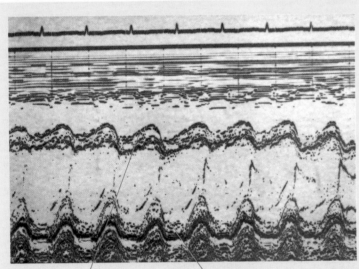

abnormal septal motion following P wave   squaring off of posterior wall

FIGURE 9.30   Cross-sectional echocardiograms in a patient with pericardial calcification demonstrating an increase in the intensity and width of the pericardial echo (opposing arrows) in each of the standard views: **(A)** parasternal long-axis view; **(B)** parasternal short-axis view; **(C)** apical four-chamber view. **(D)** M-mode echocardiogram from a patient with constrictive pericarditis following radiation to the mediastinum for malignancy. Septal motion is abnormal beginning after the P wave. The posterior wall abruptly squares off in diastole as filling of the ventricle is limited by the scarred pericardium. (LV = left ventricle; RV = right ventricle; Ao = aorta; LA = left atrium; RA = right atrium). (Reproduced with permission; see Figure Credits)

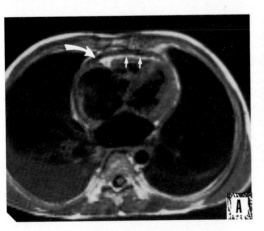
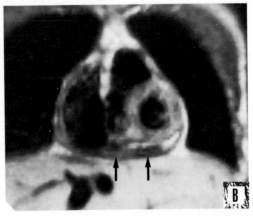

FIGURE 9.31   Transverse **(A)** and coronal **(B)** MR images of a patient with constrictive pericarditis. The thickened pericardium is visible as a low-signal intensity line (curved arrow) between the high-intensity regions produced by pericardial and epicardial fat (small arrows). There are pleural effusions bilaterally. Note the thick pericardium along the diaphragmatic surface of the heart. (Reproduced with permission; see Figure Credits)

rditis;[6,11] an exploratory thoracotomy may be necessary. Endocardial biopsy ay identify myocardial disease.[20]

NATURAL HISTORY

'ithout surgical intervention the patient with constrictive pericarditis shows ow progressive deterioration with the development of atrial filbrillation, car-ac cirrhosis, nephrosis, and all of the consequences of low cardiac output.

Congenital Absence of the Pericardium

ccasionally, partial or total absence of the pericardium occurs. The partial efects are usually left-sided; 30% of these patients will have associated con-

genital cardiac defects. Patients may complain of nonspecific, left-sided chest pain. ECG changes relate to a leftward shift of the heart. The diagnosis is often suggested by the chest x-ray (Fig. 9.32). Confirmation of the diagnosis is usually made by echocardiographic examination.

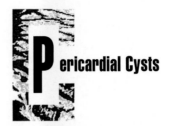

Pericardial Cysts

Pericardial cysts are rare developmental anomalies usually located at the right costophrenic angle; occasionally they are noted at the cardiac apex. The cysts are usually unilocular and filled with clear fluid. They are usually unaccompanied by any clinical symptoms and are discovered by chance during a chest x-ray. Computed tomography or magnetic resonance imaging will usually confirm the diagnosis (Fig. 9.33).

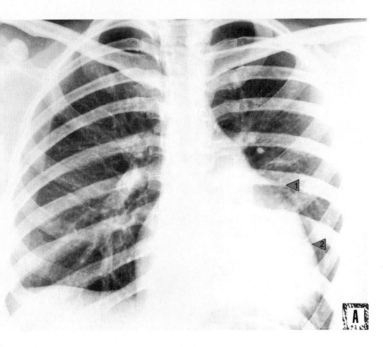

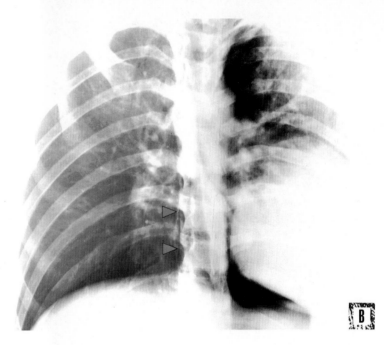

IGURE 9.32 Congenital absence of the left pericardium. **(A)** In the rontal projection, the heart is displaced to the left and the left heart border ies close to the lateral chest wall. The left atrial appendage *(arrow 1)* and left ventricular contour *(arrow 2)* are clearly seen in this decubitus projection

that was obtained after injection of air into the pleural space. Air has entered the pericardial space through the defect in the left pericardium and outlines the intact right pericardium *(arrows).* (Reproduced with permission; see Figure Credits)

FIGURE 9.33 Coronal MR image demonstrating pericardial cyst adjacent to the left ventricle (LV). A simple cyst with low protein content produces low MR signal intensity. (Reproduced with permission; see Figure Credits)

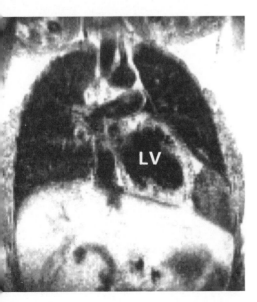

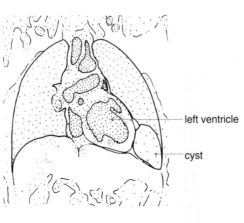

ACKNOWLEDGMENT

This chapter is based in part on Shabetai R: Diseases of the pericardium. In Hurst JW (ed): The Heart, 6th ed. McGraw-Hill, New York, 1986.

FIGURE CREDITS

Figs. 9.1, 9.11, 9.13 from Hurst JW (ed): The Heart, 6th ed. McGraw-Hill, New York, 1986. Fig. 9.1 has been modified.

Figs. 9.2–9.4, 9.19, 9.23, 9.29, 9.30A–D from Hurst JW (ed): Atlas of the Heart. Gower, New York, 1988.

Figs. 9.5, 9.9, 9.22 from Becker AE, Anderson RH: Cardiac Pathology. Raven Press, New York, 1983.

Figs. 9.6, 9.8, 9.17, 9.18, 9.28, 9.31, 9.33 from Chatterjee K, et al: Cardiology: An Illustrated Text–Reference. Gower, New York, 1992.

Figs. 9.7, 9.24, 9.25, 9.27 redrawn from Sabetai R: The Pericardium. Grune & Stratton, New York, 1981.

Fig. 9.10 redrawn from Holt JP: The normal pericardium. Am J Cardiol 26:455, 1970.

Figs. 9.12, 9.14, 9.32 from Kassner EG: Atlas of Radiologic Imaging. Gower, New York, 1989.

Fig. 9.15 redrawn from Surawicz B, Lasseter KC: Electrocardiogram in pericarditis. Am J Cardiol 26:472, 1970.

Figs. 9.12, 9.16, 9.21, 9.30A–C courtesy of Joel M. Felner, MD, Atlanta, GA.

Fig. 9.19 courtesy of Murray Baron, MD, Atlanta, GA.

Fig. 9.20 redrawn from Sabiston DC (ed): Gibbon's Surgery of the Chest, 4th ed. WB Saunders, Philadelphia, 1983.

Fig. 9.26 redrawn from Grossman W (ed): Cardiac Catheterization and Angiography, 2nd ed. Lea & Febiger, Philadelphia, 1980.

Fig. 9.29 courtesy of Stephen D. Clements, Jr, MD, and William J. Casarella, MD, Atlanta, GA.

Fig. 9.30D courtesy of Stephen D. Clements, Jr, MD.

REFERENCES

1. Anand IS, Rerrari R, Kalra GS, et al: Pathogenesis of edema in constrictive pericarditis—Studies of body water and sodium, renal function, hemodynamics, and plasma hormones before and after pericardiectomy. Circulation 83:1880, 1991.

2. Andrews GWS, Pickering GW, Sellors TH: The aetiology of constrictive pericarditis with special reference to tuberculosis pericarditis, together with a note on polyserositis. Q J Med 17:291, 1948.

3. Beck CS: Two cardiac compression triads. JAMA 104:714, 1935.

4. Burchell HB: Problems in the recognition and treatment of pericarditis. Lanc 74;465, 1954.

5. Chuttani K, Pandian NG, Mohanty PK, et al: Left ventricular diastolic collapse: A echocardiographic sign of regional cardiac tamponade. Circulation 83:1999, 1991.

6. Cohn JN, Pinkerson AL, Tristani FE: Mechanism of pulsus paradoxus in clinic shock. J Clin Invest 46:1744, 1967.

7. Gilliam LD, Guyer DE, Gibson TC, et al: Hemodynamic compression of the right atr um, a new echocardiographic sign of cardiac tamponade. Circulation 68:294, 1983.

8. Goodwin JF, Oakley CM: The cardiomyopathies. Br Heart J 34:345, 1972.

9. Haaz WS, Mintz GS, Kotler MN, et al: Two-dimensional echocardiographic recogn tion of the descending thoracic aorta: Value in differentiating pericardial from pleu effusion. Am J Cardiol 46:739, 1980.

10. Hancock EW: Subacute effusive–constrictive pericarditis. Circulation 43:183, 1971.

11. Hoit BD, Gabel M, Fowler NO: Cardiac tamponade in left ventricular dysfunctio Circulation 82:1370, 1990.

12. Holt JP: The normal pericardium. Am J Cardiol 26:455, 1970.

13. Leimgruber PP, Klopfenstein HS, Wann LS, et al: The hemodynamic derangeme associated with right ventricular diastolic collapse in cardiac tamponade: An exper mental echocardiographic study. Circulation 68:612, 1983.

14. Levine MJ, Lorell BH, Diver DJ, et al: Implications of echocardiographically assiste diagnosis of pericardial tamponade in contemporary medical patients: Detectic before hemodynamic embarrassment. J Am Coll Cardiol 17:59, 1991.

15. Meany E, Shabetai R, Bhargava V, et al: Cardiac amyloidosis, constrictive pericardi and restrictive cardiomyopathy. Am J Cardiol 38:547, 1976.

16. Reddy PS, Curtiss EI, Uretsky BF: Spectrum of hemodynamic changes in cardi tamponade. Am J Cardiol 66:1487, 1990.

17. Spodick DH: Acoustic phenomena in pericardial disease. Am Heart J 812:11 1971.

18. Spodick DH: Diagnostic electrocardiographic sequences in acute pericarditi Significance of PR segment and PR vector changes. Circulation 48:575, 1973.

19. Spodick DH: Frequency of arrythmias in acute pericarditis determined by Holte monitoring. Am J Cardiol 53:842, 1984.

20. Swanton RH, Brooksby IAB, Davies MJ, et al: Systolic and diastolic ventricul function in cardiac amyloidosis. Am J Cardiol 39:658, 1977.

21. Teicholz LE: Echocardiographic evaluation of pericardial diseases. Prog Cardiovas Dis 21:133, 1978.

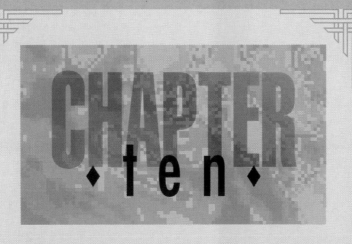

CHAPTER •ten•

HEART DISEASE DUE TO LUNG DISEASE AND PULMONARY HYPERTENSION

CHRONIC COR PULMONALE

J. WILLIS HURST, MD
JOSEPH C. ROSS, MD
JOHN F. NEWMAN, MD
ANTON E. BECKER, MD
JOSEPH S. ALPERT, MD

PULMONARY EMBOLISM

J. WILLIS HURST, MD
JAMES E. DALEN, MD
JOSEPH S. ALPERT, MD
ANTON E. BECKER, MD

PRIMARY PULMONARY HYPERTENSION

J. WILLIS HURST, MD
HIROSHI KUIDA, MD
ANTON E. BECKER, MD

This chapter deals with three pulmonary problems that may produce heart disease: chronic lung disease of various types; pulmonary embolism; and primary pulmonary hypertension.

Chronic Cor Pulmonale

The term *chronic cor pulmonale* is used to designate the effect of chronic lung disease on the right side of the heart. Many different types of chronic lung disease cause chronic cor pulmonale; the common denominator is pulmonary hypertension and its effect on the right ventricle. The term *cor pulmonale* should not be applied to right-sided heart disease due to congenital heart disease, to diseases causing elevation of the left atrial pressure, or to primary pulmonary hypertension.

ETIOLOGY AND PATHOLOGY

Emphysema and chronic bronchitis cause at least half of the cases of chronic cor pulmonale in the United States. In turn cor pulmonale is responsible for about 20% to 30% of hospital admissions for heart faillure. The condition occurs more frequently in males who smoke tobacco and who are between the ages of 50 and 60 years. The major causes of chronic cor pulmonale are shown in Figure 10.1.

In pulmonary emphysema the main pathologic features are loss of elasticity, accompanied by destruction of the wall of the terminal bronchioli in the case of centrilobular emphysema (Fig. 10.2) or of the distal terminal airways in the case of panacinar emphysema. As a result, air spaces are dilated and the total alveolar surface area is decreased. Alveolar hypoxia underlies constriction of the arterioles, which is often accompanied by a longitudinally oriented smooth-muscle cell proliferation within the intima (Fig. 10.3). Under these circumstances pulmonary hypertension may result. In long-standing disease the major pulmonary arteries often display atherosclerosis (Fig. 10.4), a hugely dilated pulmonary trunk, and a markedly enlarged right heart (Fig. 10.5). Right ventricular wall hypertrophy is often accompanied by dilation of the chamber, leading to a marked distortion of ventricular geometry (Fig. 10.6). The ventricular septum is "pushed" toward the left side, thereby distorting the left ventricular contour (Fig. 10.7). Under such circumstances myocardial ischemia and infarction may occur despite minimal obstructive coronary atherosclerotic disease.

PATHOPHYSIOLOGY
NORMAL PULMONARY CIRCULATION

The pulmonary vascular system in a healthy person receives the entire cardiac output in order to permit the exchange of O_2 and CO_2 between the capillaries and the alveolar spaces. The normal mean pulmonary arterial pressure is about 12 to 17 mmHg. The pulmonary vascular resistance is 10- to 20-fold less than the vascular resistance in the systemic circuit. This is possible because (1) the pulmonary arteries are thin-walled with little resting muscle tone, (2) there is little vasomotor control by the autonomic nervous system in adults, and (3) many arterioles and capillaries are nonperfused at rest but are recruited as needed.

FIGURE 10.1 ETIOLOGIES OF CHRONIC COR PULMONALE BY MECHANISM PULMONARY HYPERTENSION

Hypoxic vasoconstriction
Chronic bronchitis and emphysema, cystic fibrosis
Chronic hypoventilation
Obesity
Sleep apnea
Neuromuscular disease
Chest wall dysfunction
High-altitude dwelling and chronic mountain sickness

Occlusion of the pulmonary vascular bed
Pulmonary thromboembolism, parasitic ova, tumor emboli
Veno-occlusive disease
Pulmonary angiitis from systemic diseas
Collagen vascular diseases
Drug-induced lung disease

Parenchymal disease with destruction of vascular surface area
Chronic bronchitis and emphysema
Bronchiectasis, cystic fibrosis
Diffuse interstitial disease
Pneumoconioses
Sarcoid, idiopathic pulmonary fibrosis, histiocytosis X
Tuberculosis, chronic fungal infection
Collagen vascular diseases

(Reproduced with permission; see Figure Credits)

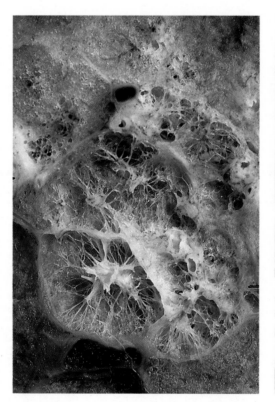

FIGURE 10.2   Gross aspect of a lung with pulmonary emphysema. Note the centrally dilated air spaces surrounded by a rim of less affected parenchyma; this is a classic example of centrilobular emphysema. (Reproduced with permission; see Figure Credits)

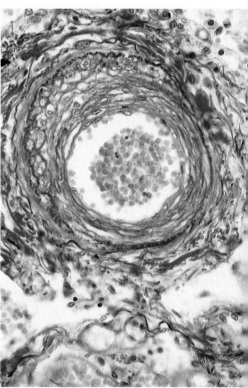

FIGURE 10.3   Histologic section of a pulmonary arteriole depicting eccentric intimal thickening due to proliferation of longitudinally oriented smooth muscle cells. This is often seen in hypoxic pulmonary hypertension (elastic tissue stain). (Reproduced with permission; see Figure Credits)

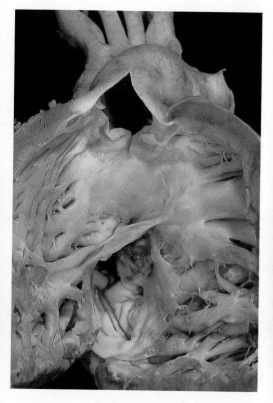

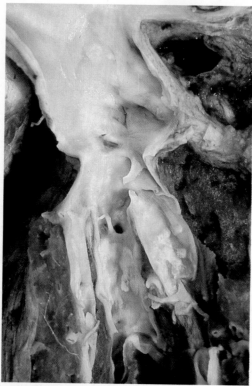

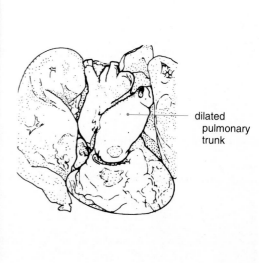

dilated
pulmonary
trunk

FIGURE 10.4   Central pulmonary artery and its main branches displaying extensive atherosclerosis due to long-standing pulmonary hypertension. (Reproduced with permission; see Figure Credits)

FIGURE 10.5   Heart–lung specimen from a patient with chronic cor pulmonale. Note the dilated pulmonary trunk and the markedly increased size of the right heart. (Reproduced with permission; see Figure Credits)

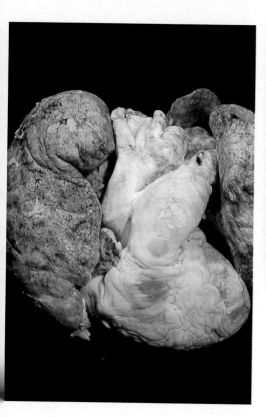

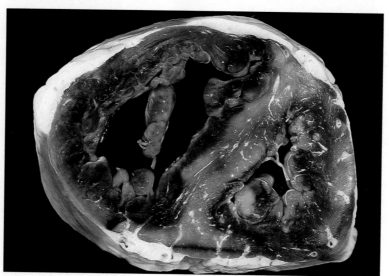

FIGURE 10.7   Cross section of a heart from a patient who had long-standing pulmonary hypertension. Note the massive right ventricular wall hypertrophy with a displaced ventricular septum, which distorts left ventricular geometry. Diffuse, patchy myocardial infarction (pale-staining areas) contrasts with the dark-blue zones of viable myocardium (macroenzyme staining technique). (Reproduced with permission; see Figure Credits)

myocardial infarction
right ventricular wall hypertrophy

displaced ventricular septum
viable myocardium

FIGURE 10.6   Right side of the heart opened to show marked right ventricular hypertrophy and a dilated right ventricular chamber in a case of chronic cor pulmonale. (Reproduced with permission; see Figure Credits)

Different factors may cause dilation and constriction of the pulmonary arterioles (Fig. 10.8). Hypoxia is the most important clinical cause of vasoconstriction (Fig. 10.9).

Other factors may elevate the pulmonary arterial blood pressure (Fig. 10.10). When a large area of the lungs is reduced because of pulmonary disease, there is an increase in cardiac output, heart rate, and blood volume, which increases the pulmonary arterial pressure. Acidosis, increased blood viscosity, and left ventricular failure also increase the likelihood of pulmonary hypertension. Pulmonary hypertension due to hypoxia leads to irreversible pulmonary hypertension due to the gradual increase in the muscular component of the arterioles; this elevates the resting pulmonary arterial pressure and also the vasoconstrictive response to stimuli.

RESPONSE OF THE HEART TO PULMONARY HYPERTENSION

The right ventricle, because of its thin wall and relatively large radius of curvature, tolerates a volume load better than it tolerates a pressure load. The hypoxia of chronic lung disease leads to chronic pulmonary hypertension, which in turn leads to right ventricular dilation, hypertrophy, and eventually heart failure. Modifying factors include alteration in ventilatory function, alteration in the degree of hypoxia, hypercapnia, acidosis, and alteration in volume load on the right ventricle.

Left ventricular dysfunction may also occur as a result of chronic lung disease. The cause is unclear and has been the stimulus for much investigation. In most

---

FIGURE 10.8 PULMONARY VASOMOTOR TONE

DILATOR	CONSTRICTOR
Beta-adrenergic agonists	Alpha-adrenergic agonists
Histamine H_2	Histamine H_1
Prostacyclin (PGI$_2$)	PGE$_2$, PGF$_{2\alpha}$, thromboxane A$_2$
Acetylcholine	Serotonin
O$_2$	Hypoxia
Bradykinin	Angiotensin II

(Reproduced with permission; see Figure Credits)

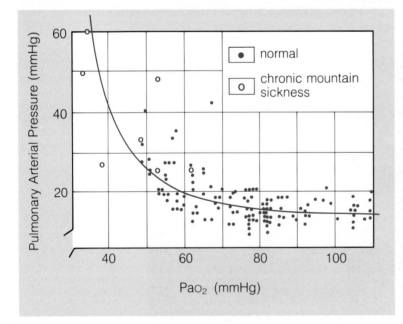

FIGURE 10.9　Pulmonary arterial pressure as a function of Pao$_2$ in healthy residents of cities of different altitudes and in patients with chronic mountain sickness. Pulmonary arterial pressure rises steeply as Pao$_2$, decreases below 55 torr. (Reproduced with permission; see Figure Credits)

FIGURE 10.10 MECHANISMS AND CAUSES OF PULMONARY HYPERTENSION

MECHANISMS	CLINICAL CAUSES
Increased pulmonary blood flow	Left-to-right shunts
	Increased cardiac output
	Bronchiectasis
Increased blood viscosity	Polycythemia
Decreased radius of pulmonary arterial bed	
Loss of vessels	Pneumonectomy
Luminal narrowing	
Anatomical	Embolism
	Emphysema
	Embolism
	Chronic hypoxia
	Thoracic deformity
	Vasculitis
	Neoplasm
	Fibrosis
	Inflammation
	Infiltration
Vasoconstrictive	Hypoxia
	Acidosis
	Toxins
	Primary pulmonary hypertension
Increased pulmonary venous pressure	Left atrial hypertension
	Venous thrombosis
	Mediastinitis
	Veno-occlusive disease
Increased intrathoracic pressure	Chronic obstructive pulmonary disease

(Reproduced with permission; see Figure Credits)

---

instances dysfunction is due to some other cause of left ventricular disease, such as unrecognized coronary artery disease. However, right ventricular dysfunction and failure alone can produce mild abnormalities in left ventricular systolic and diastolic function. Regardless of the cause, chronic left ventricular failure aggravates pulmonary arterial hypertension and right ventricular dysfunction. In the minority of patients with chronic cor pulmonale there is evidence of left ventricular dysfunction, with no evidence of primary left ventricular disease. There is some evidence that right ventricular hypertrophy and elevation of the end-diastolic pressure of the right ventricle may reduce left ventricular compliance. In addition, the wide swing in transpulmonary pressure in patients with obstructive lung disease may result in a decrease in left ventricular filling and an increase in left ventricular after load.

Peripheral edema occurs in some, but not all, patients with chronic cor pulmonale. The mechanism of production of edema is not clear, but it is related to increased venous pressure, an increase in P_{CO_2}, and a decrease in P_{O_2}. Once the liver is congested, there is a decrease in the clearance of aldosterone. Pleural effusion and pulmonary edema are not a consequence of cor pulmonale.

CLINICAL MANIFESTATIONS

The initial diagnostic problem is to identify the presence and the type of chronic lung disease. The next step is to search for clues to the diagnosis of the heart disease that results from the lung disease.

SYMPTOMS

The physician must remember that heart failure or chronic hypoxia may occur in any patient with pulmonary hypertension. Heart failure is often overlooked because it occurs gradually and imperceptibly. There is no history that is specific for heart failure in patients with cor pulmonale, but the development of heart failure should be considered whenever there is an increase in dyspnea in a patient with chronic lung disease.

PHYSICAL EXAMINATION

The pulmonary component of the second sound may be accentuated. An anterior lift of the sternum may be detected during systole, except when severe pulmonary emphysema prevents it from being observed. Abnormal right ventricular movement may be felt in the epigastrium when severe emphysema is present. The neck veins may be abnormally distended, and they may reveal the systolic wave form of tricuspid regurgitation (V waves). Peripheral edema may also be present. While cyanosis may be evident, the extremities may be warm because of peripheral arteriolar dilation due to hypercapnia.

LABORATORY STUDIES

Chest Radiography   Evidence of pulmonary disease and pulmonary hypertension is seen on chest films (Fig. 10.11). Pulmonary hypertension should be suspected when there is enlargement of the pulmonary trunk and its right and left branches, or when the right descending pulmonary artery is greater than 16 mm in diameter. The heart may not be increased in size when viewed in the anteroposterior projection, while the right ventricle may or may not appear to be enlarged when viewed in the left lateral projection.

Electrocardiography   The classic signs of right ventricular hypertrophy are usually not evident in the electrocardiogram (ECG) in patients with cor pulmonale due to parenchymal pulmonary lung disease, such as emphysema and chronic bronchitis. The classic signs of right ventricular hypertrophy are generally limited to conditions associated with an anatomic restriction of the pulmonary arteriolar vascular bed. ECGs of patients with chronic cor pulmonale due to emphysema and chronic bronchitis may reveal low QRS voltage, right atrial abnormalities of the P waves, and right-axis deviation of the mean QRS vector. Right bundle branch block may be present, and atrial and ventricular arrhythmias may occur. When the electrical field is distorted by emphysema, the mean QRS vector may be superiorly directed. Poor R-wave progression is often noted in the precordial leads.

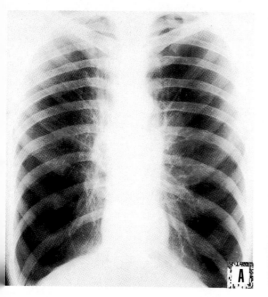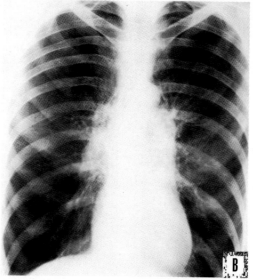

FIGURE 10.11   **(A)** Chest film of a patient with severe obstructive emphysema. Overaeration of the lungs, a centralized flow pattern, and a small heart size are present. **(B)** Three years later the same patient was in frank right-sided heart failure. The heart enlarged as the emphysema worsened, and the centralized flow pattern became more severe. (Reproduced with permission; see Figure Credits)

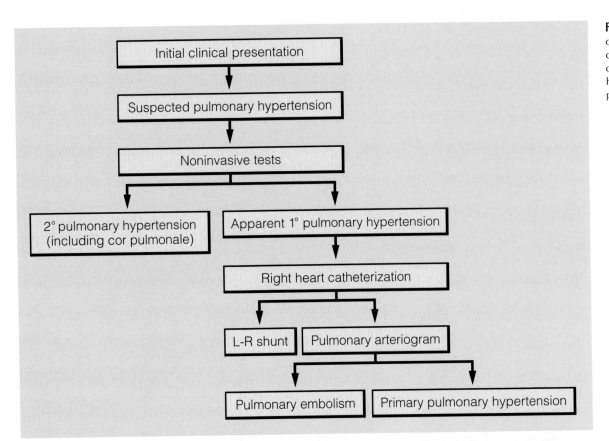

FIGURE 10.12 Interrelation of noninvasive testing and cardiac catheterization in the evaluation of patients with pulmonary hypertension. (Reproduced with permission; see Figure Credits)

FIGURE 10.13 POSSIBLE SOURCES OF PULMONARY EMBOLI

Thromboembolism
  Deep veins of the thigh
  Prostatic or pelvic veins
  Vena cava, renal veins, hepatic veins
  Right atrium or ventricle
  Right-sided artificial valves
  Venous filters, ventriculoatrial shunts
Amniotic fluid and debris
Bone marrow and fat
Right atrial myxomata and other right-sided tumors
Malignancies invading the systemic venous circuit,
  especially hypernephroma
Right-sided valvular vegetations
Parasites
Talc and other debris used in illicit intravenous drugs
Catheter fragments
Right-sided artificial valve fragments
Air introduced with central venous catheterization or
  from traumatic venous laceration

(Reproduced with permission; see Figure Credits)

FIGURE 10.14 PREDISPOSITION TO VENOUS THROMBOSIS

"VIRCHOW'S TRIAD"	PRECIPITATING CAUSES
Endothelial injury	Trauma
	Inflammation
	Infection
	Hemodynamic stress
	Ischemia
Blood stasis	Immobility
	Obesity
	Heart failure
Hypercoagulable state	Pregnancy
	Oral contraceptives
	Cancer
	Polycythemia
	Nephrotic syndrome
	Thrombocytosis
	Sickle cell disease
	Deficiencies
	Antithrombin III
	Protein C or S
	Fibrin
	Plasminogen
	Plasminogen activator
	Lupus anticoagulant
	Paroxysmal nocturnal hemoglobinuria
	Thrombotic thrombocytopenic purpura
	Heparin-induced thrombocytopenia
	Diabetes mellitus
	Hyperlipidemia
	Homocystinuria

(Reproduced with permission; see Figure Credits)

Other Laboratory Studies The *echocardiogram* is often not useful in assessing the function of the right ventricle in patients with cor pulmonale because of difficulty in visualizing the heart.

The *first-pass radionuclear angiogram* using technetium-99m (^{99m}Tc) reveals a decrease in right ventricular ejection fraction.

Cardiac catheterization reveals an increase in diastolic pulmonary arterial pressure. The wedge pressure in such patients is significantly lower than the diastolic pulmonary arterial pressure; this excludes left ventricular failure as the cause of the pulmonary hypertension. The pulmonary arterial pressure may be severely elevated when patients have obliterative arteriolar disease, but it is only moderately increased when the pulmonary hypertension is due to disease of the lung parenchyma. The pressure may rise abruptly, however, when there is superimposed hypoxemia or when the patient exercises.

An algorithm for the evaluation of a patient with pulmonary hypertension is presented in Figure 10.12.

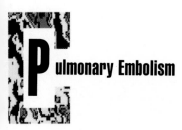

Pulmonary Embolism

Pulmonary embolism is a common problem that is often undiagnosed.

ETIOLOGY AND PATHOLOGY

Pulmonary emboli can originate from a variety of sources and conditions (Fig. 10.13). Most pulmonary emboli originate as thrombi in the proximal deep venous system of the legs. The risk factors favoring deep venous thrombosis were first identified by the 19th century pathologist Rudolph L. K. Virchow (1821–1902) (Fig. 10.14). Accordingly, the prevention of pulmonary emboli is achieved by preventing deep venous thrombosis (Fig. 10.15). Certain operative procedures are more likely to be complicated by deep venous thrombosis, including hip replacement, hip fractures, and urological procedures. The thrombi begin to develop in the venous system while the patient is anesthetized in the operating room. Accordingly, prophylactic treatment should begin prior to the use of anesthesia.[5]

DIAGNOSIS OF DEEP VENOUS THROMBOSIS

The minority of patients with deep venous thrombosis have swelling of the leg; however, physical signs of the condition are not commonly present. Venography or noninvasive tests must be used to identify the condition. Since such tests are not performed without indications, deep vein thrombosis is underdiagnosed.

Venography is the most sensitive and specific test. Scanning of the legs injected with ^{125}iodine-labeled fibrinogen, the Doppler technique, and impedance plethysmography (IPG) are also useful when properly performed.

DIAGNOSIS OF ACUTE PULMONARY EMBOLISM

Acute pulmonary embolism may produce three clinical syndromes: acute, unexplained dyspnea; acute cor pulmonale; and pulmonary infarction (Fig. 10.16).

ACUTE, UNEXPLAINED DYSPNEA

Pulmonary embolism does not produce acute cor pulmonale unless approximately 50% to 60% of the pulmonary circulation is obstructed. Accordingly, pulmonary embolism may not produce abnormalities detectable on the ECG or on physical examination of the lungs. When pulmonary infarction does not occur, pleuritic chest pain and abnormalities on the chest radiograph are absent. Pulmonary embolism may be difficult to diagnose, since the only clue to its occurrence may be an acute episode of dyspnea. The physician may consider acute left ventricular failure, pneumonia, or anxiety in the differential diagnosis of patients with acute dyspnea. The existence of a clinical setting where deep venous thrombosis is likely to occur should always stimulate the physician to consider the possibility of pulmonary embolism. Left ventricular failure and pneumonia can usually be identified by abnormalities elicited from further

---

FIGURE 10.15 PREVENTION OF DEEP VENOUS THROMBOSIS

Anticoagulation
    Low-dose subcutaneous heparin
    Warfarin
Platelet-active agents
    Aspirin
    Dextran
Other agents
    Dihydroergotamine
Prevention of venous stasis
    Graded compression stockings
    Intermittent pneumatic compression

(Reproduced with permission; see Figure Credits)

FIGURE 10.16 SYNDROMES OF ACUTE PULMON EMBOLISM

Acute, Unexplained Dyspnea
    Dyspnea, tachypnea, most
      often hypoxemia

Pulmonary Infarction
    Pleurisy, cough, hemoptysis
    Mild fever and leukocytosis
    Pulmonary infiltrate and effusion
    Usually hypoxemia

Acute Cor Pulmonale Failure
    Dyspnea, tachypnea,
      hypoxemia
    Central venous hypertension
    Angina-like chest pain
    Possible syncope or
      cardiogenic shock

(Reproduced with permission; see Figure Credits)

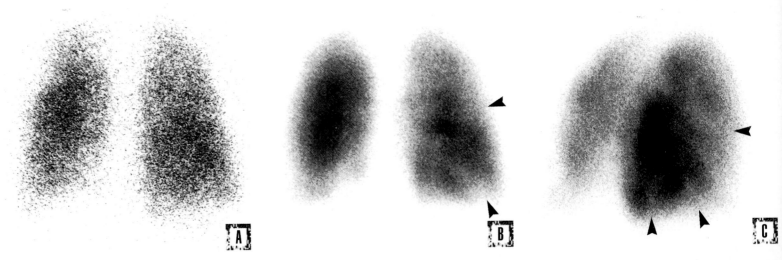

FIGURE 10.17   Ventilation/perfusion scan of a patient with chest pain. **(A)** Posterior view of a ventilation scan is normal. **(B)** Posterior view of a perfusion scan shows subsegmental defects (*arrows*). **(C)** Right posterior view of a perfusion scan shows multiple subsegmental defects (*arrows*). (Reproduced with permission; see Figure Credits)

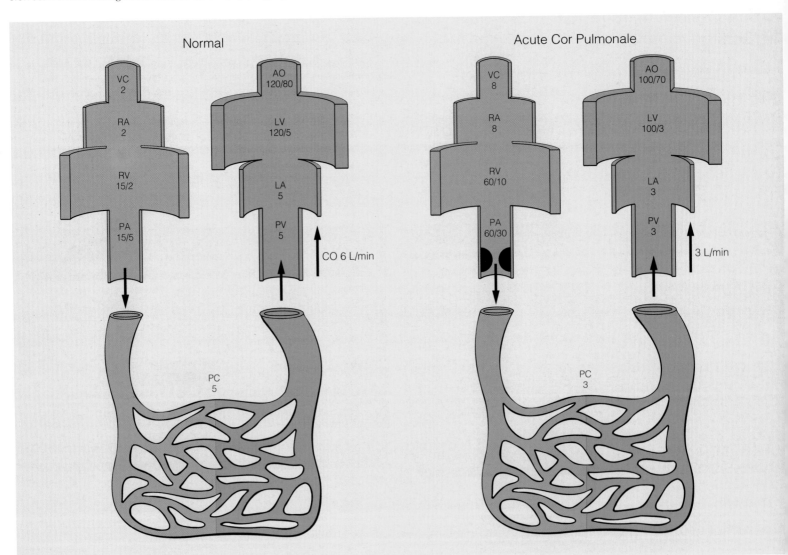

FIGURE 10.18   Pathophysiology of acute cor pulmonale secondary to pulmonary embolism. The sudden increase in pulmonary resistance, which occurs secondary to pulmonary embolism, produces marked right ventricular (RV) systolic and pulmonary arterial hypertension, increasing these pressures to approximately 60 mmHg. The RV dilates, increasing RV diastolic pressure. This rise in pressure is transmitted to the right atrium (RA) and central veins, which also exhibit an increase in pressure. There is a fall in blood flow distal to the pulmonary embolism, and consequently, left heart pressures—pulmonary capillary (PC), pulmonary venous (PV), left atrial (LA), and left ventricular (LV) diastolic pressures—decrease. The decrease in LV loading results in a fall in LV systolic pressure. RV decompensation results in a decreased RV stroke volume, which in turn produces a fall in LV stroke volume. (V = vena cava; PO = pulmonary artery; CO = cardiac output; AO = aorta) (Redrawn with permission; see Figure Credits)

history, physical examination, and chest radiography. Hyperventilation related to anxiety is associated with a decrease in arterial Pco_2 and normal Po_2. The diagnosis of pulmonary embolism can be confirmed with a ventilation/perfusion lung scan (Fig. 10.17).[6,8]

ACUTE COR PULMONALE

Acute cor pulmonale occurs when more than 60% to 75% of the pulmonary circulation is obstructed by pulmonary embolism. Such a catastrophe leads to an increase in the systolic pressure of the right ventricle, which dilates when the systolic pressure is increased beyond 50 to 60 mmHg. When this occurs, the right ventricle fails, the stroke output diminishes, and the cardiac output and the systolic blood pressure fall (Fig. 10.18).

The patient may experience acute dyspnea, syncope, or sudden death (Fig. 10.19). Tachycardia, tachypnea, and hypotension usually occur. The neck veins are distended, and a right ventricular S_3 gallop may be heard. An abnormal anterior movement of the sternal area due to dilation of the right ventricle is often present. Signs of deep venous thrombosis may or may not be apparent.

The ECG may show the $S_1Q_3T_3$ pattern described by McGinn and White[3] (Fig. 10.20). These electrocardiographic abnormalities may simulate inferior myocardial infarction. Anterior ST–T changes may be noted and may be confused with an acute coronary event. Incomplete right bundle branch block or atrial arrhythmias may occur.

When hypotension is present, the central venous pressure and the right atrial pressure are usually elevated. Myocardial infarction or hypovolemia are more likely to be present when hypotension is associated with normal right atrial and central venous pressures.

The arterial Po_2 and Pco_2 are abnormally diminished in patients with acute cor pulmonale. A ventilation/perfusion scan reveals the pulmonary embolism in almost all instances (see Fig. 10.17).[2] Pulmonary angiography may be needed when the diagnosis remains uncertain (Fig. 10.21).

FIGURE 10.19
Symptoms experienced with acute cor pulmonale.

```
Massive pulmonary embolism
        ↓
Acute right ventricular failure
        ↓
↓Stroke volume
        ↓
↓Cardiac output
        ↓
Hypotension or frank shock
        ↓
↓Cerebral blood flow
        ↓
Syncope or death
```

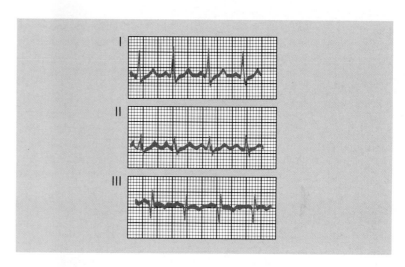

FIGURE 10.20   ECG recorded 2 hours after an attack of pulmonary embolism. Note the S wave in lead I and Q wave and inverted T waves in lead III. At times this abnormality simulates inferior myocardial infarction. (Reproduced with permission; see Figure Credits)

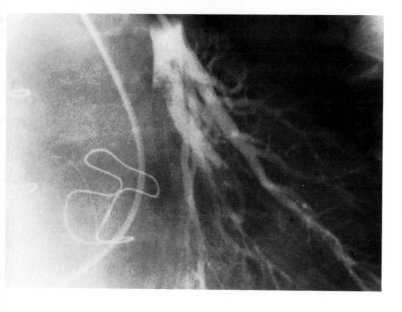

FIGURE 10.21   Balloon–occlusion pulmonary arteriogram demonstrating intraluminal filling defects and cut-offs in the lower lobe vessels. These defects were poorly demonstrated on nonselective pulmonary arteriograms. (Reproduced with permission; see Figure Credits)

PULMONARY INFARCTION

The diagnosis of pulmonary embolism is most frequently made when the complication of pulmonary infarction is recognized.

Patients with pulmonary venous congestion, such as those with mitral stenosis or following myocardial infarction, are particularly susceptible to pulmonary infarction (Fig. 10.22). Pulmonary emboli in middle-sized pulmonary arteries do not necessarily lead to infarcts because of collateral blood supply. The same mechanism underlies the hemorrhagic nature of the infarct, once it occurs. Fibrinous pleuritis is a reactive phenomenon to the infarcted lung.

Pulmonary infarction should be suspected when the patient experiences pleuritic chest pain. Dyspnea and hemoptysis may or may not be present. The physical examination may reveal tachypnea, rales, pulmonary wheezes, pleural friction rub, pleural effusion, and evidence of deep venous thrombosis. The chest radiograph may show an elevation of the diaphragm on one side, a small pleural effusion, or a pulmonary infiltrate.

This condition must be separated from pulmonary infection. The sputum examination, white blood cell count, and differential all aid in the identification of infection of the lung. The arterial Pco_2 may be diminished, while the arterial Po_2 may be normal. Pulmonary angiography may be needed when the diagnosis remains uncertain.

LABORATORY STUDIES

The chest film, the ECG, arterial blood gases, ventilation/perfusion lung scans (Fig. 10.23), and pulmonary angiography are useful in the diagnosis of pulmonary embolism and infarction. An echocardiogram should be performed on patients with pulmonary embolism; a thrombus may be lodged in the right side of the heart, and emboli may be fed to the lung from that site. Magnetic resonance imaging can, on occasion, disclose pulmonary embolism (Fig. 10.24).

PULMONARY EMBOLISM AND CANCER

The patient with pulmonary embolism, with or without infarction, should be screened for cancer of the gastrointestinal tract, pancreas, lung, breast, uterus, and prostate, since venous thrombosis and pulmonary emboli may occur as a consequence of all these diseases. Such patients may have thrombophlebitis migrans of the arms, although deep venous thrombosis is more common.

Primary Pulmonary Hypertension

Pulmonary hypertension is a secondary event in most patients. The conditions that are responsible for it include (1) lesions that produce elevated left atrial pressure, such as mitral stenosis, (2) heart failure with elevated left ventricular diastolic pressure, (3) congenital heart disease with a left-to-right shunt and pulmonary vascular disease, and (4) pulmonary disease of various types. Primary pulmonary hypertension, which affects a small percentage of patients with pulmonary hypertension, usually has no identifiable cause (see Fig. 10.10).

ETIOLOGY AND PATHOLOGY

The etiology of primary pulmonary hypertension is unknown. Predisposing factors are the female gender, pregnancy (suggesting a relationship to amniotic fluid or thromboplastin-induced fibrin emboli), Raynaud's phenomenon (suggesting a relationship to collagen disease), family history (suggesting a genetic predetermination), and ingestion of drugs, such as aminorex and colsa oil (implicating environmental factors). An unknown number of patients with primary pulmonary hypertension have silent pulmonary emboli.[4,7]

In the vast majority of patients with secondary pulmonary hypertension, a firm diagnosis can be made. In a minority of patients the clinician may have great difficulties in establishing the precise cause of the pulmonary hypertension. Three conditions should be taken into consideration. First, chronic silent pulmonary emboli may eventually lead to increased pulmonary vascular resistance and pulmonary hypertension. Since most patients with this abnormality show no signs of venous thrombosis or other signs indicative of a chronic thrombotic process, the definitive diagnosis is often difficult to ascertain. A second category to be taken into account is the rare anomaly of pulmonary veno-occlusive disease. Diffuse obliteration of small venules throughout the lungs leads to pulmonary hypertension. In the third category, there is no detectable cause for the pulmonary

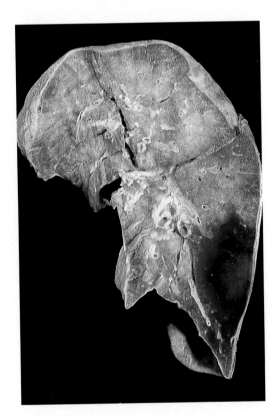

FIGURE 10.22 Infarct of the lung showing the hemorrhagic aspect due to the collateral supply. The infarct is wedge-shaped with a broad base at the pleural surface. (Reproduced with permission; see Figure Credits)

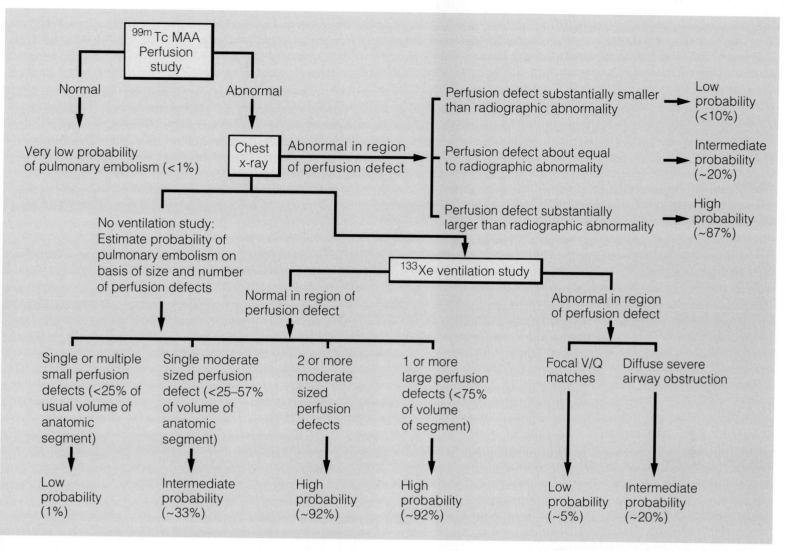

FIGURE 10.23 Relation of chest x-ray studies and ventilation/perfusion scans to the probability of pulmonary embolus. (Reproduced with permission; see Figure Credits)

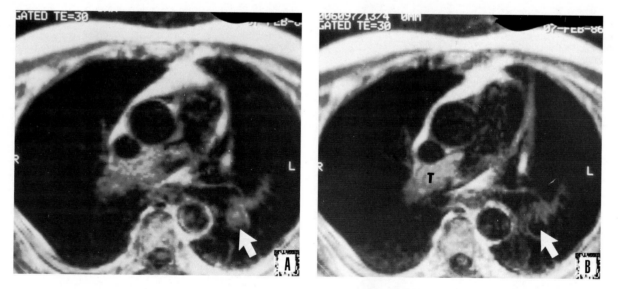

FIGURE 10.24 Magnetic resonance imaging of a patient with pulmonary arterial hypertension and pulmonary embolism. The ECG-gated images were taken during diastole (A) and systole (B). The image at late diastole demonstrates the signal in the right and descending branch of the left pulmonary artery, while the image in systole demonstrates clearing of the signal in the descending branch of the left pulmonary artery (*arrow*), indicating slow blood flow at this site. Persistence of the signal at all phases of the cardiac cycle indicates a thrombus (T) in the right pulmonary artery. (Reproduced with permission; see Figure Credits)

vascular disease, even at pathologic study. In such instances there is a diffuse and abrupt narrowing of the caliber of the smaller-sized pulmonary arteries, underlying the changes seen on the chest radiograph and the "winter-tree" aspect on postmortem pulmonary angiography (Fig. 10.25). The muscular pulmonary arteries show an edematous concentric intimal layering, often referred to as *onion skinning* (Fig. 10.26); this is the morphologic counterpart of the increased vascular resistance. In its most extreme form advanced lesions occur; these are characterized by fibrinoid necrosis of the arterial walls with plexiform lesions (Fig. 10.27). The latter form of pulmonary hypertension with unknown etiology is usually referred to as *primary pulmonary hypertension.*

CLINICAL MANIFESTATIONS

The patient with primary pulmonary hypertension may complain of dyspnea on effort, syncope, or chest pain; sudden death may occur. The physical abnormalities that may be present include a large a wave in the neck veins, anterior lift of the sternum due to right ventricular hypertrophy, palpable pulmonary trunk pulse, a loud pulmonary valve closure sound, and a diastolic murmur of pulmonary valve regurgitation.[1]

The chest radiograph reveals right ventricular hypertrophy and large pulmonary arteries that taper quickly. The ECG demonstrates evidence of right ventricular hypertrophy with prominent P waves consistent with right atrial abnormality (Fig. 10.28). Right ventricular hypertrophy and pulmonary valve regurgitation are also evident from the echocardiogram, while evidence of pulmonary hypertension and normal pulmonary wedge pressure without other evidence of disease are demonstrated at cardiac catheterization. The P_{O_2} may be diminished when there is a right-to-left shunt through the oval foramen.

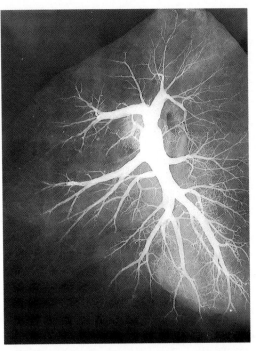

FIGURE 10.25
Postmortem angiogram of pulmonary vascular disease. Note the "winter-tree" aspect due to structural changes at the level of the smaller sized muscular pulmonary arteries. (Reproduced with permission; see Figure Credits)

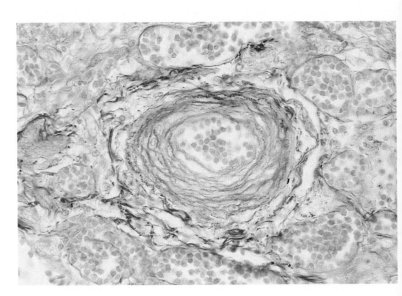

FIGURE 10.26 Histologic section of a muscular pulmonary artery from a patient with pulmonary vascular disease. Lamellar intimal fibrosis, also known as *onion skinning* (elastic tissue stain), is present. (Reproduced with permission; see Figure Credits)

FIGURE 10.27 Histologic section of a plexiform lesion from a patient with advanced pulmonary vascular disease. The lesion is characterized by multiple, often slit-like, endothelial-lined vascular spaces, most likely due to fibrinoid necrosis of the wall of pre-existing arterioles (H&E stain). (Reproduced with permission; see Figure Credits)

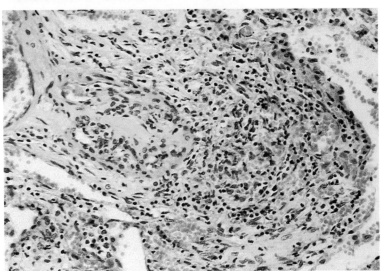

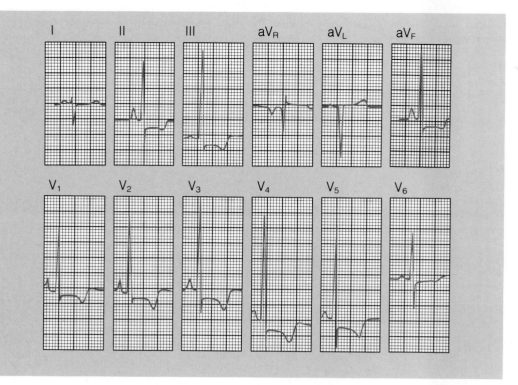

FIGURE 10.28 ECG of a patient with primary pulmonary hypertension. The mean QRS vector is directed to the right and anteriorly and there is a right atrial abnormality. The QRS voltage is larger than it usually is when the right ventricular hypertrophy is due to pulmonary emphysema. (Reproduced with permission; see Figure Credits)

ACKNOWLEDGMENTS

This chapter is based in part on Ross JC, Newman JH: Chronic cor pulmonale; Dalen JE, Alpert JS: Pulmonary embolism; Kuida H: Pulmonary hypertension: Mechanisms and recognition; and Kuida H: Primary pulmonary hypertension. In Hurst JW (ed): The Heart, 6th ed. McGraw-Hill, New York, 1986.

FIGURE CREDITS

Figs. 10.1–10.3, 10.5–10.7, 10.22, 10.25–10.27 from Hurst JW (ed): Atlas of the Heart. Gower, New York, 1988.

Fig. 10.4 from Becker AE, Anderson RH: Cardiac Pathology. Raven Press, New York, 1983.

Figs. 10.8, 10.11, 10.15, 10.17 from Hurst JW (ed): The Heart, 6th ed. McGraw-Hill, New York, 1986.

Fig. 10.9 redrawn from Reeves JT, Grover RE: High-altitude pulmonary edema. Prog Cardiol 4:105, 1975.

Figs. 10.10, 10.12–10.14, 10.16, 10.21, 10.23, 10.24 from Chatterjee K, et al: Cardiology: An Illustrated Text–Reference. Gower, New York, 1992.

Fig. 10.18 redrawn from Selzer A: Principles of Clinical Cardiology: An Analytic Approach. WB Saunders, Philadelphia, 1975.

Fig. 10.20 redrawn from McGinn S, White PD: Acute cor pulmonale resulting from pulmonary embolism. JAMA 104:1475, 1935.

Fig. 10.28 redrawn from Voelkel NF, Reeves JT: Primary pulmonary hypertension. In Moser KM (ed): Pulmonary Vascular Diseases. Marcel Dekker, New York, 1979.

REFERENCES

1. Hawkins JW, Dunn MI: Prelimary pulmonary hypertension in adults. Clin Cardiol 13:382, 1990.
2. Kelley MA, Carson JL, Palevsky HI, et al: Diagnosing pulmonary embolism: New facts and strategies. Ann Intern Med 114:300, 1991.
3. McGinn S, White PD: Acute cor pulmonale resulting from pulmonary embolism. JAMA 104:1473, 1935.
4. Miller DD: The environmental causes of pulmonary hypertension. In Hurst JW (ed): Clinical Essays on The Heart, vol 5. McGraw-Hill, New York, 1985.
5. Moser KM: Venous thromboembolism. Ann Rev Respir Dis 141:235, 1990.
6. Prediletto R, Paoletti P, Fornai E, et al: Natural history of treated pulmonary embolism—Evaluation by perfusion lung scintigraphy, gas exchange, and chest roentgenogram. Chest 97:554, 1990.
7. Robalino BD, Moodie DS: Association between primary pulmonary hypertension and portal hypertension: Analysis of its pathophysiology and clinical, laboratory, and hemodynamic manifestations. J Am Coll Cardiol 17:492, 1991.
8. Stein PD, Alavi A, Gottschalk A, et al: Usefulness of noninvasive diagnostic tools for diagnosis of acute pulmonary embolism in patients with a normal chest radiograph. Am J Cardiol 67:1117, 1991.

CHAPTER eleven

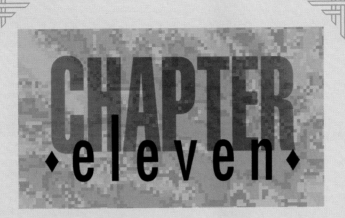

INFECTIVE ENDOCARDITIS

J. WILLIS HURST, MD

DAVID T. DURACK, MD

ANTON E. BECKER, MD

JOSEPH S. ALPERT, MD

When the endothelial surface of the heart or the arteries is infected by bacteria or fungi, the patient is said to have infective endocarditis. Noninfective endocarditis is not produced by microbes; it presents as thrombotic lesions rather than as inflammation. However, these lesions are sometimes colonized by circulating organisms, which convert this condition to infective endocarditis.

Infective endocarditis may follow a chronic, indolent course, a hectic, acute course, or an intermediate, subacute course, depending on the infectious agent and host resistance. Endocarditis remains a serious and often lethal disease.

FIGURE 11.1 FREQUENCY OF THE MAJOR PRE-EXISTING CARDIAC LESIONS IN PATIENTS WITH INFECTIVE ENDOCARDITIS

	CHILDREN		ADULTS		
	<2 Years Old (%)	*2–15 Years Old* (%)	*15–50 Years Old* (%)	*>50 Years Old* (%)	*IV Drug Abusers* (%)
No known heart disease	50–70	10–15	10–20	10	50–60
Congenital heart disease	30–50	70–80	20–30	10–20	10
Rheumatic heart disease	Rare	10–20	30–40	20–30	10
Degenerative heart disease	0	0	Rare	10–20	Rare
Previous cardiac surgery	5	10–15	10–20	10–20	10–20
Previous endocarditis	Rare	5	5	5–10	10–20

(Reproduced with permission; see Figure Credits) (Information compiled from references 1–3, 6, 13, 15, 17, 18, 20–23, 26, 30–33, 38, 40)

FIGURE 11.2 ESTIMATES OF THE RELATIVE RISK FOR INFECTIVE ENDOCARDITIS FROM VARIOUS CARDIAC LESIONS

RELATIVELY HIGH RISK	INTERMEDIATE RISK	VERY LOW OR NEGLIGIBLE
Prosthetic heart valves	Mitral valve prolapse	Atrial septal defects
Aortic valve disease	Pure mitral stenosis	Arteriosclerotic plaques
Mitral insufficiency	Tricuspid valve disease	Coronary artery disease
Patent arterial duct	Pulmonary valve disease	Syphilitic aortitis
Ventricular septal defect	Previous infective endocarditis	Cardiac pacemakers
Coarctation of the aorta	Asymmetric septal hypertrophy	Surgically corrected cardiac lesions
Marfan's syndrome	Calcific aortic sclerosis	(without prosthetic implants, more than
	Hyperalimentation or pressure-monitoring lines	6 months after operation)
	that reach the right atrium	
	Nonvalvular intracardiac prosthetic implants	

(Reproduced with permission; see Figure Credits) (Information compiled from references 5, 8–10, 14, 22, 26, 30, 39, 40)

FIGURE 11.3 FREQUENCY OF VARIOUS ORGANISMS CAUSING INFECTIVE ENDOCARDITIS*

	NATIVE VALVE ENDOCARDITIS (%)	IV DRUG ABUSERS (%)	EARLY PROSTHETIC VALVE ENDOCARDITIS (%)	LATE PROSTHETIC VALVE ENDOCARDITIS (%)
Streptococci	40–65	15	10	35
Viridans, alpha-hemolytic	35	5	<5	25
Strep. bovis (group D)	15	<5	<5	<5
Enterococcus faecalis (group D)	10	8	<5	<5
Other streptococci	<5	<5	<5	<5
Staphylococci	25–50	50–80	50	30
Coagulase-positive	23–40	50	20	10
Coagulase-negative	<5	<5	30	20
Gram-negative aerobic bacilli	<5	5	20	15
Fungi	<5	5	10	5
Miscellaneous bacteria	<5	5	5	5
Diphtheroids, propionibacteria	<1	<5	5	<5
Other anaerobes	<1	<1	<1	<1
Rickettsia	<1	<1	<1	<1
Chlamydia	<1	<1	<1	<1
Polymicrobial infection	<1	5	5	5
Culture-negative endocarditis	5–10	5	<5	<5

(Reproduced with permission; see Figure Credits) (Information compiled from references 6, 15, 16, 18, 22, 24, 26, 28, 30, 31, 35, 38, 40)

Etiology and Pathology

Most patients with infective endocarditis have pre-existing heart disease (Figs. 11.1, 11.2). The frequency of various organisms causing endocarditis is shown in Figure 11.3. In recent years, there has been a steady increase in the percentage of patients in whom staphylococci are the infecting bacteria[34] (Fig. 11.4).

The pathology of infective endocarditis is characterized by the adherence of bacteria to the surface of cardiac valves with an altered endothelium.

The approximate frequency of anatomic location of infective endocarditis is shown in Figure 11.5.[12] This process is accompanied by fibrin–platelet deposi-tions, which together with the affected valve tissue produce vegetations.

Endocarditis is a destructive disease. In semilunar valves, such as the aortic valve, the infective process is particularly prominent along the line of closure (Fig. 11.6). The mitral valve shows a distinct tendency for chordal rupture (Fig. 11.7). From a clinical point of view, therefore, valvular regurgitation is the leading complication of infective endocarditis. Complications are largely determined by the site of the primary infection.[7] Endocarditis of the aortic root may spread onto neighboring structures, such as the epicardial surface, the right ventricular outflow tract, both atria, and the mitral valve (Fig. 11.8). Aortic valve regurgitation may cause secondary and remote infection of the mitral valve as a result of the regurgitant flow (Fig. 11.9). It may also cause massive left ventricular dilation with secondary myocardial ischemia (Fig. 11.10). The vegetations may cause thromboemboli, which are often infected (Fig. 11.11). Septic myocarditis is a common complication in patients with aortic valve endocarditis (Fig. 11.12).

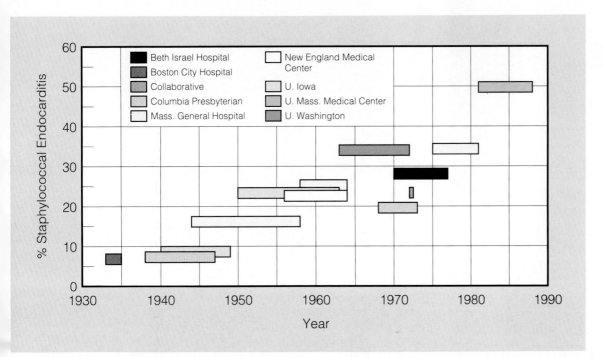

FIGURE 11.4 Incidence of staphylo-coccal infective endocarditis in reported series at various medical centers. (Data compiled; see Figure Credits)

Legend:
- Beth Israel Hospital
- Boston City Hospital
- Collaborative
- Columbia Presbyterian
- Mass. General Hospital
- New England Medical Center
- U. Iowa
- U. Mass. Medical Center
- U. Washington

FIGURE 11.5 FREQUENCY OF ANATOMIC LOCATION OF VEGETATIONS IN SUBACUTE AND ACUTE BACTERIAL ENDOCARDITIS, AND ENDOCARDITIS ASSOCIATED WITH IV DRUG ABUSE

	SUBACUTE BACTERIAL ENDOCARDITIS (%)	ACUTE BACTERIAL ENDOCARDITIS (%)	ENDOCARDITIS IN IV DRUG ABUSERS (%)
Left-sided valves	85	65	40
Aortic	15–26	18–25	25–30
Mitral	38–45	30–35	15–20
Aortic and mitral	23–30	15–20	13–20
Right-sided valves	5	20	50
Tricuspid	1–5	15	45–55
Pulmonary	1	Rare	2
Tricuspid and pulmonary	Rare	Rare	3
Left- and right-sided sites	Rare	5–10	5–10
Other sites (patent duct, VSD, coarctation, jet lesions)	10	5	5

(Reproduced with permission; see Figure Credits) **(Information compiled from references 6, 15, 22, 25, 29-31, 38, 40)**

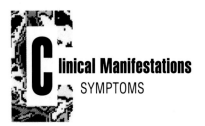

Clinical Manifestations
SYMPTOMS

The patient may give a history of dental work or a recent infection, and report fever, chills, anorexia, weakness, headache, myalgia, and arthralgia. The patient may complain of flu-like symptoms. Symptoms may relate to systemic emboli to the brain, kidney, intestinal tract, extremities, spleen, eye, coronary artery, or other areas. Symptoms of heart failure may appear; if failure was present before the infection, it may worsen due to damage to the aortic or the mitral valve, rupture of tendinous cords, or myocarditis. Figure 11.13 summarizes the major clinical manifestations of endocarditis and the investigative tests that aid in diagnosis.

PHYSICAL EXAMINATION

The patient may appear chronically or acutely ill; temperature is usually elevated. Petechial hemorrhages of the skin and the mucous membranes may be evident. Splinter hemorrhages, Osler's nodes, Janeway lesions, retinal hemorrhages, Roth's spots, endophthalmitis, clubbing of the fingers, signs of peripheral

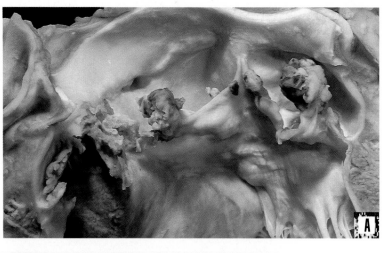

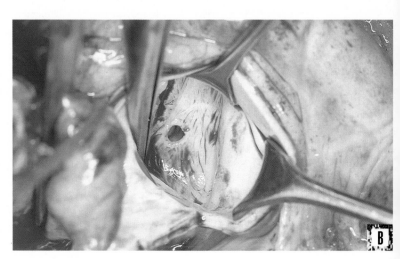

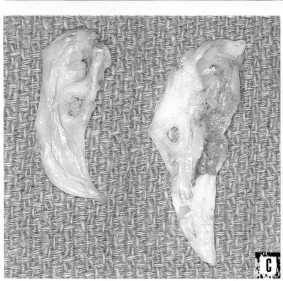

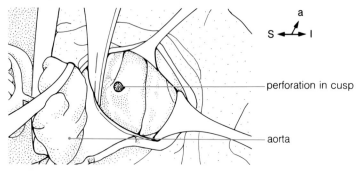

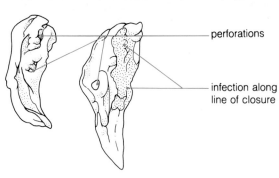

perforations

infection along
line of closure

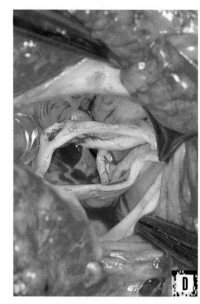

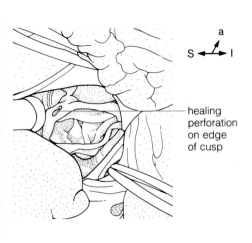

FIGURE 11.6 **(A)** Infective endocarditis of the aortic valve. There is massive destruction of the leaflets with vegetations. **(B,C)** A "healing" perforation is seen in a bicuspid aortic valve with small vegetations. **(D)** A healed perforation is exposed in this patient with a bicuspid aortic valve and congenital subaortic stenosis. (Reproduced with permission; see Figure Credits)

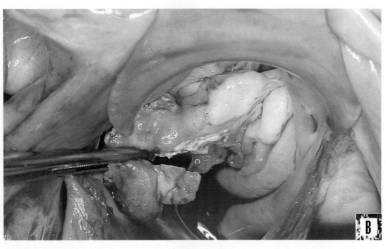

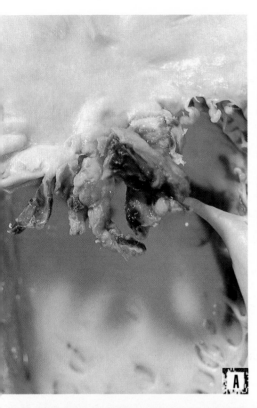

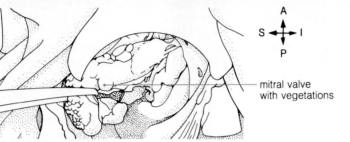

mitral valve
with vegetations

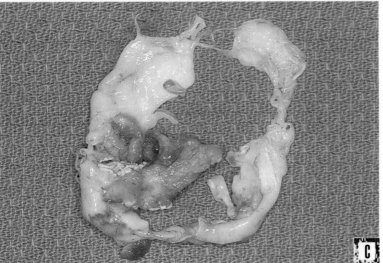

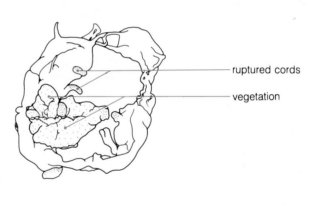

ruptured cords

vegetation

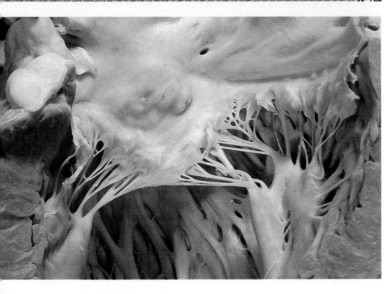

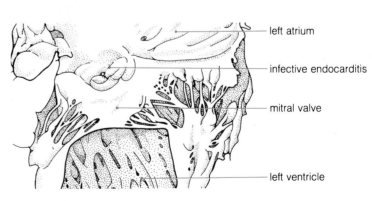

left atrium

infective endocarditis

mitral valve

left ventricle

FIGURE 11.8 Spread of infection from the aortic root onto the mitral valve in the area of aortic–mitral valve continuity, as viewed from the atrial aspect. (Reproduced with permission; see Figure Credits)

emboli, and splenomegaly may all be identified.

Most patients have a heart murmur due either to stenosis, and/or regurgitation of the aortic, mitral, pulmonary, or tricuspid valves, an interventricular septal defect, patent arterial duct, coarctation, ostium primum atrioventricular septal defect, or prosthetic valves.

The physical findings associated with heart failure, embolization or mycotic aneurysm may be detected.

LABORATORY STUDIES

Anemia develops in most patients with subacute endocarditis; in many patients with acute infection it develops after the first week. The anemia is usually normochromic and normocytic, but it may be hemolytic when acute infection occurs. Leukocytosis may develop; an extremely high white blood count suggests an abscess. The erythrocyte sedimentation rate is usually elevated. Hematuria may be present. Red cell casts and proteinuria may be found in patients with glomerulonephritis due to endocarditis.

Blood cultures should be obtained from all patients with a heart murmur and fever. Although there are reports that arterial blood is more likely to yield positive cultures than venous blood, most physicians continue to use venous blood. Durack suggests the following approach (from p. 9.7, Atlas of the Heart, Gower, 1988):

> Draw three separate venous blood cultures on the first day. If these cultures show no growth by the second day, draw two more venous cultures. If all are negative on the third day *but the diagnosis of endocarditis still seems likely*, draw two more venous cultures and one arterial blood culture. If the patient had received prior antibiotic therapy, three more venous samples may be taken over the following week, looking for a late recrudescence of bacteremia after partial treatment.

Because *Staph. epidermidis* and diphtheroids can cause endocarditis,[19,24] special care must be taken during venipuncture to avoid contamination of the specimen with these common skin organisms, which would result in diagnostic con-fusion. Cultures should be incubated for at least 3 weeks, and Gram stains made at intervals even if no growth is apparent on inspection.

RADIOLOGIC STUDIES

The electrocardiogram may be normal. However, it may reveal the anatomic features of the underlying heart disease, infarction due to a coronary embolism, or a new conduction defect caused by a small abscess involving the conduction system.

The chest film may reveal the anatomic consequences of the underlying heart disease and, with tricuspid valve endocarditis, evidence of septic pulmonary emboli.

ECHOCARDIOGRAPHY

Echocardiography may be used to identify vegetations[37](Figs. 11.14–11.17). Two-dimensional imaging with color-flow Doppler is very helpful in assessment of possible endocarditis. Vegetations less than 2 mm in size cannot be detected, and all valves cannot always be visualized. The tricuspid valve, for example, is difficult to study. False-positive echocardiograms for vegetations do commonly occur in patients with myxomatous degeneration of the mitral valve. The echocardiogram usually reveals evidence of the underlying heart disease. Transesophageal echocardiography is approximately 90% sensitive for the detection of vegetations,[11,36] and has become a vitally important test in diagnosis of endocarditis.

CARDIAC CATHETERIZATION

Cardiac catheterization is reserved for those patients in whom surgical intervention is planned.

RADIONUCLIDE STUDIES

Radionuclide imaging of the liver and spleen may reveal emboli. Computed tomographic scanning or magnetic resonance imaging may demonstrate emboli to the brain or splenic abscesses.[4]

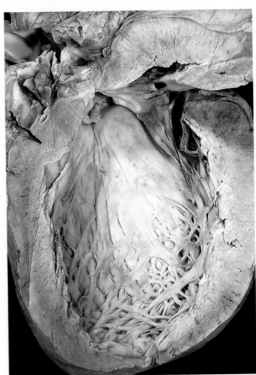

FIGURE 11.10
Aortic valve regurgitation leading to massive left ventricular chamber dilation as an adaptive phenomenon (same heart as shown in Fig. 11.9). Subendocardial ischemia and infarction are also present. (Reproduced with permission; see Figure Credits)

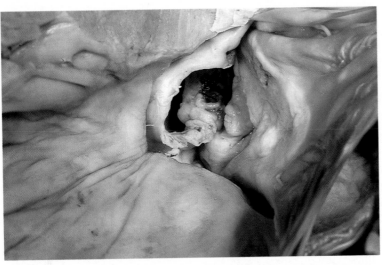

FIGURE 11.9   Infective endocarditis of the aortic valve leading to valve destruction and regurgitation. The regurgitant flow caused secondary infection of the ventricular aspect of the adjoining mitral valve leaflet. (Reproduced with permission; see Figure Credits)

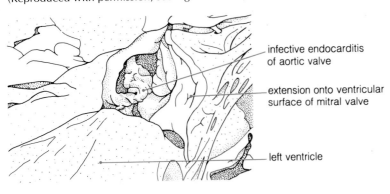

infective endocarditis of aortic valve

extension onto ventricular surface of mitral valve

left ventricle

MINIMUM DIAGNOSTIC CRITERIA

The disease should be considered whenever fever of unknown cause develops in a patient with a heart murmur. Blood cultures should be drawn; they are usually positive in the patient who has not received antibiotics. The echocardiogram may be helpful, but a negative study does not exclude the disease.

NATURAL HISTORY

The disease is usually fatal if unrecognized and untreated. Early treatment is imperative, because valve damage, fistula formation, heart failure, and emboli may limit the chances of recovery even if there is bacteriologic cure (Figs. 11.18, 11.19).

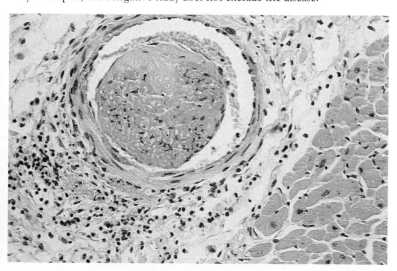

FIGURE 11.11 Histologic section of an intramyocardial coronary artery branch with an infected thromboembolus. Some inflammatory infiltrate is detectable in the immediate vicinity (H&E stain). (Reproduced with permission; see Figure Credits)

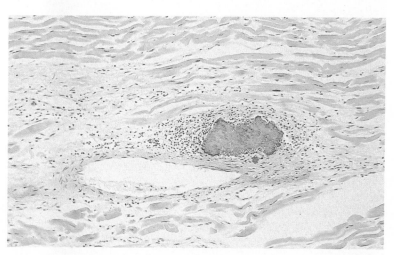

FIGURE 11.12 Septic myocarditis exemplified by a colony of bacteria surrounded by an inflammatory infiltrate (H&E stain). (Reproduced with permission; see Figure Credits)

FIGURE 11.13 MAJOR CLINICAL MANIFESTATIONS OF INFECTIVE ENDOCARDITIS

MANIFESTATIONS	HISTORY	EXAMINATION	INVESTIGATIONS
Systemic infection	Fever, chills, rigors, sweats, malaise, weakness, lethargy, delirium, headache, anorexia, weight loss, backache, arthralgia, myalgia Portal of entry: 　Oropharynx, skin 　Urinary tract 　Drug addiction 　Nosocomial bacteremia	Fever Pallor Weight loss Asthenia Splenomegaly	Anemia Leukocytosis (variable) Raised erythrocyte, sedimentation rate Blood cultures positive Abnormal cerebrospinal fluid
Intravascular lesion	Dyspnea, chest pain, focal weakness, stroke, abdominal pain, cold and painful extremities	Murmurs Signs of cardiac failure Petechiae—skin, eye, mucosae Roth's spots, Osler's nodes Janeway lesions Splinter hemorrhages Stroke Mycotic aneurysm Ischemia or infarction of viscera or extremities	Blood in urine Chest radiograph Echocardiography Arteriography Liver–spleen scan Lung scan, brain scan, CT scan Histology, culture of emboli
Immunologic reactions	Arthralgia, myalgia, tenosynovitis	Arthritis Signs of uremia Finger clubbing	Proteinuria, hematuria, casts, uremia, acidosis Polyclonal increases in gamma globulins Rheumatoid factor, decreased complement, immune complexes in serum Antistaphylococcal teichoic acid antibodies

(Reproduced with permission; see Figure Credits) (Information compiled from references 26, 27, 30, 40)

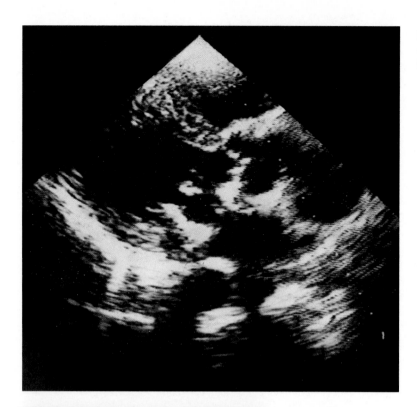

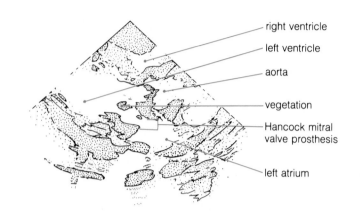

FIGURE 11.14 Cross-sectional echocardiogram in the parasternal long axis view of a patient with endocarditis. A vegetation is seen on the prosthetic (Hancock) mitral valve. (Reproduced with permission; see Figure Credits)

right ventricle
left ventricle
aorta
vegetation
Hancock mitral valve prosthesis
left atrium

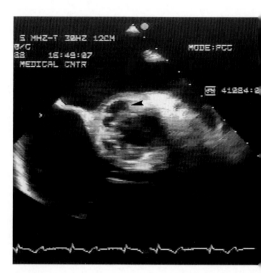

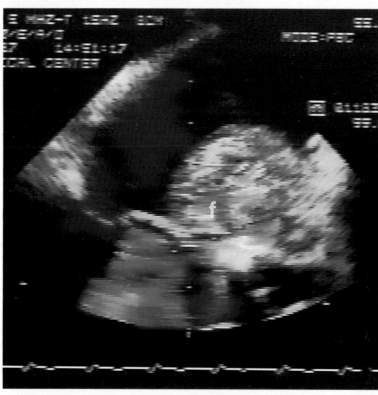

FIGURE 11.15
Echocardiogram of aortic endocarditis with bulky vegetation (veg) arising from the aortic valve. Note that the vegetation is large enough to prolapse into the left ventricular (LV) outflow tract. There is also a left atrial vegetation (*arrows*). (Reproduced with permission; see Figure Credits)

FIGURE 11.17 Transesophageal echocardiogram showing a bacterial abscess involving an aortic prosthesis. The necrotic spaces in the abscess are evident (arrow) and can potentially rupture into adjacent chambers to create fistulae. (Reproduced with permission; see Figure Credits)

FIGURE 11.16
Transesophageal echocardiogram of an aortic abscess. Color-flow Doppler demonstrates flow (f) into the cavity of the abscess. (Reproduced with permission; see Figure Credits)

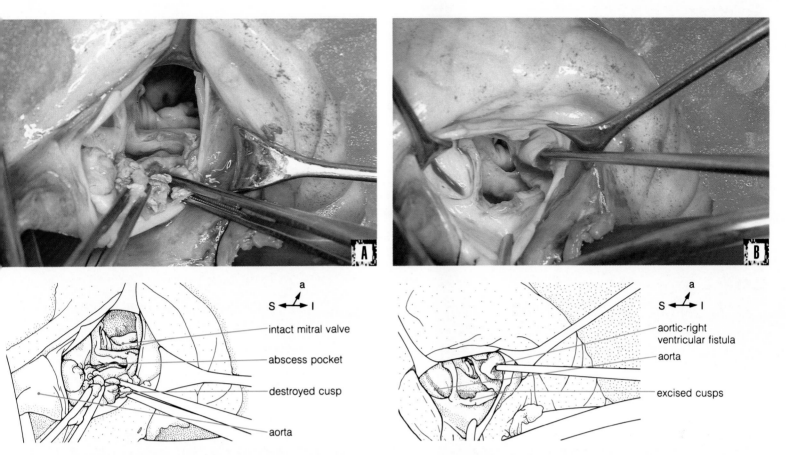

FIGURE 11.18   **(A)** Patient with extensively damaged aortic valve. A large abscess formation separates the aorta from the myocardial mass. **(B)** Sinus of Valsalva–right ventricular fistula causes left-to-right shunting. (Reproduced with permission; see Figure Credits)

intact mitral valve
abscess pocket
destroyed cusp
aorta

aortic–right
ventricular fistula
aorta

excised cusps

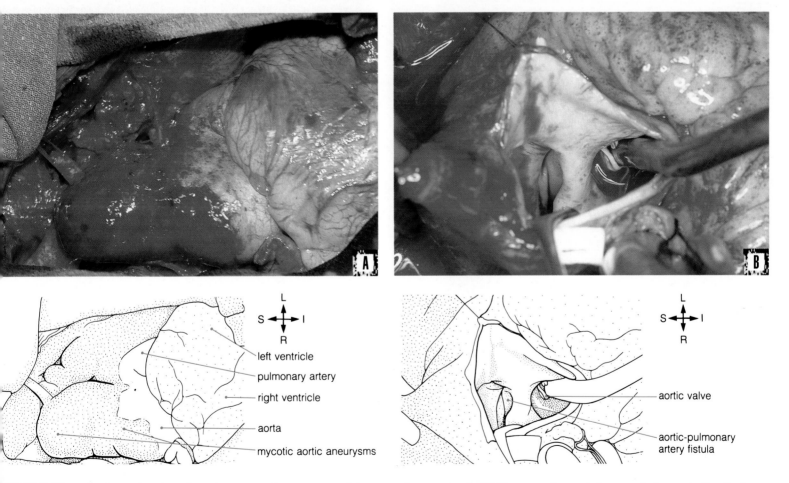

left ventricle
pulmonary artery
right ventricle
aorta
mycotic aortic aneurysms

aortic valve

aortic–pulmonary
artery fistula

FIGURE 11.19   **(A)** Operative view of two large mycotic aneurysms of the ascending aorta. One is located at the base of the brachiocephalic artery, and the other extends posteriorly, resulting in fistula formation into the pulmonary trunk. **(B)** The ascending aorta is opened, demonstrating the large posterior fistula. (Reproduced with permission; see Figure Credits)

ACKNOWLEDGMENT

This chapter is based in part on Durack DT: Infective and noninfective endocarditis. In Hurst JW (ed): The Heart, 6th ed. McGraw-Hill, New York, 1986.

FIGURE CREDITS

Figs. 11.1–11.3, 11.5, and 11.13, 11.14 from Hurst JW (ed): The Heart, 6th ed. McGraw-Hill, New York, 1986.

Fig. 11.4 data compiled from Carrol K, Cheeseman S: Infective endocarditis. In Dalen JE, and Alpert JS: Valvular Heart Disease, 2nd ed, Little, Brown and Company, Boston, 1986; and Sanabria T, Alpert JS, Goldberg R, et al: Increasing frequency of staphylococcal infective endocarditis: Experience at a university hospital, 1981 through 1988. Arch Intern Med 150:1305, 1990.

Figs. 11.6–11.12, 11.18, 11.19 from Hurst JW (ed) : Atlas of the Heart. Gower, New York, 1988.

Fig. 11.14 courtesy of Stephen D. Clemens, Jr., MD, and John Perkins, Atlanta, GA.

Figs. 11.15–11.17 from Chatterjee K, et al: Cardiology: An Illustrated Text–Reference. Gower, New York, 1991.

REFERENCES

1. Bayliss R, Clarke C, Oakley C, Somerville W, Whitfield AGW: The teeth and infective endocarditis. Br Heart J 50:506, 1983.

2. Bayliss R, Clarke C, Oakley C, Somerville W, Whitfield AGW, Young SEJ: The microbiology and pathogenesis of infective endocarditis. Br Heart J 50:513, 1983.

3. Bayliss R, Clarke C, Oakley C, Somerville W, Whitfield AGW, Young SEJ: The bowel, the genitourinary tract and infective endocarditis. Br Heart J 51:339, 1983.

4. Bertorini TE, Laster RE, Thompson BF, et al: Magnetic resonance imaging of the brain in bacterial endocarditis. Arch Intern Med 149:815, 1989.

5. Beton DC, Brear SG, Edwards JD, Leonard JC: Mitral valve prolapse: An assessment of clinical features, associated conditions and prognosis. Q J Med 52:150, 1983.

6. Cannon NJ, Cobbs CG, Infective endocarditis in drug addicts. In D Kaye(ed): Infective Endocarditis. University Park Press, Baltimore. 1977, p 111.

7. Chan P, Ogilby JD, Segal B: Tricupid valve endocarditis. Am Heart J 117:1140, 1989.

8. Clemens JD, Horwitz RI, Jaffe CG, Feinstein AR, Stanton BF: A controlled evaluation of the risk of bacterial endocarditis in persons with mitral-valve prolapse. N Engl J Med 307:776, 1982.

9. Clemens JD, Ransohoff DF: A quantitative assessment of pre-dental antibiotic prophylaxis for patients with mitral-valve prolapse. J Chronic Dis 37:531, 1984.

10. Corrigal D, Bolen J, Hancock EW, Popp RL: Mitral valve prolapse and infective endocarditis. Am J Med 63:215, 1977.

11. Daniel WG, Mugge A, Martin RP, et al: Improvement in the diagnosis of abscesses associated with endocarditis by transesophageal echocardiography. N Engl J Med 324:795, 1991.

12. Dressler FA, Roberts WC: Infective endocarditis in opiate addicts: Analysis of 80 cases studies at necropsy. Am J Cardiol 63:1240, 1989.

13. Durack DT, Petersdorf RG: Changes in the epidermiology of endocarditis: In Kaplan EL, Taranta AV (eds): Infective Endocarditis, American Heart Association, AHA Monograph no. 52, 1977, p.3.

14. Durack DT, Kaplan EL, Bisno AL: Apparent failure of endocarditis prophylaxis: analysis of 52 cases submitted to a national registry. JAMA 250:2318, 1983.

15. El-Khatib MR, Wilson FM, Lerner AM: Characteristics of bacterial endocarditis in heroin addicts in Detroit. Am J Med Sci 271:147, 1976.

16. Feldner JM, Dowell VR: Anaerobic bacterial endocarditis. N Engl J Med 283:1189, 1970.

17. Finland M, Barnes NW: Changing etiology of bacterial endocarditis in the antibacterial era: Experiences at Boston City Hospital. Ann Intern Med 72:341,1970.

18. Garvey GJ, Neu HC: Infective endocarditis–An evolving disease: A review of endocarditis at the Columbia-Presbyterian Medical Center, 1968-1973. Medicine 57:105, 1978.

19. Gerry JL, Greenough W: Diphtheroid endocarditis: Report of the nine cases and review of the literature. Johns Hopkins Med J 139:61, 1976.

20. Johnson CM, Rhodes KH: Pediatric endocarditis. Mayo Clin Proc 51:581, 1982.

21. Johnson DH, Rosenthal A, Nadas AS: A forty year review of bacterial endocarditis. Circulation 51:581, 1975.

22. Kaplan EL, Rich H, Gersony W, Manning J: A collaborative study of infective endocarditis in the 1970's: Emphasis on patients who have undergone cardiovascular surgery. Circulation 59:327, 1979.

23. Kaye D: Definitions and demographic characteristics. In Kaye D(ed): Infective Endocarditis, University Park Press, Baltimore, 1977, p.1.

24. Keys TT, Hewitt WL: Endocarditis due to micrococci and Staphylococcus epidermidis. Arch Intern Med 132:216, 1973.

25. Lepeschkin E: On the relation between the site of valvular involvement in endocarditis and the blood pressure resting on the valve. Am J Med Sci 224:318, 1952.

26. Lerner PI, Weinstein L: Medical Progress: Infective endocarditis in the antibiotic era. N Engl J Med 274:199, 1966.

27. McAnulty JH, Rahimtoola SH, Demots H, Griswold HE: Clinical features of infective endocarditis. In Rahimtoola SH (ed): Infective Endocarditis, Grune & Stratton, New York, 1978, p. 125.

28. McLeod R, Remington JS: Fungal endocarditis. In Rahimtoola SH (ed): Infective Endocarditis, Grune & Stratton, New York, 1978, p. 211.

29. Pankey GA: Acute bacterial endocarditis at the University of Minnesota Hospital 1939-1959. Am Heart J 64:583, 1962.

30. Pelletier LL, Petersdorf RG: Infective endocarditis: A review of 125 cases from the University of Washington Hospitals, 1963-72. Medicine 56:287, 1977.

31. Reisberg BE: Infective endocarditis in the narcotic addict. Prog Cardiovasc Dis 22:193, 1979.

32. Ries K: Endocarditis in the elderly. In Kaye D (ed): Infective Endocarditis, University Park Press, Baltimore, 1977, p. 143.

33. Rosenthal A, Nadas AS: Infective endocarditis in infancy and children, in Rahimtoola SH (ed): Infective Endocarditis, Grune & Stratton, New York, 1978, p 149.

34. Sanabria T, Alpert JS, Goldberg R, et al: Increasing frequency of staphylococcal infective endocarditis: Experience at a university hospital, 1981 through 1988. Arch Intern Med 150:1305, 1990.

35. Scheld WM, Sande MA: Endocarditis and intravascular infections. In Mandell GL, Douglas RG, Bennett JE (eds): Principles and Practice of Infectious Diseases, 2nd ed. John Wiley & Sons, New York, 1984.

36. Shively BK, Gurule FT, Roldan CA, et al: Diagnostic value of transesophageal compared with transthoracic echocardiography in infective endocarditis. J Am Coll Cardiol 18:391, 1991.

37. Steckelberg JM, Murphy JG, Ballard D, et al: Emboli in infective endocarditis: The prognostic valve of echocardiography. Ann Intern Med 114:635, 1991.

38. Stimmel B, Dack S: Infective endocarditis in narcotic addicts, in Rahimtoola SH (ed): Infective Endocarditis, Grune & Stratton, New York, 1978, p.195.

39. Wang K, Gobel FL, Gleason DF: Bacterial endocarditis in idiopathic hypertrophic subaortic stenosis. Am Heart J 89:359, 1975.

40. Weinstein L, Rubin RH: Infective endocarditis 1973. Prog Cardiovasc Dis 16:239, 1973.

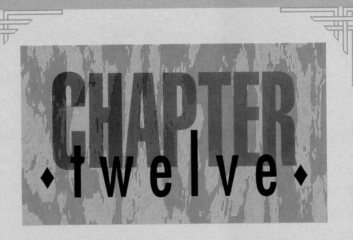

CHAPTER twelve

CARDIOVASCULAR TRAUMA

J. WILLIS HURST, MD

PANAGIOTIS N. SYMBAS, MD

ANTON E. BECKER, MD

JOSEPH S. ALPERT, MD

The incidence of traumatic disease of the cardiovascular system has increased in recent years because of the increasing number of automobile accidents and handgun injuries. The physician must consider injury to the heart and vessels whenever trauma has occurred. Traumatic heart disease may be overlooked when other more conspicuous injuries attract the physician's immediate attention, or when diagnostic clues are not immediately apparent.[1]

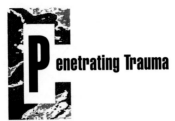

Penetrating Trauma

Almost any area of the heart and great vessels may be damaged by penetrating trauma (Fig. 12.1). Although wounds are usually considered inflicted from without, it is useful to remember that the heart wall can also be traversed from inside outward (Fig. 12.2). This danger, perhaps becoming more prevalent with the increasing number and range of procedures that are performed in the catheter laboratory and the intensive care setting. The treatment is determined by the type and the clinical manifestations of the injury; surgical intervention is often needed.

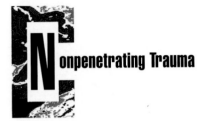

Nonpenetrating Trauma

Nonpenetrating trauma may also damage the heart and vessels (Fig. 12.3). Myocardial laceration (Fig. 12.4), injury to valve leaflets (Fig. 12.5), and coronary artery laceration (Fig. 12.6) are among the most common complications. Rupture of the aorta may also occur (Fig. 12.7). Partial rupture of the aorta can lead to chronic pseudoaneurysm or true aneurysm formation (Figs. 12.8, 12.9).

FIGURE 12.1 PENETRATING WOUNDS OF THE HEART

Pericardial damage
  Laceration or perforation
  Hemopericardium with or without cardiac tamponade
  Serofibrinous or suppurative pericarditis
  Pneumopericardium
  Constrictive pericarditis
Myocardial damage
  Laceration
  Penetration or perforation
  Retained foreign body
  Structural defects
  Aneurysm formation
  Septal defects
  Aortocardiac fistula
Valvular injury
  Leaflet injury
  Papillary muscle or tendinous cords laceration
Coronary artery injury
  Laceration or thrombosis with or without myocardial
    infarction
  Arteriovenous fistula
  Aneurysm
Embolism
  Foreign body
  Thrombus (septic or sterile)
Infective endocarditis
Rhythm or conduction disturbances

(Reproduced with permission; see Figure Credits)

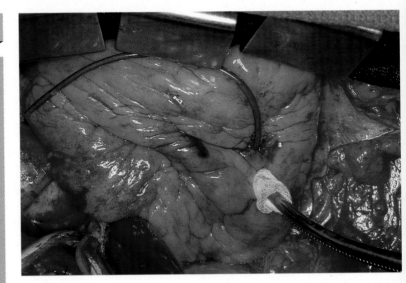

FIGURE 12.2   Operative view through a median sternotomy showing a pacing catheter that was inserted into the patient in the coronary care unit. The catheter perforated the right ventricular wall. (Reproduced with permission; see Figure Credits)

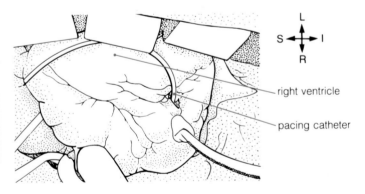

right ventricle

pacing catheter

Significant nonpenetrating or blunt trauma of the heart may result in damage to the myocardium or to the valves themselves. When valvular damage occurs, the tension apparatus of the atrioventricular valves, more frequently the tricuspid valve, is usually affected. Myocardial damage manifests itself either as a cardiac contusion, cardiac rupture, or a ventricular septal rupture. Ventricular aneurysm or pseudoaneurysm may be the result of such injury. This lesion is well illustrated in the case (Fig. 12.10) of a 9-year-old child who, 4 weeks prior to surgery, had received multiple injuries in an automobile accident. On admission to the hospital he was noted to have right bundle branch block on the electrocardiogram; cardiac enzyme analysis indicated myocardial damage. The electrocardiographic pattern evolved to show an inferior myocardial infarction; cross-sectional echocardiography demonstrated an apparent pseudoaneurysm of the right ventricle. Cardiac catheterization showed a true aneurysm of the left ventricle encroaching on the right ventricle. There was no evidence of left-to-right shunting and the cardiac valves were not damaged. Coronary angiography was not performed, but an aortic root injection demonstrated a dominant right coronary system.

At the time of operation the patient was found to have an aneurysm of the left ventricular apex that extended along the diaphragmatic surface to the base of the heart. There was no evidence of ventricular septal rupture.

Rapid diagnostic evaluation of patients with suspected cardiac trauma is essential. History, physical examination, ECG, chest x-ray, and two-dimensional echocardiography[2] are usually employed. Cardiac catheterization and angiography are often required. The natural history of cardiac traumatic injuries varies according to the nature of the injury and the age and condition of the patient.

FIGURE 12.3 NONPENETRATING TRAUMA OF THE HEART

Pericardial injury
  Hemopericardium
  Rupture or laceration
  Serofibrinous pericarditis
  Constrictive pericarditis
Myocardial injury
  Contusion
  Rupture of free cardiac wall, early or delayed
  Rupture of septum
  Aneurysm
  Laceration
Disturbances of rhythm or conduction
Valvular injury
  Rupture of valve leaflets, cusp, or tendinous cords
  Contusion of papillary muscle
Coronary artery injury
  Thrombosis with or without myocardial infarction
  Arteriovenous fistula
  Laceration with or without myocardial infarction
Great-vessel injury
  Rupture
  Aneurysm formation
  Aortocardiac chamber fistula
  Thrombotic occlusion

(Reproduced with permission; see Figure Credits)

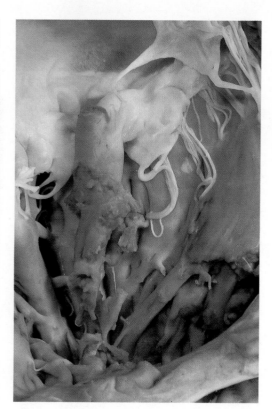

FIGURE 12.4
Laceration of the anterior papillary muscle of the tricuspid valve with complete rupture resulting from blunt chest trauma. (Reproduced with permission; see Figure Credits)

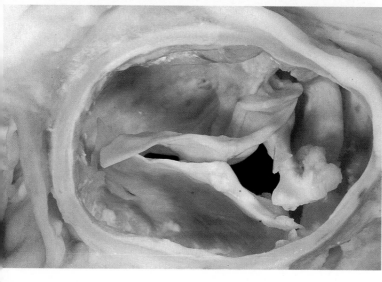

FIGURE 12.5   Torn aortic cusp resulting from blunt chest trauma. (Reproduced with permission; see Figure Credits)

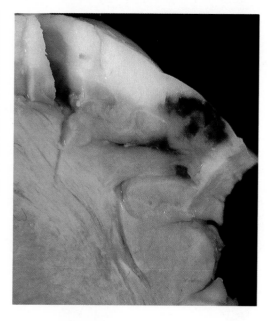

FIGURE 12.6
Laceration of the anterior descending coronary artery following nonpenetrating trauma to the heart. (Reproduced with permission; see Figure Credits)

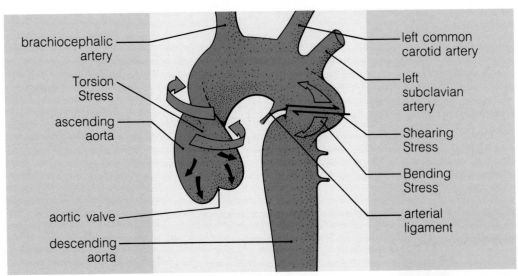

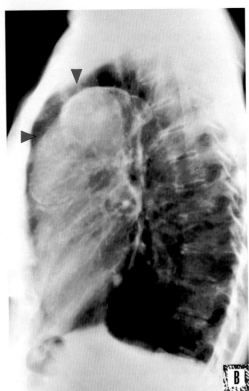

FIGURE 12.7 Forces acting upon the aortic wall during rupture of the aorta from blunt trauma. (Redrawn with permission; see Figure Credits. Also see Fig. 60-1, Hurst JW (ed): The Heart, 6th ed. Gower, New York, 1986)

brachiocephalic artery

left common carotid artery

Torsion Stress

left subclavian artery

ascending aorta

Shearing Stress

Bending Stress

aortic valve

descending aorta

arterial ligament

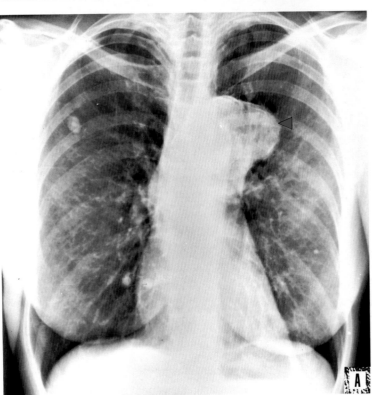

FIGURE 12.8 Calcified traumatic aneurysm of the aortic arch. (A) Posteroanterior and (B) lateral chest x-rays show deformity of the aortic arch (arrows) in a patient with a history of trauma. There is extensive linear calcification in the wall of the aneurysm. (Reproduced with permission; see Figure Credits)

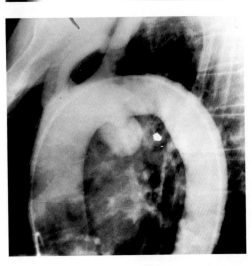

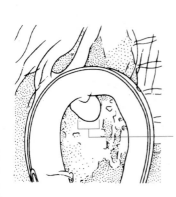

saccular aneurysm

FIGURE 12.9 Traumatic aneurysm of the aortic arch. Lateral aortogram shows a sharply demarcated saccular aneurysm arising from the inferior wall of the aortic arch. Most traumatic aneurysms are actually pseudoaneurysms. (Reproduced with permission; see Figure Credits)

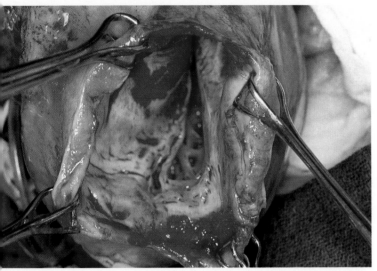

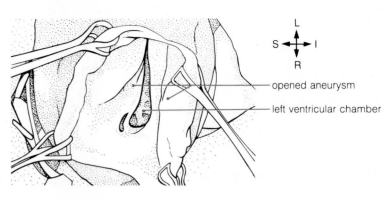

opened aneurysm

left ventricular chamber

FIGURE 12.10   Operative view of the heart in repair of a true ventricular aneurysm caused by blunt trauma. The opened aneurysm shows a smooth, thin-walled accular deformity extending from the apex to the base of the heart. (Reproduced with permission; see Figure Credits)

ACKNOWLEDGMENT

This chapter is based in part on Symbas PN, Arensberg D: Traumatic heart disease. In Hurst JW (ed): The Heart, 6th ed. McGraw-Hill, New York, 1986.

FIGURE CREDITS

Figs. 12.1, 12.3 from Symbas PN, Arensberg D: Traumatic heart disease. In Hurst JW (ed): The Heart, 6th ed. McGraw-Hill, New York, 1986.
Figs. 12.2, 12.4–12.6, and 12.10 from Hurst JW (ed): Atlas of the Heart. Gower, New York, 1988.
Fig. 12.7 redrawn from Symbas PN: Traumatic Injuries of the Heart and Great Vessels. Charles C Thomas, Springfield, IL, 1971.
Figs. 12.8, 12.9 from Kassner EG: Atlas of Radiologic Imaging. Gower, New York, 1989.

REFERENCES

1. Miller FA, Seward JB, Gersh BJ, et al: Two-dimensional echocardiographic findings in cardiac trauma. Am J Cardiol 50:1022, 1982.
2. Symbas PN: Cardiac trauma. Am Heart J 92:387, 1976.

CHAPTER

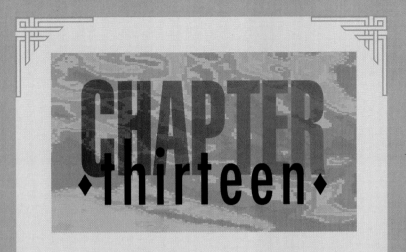

thirteen

DISEASES OF THE AORTA

JOSEPH S. ALPERT, MD

Aortic diseases are either congenital or acquired and include a number of common pathologic entities such as dissection and arteriosclerotic aneurysms (Fig. 13.1). Abdominal arteriosclerotic aneurysms are dealt with in Chapter 14. This chapter will describe two of the most common diseases of the aorta: dissection and thoracic aneurysms.

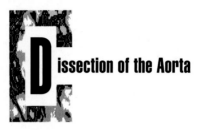

issection of the Aorta

Dissection of the aorta is not the same as an aneurysm. It is actually a hematoma that dissects for a variable distance along the aortic media following disruption of the aortic intima.

ETIOLOGY AND PATHOLOGY

Aortic dissection is a moderately common disease affecting approximately 2,000 patients each year in the United States. Dissection develops when there is a sudden disruption of the aortic intima, allowing blood at systemic arterial pressure to gain access to the aortic media. The force applied results in dissection blood for a variable distance along the aortic media. The primary event may l a tear in the aortic intima by forces applied from within the aortic lumen. C the other hand, disruption of the intima may be the result of hemorrhage with the media, with secondary rupture of the intima[2,13,17] (Fig. 13.2).

The clinical expression of aortic dissection depends on the route taken l the dissecting hematoma. If arch vessels are interrupted, cerebral or upp extremity ischemia/infarction may develop. Similarly, interruption of descend ing aortic branches may lead to renal, mesenteric, or limb ischemia. The di secting hematoma may involve the aortic root, disrupting the annulus of th aortic valve and producing acute aortic regurgitation. The hematoma may als rupture through the aortic adventitia and thereby gain access to the pericardi or left pleural space. Tamponade or fatal intrathoracic hemorrhage may result.

Factors associated with aortic dissection are listed in Figure 13.3. Degener tive alterations, known as *cystic medial degeneration*, must develop in the aort media in order for dissection to occur. Cystic deterioration of medial collage and elastic tissue is almost invariably found when aortic tissue from a patier with dissection is examined. The combination of cystic medial degeneratio and one or more of the factors listed in Figure 13.3 produce the dissectir hematoma. Cystic medial degeneration is either congenital (e.g., Marfan's Ehlers-Danlos syndromes) or acquired (e.g., long-standing hypertension).

FIGURE 13.1 DISEASES OF THE AORTA

Aortic dissection
Arteriosclerotic aortic aneurysm
Annuloaortic ectasia
Aortic arteritis
Takayasu's arteritis
Giant-cell arteritis
Ankylosing spondylitis
Psoriatic arthritis
Relapsing polychondritis
Reiter's syndrome
Behçet's syndrome
Luetic involvement of the aorta
Traumatic injuries of the aorta
Aortic thromboembolic disease
Aortic bacterial infection
Aortic tumors
Coarctation and pseudo-coarctation
Hypoplastic aorta syndromes

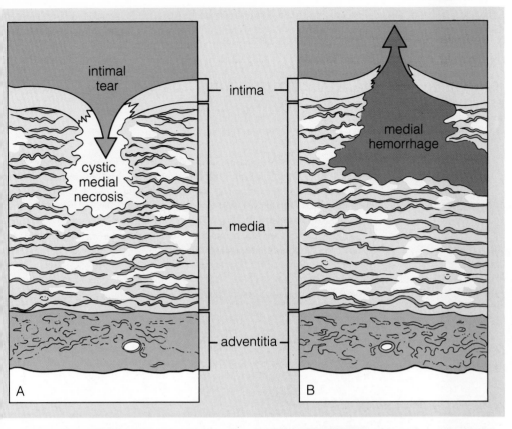

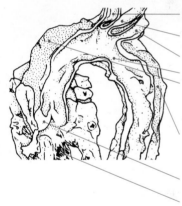

FIGURE 13.2 Potential mechanisms of aortic dissection. (A) An intimal tear allows blood to enter the media. (B) Hemorrhage present in the media, with secondary rupture of the overlying intima. (C) Arterial blood gains access to the media. (D) Hematoma dissects antegrade and retrograde along the aortic wall. (E) Pathologic specimen displaying the ascending aorta, the aortic arch, and the descending arch in a patient with an ascending aortic dissection. The blood-filled false lumen is clearly seen. (E reproduced with permission; see Figure Credits)

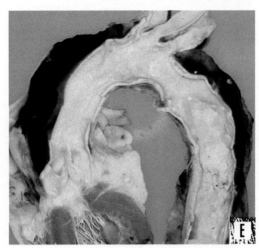

innominate artery
left carotid artery
left subclavian
aortic arch
false lumen of dissection filled with clotted blood
false lumen of dissection filled with clotted blood
aortic valve leaflets
left ventricular cavity

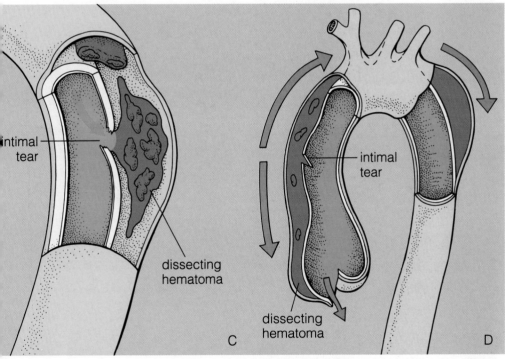

FIGURE 13.3 FACTORS PREDISPOSING TO AORTIC ISSECTION

Cystic medial degeneration, primary or secondary, usually combined with one or more of the following:
    Advanced age
    Hypertension
    Pregnancy

Atherosclerosis
Aortic valve disease
Coarctation of the aorta
Aortic trauma including iatrogenic trauma (e.g., angiographic catheter)

More than 95% of dissections begin either just above the aortic valve or just beyond the origin of the left subclavian artery. A few dissections remain localized to the aortic arch. Aortic dissections were originally classified as type I, II, or III (Fig. 13.4). Type I dissections originate just above the aortic valve and extend to the descending thoracic aorta or beyond. Type II dissection, which is quite uncommon, is localized to the aortic arch. Type III dissection begins just beyond the origin of the left subclavian artery and extends into the abdominal aorta or beyond. Current terminology classifies type I and II dissections together under the term *ascending aortic dissection*, while type III dissection is known as *descending aortic dissection*[7,10,12,12a,12b] (see Fig. 13.4).

CLINICAL MANIFESTATIONS
MEDICAL HISTORY

Most patients complain of severe chest pain that attains maximal severity at onset. This often helps to distinguish the pain of dissection from that of myocardial ischemia/infarction, which builds over some minutes. The pain felt from dissection is often described as tearing, ripping, or stabbing. It frequently migrates along the course of the dissection. For example, pain associated with ascending aortic dissection might begin in the anterior chest and then migrate to the mid or lower back. Anxiety, diaphoresis, nausea and vomiting, and faintness often accompany the pain. In an occasional patient, dissection is painless or presents with atypical symptoms such as syncope or heart failure secondary to acute aortic regurgitation. Patients with descending aortic dissection tend to be older and to have more associated medical diseases (hypertension, diabetes, heart disease) than individuals with ascending aortic dissection.[11]

PHYSICAL EXAMINATION

The diagnosis of aortic dissection is often strongly inferred from the physical findings. Pulse and blood pressure inequalities and hypotension are commonly observed. The murmur of aortic regurgitation, neurologic deficits, and/or findings associated with cardiac tamponade (hypotension, jugular venous distension, distant heart sounds) may be present in patients with ascending aortic dissection. Pulse deficits are less commonly noted in patients with descending aortic dissection. Heart failure secondary to acute aortic regurgitation may lead to pulmonary rales and a third heart sound. Unusual routes of dissection may produce unexpected findings, such as a continuous murmur secondary to rupture of the dissection into a right heart chamber.[14]

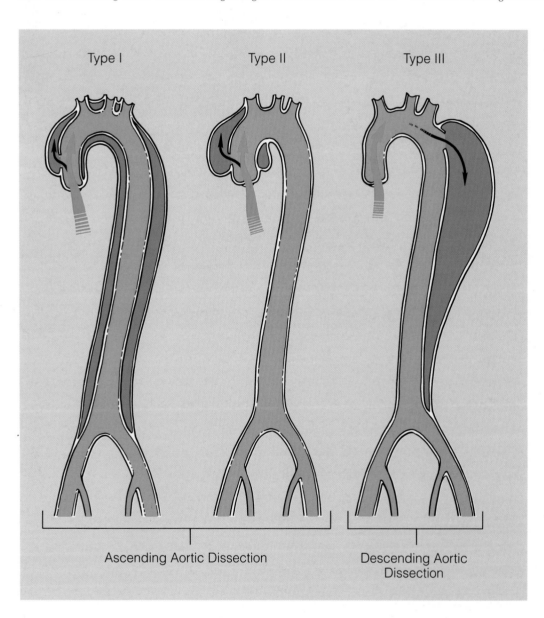

Type I Type II Type III

Ascending Aortic Dissection

Descending Aortic Dissection

FIGURE 13.4 Classification of the three types of aortic dissection. (Modified from ref. 12a, and reproduced with permission; see Figure Credits.)

Chest Radiography The chest x-ray often suggests the diagnosis of dissection. Mediastinal widening on the posteroanterior roentgenogram is usually observed (Fig. 13.5). Progressive widening of the aortic shadow and an increased distance (>1.0 cm) from aortic intimal calcification to the outer edge of the aortic shadow are specific for dissection.[4]

Electrocardiography The ECG in dissection is usually unremarkable. Thus, it is helpful in excluding myocardial infarction as the cause of the chest pain. Rarely, the dissection compromises a coronary artery, thereby producing a myocardial infarction that is seen on the ECG tracing. Left ventricular hypertrophy from pre-existing hypertension is often noted on the ECG tracing.

Echocardiography Transthoracic M-mode and two-dimensional echocardiography are often helpful in confirming the diagnosis of dissection.[5,6] The disrupted intimal flap and the false lumen created by the dissecting hematoma are observed (Fig. 13.6). Transesophageal echocardiography is particularly useful in visualizing these diagnostic features of aortic dissection. Most patients with dissection will have a diagnostic transesophageal echocardiogram.

Cardiac Catheterization Angiography is a highly accurate diagnostic technique for delineating dissection and its consequences.[9] The intimal flap, the location and extent of the false lumen, and compromised arteries are all well defined on the angiogram (Fig. 13.7).

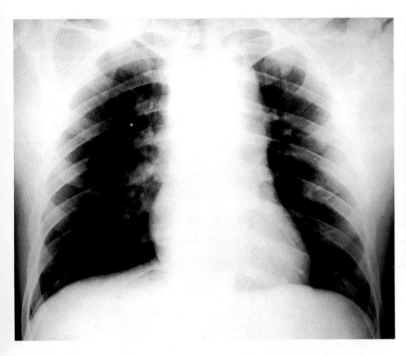

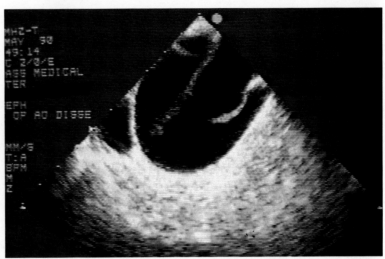

FIGURE 13.6 Transesophageal echocardiogram of the aortic root in a patient with an ascending aortic dissection. Note the clearly visible intimal flaps. (Reproduced with permission; see Figure Credits)

FIGURE 13.5 Posteroanterior projection of a 64-year-old hypertensive man with sudden severe back pain. Note the widened mediastinum and large aortic knob with indistinct superior border. On angiography, the patient had a descending aortic dissection. (Reproduced with permission; see Figure Credits)

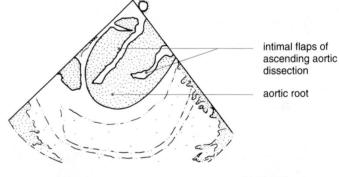

intimal flaps of ascending aortic dissection

aortic root

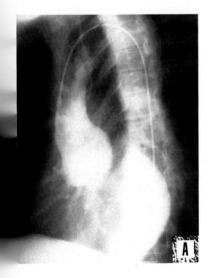
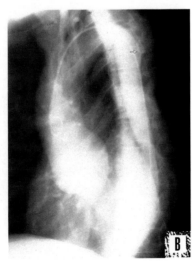

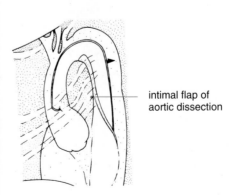

intimal flap of aortic dissection

FIGURE 13.7
(A,B) Thoracic aortic angiograms in a patient with a proximal aortic dissection. Note the intimal flap seen best in the distal thoracic aorta. The arrow points to irregularities in the true aortic lumen created by pressure from the false lumen. Note the irregular aortic contrast stream proximal and distal to this point.

Other Imaging Modalities Both CT and MRI scans are capable of visualizing aortic dissections with considerable accuracy.[15,16] The intimal tear and the extent of the dissection are both seen (Figs. 13.8, 13.9).

NATURAL HISTORY

Aortic dissection occurs more commonly in men than in women. The peak incidence is during the sixth and seventh decades. Patients with ascending aortic dissection tend to be younger than individuals with descending dissection. The prognosis for patients with untreated dissection is poor. Approximately 70% of patients with untreated dissection die within the first week following the onset of the disease, and 90% within the first month.[1]

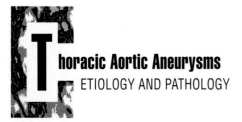

Thoracic Aortic Aneurysms
ETIOLOGY AND PATHOLOGY

Thoracic aortic aneurysms are most commonly the result of arteriosclerosis of the aorta (Fig. 13.10). Less common etiologies include annuloaortic ectasia (e.g.,

Marfan's Syndrome), aortic valve disease, and syphilis.[7,11] Seventy-five percent of arteriosclerotic aortic aneurysms develop in the abdomen; 25% occur in the chest. Abdominal aortic aneurysms are discussed in Chapter 14. Arteriosclerotic thoracic aortic aneurysms can develop in any segment of the thoracic aorta. Luetic aneurysms, on the other hand, are located predominantly in the ascending aorta. Similarly, annuloaortic ectasia usually leads to aneurysmal dilatation of the aortic root and ascending aorta. The aortic arch may also be involved. Aortic valve disease (aortic regurgitation, aortic stenosis, prosthetic aortic valve) occasionally produces aneurysmal dilatation of the aortic root and ascending aorta.

Aortic aneurysms develop secondary to weakening of structural elements in the aortic wall. Arteriosclerosis, luetic arteritis, or cystic medial degeneration (annuloaortic ectasia) each lead to thoracic aortic aneurysm by this process. Once an aortic segment is dilated, the law of Laplace (wall tension = pressure x radius) predicts that wall tension in that segment will increase. Increased wall tension leads to further aortic dilatation and hence to even greater wall tension. This upward spiral of aortic wall tension and diameter leads to aneurysmal formation and eventually to aortic rupture.

CLINICAL MANIFESTATIONS
MEDICAL HISTORY

Symptoms related to thoracic aortic aneurysms are often the result of impinge-

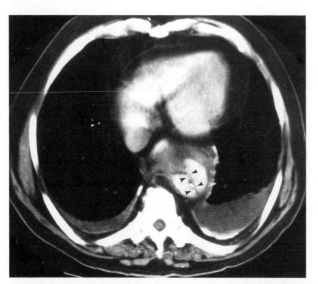

FIGURE 13.8 CT scan identifying the intimal flap *(arrows)* of a thoracic aortic dissection. There is a hematoma surrounding the aorta and a left pleural effusion. (Reproduced with permission; see Figure Credits)

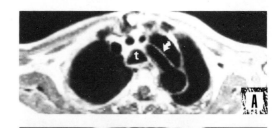

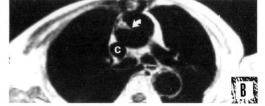

FIGURE 13.9 Aortic dissection. MR images through the ascending aorta **(A)** and aortic arch **(B)** show the intimal flap in the aortic lumen *(curved arrow)*. (c = superior vena cava; t = trachea) (Reproduced with permission; see Figure Credits)

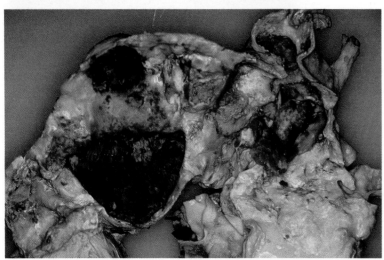

FIGURE 13.10 Pathologic specimen displaying the aortic arch in a patient with a large ascending aortic atherosclerotic aneurysm. Note the severe atherosclerosis of the aorta and the blood-filled aneurysm. (Reproduced with permission; see Figure Credits)

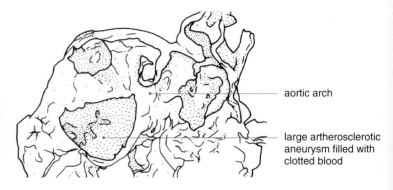

aortic arch

large artherosclerotic aneurysm filled with clotted blood

ent of the aneurysm on contiguous structures. Wheezing, cough, dyspnea, stridor, and hemoptysis are the result of tracheal/bronchial and pulmonary compression. Hoarseness can result from compression of the recurrent laryngeal nerve. Patients may complain of dysphagia secondary to aneurysmal compression of the esophagus. Anterior chest pain may be described. This discomfort is often constant and may be quite severe. It is the result of aneurysmal compression and erosion of adjacent thoracic musculoskeletal components.

PHYSICAL EXAMINATION

If the aneurysm is large, visible and palpable pulsations may be observed on the anterior chest wall along either sternal border or at either sternoclavicular joint. The aneurysm may also be palpable in the suprasternal notch. A systolic tracheal tug may be felt or tracheal deviation may be noted. Superior vena cava syndrome may be observed in individuals with aneurysmal compression of the superior vena cava or innominate veins. Hypotension or frank shock may be seen in patients with ruptured thoracic aortic aneurysms although this is a less common presentation than is observed with abdominal aortic aneurysm. Blood pressure readings may differ between the two arms. Patients with luetic aortic aneurysms may have coexisting ostial coronary arterial obstruction with signs and symptoms of severe myocardial ischemia, as well as other findings associated with tertiary syphilis. Patients with annuloaortic ectasia often have physical signs of Marfan's syndrome, including arachnodactyly, ectopia lentis, high

arched palate, tall stature, and kyphoscoliosis. Aortic insufficiency is often present, producing its characteristic diastolic murmur.[3,11]

LABORATORY STUDIES

Chest Radiography   Most thoracic aortic aneurysms are clearly visible on routine posteroanterior and lateral chest x-rays (Figs. 13.11–13.13). At times it may be difficult to distinguish a thoracic aortic aneurysm from a mediastinal mass secondary to tumor by means of chest x-ray alone. CT or MR imaging is often helpful in diagnosing these patients. Characteristic linear, "egg-shell" calcifications of the ascending aorta may be observed in patients with syphilitic thoracic aortic aneurysms.[7]

Electrocardiography   Thoracic aortic aneurysms produce no characteristic ECG alteration. Left ventricular hypertrophy secondary to coexisting hypertension and infarct patterns secondary to coexisting coronary artery disease are frequently observed. Bundle branch block is often noted in older individuals.

Echocardiography   Two-dimensional echocardiographic examination usually demonstrates thoracic aortic aneurysms quite clearly.[8] This is particularly the case if a transesophageal echocardiographic study is employed. A transthoracic echocardiogram can delineate ascending aortic aneurysms. However, arch or descending aortic aneurysms are poorly seen with transthoracic studies. Most of these latter aneurysms can be visualized by transesophageal echocardiography.

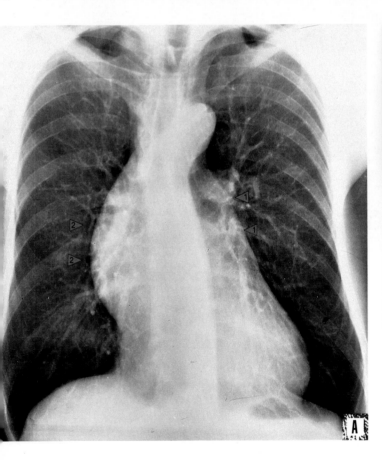

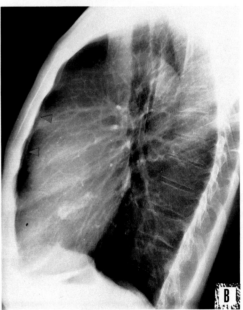

FIGURE 13.11   Chest x-rays depicting aortic root aneurysm in a 20-year-old man with Marfan's syndrome. **(A)** On the posteroanterior projection, the enlargement of the ascending aorta to the left *(arrows 1)* and right *(arrows 2)* produces a widened mediastinal image. **(B)** On the lateral projection, the dilated aortic root *(arrows)* fills the retrosternal space. (Reproduced with permission; see Figure Credits)

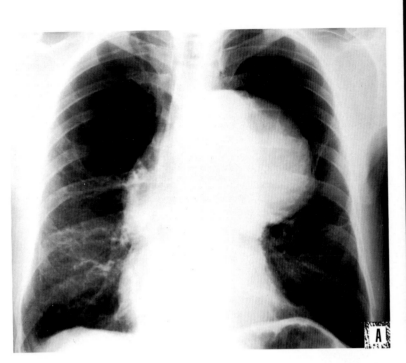

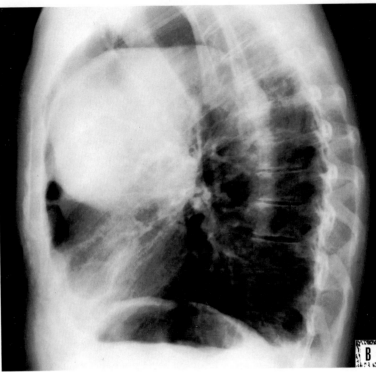

FIGURE 13.12 Chest x-rays of a massive aortic aneurysm of unknown etiology arising from the superior portion of the ascending aorta and transverse aorta. (A) Posteroanterior projection. A large upper left mediastinal mass is seen adjacent to the cardiac silhouette. The aortic arch is clearly seen through the mass. (B) Left lateral projection showing the superior mediastinal mass associated with the upper part of the ascending aorta. (Reproduced with permission; see Figure Credits)

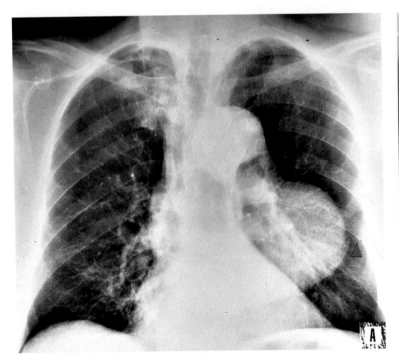

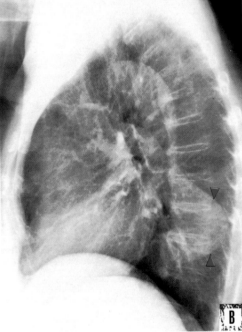

FIGURE 13.13 Chest radiographs of an aneurysm of the descending thoracic aorta. Posteroanterior (A) and lateral (B) views show a mass contiguous with the thoracic aorta (arrows) projecting into the left lung. (Reproduced with permission; see Figure Credits)

Cardiac Catheterization   Aortic angiography is the definitive procedure for outlining a thoracic aortic aneurysm (Figs. 13.14–13.16). Aneurysmal involvement of various arterial branches is also clearly depicted. All patients who are being considered for surgical therapy should undergo angiography. If surgery is not being considered, noninvasive diagnostic measures such as echocardiography, CT, or MRI are sufficient.

Other Imaging Modalities   Both CT and MRI scans can delineate thoracic aortic aneurysms with considerable accuracy (Fig. 13.17).

Laboratory Tests   Approximately 70% to 90% of patients with syphilitic aortic aneurysms will have a positive serologic test for syphilis (Wassermann, Hinton, VDRL). An even higher percentage of these individuals will have a positive fluorescent treponemal antibody absorption test or a Reiter's protein complement fixation test. Patients with arteriosclerotic thoracic aortic aneurysms usually have elevated serum cholesterol levels.

NATURAL HISTORY

Less is known about the natural history of thoracic aortic aneurysm than is the case with abdominal aortic aneurysm. Nevertheless, survival is related to the size of the aneurysm regardless of location. Thoracic aortic aneurysms greater than 7 cm in diameter are more prone to rupture than are smaller aneurysms. The natural history of arteriosclerotic aortic aneurysm is often determined by associated coronary artery and cerebrovascular disease. Two thirds of the deaths in patients with arteriosclerotic thoracic aortic aneurysm are due to associated vascular disease. Symptomatic aneurysms are twice as likely to rupture compared to asymptomatic aneurysms.

Patients with annuloaortic ectasia frequently develop aortic dissection. Luetic thoracic aortic aneurysms greater than 7 cm in diameter are also prone to rupture. The natural history of luetic aortic aneurysm may be complicated by coexisting aortic regurgitation and/or ostial coronary arterial stenoses.

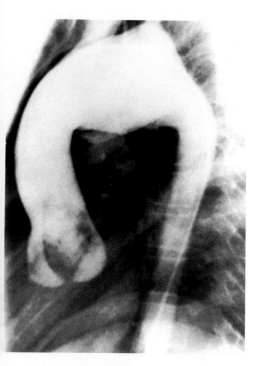

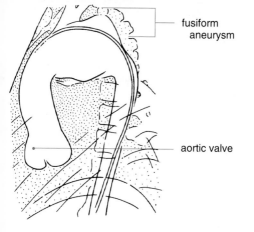

fusiform aneurysm

aortic valve

FIGURE 13.14   Lateral aortogram of an arteriosclerotic aneurysm of the aortic arch. The film reveals a fusiform aneurysm involving the entire aortic arch. (Reproduced with permission; see Figure Credits)

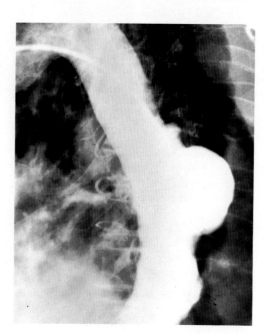

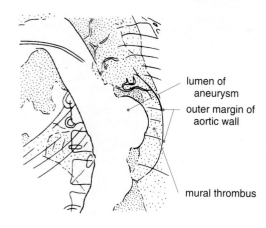

lumen of aneurysm

outer margin of aortic wall

mural thrombus

FIGURE 13.15
Lateral aortogram of an aneurysm of the descending thoracic aorta. The projection shows a saccular aneurysm arising from the posterior wall of the descending aorta in a 60-year-old patient. The gap between the opacified lumen of the aneurysm and the outer margin of the aortic wall represents mural thrombus. (Reproduced with permission; see Figure Credits)

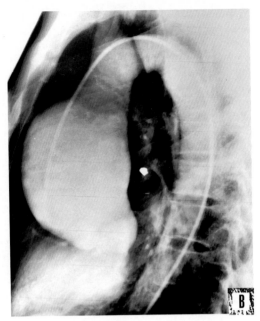

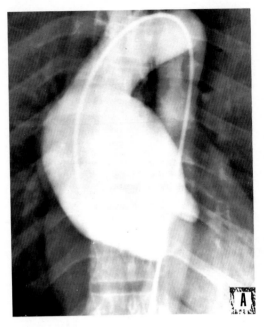

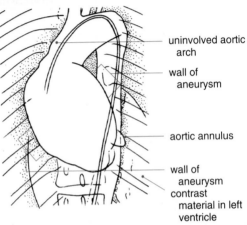

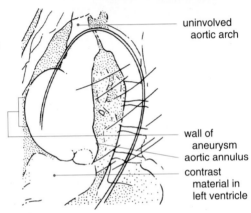

FIGURE 13.16 Aortogram (injection into the aortic root) of an aneurysm of the aortic root. A large aneurysm of the ascending aorta is seen protruding anteriorly and more to the right than to the left. The aortic annulus is involved, resulting in severe aortic insufficiency (note the opacification of the left ventricle). The aortic arch is not involved. (Reproduced with permission; see Figure Credits)

uninvolved aortic arch

wall of aneurysm

aortic annulus

wall of aneurysm
contrast material in left ventricle

uninvolved aortic arch

wall of aneurysm
aortic annulus

contrast material in left ventricle

FIGURE 13.17 Contrast-enhanced CT scan demonstrating a thoracic aortic aneurysm. A large aneurysm of the ascending aorta protrudes anteriorly and to the right. The large filling defect in the aneurysm represents mural thrombus. The descending thoracic aorta is normal. (Reproduced with permission; see Figure Credits)

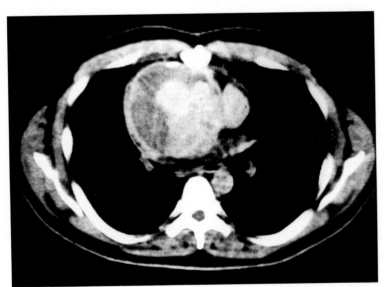

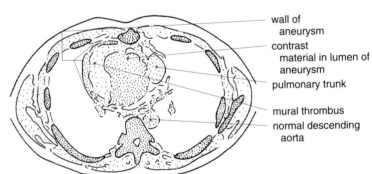

wall of aneurysm

contrast material in lumen of aneurysm

pulmonary trunk

mural thrombus

normal descending aorta

FIGURE CREDITS

gs. 13.2E, 13.10 courtesy of Henri Cuenoud, MD.

g. 13.4 modified from DeBakey ME, Henley WS, Cooley DA, et al: Surgical management of dissecting aneurysm of the aorta. J Thorac Cardiovasc Surg 49:130, 1965.

gs. 13.5, 13.12 from Chatterjee K, et al: Cardiology: An Illustrated Text–Reference. Gower, New York, 1992.

g. 13.6 courtesy of Linda A. Pape, MD.

g. 13.8 from White RD, et al: Noninvasive evaluation of suspected thoracic aortic disease by contrast enhanced computed tomography. Am J Cardiol 57:282, 1986.

g. 13.9 from Amparo EG, et al: Aortic dissection: Magnetic resonance imaging. Radiology 155:399, 1985.

gs. 13.11, 13.13–13.17 from Kassner EG: Atlas of Radiologic Imaging. Gower, New York, 1989.

REFERENCES

Anagnostopoulos CE, Prabhakar MJS, Kittle CF: Aortic dissections and dissecting aneurysms. Am J Cardiol 30:263, 1972.

Dalen JE, Pape LA, Cohn LH, et al: Dissection of the aorta: Pathogenesis, diagnosis and treatment. Prog Cardiovasc Dis 23:237, 1980.

Eagle KA, Quertermous T, Kritzer GA, et al: Spectrum of conditions initially suggesting acute aortic aneurysm. Am J Med 59:171, 1975.

Earnest F IV, Muhm JR, Sheedy PF II: Roentgenographic findings in thoracic aortic dissection. Mayo Clin Proc 54:43, 1979.

Fox R, Ren J, Pandis JP, et al: Annuloaortic ectasia: A clinical and echocardiographic study. Am J Cardiol 54:177, 1984.

6. Granato JE, Dee P, Gibson RS: Utility of two-dimensional echocardiography in suspected ascending aortic dissection. Am J Cardiol 56:123, 1985.

7. Heggtveit HA: Syphilitic aortitis: A clinicopathologic autopsy study of 100 cases, 1950 to 1960. Circulation 29:346, 1964.

8. Iliceto S, Antonelli G, Biasco G, et al: Two-dimensional echocardiographic evaluation of aneurysms of the descending thoracic aorta. Circulation 66:1045, 1982.

9. Lemon DK, White CW: Annuloaortic ectasia: Angiographic, hemodynamic and clinical comparison with aortic valve insufficiency. Am J Cardiol 41:482, 1978.

10. Moreno-Cabral CE, Miller C, Mitchell S, et al: Degenerative and atherosclerotic aneurysms of the thoracic aorta. J Thorac Cardiovasc Surg 88:1020, 1984.

11. Pyeritz RE, McKusick VA: The Marfan syndrome: Diagnosis and management. N Engl J Med 300:772, 1979.

12. Roberts WC: Aortic dissection: Anatomy, consequences, and causes. Am Heart J 101:195, 1981.

12a. DeBakey ME, Henley WS, Cooley DA, et al: Surgical management of dissecting aneurysm of the aorta. J Thorac Cardiovasc Surg 49:130, 1965.

12b. Lindsay J Jr, Hurst JW (eds): The Aorta. Grune and Stratton, New York, 1979:241.

13. Schlatmann TJM, Becker AE: Pathogenesis of dissecting aneurysm of the aorta. Am J Cardiol 39:21, 1977.

14. Slater EE, DeSanctis RW: The clinical recognition of dissecting aortic aneurysm. Am J Med 60:625, 1976.

15. Thorsen MK, San Dretto MA, Lawson TL, et al: Dissecting aortic aneurysms: Accuracy of computed tomographic diagnosis. Radiology 148:773, 1983.

16. Vasile N, Mathieu D, Keita K, et al: Computed tomography of thoracic aortic dissection: Accuracy and pitfalls. J Comp Assist Tomogr 10:211, 1986.

17. Wheat MW Jr: Acute dissecting aneurysms of the aorta: Diagnosis and treatment—1979. Am Heart J 99:373, 1980.

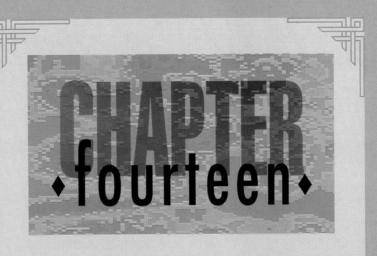

CHAPTER fourteen

PERIPHERAL ARTERIAL DISEASE

STEPHEN L. KEITH, MD

MICHAEL J. ROHRER, MD

The number of techniques available for the diagnosis of peripheral arterial disease has increased significantly over the last three decades. However, a thorough history and physical examination remains the cornerstone of the vascular diagnostic evaluation. Noninvasive testing usually serves to confirm the initial diagnostic impression gained from the history and physical examination and to quantitate the severity of the disease process. Invasive testing is rarely warranted as a diagnostic procedure to determine the presence of peripheral arterial disease; rather its primary value is to provide further anatomic detail as a prelude to therapeutic intervention.

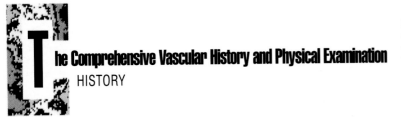

The Comprehensive Vascular History and Physical Examination

HISTORY

Lower extremity claudication or ischemic rest pain is the most common presenting complaint in the patient with peripheral arterial disease. As with pain of any etiology, it is important to determine the location, quality, time of onset, duration, magnitude, and factors that reduce or exacerbate the symptom. Additional points to establish include a history of pulsatile masses, ulcerated skin lesions, extremity swelling, and alterations in sexual function (which may occur in men with aortoiliac occlusive disease). The patient should be questioned about prior arterial surgery and about symptoms of atherosclerotic occlusive disease involving other organ systems, such as a history of myocardial infarction or angina, transient ischemic attacks or stroke, postprandial abdominal pain and weight loss, and hypertension.

PHYSICAL EXAMINATION

Atherosclerotic occlusive disease is a diffuse process that can effect the entire arterial system. Therefore, the comprehensive vascular examination should include investigation of the entire arterial system to identify disease that may have been previously unrecognized. The heart rate and rhythm should be noted by palpation and auscultation, and blood pressures should be measured in both upper extremities. A difference in systolic pressures of greater than 20 mmHg is indicative of a hemodynamically significant proximal arterial stenosis.

The neck should be palpated just anterior to the sternocleidomastoid muscle to identify the carotid pulse, and the neck near the angle of the mandible should be auscultated with a stethoscope to detect the presence of a carotid bruit. A carotid bruit may be the only physical finding indicative of a stenosis of the internal carotid artery at the carotid bifurcation.

Inspection of the feet may reveal information about the arterial perfusion of the lower extremities. The extremity with mild ischemia may appear normal, but as chronic ischemia progresses, patients develop dependent rubor in the distal forefoot and toes that blanches with leg elevation. If ischemia continues to worsen, patients will eventually develop dry gangrene or ulceration, which typically involves the toes or distal forefoot. Trivial wounds may not heal in the setting of arterial occlusive disease due to insufficient foot perfusion.

Palpation of the peripheral pulses is the most direct means of assessing the peripheral arterial circulation. The carotid, brachial, radial, femoral, popliteal, dorsalis pedis, and posterior tibial pulses are all normally palpable. The common femoral artery pulse is located just below the inguinal ligament at the point halfway between the pubic tubercle and the anterior superior iliac spine. Auscultation of the groin may reveal evidence of a bruit because of turbulent arterial flow secondary to occlusive disease. The presence of a continuous "machinery murmur," which is heard throughout systole and diastole, is indicative of an *arteriovenous fistula*. The popliteal pulse is often difficult to feel because of the artery's location deep within the popliteal space. It is best assessed with the fingertips of both hands placed at the popliteal space while the patient lies in the supine position with the leg relaxed and knee slightly flexed. The dorsalis pedis pulse is found on the dorsum of the foot just lateral to the extensor hallucis longus tendon. The posterior tibial pulse is located in the groove behind the medial malleolus.

Pulse intensity is graded on a scale of 0 to 4. An absent pulse is denoted as 0. A 1+ pulse is barely palpable, a 2+ pulse is palpable but clearly diminished, a 3+ pulse is easily palpable but slightly diminished, and a 4+ pulse is normal.

Patients with peripheral arterial disease commonly do not have pulses in their feet. Under these circumstances, the adequacy of the circulation can be quantified by using a Doppler ultrasonic flow detector to identify blood flow in the dorsalis pedis and posterior tibial arteries. If flow is detected, then an *ankle-brachial index* (ABI) can be calculated for each leg. This test is performed by placing a blood pressure cuff around the ankle and slowly inflating it while listening to the arterial flow with the Doppler probe. The pressure at which flow ceases is the ankle occlusion pressure. The equation for the calculation of ABI is: ABI = ankle systolic pressure/brachial systolic pressure.

The higher of the two brachial artery systolic pressures is used in the denominator. For each leg, the artery with the highest pressure (i.e., dorsalis pedis or posterior tibial) should be used in the numerator. The ABI in normal individuals is slightly greater than 1.0.

FIGURE 14.1   True aneurysms are bounded by all three layers of the arterial wall demonstrating generalized arterial dilatation. False aneurysms are contained by the soft tissues surrounding an area of arterial disruption.

True Aneurysm

False Aneurysm

soft
tissue

blood
flow

turbulent
blood
flow

Media

Intima

Adventitia

The abdomen should be palpated to detect the presence of an abdominal aortic aneurysm (AAA). The aortic pulsation is noted primarily in the epigastrium since the aortic bifurcation is at the level of the umbilicus. The size of the aorta can be estimated by simultaneously noting the two lateral boundaries of the pulsatile mass. With experience, the diameter of the abdominal aorta can be determined with a high degree of accuracy. The typical AAA originates below the level of the renal arteries and, in a thin patient, can usually be felt to converge to a relatively normal aortic diameter below the costal margin. If the aortic impulse is still wide high in the abdomen, it is possible that the AAA extends above the level of the renal arteries. A tender AAA or the elicitation of referred back pain with palpation of the aneurysm may indicate that aneurysm rupture is imminent and is therefore an important physical finding.

It is crucial for patients with peripheral arterial disease to have a thorough vascular examination prior to undergoing invasive diagnostic and therapeutic interventions, such as arteriography, cardiac catheterization, or insertion of an intra-aortic balloon pump. An assessment of the patient's vascular disease prior to these procedures will help to direct the clinician when he performs the test (such as cannulating the left femoral artery when the right femoral pulse is diminished). Furthermore, physical findings are useful to the vascular surgeon should the patient suffer a complication following the procedure, such as arterial thrombosis with resultant limb ischemia.

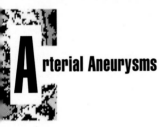

Arterial Aneurysms

An artery is considered to be aneurysmal when it has a focal dilatation that is at least 50% greater than the adjacent normal artery.[12] Aneurysms are clinically important because of their potential for multiple complications, the most well recognized being rupture which can lead to life-threatening hemorrhage.

Alternatively, aneurysms may also acutely thrombose or be a source of distal embolization and therefore cause acute limb ischemia. Aneurysms can also cause local compression of surrounding structures such as veins, nerves, or ureters, which can lead to lower extremity swelling and DVT, peripheral neurologic sequelae, and hydronephrosis.

An aneurysm can be classified as either *true* or *false*. A true aneurysm is contained by the three layers of the arterial wall—the intima, media, and adventitia—and represents generalized arterial dilatation. In contrast, a false aneurysm or *pseudoaneurysm* is contained only by periarterial soft tissues (Fig. 14.1). Such an aneurysm is usually the result of arterial trauma in which the arterial wall has not completely sealed. The resulting arterial defect permits the escape of pulsatile blood from the artery, which dissects into the surrounding soft tissues and promotes the formation of a surrounding fibrous capsule.

True aneurysms are morphologically described as being either *fusiform* or *saccular*. Fusiform aneurysms are more common and are characterized by circumferential dilatation of the vessel. Saccular aneurysms are characterized by a localized outpouching of the vessel wall and are often the result of congenital arterial abnormalities or focal arterial infection (Fig. 14.2).

A *dissecting aortic aneurysm* represents an entirely different pathologic entity, developing when a tear in the intima allows the blood to separate the layers of the aorta (Fig. 14.3) The tear may extend proximally and distally through the diseased media, creating a "false lumen" in which blood is able to flow. Aortic dissections occur most frequently in the ascending or proximal descending thoracic aorta, whereas fusiform atherosclerotic aneurysms occur most often in the infrarenal abdominal aorta.

ABDOMINAL AORTIC ANEURYSMS

Abdominal aortic aneurysms are the most commonly found aneurysms in the body. These aneurysms typically involve the infrarenal aorta and iliac arteries, although they occasionally extend proximally to involve the origin of the renal and visceral arterial branches. Aneurysms inevitably enlarge with time, albeit at widely variable rates in different individuals. The size of the aneurysm is a concern because the risk of rupture and the threat of exsanguinating hemorrhage increases exponentially with increasing aneurysm diameter.[10]

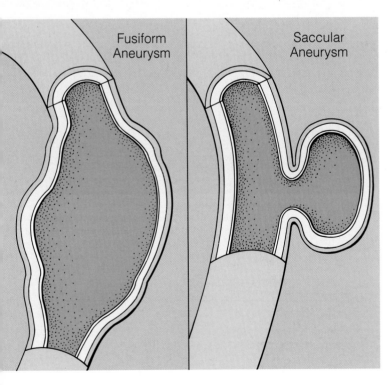

FIGURE 14.2   Fusiform aneurysms result from diffuse arterial degeneration. Saccular aneurysms result from focal arterial defects.

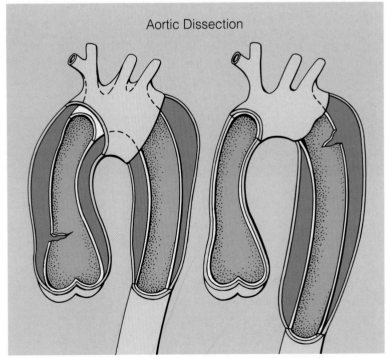

FIGURE 14.3   Aortic dissection resulting from blood dissecting the arterial media to separate the intimal and medial layers of the aorta. Most aortic dissections originate in the ascending aorta, but dissections beginning in the descending thoracic aorta are not unusual.

HISTORY AND PHYSICAL EXAMINATION

Although patients may occasionally recognize the presence of a pulsatile abdominal mass, most AAAs are asymptomatic. In rare cases, patients may describe epigastric fullness or alteration in appetite. A much more ominous symptom is pain, which may present in the epigastrium, groin, hip, or, most commonly, low back. Acute pain or aneurysmal tenderness usually represents either rupture or acute expansion of the aneurysm with impending rupture. Most aneurysms are initially detected as asymptomatic pulsatile masses in the epigastrium during routine physical examination. Aneurysms are also occasionally identified incidentally by the finding of a calcified perimeter on abdominal radiographs.

LABORATORY STUDIES

The size of an AAA identified by physical examination should be determined since the risk of rupture increases substantially with increasing cross sectional diameter.[10] The most common method in use both for confirming the presence of an AAA and for establishing its size is abdominal ultrasound[7,9] (Fig. 14.4). This diagnostic technique is accurate, noninvasive, relatively inexpensive, easily repeated, and free of radiation exposure. A second method in common use for the evaluation of an AAA is CT scanning[19] (Fig. 14.5). In addition to confirming the diagnosis and measuring the size of the AAA, the CT scan may provide valuable information about surrounding venous and retroperitoneal anomalies and can evaluate coincident intra-abdominal pathology.[14] CT scanning is also able to detect the presence of extraluminal retroperitoneal blood, which is diagnostic of aneurysm rupture.[20]

Angiography also plays an important role in the management of a patient with an AAA. This tool can delineate the proximal and distal extent of the aneurysm, as well as define associated renal and visceral artery anomalies and occlusive disease (Fig. 14.6) It is important to emphasize, however, that angiography is not used to establish the diagnosis of AAA but rather to plan the strategy of operative repair. In fact, it is possible for even large AAAs to elude angiographic diagnosis since the aneurysm sac is often filled with laminated thrombus, and the actual channel through which the contrast-containing blood flow may have a relatively normal caliber (Fig. 14.7).

ANEURYSMS OF THE EXTREMITIES

Although aneurysms have been described in each of the upper and lower extremity arteries, the two most common locations for peripheral arterial aneurysms are, in order of frequency, the popliteal and common femoral arteries. There is a high incidence of multiple aneurysms in patients with peripheral aneurysms. Almost 60% of patients with one popliteal aneurysm will have a second in the other leg, and 55% of patients with a popliteal aneurysm will have another aneurysm in a different location, usually the abdominal aorta.[5] Because of this high incidence of multiple aneurysms in patients discovered to have at least one extremity aneurysm, diligent screening for additional aneurysms by physical examination followed by ultrasound examination of the abdominal aorta, iliac and femoral arteries, and popliteal arteries is warranted.[4,8]

In contrast to intra-abdominal aneurysms, peripheral arterial aneurysms rarely rupture. Instead, they typically produce acute limb ischemia secondary to either acute thrombosis or distal embolization. This diagnosis is often overlooked as a cause of acute limb ischemia since, once thrombosed, the aneurysm is no longer detectable as a pulsatile mass. The only clinical clue may be the presence of a contralateral aneurysm since they are so often found bilaterally. The rate of limb loss secondary to this problem is high because aneurysm thrombosis is often precipitated by prior embolization which obliterates the arterial outflow, thus precluding limb-salvaging vascular reconstruction.

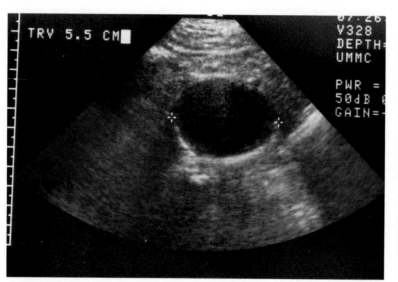

FIGURE 14.4   Ultrasound of an abdominal aortic aneurysm (AAA) measuring 5.5 cm in transverse diameter.

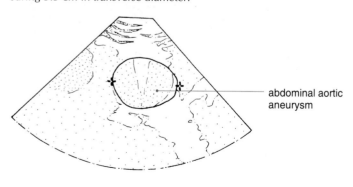

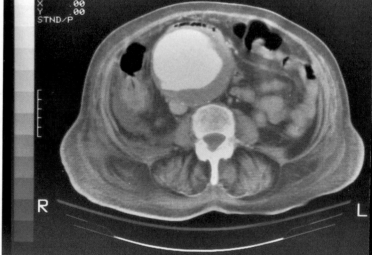

FIGURE 14.5   CT scan of an infrarenal AAA using intravenous contrast. This aneurysm is 8 cm in transverse diameter. Laminated thrombus within the lumen of the aorta is a common finding in aneurysms.

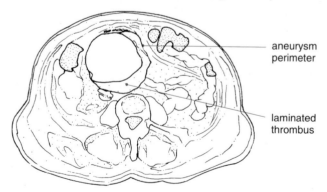

Peripheral aneurysms are usually asymptomatic, but may occasionally be noted by the patient as a pulsatile mass. On rare occasions peripheral aneurysms may enlarge to the point of causing compression of the adjacent nerves and veins and result in extremity pain or swelling. On physical examination, an aneurysm in the extremity is most often detected as a pulsatile mass[1] (Fig. 14.8). In the femoral triangle or the popliteal fossa, a thrombosed aneurysm may be detected as a nonpulsatile mass.

Aneurysms in the extremities can be detected and their size quantified by ultrasound or CT scanning. Arteriography is necessary prior to aneurysm resection to

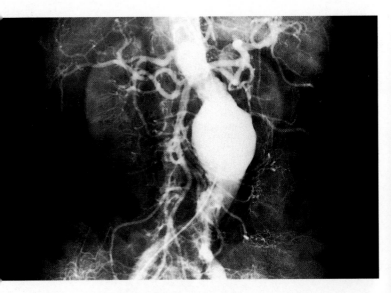

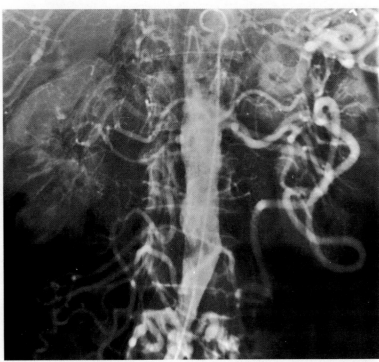

IGURE 14.6 Arteriogram demonstrating an infrarenal abdominal aortic aneurysm (AAA). The renal arteries can be seen originating above the aneurysm. Note that the aneurysm converges to a normal arterial diameter proximal to the aortic bifurcation.

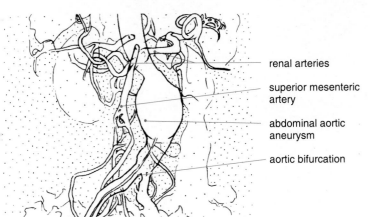

renal arteries

superior mesenteric artery

abdominal aortic aneurysm

aortic bifurcation

FIGURE 14.7 Aortogram of abdominal aortic aneurysm measuring 5 cm in diameter by ultrasound. The laminated thrombus within the aneurysm gives the false impression that no aneurysm is present.

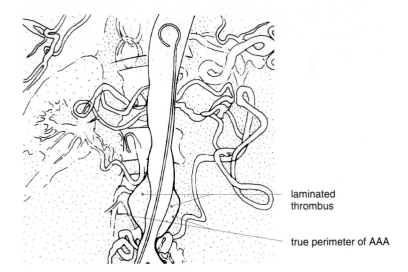

laminated thrombus

true perimeter of AAA

FIGURE 14.8 DIFFERENTIAL DIAGNOSIS OF THE PULSATILE GROIN MASS	
True aneurysm	Arteriovenous fistula
False aneurysm	Arteriovenous malformation
Traumatic	Hematoma
Anastomotic	Lymphocele
	Lymphadenopathy

identify the proximal and distal extent of the arterial dilatation, as well as to identify any associated occlusive lesions.

FALSE ANEURYSMS

The most common form of false aneurysms encountered in medical practice today is iatrogenic, occurring in the femoral artery after an invasive procedure such as arteriography, angioplasty, or intra-aortic balloon placement. Infected false aneurysms are found in drug abusers who inject drugs intra-arterially. Focal infection with arterial wall degeneration is important in the development of these false aneurysms, which are referred to as *mycotic aneurysms*.

Another type of false aneurysm is the *anastomotic false aneurysm*, which occurs at the site of a previous arterial anastomosis. These aneurysms usually represent disruption of an anastomotic suture line secondary to arterial degeneration, although infection may occasionally play a role in their development. Anastomotic false aneurysms are most commonly identified in the groin following aortofemoral or axillofemoral bypass grafting.

Although some small false aneurysms may spontaneously thrombose, most will enlarge with time and are capable of producing the same complications as these found with true aneurysms.[11]

HISTORY AND PHYSICAL EXAMINATION

False aneurysms frequently present as pulsatile masses. When there is a history c recent needle puncture or prior operation, there should be a high degree of sus picion that the pulsatile mass represents a pseudoaneurysm. The patient with fever as well as local and systemic signs of sepsis probably has a mycoti aneurysm.

LABORATORY STUDIES

When the lesion is located in an extremity, duplex ultrasound scanning ha proven to be highly accurate at identifying the presence of a false aneurysm. Th duplex scan is able to image the origin and extent of the pseudoaneurysm, and i is also able to document the presence of blood flow in this collection. This diag nostic modality has been proven to be so reliable that it is often the only tes obtained prior to undertaking pseudoaneurysm repair[6] (Fig. 14.9). In cases wher the false aneurysm is associated with a previous grafting procedure, arteriograph is generally required to define the origin and extent of the lesion (Fig. 14.10).

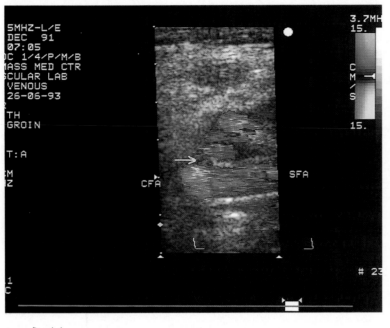

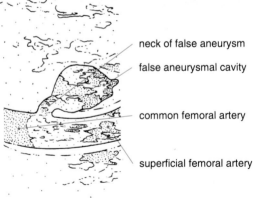

FIGURE 14.9   Color duplex scan of a pseudoaneurysm arising from the common femoral artery following cardiac catheterization. The arrow indicates site of hole in the artery, which communicates with the pseudoaneurysm cavity.

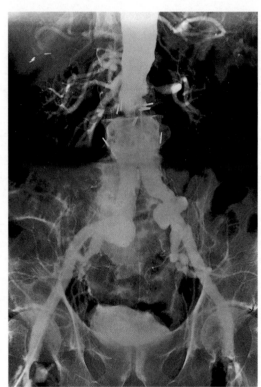

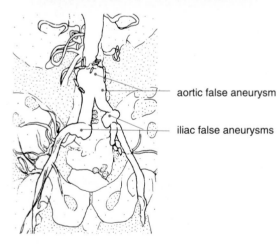

FIGURE 14.10
Arteriogram demonstrating proximal aorti and bilateral iliac anastomotic false aneurysms. At the time of the operation to repair these false aneurysms, the proximal graft was found to have completely separated from the proximal aorta, and the graft limbs had pulled away from the iliac arteries bilaterally.

Arterial Occlusive Disease

The symptoms produced by arterial occlusion are largely determined by the rapidity of onset of the occlusive process. Acute arterial occlusion tends to produce more profound signs and symptoms than occlusions that develop over a more prolonged period. In general, acute arterial occlusion produces limb-threatening ischemia, which must be urgently treated. Chronic arterial occlusions, however, usually do not result in immediate limb-threatening ischemia and thus may be evaluated under less urgent circumstances.

ACUTE ARTERIAL OCCLUSION

Excluding trauma, the most common etiologies of acute arterial occlusion are peripheral embolization and acute arterial thrombosis. Peripheral emboli have multiple potential sources, the most common being the heart (Fig. 14.11). Emboli tend to lodge at points of bifurcation in the arterial tree where there is an abrupt decrease in vessel size, such as the bifurcation of the aorta or the common femoral artery. In contrast, acute arterial thrombosis usually occurs in arteries that already have a significant stenotic lesion secondary to atherosclerosis. This clot develops in situ in the affected artery, as opposed to an embolus, which forms in a remote location and is transported to the affected artery through the circulation.

HISTORY AND PHYSICAL EXAMINATION

The symptoms produced by an acute arterial occlusion are dictated by the magnitude of the ischemia, which in turn is influenced by the adequacy of collateral arteries and the location of the occlusion. The most dramatic presentations are accompanied by the "5 p's" of acute limb ischemia: severe limb **p**ain, **p**aralysis, and **p**aresthesias, as well as the findings of **p**allor and **p**ulselessness. Not all of these findings may be simultaneously present in a patient with acute limb ischemia.

It is important to ascertain if there is a history of atrial fibrillation or myocardial infarction, both of which are major risk factors for embolization. Acute limb ischemia in a patient with a history of claudication suggests acute thrombosis of a previously stenotic artery.

On physical examination particular attention should be given to the status of the distal extremity pulses. If pulses are not palpable, then an ABI should be measured. Capillary refill will typically be sluggish or absent. The absence of motor or sensory function on physical examination indicates that the extremity is nonviable and that immediate intervention is mandatory.

LABORATORY STUDIES

After the history and physical examination have yielded a tentative diagnosis, a decision must be made whether additional diagnostic studies are necessary before instituting therapy. The patient with no prior symptoms of arterial occlusive disease who presents with atrial fibrillation and acute limb ischemia has almost certainly suffered an arterial embolus and should be taken directly to the operating room without additional diagnostic studies. If the diagnosis remains in doubt, then arteriography can yield information about both the etiology and the extent of the acute arterial occlusion (Fig. 14.12).

CHRONIC ARTERIAL OCCLUSIVE DISEASE

Chronic arterial occlusive disease is characterized by a gradual onset and progression of symptoms. The initial symptom of lower extremity occlusive disease is usually claudication. This phenomenon is manifest by a cramping or aching pain in the buttock, thigh, or calf, which is reproducibly brought on by exertion and relieved by rest. In patients with claudication, the blood flow to the distal extremity is adequate to meet the metabolic demands of the tissues at rest. However, when exertion increases these demands, the blood flow cannot increase to a commensurate level secondary to the proximal arterial stenosis or occlusion. A nutrient and oxygen deficit results and produces the symptoms of claudication.

As the atherosclerotic occlusive disease progresses, claudication occurs at lower levels of exertion. Eventually, the severity of the occlusive process may advance to the point that ischemic pain occurs at rest. Rest pain typically presents in the most distal portion of the extremity and indicates that the arterial perfusion is inadequate to meet the metabolic demands of the tissue, even when the patient is at rest.

FIGURE 14.11 SOURCES OF ARTERIAL EMBOLI

CARDIAC
Atrial fibrillation
Mural thrombus after myocardial
 infarction
Atrial myxoma
Valvular vegetation
Prosthetic valve vegetation

PROXIMAL ARTERY
Aneurysms
Ulcerated atherosclerotic plaque

FOREIGN BODY
Indwelling catheter
Arteriography
Intra-aortic balloon pump

VENOUS SYSTEM
Paradoxical embolus

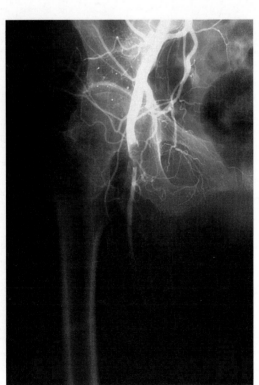

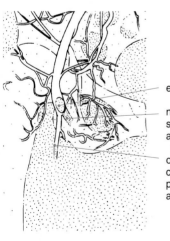

FIGURE 14.12 Embolus lodged at the femoral arterial bifurcation. The abrupt interruption of the contrast column is characteristic of an embolus.

embolus

no contrast filling superficial femoral artery

only trace of contrast opacifies profunda femoris artery

There are several disease entities that may mimic the symptoms of chronic arterial occlusive disease, including osteoarthritis, nerve root compression, peripheral neuritis, and gout. Many of these entities in the differential diagnosis can be ruled out during the physical examination and by simple noninvasive vascular testing.

HISTORY AND PHYSICAL EXAMINATION

The muscle group in which the symptoms occur provides a clue as to the level of the arterial obstructive process. In general, the symptomatic muscle group is distal to the predominant arterial occlusive lesion. For example, patients with thigh claudication usually have aortoiliac occlusive disease, and patients with calf claudication typically have superficial femoral artery occlusions.

In general, claudication results from a single level of chronic arterial occlusive disease. In these instances, the collateral circulation is almost always adequate enough so that the limb is not in jeopardy of developing gangrenous changes. Ischemic rest pain and tissue loss usually result from the development of a second level of occlusive disease in series, such as combined iliac artery and superficial femoral artery occlusions (Fig. 14.13). Symptoms of rest pain are usually first noted at night, when heart rate, blood pressure, and cardiac output are reduced. Patients often intuitively place the affected foot in a dependent position to improve the arterial blood flow, which decreases the pain. Critically ischemic extremities often become edematous because of this practice.

Limb-threatening ischemic ulceration and infection inevitably follow untreat rest pain. It is not unusual for such ulcers to be initiated by mild trauma. As w rest pain, the most common location of these lesions are the distal foot and toes.

Physical examination of the vascular system begins with a complete pul examination. If the distal pulses are not palpable, then an ABI should obtained. Patients with claudication typically have an ABI ranging between C and 0.4, and those with rest pain usually have an ABI less than 0.4. Patier with ischemic ulceration generally have an ABI less than 0.3[21] (Fig. 14.14).

Additional stigmata of chronic arterial occlusive disease include the presen of atrophic skin changes, such as hair loss and thinning of the skin, and depe dent rubor. Dependent rubor is characterized by a dark reddish discoloration the foot and toes when the leg suffering from serious occlusive disease is put in a dependent position. These extremities characteristically develop a marked pa lor with elevation.

LABORATORY STUDIES

Noninvasive Testing   There are instances in which t ABI can be spuriously elevated, despite the presence of significant arterial occ sive disease and ischemia. Arteries with medial calcinosis, usually seen patients with longstanding diabetes mellitus, may not be compressible, and blood pressure cuff around the ankle can often be inflated as high as 300 mmH without obliterating the distal Doppler arterial signal. The severity of t

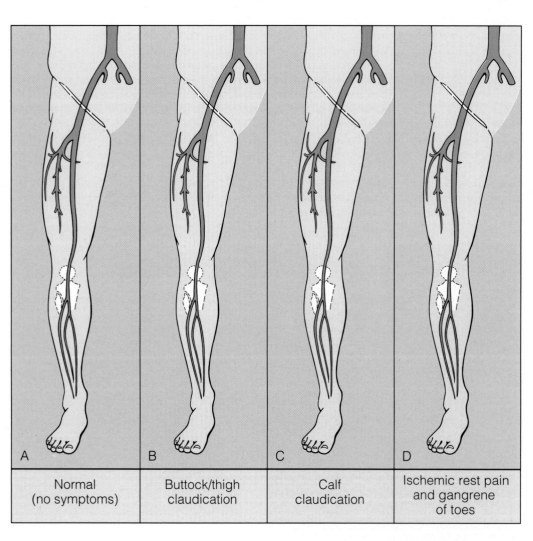

| Normal (no symptoms) | Buttock/thigh claudication | Calf claudication | Ischemic rest pain and gangrene of toes |

FIGURE 14.13   Relationship of levels of occl sive disease to symptomatology. **(A)** In the absence of any significant occlusive disease, there are no symptoms of claudication and the ankle-brachial index is slightly greater than 1.0. **(B)** A single level of occlusive disease in the iliac arter typically results in thigh and buttock claudicatio **(C)** Isolated superficial femoral artery occlusion often causes calf claudication. In each of these cases **(B,C)**, the ankle–brachial index is typically approximately 0.5. **(D)** When two occlusive lesions are present in series, there is more profound ischemia of the lower extremities with res pain and ulceration. In these cases, the ankle–brachial index is typically less than 0.25.

ischemic process can therefore be masked by artificially high ABIs in these cases. In order to better quantify the extent of the occlusive disease under such conditions, systolic toe pressures can be measured using an appropriately sized blood pressure cuff.[15] Normal toe pressures range from 90 to 110 mmHg. Patients with claudication typically have toe pressures from 40 to 60 mmHg, and patients with ischemic rest pain or ulceration often have digital pressures less than 20 mmHg.

The location of arterial occlusive lesions of the lower extremities may be objectively identied by using segmental arterial pressures. Blood pressure cuffs are placed around the thigh, upper calf, and ankle. The systolic occlusion pressure can be determined at each of these locations. The presence of hemodynamically significant arterial stenoses or occlusions is noted by a fall in the systolic blood pressure measured between the cuffs[16] (Fig. 14.15).

Another useful test, pulse volume recording (PVR), utilizes segmental plethysmography to detect the amplitude of the arterial impulse.[17] To perform this test, pneumatic cuffs are placed around the thigh, calf, and ankle. The plethysmograph then records volume changes in the leg with each heart beat. In normal individuals, the PVR tracing looks remarkably similar to an arterial pressure waveform with a dicrotic notch. In the presence of proximal occlusive lesions, the PVR becomes blunted. This test thus assists in localizing the arterial lesion and assessing its severity (Fig. 14.16).

Occasionally, patients will present with symptoms that are not concordant with the findings noted on physical examination. For example, a patient may have symptoms suggestive of claudication, but the pulse examination is normal. In these cases there are physiologic tests available, such as exercise testing.[2,17,18] The standard exercise test is performed with the patient walking 2 miles/hr at a 10° incline on a treadmill. The patient is instructed to continue as long as he is able and to report the first symptoms of claudication. Most patients with hemodynamically significant lesions will experience claudication before 5 min have elapsed. Useful information obtained from exercise testing includes the distance walked, as well as the ankle pressure before and after the exercise period. A normal individual without atherosclerotic occlusive disease will experience no fall in ankle blood pressure with exercise.[2,17] In the setting of a significant arterial stenosis, flow will not be able to increase sufficiently to meet the metabolic demands of the tissues and thus lower ankle blood pressures will be recorded. Occasionally, the response can be so pronounced ankle pressures may be unobtainable when the patient first completes the exercise test. As the patient recovers during the subsequent rest period, ankle pressures return and gradually increase to baseline levels. In the patient with multilevel disease, up to 15 min may elapse before a Doppler arterial signal becomes detectable at the ankle (Fig. 14.17).

Duplex scanning combines B-mode ultrasound and Doppler spectral analysis

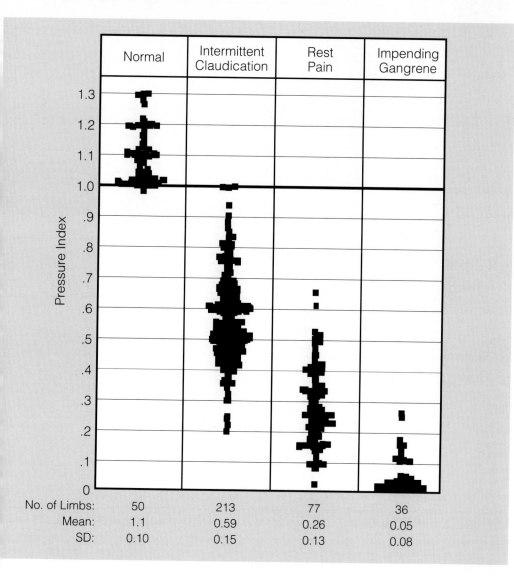

FIGURE 14.14   Range of ankle–brachial index associated with symptoms commonly experienced by the patients with arterial occlusive disease. (Reproduced with permission; see Figure Credits)

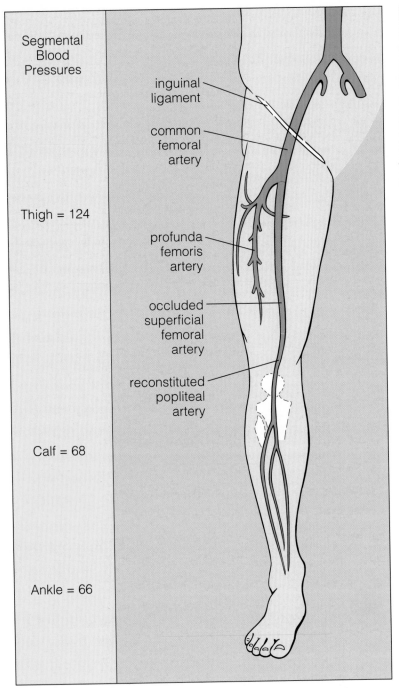

Segmental Blood Pressures

inguinal ligament

common femoral artery

Thigh = 124

profunda femoris artery

occluded superficial femoral artery

reconstituted popliteal artery

Calf = 68

Ankle = 66

FIGURE 14.15   Segmental arterial pressures. In this case the primary level of atherosclerotic occlusive disease is found in the superficial femoral artery. Note the drop in pressure between the thigh and calf determinations.

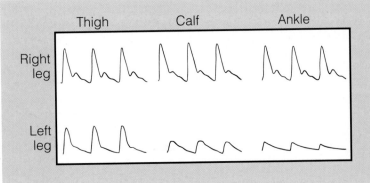

Thigh   Calf   Ankle

Right leg

Left leg

FIGURE 14.16   Pulse volume recording of a patient with a normal arterial study in the right leg and a superficial femoral artery occlusion in the left leg. Distal to the occlusion, the pulse volume is dampened. Note the decreased amplitude and loss of dicrotic notch in the left leg.

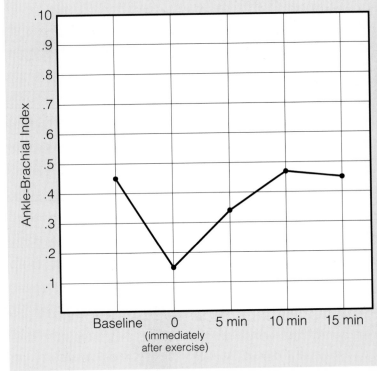

Ankle-Brachial Index

Baseline   0 (immediately after exercise)   5 min   10 min   15 min

FIGURE 14.17   Response of the ankle blood pressure produced by exercise treadmill test. Note the fall in ankle–arm index to 0.15, with gradual recovery over 10 min.

In a single unit to examine the characteristics of blood flow in a vessel. This technique is capable of grading the extent of an arterial stenosis with a high degree of accuracy. Duplex scanning has been especially useful in providing follow-up screening of arterial grafting procedures. In this setting, duplex imaging can measure the velocity of blood flow through the graft and locate focal graft stenoses that, if left untreated, can lead to graft failure[21] (Fig. 14.18).

Invasive Testing With a thorough history and physical examination and the previously discussed noninvasive diagnostic tests, the physician is usually able to reliably establish the presence of significant arterial occlusive disease. When intervention is considered for arterial reconstruction,

arteriography is indicated. This procedure serves to define the exact extent and anatomic details of the arterial occlusive disease so that appropriate corrective measures can be undertaken.

Arteriography involves the injection iodinated contrast proximal to the arteries being examined. During the injection, a rapid sequence of radiographs are taken, that are appropriately timed with the contrast injection (Figs. 14.19–14.21). Computer-assisted digital subtraction arteriography enables the use of reduced amounts of radiographic contrast and more clearly images faintly opacified arteries. This technique digitally "subtracts" overlying soft tissue and bone, thereby enhancing the imaging of the arteries (Fig. 14.22).

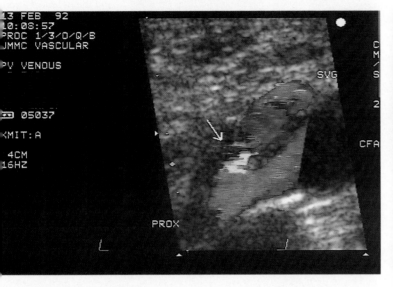

FIGURE 14.18 Duplex scan of bypass graft stenosis. Just beyond the anastomosis the stenosis is identified by the narrowing of the graft and the presence of turbulent blood flow imaged in yellow and white.

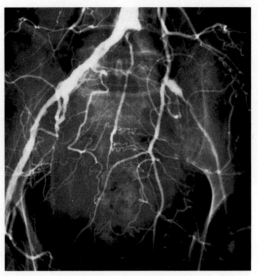

FIGURE 14.19 Arteriogram demonstrating chronic atherosclerotic occlusion of the left common iliac artery.

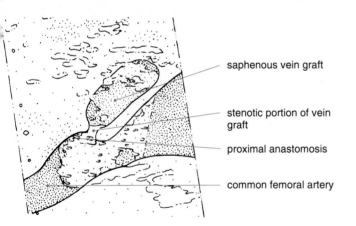

saphenous vein graft

stenotic portion of vein graft

proximal anastomosis

common femoral artery

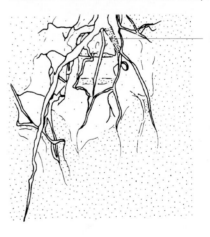

iliac artery occlusion

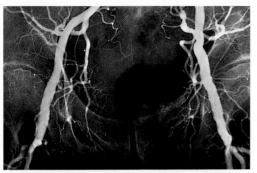

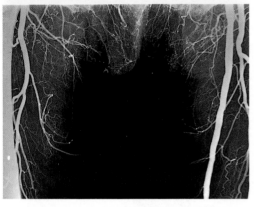

FIGURE 14.20
Arteriogram demonstrating chronic atherosclerotic occlusion of the right superficial femoral artery (SFA). The profunda femoris artery (PFA) is patent. Both the superficial femoral and profunda femoris arteries are patent on the left.

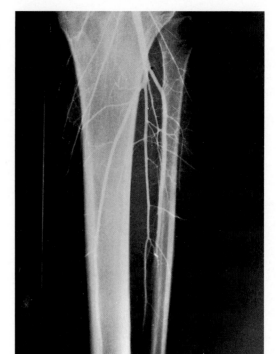

FIGURE 14.21
Arteriogram demonstrating trifurcation of the left popliteal artery. The anterior tibial artery is the first branch, heading in a lateral direction. The tibioperoneal trunk remains for a short distance before bifurcating into the posterior tibial artery medially and the peroneal artery laterally.

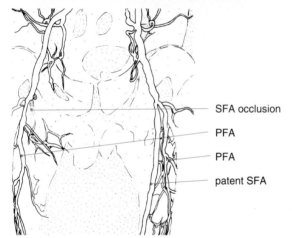

SFA occlusion

PFA

PFA

patent SFA

popliteal artery

tibia-peroneal trunk

anterior tibial artery

peroneal artery

tibia

posterior tibial artery

fibula

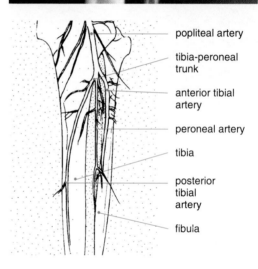

FIGURE 14.22
Digital subtraction image of the right iliac and femoral arteries. There is faint opacification of the external iliac vein medially, indicating the presence of a small arteriovenous fistula. The background structures have been "subtracted" to produce a clearer image of the opacified artery.

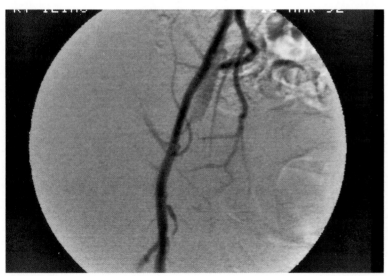

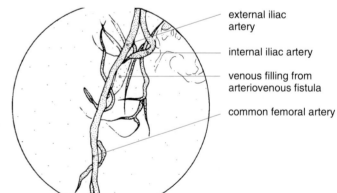

external iliac artery

internal iliac artery

venous filling from arteriovenous fistula

common femoral artery

FIGURE CREDIT

g. 14.14 from Yao ST: Haemodynamic studies in peripheral arterial disease. Br J Surg 57:761, 1970.

REFERENCES

1. Cardullo PA, Keith SL, Cutler BS: Color flow imaging of the pulsatile mass. J Vasc Tech 15:144, 1991.
2. Carter SA: Response of ankle systolic pressure to leg exercise in mild or questionable arterial disease. N Engl J Med 287:578, 1972.
3. Darling RC, Raines JK, Brener BJ, et al: Quantitative segmental pulse volume recorder: A clinical tool. Surgery 72:873, 1972
4. Davis RP, Neiman HL, Yao JST, et al: Ultrasound scan in diagnosis of peripheral aneurysms. Arch Surg 112:55, 1977.
5. Evans WE: Popliteal and femoral aneurysm. In Cameron JL (ed): Current Surgical Therapy. B.C. Decker, Toronto, 1989.
6. Fernando CC, Letourneau JG: Conventional duplex and color Doppler ultrasonography of pseudoaneurysms. Sem Intervent Radiol 7:185, 1990.
7. Gomes MN, Choyke PL: Pre-operative evaluation of abdominal aortic aneurysms: Ultrasound or computed tomography? J Cardiovasc Surg 28:159, 1987.
8. Gooding GAW, Effeney DJ: Ultrasound of femoral artery aneurysms. AJR 134:477, 1980.
9. Hattery RR, Williamson B Jr, Wallace RB: Ultrasonic and computed tomographic imaging of the abdominal aorta. World J Surg 4:511, 1980.
10. Hollier LH, Rutherford RB: Infrarenal aortic aneurysms. In Rutherford RB (ed): Vascular Surgery, 3rd ed. W. B. Saunders Philidelphia, 1989.
11. Johns JP, Pupa LE, Bailey SR: Spontaneous thrombosis of iatrogenic femoral artery pseudoaneurysms: Documentation with color Doppler and two-dimensional ultrasonography. J Vasc Surg 14:24, 1991.
12. Johnston KW, Rutherford RB, Tilson MD, et al: Suggested standards for reporting on arterial aneurysms. J Vasc Surg 13:444, 1991.
13. Mills JL, Harris EJ, Taylor LM, et al: The importance of routine surveillance of distal bypass grafts with duplex scanning: A study of 379 reversed vein grafts. J Vasc Surg 12: 379, 1990.
14. Ramirez AA, Riles TS, Imparato AM, et al: CAT scans of inflammatory aneurysms: A new technique for preoperative diagnosis. Surgery 91:390, 1982.
15. Ramsey DE, Manke DA, Sumner DS: Toe blood pressure: A valuable adjunct to ankle pressure measurement for assessing peripheral arterial disease. J Cardiovasc Surg 24:43, 1983.
16. Rutherford RB, Lowenstein DH, Klein MF. Combined segmental systolic pressures and plethysmography to diagnose arterial occlusive disease of the legs. Am J Surg 138:211, 1979.
17. Strandness DE Jr, Bell JW. An evaluation of the hemodynamic response of the claudicating extremity to exercise. Surg Gynecol Obstet 119:1237, 1964.
18. Sumner DS, Strandness DE Jr: The relationship between calf blood flow and ankle blood pressure in patients with intermittent claudication. Surgery 65:763, 1969.
19. Todd GJ, Nowygrod R, Benvenisty A, et al: The accuracy of CT scanning in the diagnosis of abdominal and thoracoabdominal aortic aneurysms. J Vasc Surg 13:302, 1991.
20. Weinbaum FI, Dubner S, Turner JW, et al: The accuracy of computed tomography in the diagnosis of retroperitoneal blood in the presence of abdominal aortic aneurysm. J Vasc Surg 6:11, 1987.
21. Yao JST: Haemodynamic studies in peripheral arterial disease. Br J Surg 57: 761, 1970.

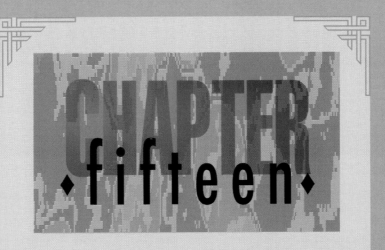

CHAPTER ·fifteen·

VENOUS DISEASES

MICHAEL J. ROHRER, MD

Acute deep venous thrombosis (DVT) is a major source of morbidity and mortality, resulting in 300,000 to 600,000 hospitalizations per year in the United States and as many as 50,000 deaths from pulmonary embolism (PE) annually.[24] When iliofemoral DVT is left undiagnosed, the afflicted have approximately a 50% chance of having a PE and an 18% to 26% risk of death from pulmonary embolization.[2,9] The incidence of PE in patients therapeutically anticoagulated falls to 2% to 12%,[1,6,12,20] with a risk of fatal PE of less than 2%.[1,6,12,18,20] Accurate diagnosis of acute DVT is therefore extremely important.

CLINICAL MANIFESTATIONS

Traditionally, physicians have relied on physical findings such as unilateral leg swelling or calf tenderness to establish the diagnosis of DVT. However, the classic physical findings of unilateral leg swelling and calf tenderness occur late in the disease process and are frequently completely absent.[14,24,28] Furthermore, none of the clinical signs or symptoms are pathognomonic, and patient complaints are often due to musculoskeletal pathology or other causes of leg swelling and tenderness. Several investigators have shown that only 20% to 50% of patients with clinically suspected DVT are found to have acute thrombus present when tested objectively.[8,10,13]

Even though physical examination does not reliably detect DVT, one should not overlook the importance of clinical risk assessment to identify patients who may develop the disease (Fig.15.1).[28] Since risk factors are additive,[5,24,28] the more risk factors present, the more likely the development of DVT. Physicians caring for patients with multiple risk factors should prescribe prophylactic measures to prevent DVT and obtain periodic objective screening tests.

The difficulty in establishing an accurate diagnosis on clinical grounds alone and the potential hazard of treatment-induced hemorrhagic complications make objective testing for DVT essential. Several objective diagnostic tests are available to clinicians to help make an accurate diagnosis of DVT.

LABORATORY STUDIES

Venography   Ascending venography using iodinated radiopaque contrast material is the reference diagnostic test against which the accuracy of all other forms of testing is compared. A vein on the dorsum of the foot is cannulated with a small needle, and contrast is injected using fluoroscopic control with the patient tilted upward at a 45°-to-60° angle to allow filling of the distal veins with the dense contrast. Venous filling is improved if the leg being examined is not bearing weight, and a tourniquet is placed at the ankle level to prevent preferential filling of the superficial veins of the leg (Fig. 15.2). Films are taken to illustrate the venous anatomy and to provide material for later review.

Criteria for the venographic diagnosis of DVT include the imaging of an intraluminal filling defect, abrupt termination of a column of contrast material, or repeated nonfilling of a deep venous segment[25] (Fig. 15.3).

Despite the fact that venograms represent the "gold standard" of DVT diagnosis, interpretation requires considerable skill and experience, and there is a surprisingly high incidence of interobserver variability.[23] Good technique in performing the study is important. The absence of filling of a venous segment may imply that the vein is completely occluded with thrombus, but there is also the possibility that the vein in question may simply not have been opacified adequately with contrast. Errors in evaluation also arise when nonopacified blood from contributing venous branches create a "washout" appearance, which may be misinterpreted as a filling defect by an inexperienced evaluator (Fig. 15.4).

Although venography represents the standard of diagnostic accuracy for diagnosing DVT, it is not a practical technique to use to identify all cases of suspected DVT. Cost factors, physician involvement, repeated contrast exposure, and potential side effects, such as contrast allergy, renal toxicity, and even contrast-induced DVT,[4] make the test impractical to use for routine screening.

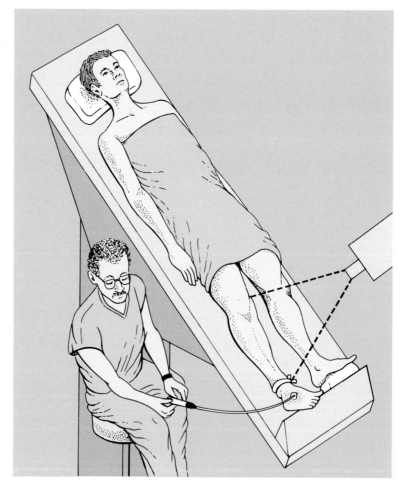

FIGURE 15.1 RISK FACTORS FOR DEVELOPING DVT

History of DVT
Major operation
Obesity
Trauma
Prolonged bedrest
Advanced age
Cancer
Sepsis
Estrogen therapy
Congenital hypercoagulable state
Acquired hypercoagulable state
Inflammatory bowel disease
Stroke

FIGURE 15.2
Lower extremity venography. Contrast is injected into a vein on the dorsum of a non-weightbearing foot while the patient is maintained upright at a 45°-to-60° angle on a tilt table. A tourniquet around the ankle prevents preferential filling of the superficial veins of the leg. Once the contrast has been injected, the patient can be gradually lowered to the horizontal position. Roentgenograms are taken of the leg as the contrast within the deep veins moves proximally.

Noninvasive diagnostic tests have therefore been developed to circumvent the practical limitations of the routine use of venography for the diagnosis of DVT.

Impedance Plethysmography

The multiple plethysmographic techniques that have been developed for the detection of DVT all rely on assessing changes in blood volume in the leg with proximal pneumatic cuff obstruction of the deep veins of the thigh. Impedance plethysmography (IPG) is the technique most widely applied clinically and most critically studied.[14]

IPG testing is performed with the resting patient in the supine positions, with the lower extremities elevated 30° and the knees gently flexed. A pneumatic cuff is inflated around the proximal thigh to a pressure of 45 cm H₂O, which functions to temporarily occlude the superficial and deep venous outflow of the extremity. The decrease in electrical impedance of the leg, resulting from the increase in blood volume of the leg during proximal venous compression, is measured by electrodes placed around the calf (Fig. 15.5). Once a stable impedance is achieved with the cuff inflated, the pressure in the cuff is abruptly released and the return to pretest levels of impedance is noted on a strip chart. In the normal leg, proximal venous occlusion by the inflated cuff leads to a substantial increase in the blood volume of the leg and a corresponding decrease in the impedance. When the cuff is deflated, the unobstructed normal veins allow the rapid egress of venous blood and the fall in impedance is prompt. In the leg with proximal DVT, inflation of the proximal thigh cuff does little to change the already obstructed venous outflow. Similarly, the release of the pressure-in the cuff is followed by only a modest decrease in venous volume (Fig. 15.6). The total change of the impedance on the strip chart recording is measured, as is the change during the 3 sec following the release of the thigh cuff, and the data are plotted on a graph. A positive test result falls below the discriminant line, while a normal test is noted above[16] (Fig. 15.7).

IPG testing has been correlated with venography and has been proven to be both sensitive and specific for detection of acute proximal DVT. A combined analysis of 16 studies in which venograms were compared to IPG results in 2561 extremities showed IPG to be 94% specific and 93% sensitive for the detection of proximal DVT.[26]

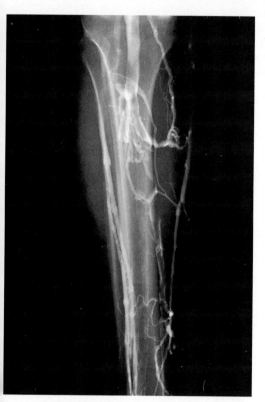

FIGURE 15.3
Venogram showing acute DVT. The tracking of contrast around intraluminal calf vein and popliteal vein thrombus is characteristic of acute DVT.

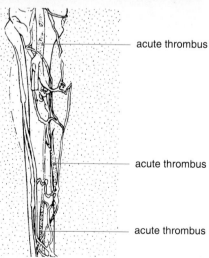

acute thrombus

acute thrombus

acute thrombus

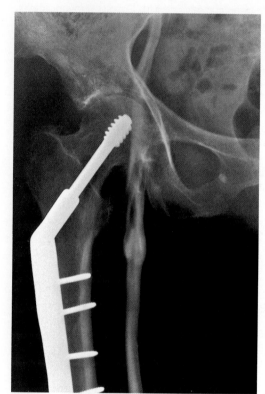

FIGURE 15.4
Venogram that could be misinterpreted by an inexperienced observer as demonstrating acute thrombus. Nonopacified blood from the profunda femoris vein dilutes the contrast-rich blood ascending in the superficial femoral vein. The resulting "washout" of contrast by contrast-free blood creates the illusion of the presence of intraluminal thrombus. Clues to help make the correct diagnosis include the typical "flame" shape of the pseudothrombus and the location of the contrast void at the confluence of the profunda femoris and superficial femoral veins.

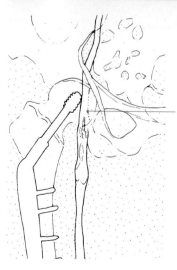

contrast void due to non-opacified blood from vein branches

IPG is a simple, noninvasive, objective test for the detection of DVT. The procedure is performed at the bedside, is well tolerated, and is easily repeatable. Furthermore, it is a test easily learned by a technician, and since the results of the test require no special interpretation, the findings are available immediately upon completion of the examination. These features make it an ideal screening test for patients at high risk for the development of proximal leg vein DVT.

There are several disadvantages associated with the use of IPG, however. Since IPG is a functional test, it is relatively insensitive to the presence of isolated tibial vein thrombosis; parallel venous channels without thrombus can provide excellent venous emptying. Fortunately, significant propagation of calf vein thrombus is unusual[19] and rarely leads to significant pulmonary embolization.[28] False-positive IPG tests occasionally occur in patients with physiologic reasons for having relative obstruction to lower extremity venous outflow, such as right heart failure and increased abdominal pressure.[27] Also, IPG testing is occasionally impossible to perform because of the presence of a lower extremity cast or orthopedic hardware precluding placement of the proximal pneumatic cuff or distal electrodes.

Venous Duplex Scanning   Duplex ultrasonography combines real-time B-mode ultrasonic imaging with Doppler ultrasonography. The veins are therefore imaged with the B-mode scanner, and flow within the vein is documented with the Doppler. The recently developed Doppler color scanner, which assigns color to different Doppler velocity shifts, provides greater feedback about intraluminal flow to the examiner (Fig. 15.8). Criteria used to establish the diagnosis of acute DVT include the imaging of thrombus within the vein, as well as finding the vessel to be focally noncompressable with gentle ultrasonic probe pressure at the site of thrombosis (Fig. 15.9).

Venous duplex scanning has been shown to have excellent sensitivity and specificity, as determined by aggregate data from studies comparing venous duplex scanning to contrast venography. It carries an overall accuracy of 94%.[14] Although duplex scanning requires more sophisticated and expensive instrumentation and more advanced technologist training and judgment than IPG

testing, it provides anatomic information about the location and extent of thrombus formation. Duplex scanning is also more widely applicable than IPG since it can be used in cases with false-positive IPGs and in cases where IPGs cannot be done because of distal leg wounds, casts, or orthopedic hardware.

SPECIAL CLINICAL PROBLEMS
RECURRENT ACUTE DVT

The patient who has a history of DVT and new leg swelling presents a diagnostic dilemma. Symptoms may be secondary to the development of the postphlebitic syndrome, with persistent venous obstruction and/or progressive venous valvular insufficiency, or they may be due to recurrent acute DVT. Since collateral circulation around the location of acute DVT improves with time and recanalization of obstructed venous segments almost always occurs,[21] IPG test results returns to normal in 95% of cases during the 12 months following the initial episode of DVT.[15] Therefore, if the initially abnormal IPG has returned to normal, IPG can be used again to assess the recurrence of proximal venous thrombosis. Unfortunately, a positive IPG is not helpful in diagnosing cases where normalization has not been documented after an initial episode of DVT.

Since venous duplex scanning localizes areas of thrombosis and recanalization, repeated scanning may identify new areas of venous obstruction and noncompressability not present on the initial duplex scan. These subsequent scans may help in the differentiation of new DVT from swelling secondary to the postphlebitic syndrome.

Venography remains the standard diagnostic method to differentiate new DVT from old. Such determinations can occasionally be quite difficult and subtle, even to an experienced radiologist (Fig. 15.10).

RECURRENT PE AFTER VENA CAVA FILTER PLACEMENT

Pulmonary embolization after placement of an inferior vena cava (IVC) filter

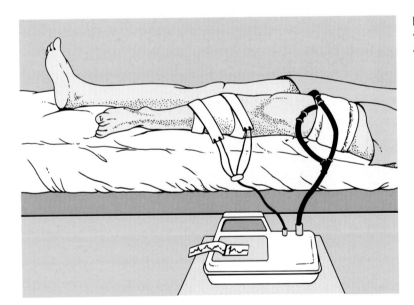

FIGURE 15.5   Correct patient positioning for IPG. The leg is slightly elevated and the knee gently flexed. The electrodes are placed around the calf and a cuff is located around the thigh.

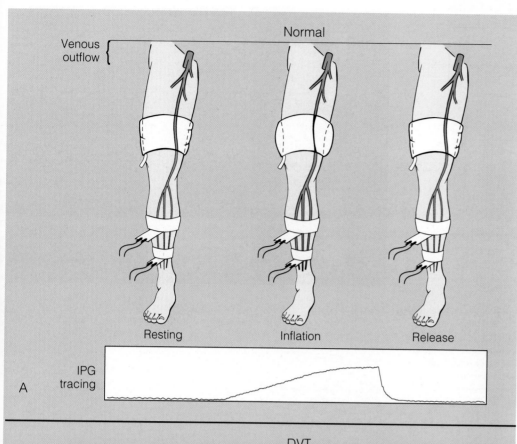

Normal

Venous outflow {

Resting   Inflation   Release

A   IPG tracing

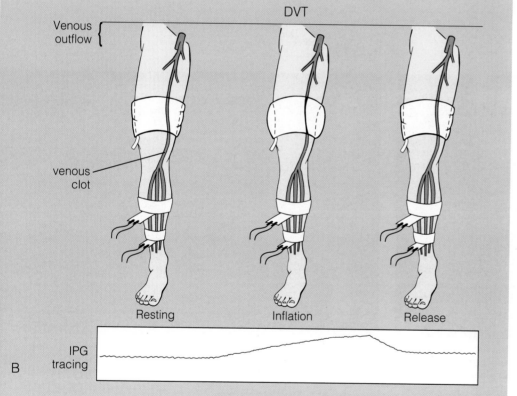

DVT

Venous outflow {

venous clot

Resting   Inflation   Release

B   IPG tracing

FIGURE 15.6   IPG detection of DVT.
(A) When no DVT is present, inflation of the thigh cuff obstructs venous outflow of the leg. The resulting increase in leg venous volume decreases leg impedance, which is represented on the graphic strip as an increasing line. When the cuff is abruptly deflated, there is prompt egress of blood from the leg, a prompt fall in venous volume, and a return to baseline electrical impedance. **(B)** When proximal DVT obstructs the venous outflow of the leg, inflation of the thigh cuff does little to change the pre-existing venous distention. There is therefore little change documented in the leg impedance. When the cuff is released, the obstructed venous system prevents rapid flow of blood out of the leg, so there is a characteristic slow rise in the leg impedance, represented by the gradual decrease in the strip chart tracing.

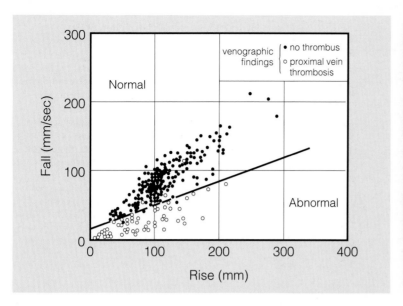

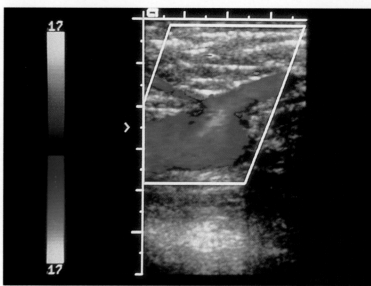

FIGURE 15.7   The discriminant line that serves to differentiate normal from abnormal IPG test results. Patients who underwent IPG and venogram testing were plotted according to their IPG rise and fall during testing. Venograms were also obtained from each patient. Venograms showing proximal DVT are identified by open circles, and normal venograms are designated by closed circles. A discriminant line is able to separate venographically proven positives from normals with a high degree of accuracy. (Reproduced with permission; see Figure Credits)

FIGURE 15.8   Duplex scan of the normal saphenofemoral junction demonstrating resolution and color representation of flow. (Reproduced with permission; see Figure Credits)

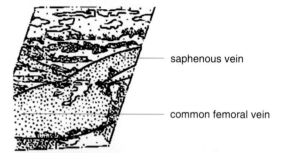

— saphenous vein

— common femoral vein

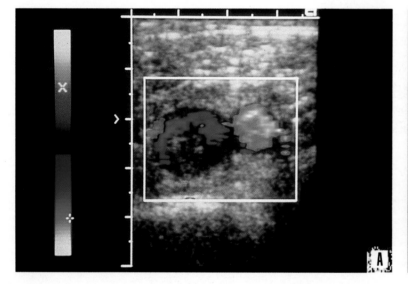

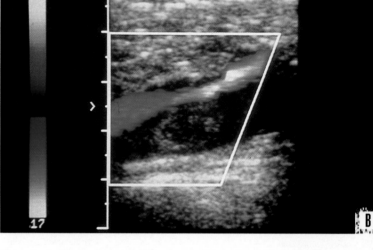

FIGURE 15.9   Duplex scan demonstrating the presence of nonocclusive thrombus in both the transverse **(A)** and longitudinal **(B)** planes.

The color void represents a localized area of thrombus with venous flow (imaged in blue) around the clot. (Reproduced with permission; see Figure Credit)

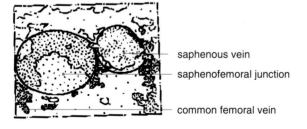

— saphenous vein
— saphenofemoral junction

— common femoral vein

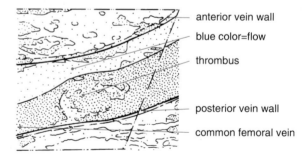

— anterior vein wall
— blue color=flow

— thrombus

— posterior vein wall

— common femoral vein

ould prompt a venacavagram. Occasionally a large thrombus will be captured y the IVC filter and lead to IVC occlusion, or proximal propagation of thrombus occurs up to and through the legs of the filter. Pulmonary emboli can occur hen thrombus dislodges from above the level of the clotted filter (Fig. 15.11) lternatively, an unsuspected, congenitally duplicated IVC may provide an ninterrupted route for a pulmonary embolus to bypass the right-sided filter. he anomalous left-sided IVC crosses over to a single suprarenal cava through ue left renal vein (Fig. 15.12). A cavagram should be performed from the left moral approach to identify the possible presence of a congenitally duplicated ft-sided vena cava, which occurs in up to 3% of individuals.[11] The absence of ny lower extremity DVT at the time of venography should prompt the clini-an to look for other unusual sources of pulmonary emboli, such as upper xtremity DVT or right heart thrombus.

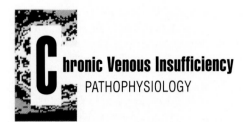

Chronic Venous Insufficiency
PATHOPHYSIOLOGY

The long-term sequelae of DVT may not become apparent until many years after the initial episode.[3] In the lower extremities, recanalization of the occluded venous segment almost always occurs,[21] and the predominant pathologic abnormality, venous valvular insufficiency, occurs because of ongoing fibrosis of

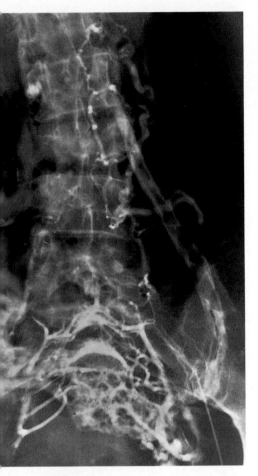

FIGURE 15.10
Venacavagram demonstrating chronic thrombosis of the vena cava with multiple collateral venous channels. The left gonadal vein contains acute thrombus that is typical in appearance and outlined by contrast.

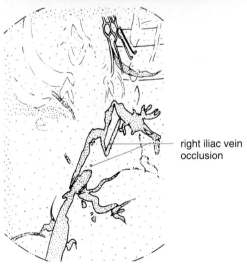

FIGURE 15.11
(A) Thrombosed vena cava seen on venograms that were performed from both a right and left femoral approach, although the relationship of the thrombus to the filter is not identified. A venacavagram performed from a jugular approach allows the definition of the thrombus at its most proximal extent.

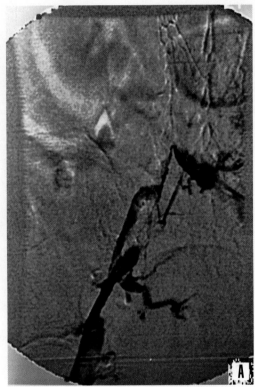

acute thrombus in gon-adal vein

collaterals

right iliac vein occlusion

the deep venous valves, which progresses for many years after the initial thrombosis (Fig. 15.13). Valvular incompetence leads to venous reflux and more distal venous distention, as well as the dilatation of the perforating veins which also have unidirectional valves intended to direct flow from the superficial to deep veins. Once the perforating vein valves are rendered incompetent by chronic fibrosis and dilatation, the elevated venous pressure is transmitted to the superficial venous system and the skin. This elevation in pressure is responsible for the development of the symptoms complex seen in chronic venous insufficiency: leg pain, swelling, cutaneous ulceration, and secondary varicose veins (Fig. 15.14).

Chronic venous valvular insufficiency is an extremely common finding following acute DVT although symptoms may take years to develop. Approximately 80% of patients with a history of DVT will eventually have the symptoms and abnormal venous hemodynamics, regardless of the initial site of DVT.[3,22] The resulting leg pain, swelling, and ulceration are frequently disabling.

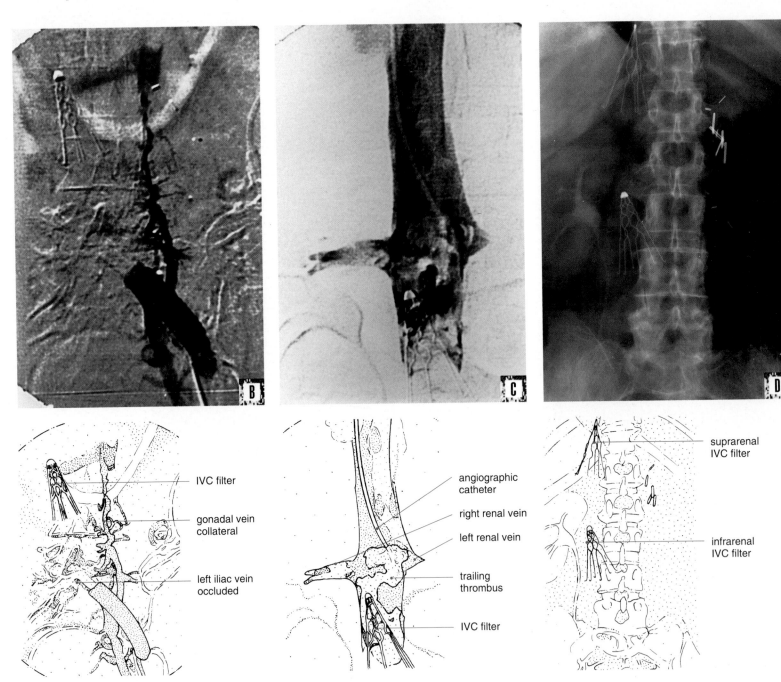

FIGURE 15.11   **(B)** Thrombosed vena cava seen on venograms that were performed from both a right and left femoral approach, although the relationship of the thrombus to the filter is not identified. A venacavagram performed from a jugular approach allows the definition of the thrombus at its most proximal extent. **(C)** A large thrombus is demonstrated to trail from the clot trapped beneath the filter. This patient suffered a recurrent pulmonary embolus in spite of therapeutic anticoagulation. **(D)** A second vena cava filter was placed above the level of the renal veins.

The physical findings of leg swelling, brawny edema, and skin pigmentation are

characteristic of the postphlebitic syndrome (Fig. 15.15). Ulceration typically occurs in the "gaiter area," especially overlying the perforating veins in skin previously affected by stasis dermatitis and pigmentation (Fig. 15.16). Venous stasis ulcers are usually shallow with a granulating base and are most often found on the medial lower third of the calf.

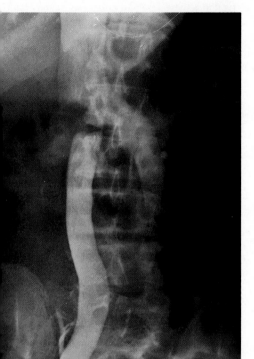

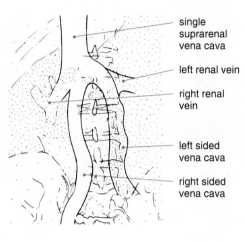

FIGURE 15.12   Venacavagram demonstrating the presence of a persistent left-sided vena cava. If a parallel left-sided vena cava system goes unrecognized and untreated, a thrombus could bypass a properly placed right-sided IVC filter and reach the suprarenal IVC through the left renal vein. (Reproduced with permission; see Figure Credits)

single suprarenal vena cava

left renal vein

right renal vein

left sided vena cava

right sided vena cava

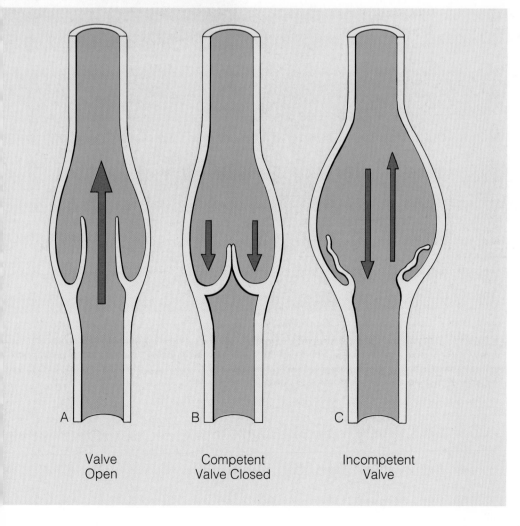

A Valve Open

B Competent Valve Closed

C Incompetent Valve

FIGURE 15.13   Normal venous valve in the open (**A**) and closed (**B**) positions. Once the valve has been damaged by the presence of deep vein thrombi, the valve cusps are unable to coapt and venous reflux is able to occur (**C**).

Objective vascular testing is directed at discerning the presence and extent of venous valvular incompetence and persistent venous occlusive disease.

LABORATORY STUDIES

Venography Ascending venography can assess the degree and location of persistent venous occlusive disease (Fig. 15.17), but it cannot be used to determine the degree of venous valvular insufficiency. In descending venography, contrast material is injected at the level of the common femoral vein while the patient performs a Valsalva maneuver. The reflux of contrast down the extremity through the incompetent venous valves to the level of the most

proximal competent valve is then radiologically assessed. The availability of oth[...] less invasive tests to assess the presence of venous valvular insufficiency limits t[...] use of descending venography to cases in which the knowledge of the precise loc[...] tion and morphology of the venous valves is essential, such as prior to surgic[...] venous valvular repair, valve replacement, or deep venous transposition.

Photoplethysmography Noninvasive assessment [...] venous valvular competence can be achieved by photoplethysmography (PPG[...] The recordings are made with the patient sitting; the legs are in a depende[...] position bearing no weight, and the PPG transducer is attached to either t[...] skin of the foot or distal leg. The transducer emits infrared light from a ligh[...] emitting diode into the underlying tissue, and the back-scattered light [...]

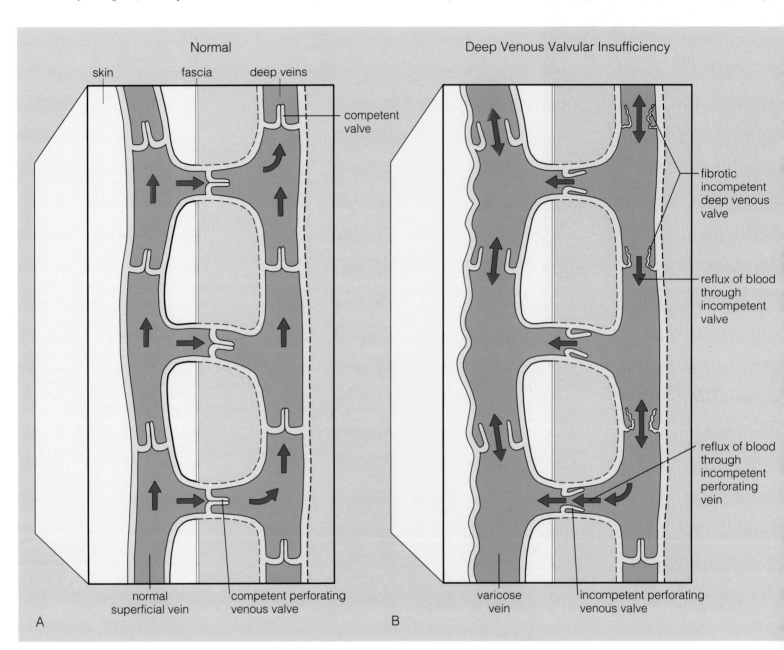

FIGURE 15.14 Normal and abnormal venous flow patterns in the lower extremity. **(A)** When deep venous valves are competent, flow moves proximally in the superficial and deep systems from the superficial system to the deep. **(B)** When deep venous valves are incompetent, the high deep venous pressures secondary to deep venous valvular insufficiency cause the perforating veins to become distended and incompetent. Elevated deep venous pressures are therefore transmitted to the superficial veins and skin of the leg, causing chronic skin changes and ulceration.

ceived by an adjacent photodetector. The patient is instructed to vigorously dorsiflex the foot four times using the calf muscle pump to forcibly eject blood from the leg, then the foot is relaxed. In patients with competent venous valves, there is no venous reflux and the blood volume of the leg, which was ejected by the calf muscle pump during exercise, is restored only by continued arterial inflow over approximately 30 sec. If the venous valves are incompetent, the blood ejected proximally by foot dorsiflexion is able to reflux distally promptly through the ineffective valves (Fig. 15.18). A refilling time of less than 20 sec is abnormal, and in clinically obvious cases of the postphlebitic syndrome, refilling times of under 6 sec are not uncommon.

Venous reflux can occur through both the superficial and deep venous system. The location of the incompetent valves can be localized to either the superficial or deep venous system by repeating the PPG after the application of a superficial tourniquet, which occludes the superficial veins and prevents the distal reflux of blood through them. If the refilling time is restored to normal after application of the tourniquet, then the deep venous valves have been shown to be competent and the reflux can be attributed to superficial venous valvular insufficiency. If the PPG refilling time is still abnormal after application of superficial tourniquets, then the valves of the the deep veins of the leg have been shown to be incompetent (Fig. 15.19).

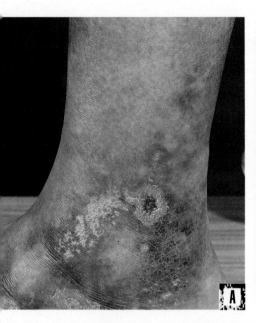
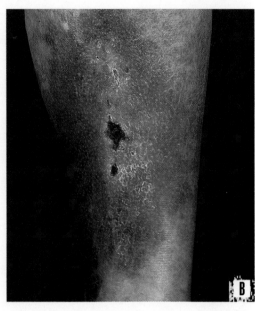

FIGURE 15.15 (A,B) Typical appearance of postphlebitic skin changes and brawny edema associated with chronic postphlebitic deep venous valvular insufficiency.

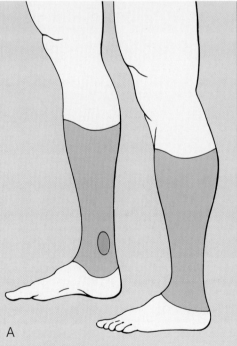
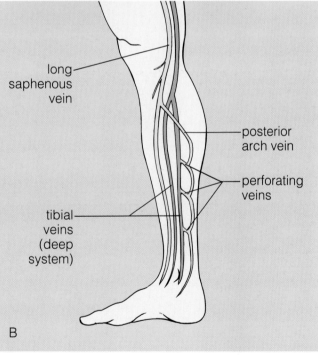

FIGURE 15.16 (A) "gaiter" area where venous stasis skin changes and ulceration are most commonly seen. (B) The location of the perforating veins explains the site of the postphlebitic skin changes and ulceration.

long saphenous vein

posterior arch vein

perforating veins

tibial veins (deep system)

A

B

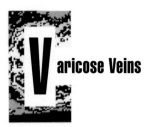

Varicose Veins

The elongation and dilatation of the superficial leg veins, which lead to the development of varicose veins, are estimated to occur in up to 15% of the adult population.[7] Although varicose veins can cause significant discomfort and disability, the varicose veins themselves are not life- or limb-threatening. Varicose veins may also represent a manifestation of deep venous disease.

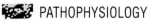 PATHOPHYSIOLOGY

Functional failure of the venous valves is the underlying pathophysiologic etiology of both primary and secondary varicose veins. In the case of primary varicose veins, the pathologic abnormality lies solely within the involved superficial vein. Classically, dilatation of the most proximal saphenous vein valve at the level of the saphenofemoral junction in the groin results in the inability of the two opposing valve cusps to coapt. The valve therefore becomes incompetent and is no longer able to prevent the reflux of blood to the more distal saphenous vein. This mechanism establishes a self-perpetuating sequence in which further venous dilatation results in even more distal superficial venous valves becoming incompetent (Fig. 15.20).

Secondary varicose veins are a superficial manifestation of incompetence of the deep venous valves. The increased venous pressure from the reflux of blood in the deep veins is transmitted to the perforating veins rendered incompetent

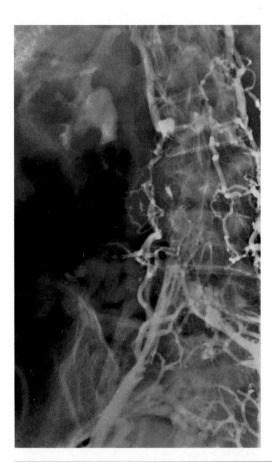

FIGURE 15.17 Chronic occlusion of the vena cava. Note the numerous collateral venous vessels.

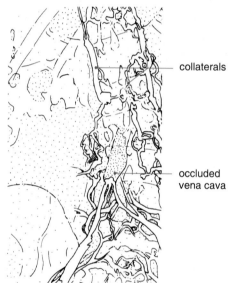

collaterals

occluded
vena cava

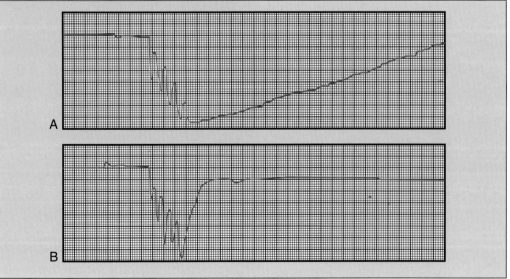

FIGURE 15.18 Assessment of venous valvular insufficiency using PPG. Active dorsiflexion of the calf ejects the blood from the deep venous circulation proximally in the leg because of the high calf pressure transiently generated by exercise. **(A)** In the normal individual, competent venous valves prevent reflux of blood. Therefore, refilling of the leg occurs only through continued arterial inflow, a process requiring approximately 30 sec. **(B)** Incompetent venous valves allow reflux of the ejected blood back into the leg, resulting in a return to baseline in a matter of several seconds.

y the distention. Once the perforating veins are rendered incompetent, the increased venous pressure is further transmitted to the superficial veins of the leg that dilate and become varicose (see Fig. 15.14).

CLINICAL MANIFESTATIONS
PHYSICAL EXAMINATION

The appearance of varicose veins is quite characteristic and their presence can be diagnosed by inspection and palpation (Fig. 15.21). The varices can often be classified as limited to either the greater saphenous vein and its branches, the lesser saphenous vein and its branches, or other territories, which are usually in the distribution of the perforating veins of the leg.

Primary and secondary varicose veins can often be differentiated on clinical grounds. The young patient with no history of or risk factors for developing DVT almost certainly has primary varicose veins. Conversely, an elderly patient with a remote history of DVT and associated edema, stasis dermatitis, and ulceration almost certainly has secondary varicose veins.

Although secondary varicose veins almost always result from a remote history

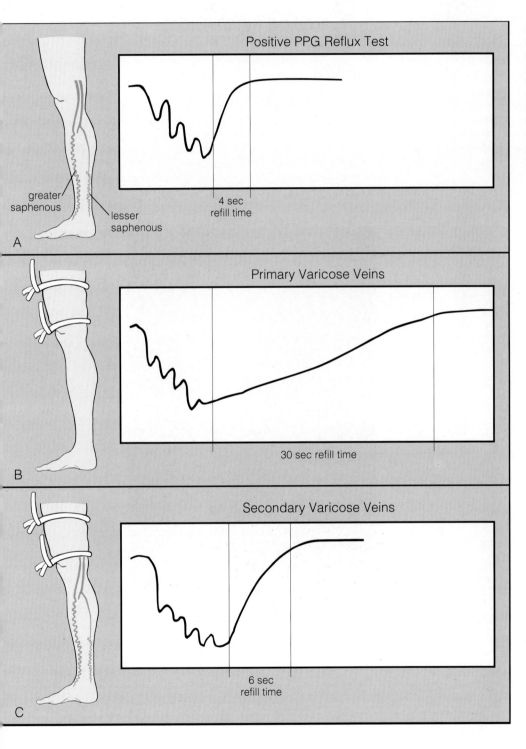

FIGURE 15.19 Differentiation of deep and superficial venous insufficiency through application of a superficial tourniquet. **(A)** An abnormal PPG tracing is obtained. **(B)** If the refilling time of the leg is extended to normal after placing a tourniquet occluding the superficial veins, it may be deduced that the source of the reflux is only the superficial veins of the leg. **(C)** If the refilling time is not changed after tourniquet occlusion of the superficial veins, the source of the venous reflux is deep venous valvular insufficiency.

of DVT, it is not unusual for there to be no recognized history of DVT. The physician may frequently be told of a hip replacement or other major operation associated with a high risk of DVT, which probably was not diagnosed at the time of its original presentation.

LABORATORY STUDIES

Although the presence of varicose veins is obvious on physical examination, the etiology of the varices is important to establish since this information has prognostic value when considering surgical excision or injection sclerotherapy.

Trendelenburg Test   Objective physical findings can be used to differentiate primary from secondary varicose veins. In the Trendelenburg test, the patient is examined while manual pressure or a superficial tourniquet is applied to the region of the origin of the greater saphenous vein at the fossa ovalis. The pressure is maintained on the saphenous vein while the patient stands. If the varicose veins do not refill, the only abnormality is the incompetent valves of the superficial venous system. On the other hand, if prompt refilling of the varices is noted, the examiner can infer that the venous dilatation pressure is being transmitted from the deep venous system to the superficial veins of the legs through the incompetent deep venous valves and perforators; therefore the varicose veins are secondary to deep venous valvular insufficiency (Fig. 15.22).

Photoplethysmography   Vascular laboratory tests can

also be performed to classify varicose veins as primary or secondary. If an abnormal PPG refilling time is normalized by the placement of a superficial tourniquet, then the patient has primary varicose veins. If venous distention occurs promptly even after placement of the superficial tourniquet and the refilling time does not normalize, then the varicose veins are considered to be secondary to the underlying deep venous valvular insufficiency (see Fig. 15.19).

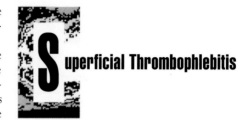

Superficial Thrombophlebitis

The diagnosis of superficial thrombophlebitis is made clinically. Thrombus formation within a superficial vein is detected in conjunction with local warmth, erythema, and tenderness along the path of the palpable subcutaneous venous cord. Such cases usually occur in patients with pre-existing varicose veins and frequently follow some type of local injury. Progression of the erythema, tenderness, and palpable cord occasionally extend proximally toward the saphenofemoral junction.[17]

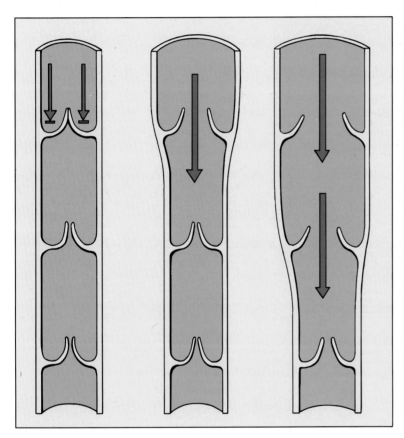

FIGURE 15.20   Venous valvular insufficiency at the saphenofemoral junction resulting in vein distention and further venous valvular insufficiency. This distal progression of venous distention leads to further venous dilation and venous valvular insufficiency.

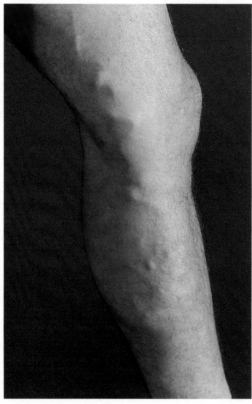

FIGURE 15.21
Varicose veins have a characteristic appearance and are obvious during inspection.

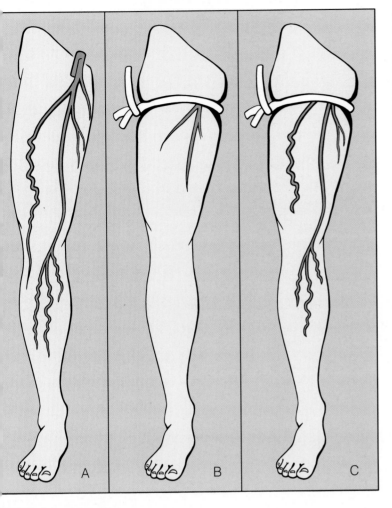

FIGURE 15.22 The Trendelenburg test differentiates primary from secondary varicose veins. **(A)** The extremity with superficial varicose veins is elevated beyond the point at which the veins empty. **(B)** A tourniquet is placed around the thigh just distal to the saphenofemoral junction. If the veins remain empty when the limb is lowered, reflux in the greater saphenous vein is the etiology of the varicose veins. **(C)** If the varicose veins become immediately apparent when the leg is lowered with the tourniquet in place, they are filling from the deep venous system as a result of deep venous valvular insufficiency and incompetent perforating veins.

FIGURE CREDITS

Fig. 15.7 redrawn from Hull R, et al: Impedance plethysmography using the occlusive cuff technique in the diagnosis of venous thrombosis. Circulation 53:696, 1976.

Figs. 15.8, 15.9 courtesy of Paul Cardullo, RN, BSN, RVT.

Fig. 15.12 from Rohrer MJ, Cutler BS: Two Greenfield filters in duplicated vena cava. Surgery 104:573, 1988.

REFERENCES

1. Adar R, Salzman EW: Treatment of thrombosis of veins of lower extremities. N Engl J Med 292:348, 1975.
2. Barritt DW, Jordan SC: Anticoagulant drugs in the treatment of pulmonary embolism: A controlled trial. Lancet 1:1309, 1960.
3. Bauer G: Roentgenological and clinical study of the sequelae of thrombosis. Acta Chir Scand 86(Suppl 74):1, 1942.
4. Bettmann MA, Robbins A, Braun SD, et al: Contrast venography of the leg: Diagnostic efficacy, tolerance, and complication rates with ionic and nonionic contrast media. Radiology 165:113, 1987.
5. Caprini JA, Arcelus JI, Hasty JH, et al: Clinical assessment of venous thromboembolic risk in surgical patients. Semin Thromb Hemost 17 (Suppl 3):304, 1991.
6. Coon WN, Willis PW III, Symons MJ: Assessment of anticoagulant treatment of venous thromboembolism. Ann Surg 170:559, 1969.
7. Crane C: The surgery of varicose veins. Surg Clin North Am 59:737, 1979.
8. Cranley JJ, Canos AJ, Sull WJ: The diagnosis of deep vein thrombosis: Fallibility of clinical symptoms and signs. Arch Surg 111:34, 1976.
9. Einarsson E, Eklof B: Acute iliofemoral venous thrombosis. In Eiseman B (ed): Prognosis of Surgical Disease. WB Saunders, Philadelphia, 1980.
10. Gallus AS, Hirsh J, Hull RD, et al: Diagnosis of venous thromboembolism. Semin Thromb Hemost 2:203, 1976.
11. Giordano JM, Trout HH III: Anomalies of the inferior vena cava. J Vasc Surg 3:924, 1986.
12. Greenfield LJ, Alexander EL: Current status of surgical therapy for deep vein thrombosis. Am J Surg 150(4A):64, 1985.
13. Haeger K: Problems of acute deep venous thrombosis: 1. The interpretation of signs and symptoms. Angiology 20:219, 1969.
14. Heijboer H, Ten Cate JW, Buller HR: Diagnosis of venous thrombosis. Semin Thromb Hemost 17 (Suppl 3):259, 1991.
15. Huisman MV, Buller JR, Ten Cate JW: Utility of impedance plethysmography in the diagnosis of recurrent deep-vein thrombosis. Arch Intern Med 148:681, 1988.
16. Hull R, van Aken WG, Hirsh J, et al: Impedance plethysmography using the occlusive cuff technique in the diagnosis of venous thrombosis. Circulation 53:696, 1976.
17. Johnson G Jr: Superficial venous thrombosis. In Rutherford RD (ed): Vascular Surgery, 3rd ed. WB Saunders, Philadelphia, 1989.
18. Jones RH, Sabiston DC Jr: Pulmonary embolism. Surg Clin North Am 56:891, 1976.
19. Kakkar VV, Howe CT, Flanc C, et al: Natural history of postoperative deep-vein thrombosis. Lancet 2:230, 1969.
20. Kernohan RJ, Todd C: Heparin therapy in thromboembolic disease. Lancet 1:621, 1966.
21. Killewich LA, Bedford GR, Beach KW, et al: Spontaneous lysis of deep venous thrombi: Rate and outcome. J Vasc Surg 9:89, 1989.
22. Lindner DJ, Edwards JM, Phinney ES, et al: Long-term hemodynamic and clinical sequelae of lower extremity deep vein thrombosis. J Vasc Surg 4:436, 1986.
23. McLachlan MSF, Thompson JG, Taylor DW, et al: Observer variation in the interpretation of lower limb venograms. AJR 132:227, 1979.
24. National Institutes of Health: Prevention of venous thrombosis and pulmonary embolism. JAMA. 256:744, 1986.
25. Rabinov K, Paulin S: Roentgen diagnosis of venous thrombosis in the leg. Arch Surg 104:134, 1972.
26. Wheeler HB, Anderson FA Jr: Can noninvasive tests be used as the basis for treatment of deep vein thrombosis? In Bernstein EF (ed): Noninvasive Diagnostic Techniques in Vascular Disease, 3rd ed. CV Mosby, St. Louis, 1985.
27. Wheeler HB, Anderson FA Jr: The diagnosis of venous thrombosis by impedance plethysmography. In Bernstein EF (ed): Noninvasive Diagnostic Techniques in Vascular Disease, 3rd ed. CV Mosby, St. Louis, 1985.
28. Wheeler HB, Rohrer MJ: Diagnosing and preventing venous thromboembolism. J Respir Dis 9:25, 1988.

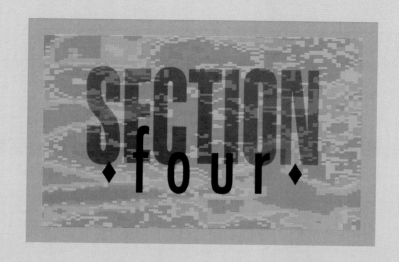

SECTION ·four·

THE HEART AND OTHER CONDITIONS

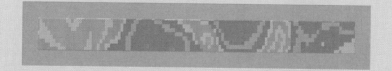

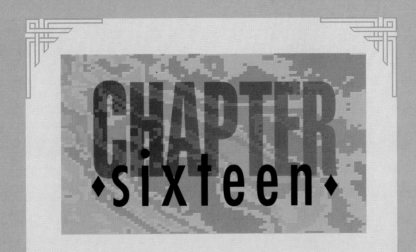

CHAPTER
◆sixteen◆

HYPERTENSION

ANDREW J. COHEN, MD

Hypertension is a group of conditions that share the property of elevated hydrostatic pressure in the systemic arterial vascular tree. Over time hypertension-induced "target organ" damage leads to significant morbidity and mortality in humans. The numerical definition of elevated blood pressure has been elusive for several reasons. First, blood pressure tends to increase with age.[31] Hence, "normal" blood pressure in an adult would be unacceptably high in a child. Second, epidemiologic studies have determined that the risk of cardiovascular disease increases over a continuum of blood pressure readings, instead of increasing at a specific breakpoint.[28] Third, elevations in blood pressure may be episodic rather than persistent. The term *labile hypertension* has been applied to this subgroup of patients.

In setting guidelines for the treatment of hypertension in adults, the fourth Joint National Committee (JNC IV) on the detection, evaluation and treatment of hypertension wrote the definitions described in Figure 16.1.[26] Since diastolic blood pressure elevation is usually accompanied by increased systolic readings, diastolic readings will usually suffice. However, since isolated systolic hypertension (diastolic BP <90 mmHg) confers risk of cardiovascular mortality and morbidity, specific categories for this condition have been devised.

Since the reliability of the blood pressure measurement is crucial in the diagnosis of hypertension, the JNC IV recommended specific guidelines for taking recordings (Fig. 16.2). Particularly in the office setting, patient anxiety and other factors may affect the blood pressure readings. The phenomenon of "white coat" hypertension has been well-documented.[52] Hence, follow-up visits to validate the initial readings are strongly recommended. In addition, determi-

nations of blood pressure at home or at work may provide further validation of the initial office readings. In some cases, repeated ambulatory blood pressure measurement may be desirable (see discussion below).

Blood pressure evaluation must commence with a complete history (Fig 16.3). In general, the history should begin with a review of any previous knowledge of hypertension (as might be found in a routine school, pre-employment or military physical examination). The known duration and severity of hypertension, as well as response to any previous therapy, should be assessed. A history of cardiovascular, renal, or cerebrovascular disease or diabetes mellitus anticipates an assessment of cardiovascular risk or target organ involvement. Any family history of hypertension, diabetes, or cardiovascular disease should be thoroughly researched. Symptoms suggestive of secondary hypertension (e.g., headache, flushing, palpitations in pheochromocytoma) should be investigated. Psychologic and environmental factors (e.g., stress, dietary sodium intake) require questioning. Finally, cardiovascular risk factors (e.g., obesity, smoking, hyperlipidemia) need to be assessed.

The necessary objective data collected in the physical and laboratory examinations are listed in Figure 16.4. As is the case in the history, the physician looks for concordant cardiovascular disease (e.g., bruits, S₃, rales,) concordant target organ damage (retinopathy, proteinuria), and signs of secondary hypertension (e.g., striae and truncal obesity in Cushing's syndrome; sweating, pallor, tachycardia, and orthostasis in pheochromocytoma or azotemia and urinary sediment abnormalities in renal disease). The presence of other cardiovascular risk factors (e.g., hyperlipidemia, diabetes mellitus) are necessary components in deciding the urgency, intensity, and type of antihypertensive therapy.

FIGURE 16.1 DEFINITIONS OF HYPERTENSION IN ADULTS*

BLOOD PRESSURE (MMHG)	CATEGORY
Diastolic BP	
<85	Normal BP
85–89	High-normal BP
90–104	Mild hypertension
105–114	Moderate hypertension
≥115	Severe hypertension
Systolic BP†	
<140	Normal BP
140–159	Borderline isolated systolic hypertension
≥160	Isolated systolic hypertension

*Proposed by the fourth Joint National Committee on the detection, evaluation and treatment of hypertension.
†When diastolic blood pressure is less than 90.

(Reproduced with permission; see Figure Credits)

FIGURE 16.2 GUIDELINES FOR THE MEASUREMENT OF BLOOD PRESSURE*

1. No caffeine or tobacco 30 minutes prior to reading.
2. BP is measured after 5 minutes of quiet rest.
3. Patient is seated with arm at heart level.
4. Appropriate cuff size: rubber bladder should encircle at least two thirds of the arm.
5. Measurements are performed with mercury sphygomanometer, recently calibrated aneroid manometer, or validated electronic device.
6. Both systolic and diastolic BP are recorded. The disappearance of sound (Phase V Korotkoff sounds) should be used for the diastolic reading.
7. Two or more readings should be averaged. If the first two readings differ by more than 5 mmHg, additional determinations should be recorded.

*Proposed by the fourth Joint National Committee on the detection, evaluation and treatment of hypertension.

(Reproduced with permission; see Figure Credits)

FIGURE 16.3 KEY ITEMS IN THE HISTORY OF PATIENTS WITH MILD OR MODERATE HYPERTENSION

SYMPTOMS	DIET AND DRUG HISTORY	DISEASE HISTORY	FAMILY HISTORY
Blurred vision	Alcohol	Angina	Coronary heart
Bronchospasm	Analgesics	Asthma	disease
Chest pain	Blood pressure medications	Diabetes	Diabetes
Claudication	Cigarettes	Glomerulonephritis	Hereditary nephritis
Depression	Cold remedies	Gout	Hyperlipidemia
Dizziness	Chewing tobacco	Hepatitis	Hyperparathyroidism
Dyspnea	Licorice	Hypertension	Hypertension
Fatigue	Nasal sprays	Lupus erythematosus	Pheochromocytoma
Flushing	Nonsteroidal anti-inflammatory	Myocardial infarction	Polycystic kidney disease
Headaches	agents	Peptic ulcer	Renal hypoplasia
Hematuria	Oral contraceptives	Pyelonephritis	Thyroid disorders
Impotence	Potassium (dietary)	Toxemia	
Joint pains	Salt (dietary or tablets)	Transient ischemic attacks	
Muscle cramps	Tricyclic antidepressants		
Nocturia			
Palpitations			
Polyuria			
Skin rash			
Sweating			
Tingling/cold extremities			
Unsteadiness			
Weakness			
Weight loss or gain			

(Reproduced with permission; see Figure Credits)

FIGURE 16.4 KEY ITEMS IN THE PHYSICAL AND LABORATORY EXAMINATIONS OF PATIENTS WITH MILD OR MODERATE HYPERTENSION

PHYSICAL EXAMINATION

GENERAL	HEENT	CHEST	ABDOMEN	EXTREMITIES	NEUROLOGIC
Appearance	Carotid bruit	Breast	Bruit	Edema	Focal signs
Blood pressure	Fundi	Diastolic murmur	Femoral pulses	Peripheral pulses	Proximal muscle
(supine or sitting;	Neck veins	Rales	Palpable kidneys	Peripheral bruits	Strength
standing; both	Ocular bruits	S_3	Truncal obesity		
arms; one leg)	Temporal arteries	S_4	Striae		
Heart rate (supine		Systolic murmur			
or sitting;		Wheezes			
standing)					

LABORATORY EXAMINATION
GENERAL

Hemoglobin	Blood urea nitrogen	Calcium	Chest radiograph
Hematocrit	Creatinine	Cholesterol	Electrocardiogram
White blood cell count	Urine dipstix	Glucose (fasting)	
	Urine sediment	HDL cholesterol	
		Potassium	
		Uric acid	

(Reproduced with permission; see Figure Credits)

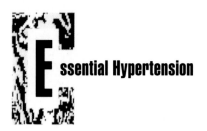

Essential Hypertension

Hypertension without a clearly definable etiology is called *essential hypertension*, accounting for well over 90% of all cases of high blood pressure (Fig. 16.5). Its existence is likely due to both genetic and environmental factors. The majority of patients with essential hypertension have a family member (usually a parent or a sibling) with high blood pressure. Presumably, the hereditary element provides the background for an environmental factor, such as salt intake.

NA, CA, AND AUTOREGULATION

While a single cause for the pathogenesis of essential hypertension has eluded researchers, several theories have emerged. Blood pressure is the arithmetic product of cardiac output and peripheral vascular resistance. Hence, hypertension may represent an increase in one or both of these factors. It has been proposed that increases in cardiac output occur early in the genesis of hypertension whereas a high, steady-state peripheral vascular resistance maintains high blood pressure later in the disease process. This phenomenon is demonstrated in Guyton's experiment of partially nephrectomized dogs (Fig. 16.6).[23] In the

FIGURE 16.5 FREQUENCY OF VARIOUS FORMS OF HYPERTENSION

TYPES	% OF FREQUENCY
Essential (primary) hypertension	89–95
Secondary hypertension	2–5
Renal parenchymal disease	0.2–4
Renovascular disease	0.1–1
Coarctation of the aorta	0.1–0.5
Hyperaldosteronism	0.1–0.2
Cushing's syndrome	0.1–0.2
Pheochromocytoma	0.2–4

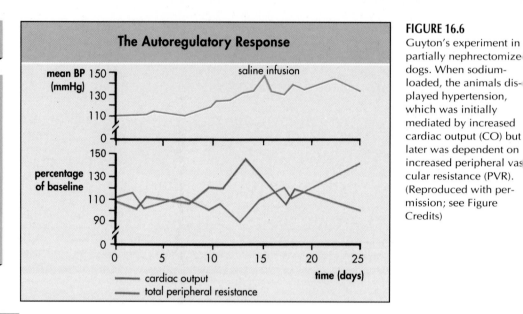

The Autoregulatory Response

FIGURE 16.6
Guyton's experiment in partially nephrectomized dogs. When sodium-loaded, the animals displayed hypertension, which was initially mediated by increased cardiac output (CO) but later was dependent on increased peripheral vascular resistance (PVR). (Reproduced with permission; see Figure Credits)

FIGURE 16.7 Effects of hypothetical sodium-transport inhibitor and its role in the pathogenesis of hypertension. (Reproduced with permission; see Figure Credits)

The Circulating Sodium-Transport Inhibitor Hypothesis

Na⁺ intake > 50 mmol/day

Na⁺ excretion inadequate

extracellular fluid volume increased

sodium transport inhibitor increased

Na⁺ ⇌ K⁺ transport decreased

artery

leucocyte lymphocyte erythrocyte

essential hypertension

tudy, isotonic saline expansion led to an increase in cardiac output within 2 weeks, followed by an increase in peripheral vascular resistance. The subsequent all in cardiac output to baseline presumably reflects the higher afterload.

Both of these phenomena can be linked by a putative sodium-transport inhibitor in hypertension (Fig. 16.7). Guyton[23] and others have held the primacy of the kidney in hypertension. A postulated defect in renal sodium excretion would lead initially to volume expansion. However, the response to this initial perturbation might be the elaboration of the sodium-transport inhibitor, which would counteract the renal defect[5] (Fig. 16.8). The hypothalamically produced transport inhibitor, which has properties similar to the cardiac glycoside digitalis, inhibits sodium–potassium ATPase. In the nephron, this results in reduced sodium reabsorption and enhanced excretion. The extrarenal results, however, augment vascular reactivity and tone, particularly in cells in the vascular wall. Regulation of vascular smooth muscle calcium is linked to intracellular sodium since cellular calcium extrusion is dependent on sodium–calcium exchange. This process is driven by an inward gradient for sodium, which, in turn, is maintained by sodium–potassium ATPase. Inhibition of sodium–potassium ATPase, it follows, leads to increased intracellular sodium, dissolution of the inward sodium gradient, and diminished sodium–calcium exchange. The resultant rise in intracellular calcium increases vascular smooth muscle contractility. The increase in vascular reactivity results in a shift of the autoregulatory relationship between tissue perfusion and arterial pressure.

THE RENIN–ANGIOTENSIN–ALDOSTERONE SYSTEM

The renin–angiotensin–aldosterone system (RAAS) has been implicated in the control of blood pressure and the genesis of hypertension since the pioneering work of Goldblatt[22] and others in the 1930s. These workers demonstrated that hypertension resulted from a renal factor produced when the kidney was subjected to constriction of the renal artery. During the 1960s, Laragh and others proposed a bipolar construct of hypertension based upon the relationship between plasma renin activity (PRA) and renal sodium excretion, the latter being a reflection of sodium intake.[37] According to this hypothesis, patients with high renin activity (i.e., above the normal range for the sodium/PRA nomogram) had a vasoconstrictive form of hypertension, owing to the effects of increased angiotensin II production. Patients with low renin essential hypertension had primarily an extracellular volume-mediated hypertension. This theory seemed to be supported by the response of patients with essential hypertension to antagonists of the RAAS. When they were given the competitive inhibitor of angiotensin II, saralasin, high renin essential hypertensive patients had marked lowering of blood pressure, whereas low renin essential hypertensives failed to display a drop in blood pressure. Similar effects were observed when oral con-

verting enzyme inhibitors were given. In recent years, however, this view of the role of the RAAS in the causation of high blood pressure has been considered overly simplistic. Measurements of PRA, coupled with hemodynamic data, have consistently shown results opposite to those predicted by the volume/vasoconstrictor bipolar analysis, namely, that the higher the plasma renin, the lower the peripheral vascular resistance. Moreover, while it is true that converting enzyme inhibitors and other agents that interrupt the RAAS lower blood pressure in some individuals, not all subjects with hypertension are responsive to these agents. In addition, the converting enzyme inhibitors may exert actions to lower blood pressure are independent of the RAAS (e.g., inhibition of kininases and increased levels of bradykinin).

Under normal conditions, the RAAS is regulated by sodium intake. A high sodium intake reduces renin release, which permits an increase in renal blood flow and a consequent rise in sodium excretion. The adrenal response to angiotensin II (i.e., the synthesis of aldosterone) is reduced in the sodium-loaded state. In contrast, with sodium restriction, the increase in the activity of the RAAS leads to a rise in angiotensin II, with consequent renal vasoconstriction and an augmented adrenal response. Hollenberg and coworkers[24] have recently found that approximately one half of hypertensive patients with normal or high PRA demonstrate failure of the normal feedback regulation of the RAAS. During sodium restriction, these individuals demonstrate a blunted aldosterone response to angiotensin II and higher PRA values. With sodium loading, they demonstrated an attenuated renal blood flow response, failure to excrete the sodium, and an increase in blood pressure. In both circumstances, the failure to regulate the local RAAS in these non-modulators might account for the hypertension. In the sodium-loaded patients, failure to reduce local angiotensin II would prevent the increase in renal blood flow necessary to accommodate volume expansion and the subsequent increment in sodium excretion. The retained sodium would increase plasma volume and, perhaps, lead to the elaboration of a sodium transport inhibitor, as described above. With sodium restriction, the failure to mount an appropriate aldosterone response causes continued volume contraction and tonic stimulation of the RAAS and an inability to close the feedback loop.

Low renin essential hypertension accounts for 20% to 30% of primary hypertension and probably includes a large number of African-American and elderly patients, both groups being more prone to this condition. While low renin hypertension still defies a single pathophysiologic explanation, several theories have arisen. It seems likely that some patients have expanded extracellular fluid volume, which diminishes renin release. This may be a primary defect or may be the result of other mechanisms, such as mineralacorticoid excess (aldosterone, deoxycorticosterone, 18-OH-DOC, or other steroids). Some forms of chronic

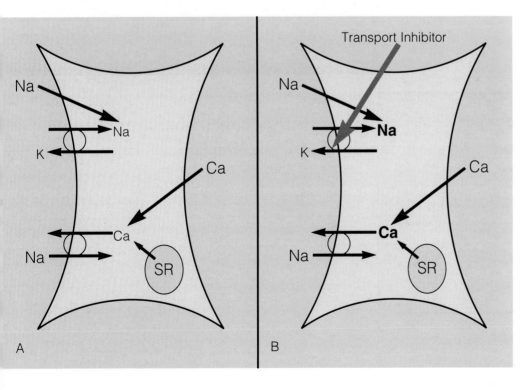

FIGURE 16.8 Effects of transport inhibitor on cytosolic calcium (Ca). **(A)** In the normal resting cell, cytosolic Ca represents the contribution of intracellular sources, such as the sarcoplasmic reticulum (SR), and inward movement from the extracellular space. This is balanced by outward movement of Ca by sodium-calcium exchange, driven by a favorable electrochemical gradient for the inward movement of sodium. The inward movement of sodium, in turn, is fueled by sodium–potassium ATPase. **(B)** A putative inhibitor of this Na–K pump leads to increased intracellular Na, a less favorable gradient for inward Na movement, and a resultant increase in intracellular Ca.

renal failure, particularly diabetic nephropathy, have been associated with a defective renin release mechanism. This may be the result of injury and sclerosis of the juxtaglomerular apparatus or a defect in juxtaglomerular cell responses to the appropriate signals for renin release (such as beta–adrenergic catecholamine). It is possible that similar mechanisms may exist in some patients with low renin essential hypertension.

There has been considerable recent interest in potential linkages among obesity, hypertension, and hyperinsulinemia.[11,18,25,30,47,49,53] Hypertension is common among diabetic patients and insulin resistance with hyperinsulinemia is frequently observed in hypertensive patients. One potential mechanism may be insulin-driven antinatriuresis,[6,12,25,42,48,50] which leads to volume expansion, or an increase in responsiveness to vasoconstrictors, as shown in Figure 16.9.

SYMPATHETIC NERVOUS SYSTEM

Overactivity of the sympathetic nervous system has long been suspected to be a cause of hypertension. The presumed association between psychologic stress and hypertension certainly applies to acute models of high blood pressure. However, the evidence supporting a role for the sympathetic nervous system in mediating sustained human hypertension remains sketchy and uncertain. Most of the data examining plasma norepinephrine and epinephrine have been criticized since plasma catecholamine levels may not reflect local activity at the neuromuscular junction. They may, instead, reflect alterations in plasma entry or metabolism of catecholamine. On the other hand, there is compelling evidence to suggest a role for the sympathetic nervous system in hypertension (Fig. 16.10). However its primacy may yet be contested.

ENDOTHELIAL AND OTHER LOCALLY ACTING FACTORS

Attention has focused increasingly on the role of vascular autocrine and paracrine factors in the control of blood pressure. These may be divided into predominantly vasodilatory and vasocontrictive substances.

VASODILATORS

The ability of the vasculature to relax in response to acetylcholine, bradykinin and other vasodilators is dependent on the presence of endothelium. With an intact endothelium, rabbit aortic strips, preconstricted with norepinephrine undergo vasorelaxation when acetylcholine is applied (Fig. 16.11). However, the aorta, denuded of endothelium, fails to display vasorelaxation with acetylcholine. The endothelial substance responsible for this property, first called *endothelial-derived relaxing factor* (EDRF), is nitric oxide derived from the metabolism of the amino acid arginine.[45] Nitric oxide appears to be released from endothelium, but with a half-life of only 5 seconds, it quickly passes into the subjacent smooth muscle where it induces cyclic GMP formation resulting in relaxation.

The importance of nitric oxide, as of this writing, seems to be limited to it

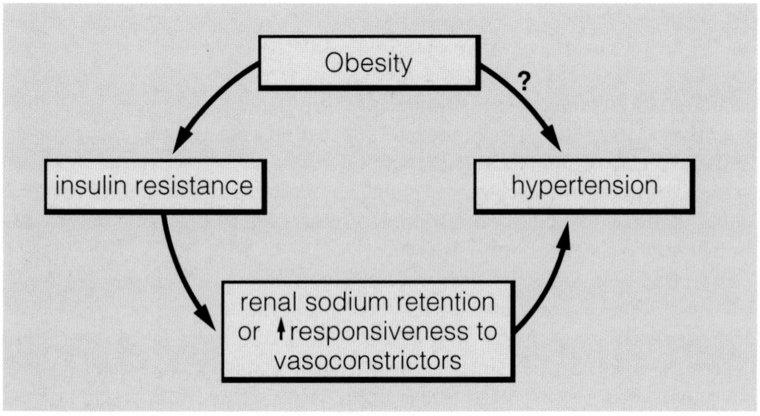

FIGURE 16.9 Possible mechanism linking insulin resistance, obesity, and hypertension.

FIGURE 16.10 EVIDENCE SUPPORTING SYMPATHETIC HYPERACTIVITY AS A CAUSATIVE FACTOR IN HYPERTENSION

1. Plasma catecholamine levels are elevated in hypertensive patients.
2. There is a higher prevalence of hypertension in high-stress occupations.
3. Sympatholytic drugs (e.g., clonidine) lower both blood pressure and plasma catecholamine levels in a correlated manner.
4. Pharmacologic blockade of the sympathetic nervous system α and β blockers) lowers blood pressure, as does surgical sympathectomy.
5. Lesions of the hypothalamic nuclei involved in blood pressure control cause hypertension.
6. Spontaneously hypertensive rats and humans with "pre-hypertension" demonstrate augmented autonomic responses.

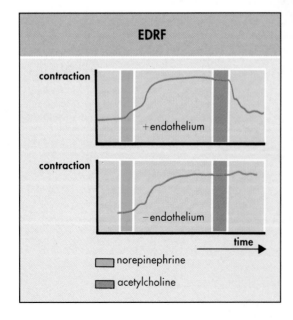

FIGURE 16.11 Effect of endothelial denudation on contraction of rabbit aorta. Intact endothelial aortic strips, preconstricted with norepinephrine, show relation when acetylcholine is applied. However, when endothelium is removed relaxation is not observed with acetylcholine. (Reproduced with permission; see Figure Credits)

unter-regulatory role in hypertension. Administration of an acetylcholine, a imulus of nitric oxide formation in hypertensive patients,[46] yields a subnormal sponse in hypertensive patients. Nitric oxide, therefore, may serve to modulate ypertension in susceptible individuals, but there is no evidence to date that npaired nitric oxide formation is a primary mechanism of high blood pressure.

A variety of eicosanoid substances appear to exhibit vasodilatory properties. owever, only *prostacyclin* appears to be produced by the endothelium in abun nce. A variety of vasodilatory substances, including bradykinin, appear to duce prostacylin synthesis, which begins with the release of arachidonic acid om cell membrane phospholipids (Fig. 16.12). Arachidonic acid is transformed a the cyclo-oxygenase enzyme into endoperoxide intermediates and subse ently into prostanoids, including prostacylin. Aspirin, indomethacin, and her nonsteroidal anti-inflammatory drugs (NSAIDs) inhibit cyclo-oxygenase d thereby impair prostacylin biosynthesis. Hence, the administration of SAIDs, particularly to hypertensive patients, causes elevations in blood pres re. (Renal sodium retention caused by the blockade of natriuretic rostaglandins may also contribute to the increase.) As in the case of nitric xide, however, it remains uncertain whether impaired prostacylin synthesis rimarily causes hypertension.

The *kallikrein–kinin* system is another local vasodilatory mechanism. allikreins, found in kidney, pancreas, and salivary glands, are enzymes that cat yze the synthesis of kinins from inactive kininogens. While the kinins exhibit otent vasodepressor activity, there is little evidence that they assume a funda ental role in the pathogenesis of hypertension. On the other hand, the kinins re destroyed by the action of kininases, which are identical to angiotensin-con erting enzymes. The blood pressure lowering action of converting enzyme nhibitors might, in part, reflect the inhibition of kininases and the resultant ugmentation of local kinins, such as bradykinin.

ASOCONSTRICTORS

he activity of the *renin–angiotensin system* (RAS) had been thought to reside rgely in the specialized juxtaglomerular apparatus of the kidney. However, ccruing evidence supports the notion that the vascular wall may contain all

the elements of the RAS.[44] Aortic tissue possesses renin mRNA, and angiotensin II is assayable in vascular tissue perfused with non-substrate-con taining medium. These findings suggest that an autocrine–paracrine action of RAS may account for some of the actions of angiotensin II rather than a circu lating form of renin or angiotensin. Thus, the antihypertensive efficacy of con verting enzyme inhibitors in some patients with low renin hypertension may be based on this phenomenon.

Recent data also suggest that angiotensin may behave as a cellular mitogen or hypertrophy factor for vascular smooth muscle,[3,39] an effect that may be impor tant in the pathologic changes accompanying hypertension or atherosclerosis (see discussion below). These actions might be seen with smaller concentrations of angiotensin than are observed with the circulating form and therefore might be due to local activity of the RAS.

The *endothelins* are a group of very potent vasoconstrictive peptides that are produced by the endothelial cell.[35,54] Endothelins are synthesized from a large precursor peptide by the action of specific endopeptidases and are subsequently cleaved from a largely inactive "big endothelin" by a putative converting enzyme (Fig. 16.13). Endothelin 1, which is a 21-amino acid peptide, appears to be the predominant species in man and, on a molar level, is the most potent vasoconstrictor isolated so far. The importance of this family of peptides in the

Secondary Hypertension
RENAL PARENCHYMAL DISEASE

pathogenesis of hypertension is largely speculative at present.

Renal parenchymal disease constitutes the most common form of secondary hypertension. However, hypertension coexisting with renal disease poses a diag nostic dilemma for the clinician: "Which came first—the chicken or the egg?"

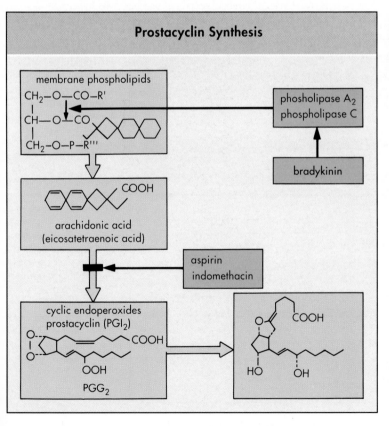

FIGURE 16.12   Biosynthesis of prostacyclin from membrane phospho lipids. (Reproduced with permission; see Figure Credits)

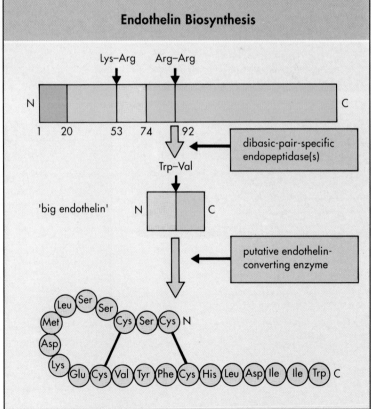

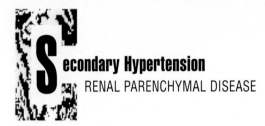

FIGURE 16.13   Biosynthetic pathway for endothelin. (Reproduced with permission; see Figure Credits)

phenomenon. Hypertension is a common manifestation of most renal diseases. However, renal insufficiency commonly complicates long-standing hypertension. Hence, recognition of which disease is primary may be difficult or, in some cases, impossible.

HYPERTENSION WITH UNILATERAL PARENCHYMAL DISEASE OR A SOLITARY KIDNEY

Hypertension may occur in a variety of conditions affecting only one kidney or in subjects with a solitary kidney (Fig. 16.14). Renin-producing juxtaglomerular cell tumors are usually unilateral, demonstrating that hypertension can arise from over-secretion of renin without renovascular disease. The elevated blood pressure is usually cured by unilateral nephrectomy or partial nephrectomy to remove the tumor.

Other conditions, such as hydronephrosis and unilateral renal cysts, appear to be renin-mediated, as suggested by the following observations: (1) renal vein renins on the affected side are usually greater than 1.5 times the contralateral values;[55] and (2) in the case of hypertension associated with isolated cysts, aspiration and collapse of the cyst often corrects both the hypertension and the hyper-reninemia, suggesting that renal ischemia and renin production may be due to compression of the renal vasculature.[2]

HYPERTENSION ASSOCIATED WITH ACUTE RENAL FAILURE

High blood pressure often complicates acute renal failure. Vascular diseases that produce injury to the renal microcirculation, such as polyarteritis nodosa or scleroderma, are usually associated with hypertension. In the latter case, malignant hypertension may be observed. Most likely this represents activation of the RAS, since blood pressure reduction usually occurs with administration of converting enzyme inhibitors.

The hypertension observed with acute inflammatory glomerular diseases, such as post-streptococcal glomerulonephritis, is accompanied by sodium and water retention. However, administration of converting enzyme inhibitors may reduce blood pressure in these cases as well, suggesting a role for RAS. Despite low determinations of PRA in acute glomerulonephritis, these levels may actually be relatively high, considering the state of volume expansion, and thus add a component of vasoconstriction (Fig. 16.15).

HYPERTENSION IN CHRONIC RENAL FAILURE

Given the perturbations in sodium and water excretion that accompany chronic renal disease, it is logical to assume that hypertension occurs as a consequence of a swollen blood volume. In fact, exchangeable sodium is expanded in chronic renal failure and blood pressure elevation correlates with both extracellular volume and exchangeable sodium. Moreover, the observation that blood pressure in most patients with end stage renal disease (ESRD) falls following hemodialysis and ultrafiltrative fluid removal substantiates the notion that their hypertension is volume-dependent.

On the other hand, there are considerable data supporting the role of vasoconstrictive factors in chronic renal failure. While early studies reported normal or even low peripheral vascular resistance, it now appears that this is most likely due to the anemia that inevitably accompanies azotemia. When anemia is corrected (as, for example, with transfusion or erythropoietin administration), an increased vascular resistance is unmasked.[36] The increase in vascular resistance has been attributed to a variety of vasopressors, including postganglionic norepinephrine release, stimulation of the RAS, and elevation of arginine vasopressin (AVP) levels. The RAS has been implicated, particularly in glomerular diseases which often are associated with more resistant hypertension.

In addition to overactivity of vasoconstrictors, diminution of vasodilatory substances has been suggested to play a role in the hypertension of chronic renal failure, particularly since some depressor compounds are produced by the kidney. Hence, the concept of renoprival hypertension postulates that the loss of renal vasodilators leads to hypertension. Vasodilatory prostaglandins (PGE2 and prostacyclin) produced in the kidney, however, are more often increased than decreased in renal hypertension. Likewise there are little data showing that a lack of antihypertensive renomedullary lipid contributes to the hypertension. The evidence showing a decrease in the kallikrein–kinin system in renal parenchymal disease fails to establish a link between this observation and the hypertension.

Rather than being mediated purely by volume or vasoconstriction, hypertension in chronic renal diseases is probably due to a mix of both factors. In the more resistant forms of hypertension associated with glomerulonephritis, vasculitis, and scleroderma, activation of the RAS leads to a predominantly vasoconstrictive type of hypertension. In the tubulointerstitial diseases, mild hypertension is often volume-dependent and sensitive to diuresis or ultrafiltrative fluid removal.

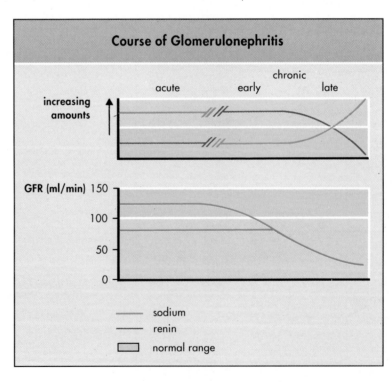

FIGURE 16.14 HYPERTENSION IN UNILATERAL RENAL DISEASE

Juxtaglomerular cell (renin-secreting) tumor
Hydronephrosis
Bacterial pyelonephritis
Vesicoureteral reflux
Solitary or unilateral cysts
Unilateral agenesis

Course of Glomerulonephritis

FIGURE 16.15
Evolution of hypertension in acute and chronic glomerulonephritis. In the acute phase, sodium and water retention are the predominant factors, while renin secretion is normal. In early chronic glomerulonephritis, activation of RAS accompanies hypertension, and in late stages, as GFR declines, sodium and water retention may again predominate (Reproduced with permission; see Figure Credits)

A theory unifying the roles of extracellular fluid volume and peripheral vaso-constriction relies on the pathophysiology of essential hypertension (as discussed above). During the early phase of chronic renal failure, small reductions in the glomerular filtration rate (GFR) may lead to transient extracellular volume expansion. This inevitably causes increased cardiac output and hypertension. The autoregulatory response to this perturbation, perhaps mediated by a hypo-thalamic digoxin-like natriuretic substance,[14] manifests itself as increased peripheral vascular resistance. Hence, in all forms of renal failure, a combination of volume expansion and vasoconstriction accounts for the hypertension, although one factor may be dominant.

RENOVASCULAR DISEASE
PATHOPHYSIOLOGY

In 1934, Harry Goldblatt first demonstrated that partial constriction of a single renal artery induced hypertension.[21,22] The experiment showed that the hypop-erfused kidney enhanced a substance, later identified as renin, that raised blood pressure. Goldblatt subsequently developed two models (Fig. 16.16). The two-kidney, one-clip model (analogous to unilateral renal artery stenosis with a con-tralateral normal kidney) induces hypertension by an angiotensin II-dependent mechanism. The contralateral kidney undergoes a pressure natriuresis that caus-es mild volume contraction (Fig. 16.17). However, the sensitivity to angiotensin

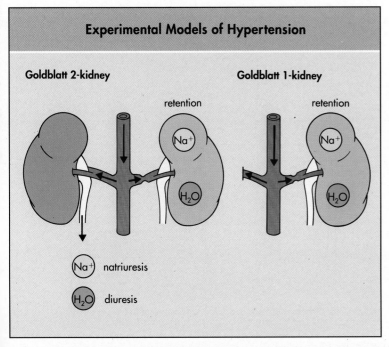

FIGURE 16.16 Models of hypertension developed by Goldblatt. (Reproduced with permission; see Figure Credits)

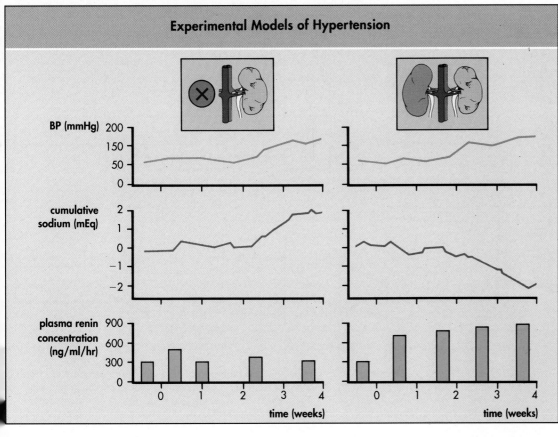

FIGURE 16.17 Relationships between cumulative sodium balance, plasma renin, and hypertension in the one- (left panel) and two-kidney (right panel) Goldblatt models. In the one-kidney model, renal ischemia in the clipped kid-ney leads to activation of renin and sub-sequent angiotensin and aldosterone secretion followed by renal sodium reten-tion. The hypertension is volume-depen-dent and renin levels are low or normal. In the two-kidney model, activation of renin–angiotensin leads to vasoconstric-tion and hypertension but a pressure natriuresis through the contralateral kid-ney prevents volume expansion. Renin levels are elevated. (Reproduced with permission; see Figure Credits)

blockade (with the competitive antagonist saralasin) is present only during early phases of hypertension (Fig. 16.18). Chronic renovascular hypertension, presumably dependent on other mechanisms, fails to respond to saralasin. The sequence of events leading to chronic renovascular hypertension is shown in Figure 16.19.

In the one-kidney, one-clip model (analogous to renovascular disease with a solitary functioning kidney) plasma renin levels do not rise. The absence of the contralateral kidney does not permit a pressure natriuresis to take place, and a gradual increase in sodium balance participates in the pathogenesis of so-called volume-mediated hypertension.[37]

While the kidney models developed by Goldblatt provide a theoretic basis for understanding renovascular disease, they do not provide a complete understanding of the response to nephrectomy or pharmacologic therapy. As discussed above, after a period of weeks to months, renin–angiotensin dependency may be superseded by other hypertensive mechanisms. Hypertrophy or nephrosclerosis of the contralateral kidney may prevent appropriate pressure natriuresis from taking place and an increase in sodium balance may result .

In addition, the response to converting enzyme inhibitors does not clearly correlate with renin-dependent hypertension. As described above, other mecha-

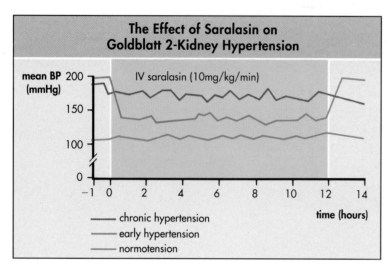

FIGURE 16.18   Effects of competitive angiotensin II blockade with saralasin in two-kidney Goldblatt hypertension. Saralasin produces a sharp reduction in blood pressure in early hypertension but no response is seen in chronic hypertension. (Reproduced with permission; see Figure Credits)

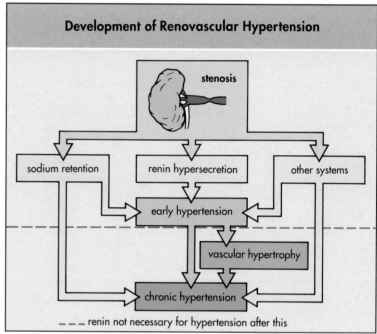

FIGURE 16.19   Pathogenesis of early and chronic hypertension in renovascular stenosis. (Reproduced with permission; see Figure Credits)

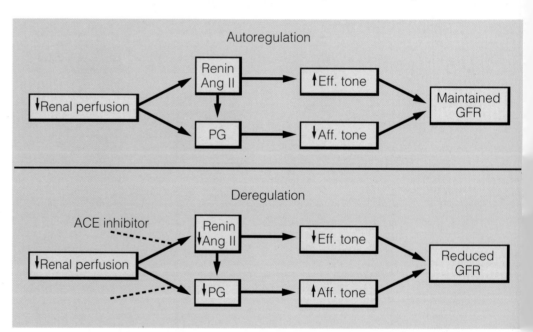

FIGURE 16.20 CHARACTERISTICS OF PATIENTS WITH RENOVASCULAR DISEASE

1. Onset of hypertension before age 25 or after age 60
2. Abdominal vascular bruit, particularly radiating to flank
3. Grade III or IV hypertensive retinopathy (in males)
4. Azotemia, particularly when aggravated by ACE inhibitors
5. Hypotensive response to low-dose ACE inhibitors

FIGURE 16.21   Mechanism of ACE inhibitor-induced diminution in GFR. Under ordinary circumstances renal hypoperfusion leads to activation of both the renin–angiotensin and prostaglandin systems. The former induces vasodilation of the afferent arteriole, while the latter promotes vasoconstriction of the efferent sphincter. The combination of the two preserves glomerular capillary pressure and GFR. With the use of an ACE inhibitor, blockade of angiotensin II formation causes diminution in efferent arteriolar tone and GFR falls. Similarly, if prostaglandin formation is blocked by nonsteroidal anti-inflammatory agents (NSAIDs), afferent vasodilation is prevented and GFR falls.

nisms, such as kininase inhibition, may account for a fall in blood pressure following converting enzyme inhibition.

DIAGNOSIS

After renal parenchymal disease, renovascular disease is the most common form of secondary hypertension. The table in Figure 16.20 lists the clinical characteristics of patients likely to have this diagnosis. Several features are worthy of mention. Although the age range given is typical of patients with renovascular disease, the disease can occur in any adult and is sometimes found in children. Azotemia, occurring within a few days of starting angiotensin converting enzyme (ACE) inhibitors, is strongly suggestive of either bilateral renovascular disease or renal artery stenosis in a solitary kidney (Fig. 16.21). During reductions in renal plasma flow (as in high-grade renal artery stenosis), maintenance of GFR requires dilatation of the afferent arterials and constriction of the efferent arterioles to maintain glomerular capillary pressure. The latter process requires angiotensin II since the predominant effect of the peptide is at the efferent sphincter. Use of ACE inhibitors under these conditions robs the kidney of its autoregulatory response, resulting in a sharp drop in GFR. (This effect is the basis for the captopril renogram, which is described below.)

Renal vascular lesions in older adults are almost always the result of atherosclerotic plaque formation at the renal artery ostium or in the proximal vessel. Patients with these lesions usually have vascular disease elsewhere, particularly in the ileac or femoral arteries and, therefore, may complain of claudication.

Fibromuscular dysplasias are usually seen in younger patients. Medial fibromuscular dysplasia, by far the most common type, is found more often in young women. Unlike atherosclerotic disease, it is generally seen in the mid or distal renal artery and can be recognized by a typical "string of beads" appearance. Figures 16.22 and 16.23 demonstrate the radiographic differences between atherosclerotic and medial fibroplastic lesions, and the table in Figure 16.24 summarizes their clinical differences.

Diagnosis of renovascular disease rests on a gold standard test, selective renal angiography. Although a variety of screening tests have been advocated in the past, none offers the sensitivity, specificity, and predictive value of angiography. Nonetheless, this invasive test represents a substantial risk for some patients (e.g., those with severe peripheral vascular disease or friable aortic atherosclerotic disease in whom arteriography poses hazards of thrombosis or atheroembolism). In these cases, screening tests may be considered.

In the 1960s, rapid-sequence intravenous pyelography became a popular modality for identifying probable renal artery disease. More recent evidence, however, suggests that its sensitivity and specificity are inferior to newer tests, which do not require exposing the patient to radiocontrast material. The modern screening tests used today are either renin secretion testing or radioisotopic scanning.

Radioisotopic scanning utilizes one of several agents: ^{99}Tc-DTPA, ^{131}I-hippurate, or Mag-3. Hippurate is predominantly secreted and 80% is removed by a single passage through the kidney; hence, the clearance of this agent is equivalent to renal blood flow. DTPA is cleared principally by glomerular filtration. Mag-3 has elements of both agents, being nearly equally cleared by tubular secretion and glomerular filtration. When rapid scintigrams are taken, the

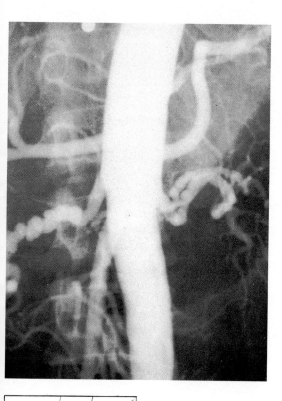

FIGURE 16.22
Aortogram demonstrating typical "string of beads" appearance of bilateral fibromuscular dysplasia.
(Reproduced with permission; see Figure Credits)

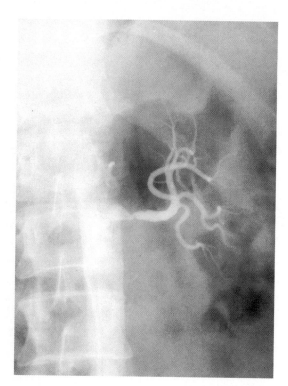

FIGURE 16.23
Aortogram showing typical appearance of a proximal atherosclerotic renal artery lesion with post-stenotic dilatation.
(Reproduced with permission; see Figure Credits)

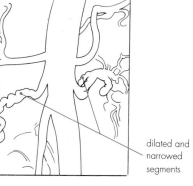

dilated and narrowed segments

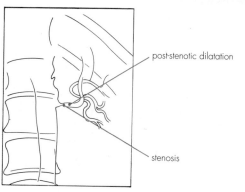

post-stenotic dilatation

stenosis

FIGURE 16.24 CLINICAL FEATURES OF ATHEROSCLEROTIC AND MEDIAL FIBROMUSCULAR DYSPLASTIC RENAL ARTERY LESIONS

		ATHEROSCLEROSIS	**FIBROMUSCULAR DYSPLASIA**
>60	Age		25–50
Male > female	Gender		Female > male
Proximal	Location		Mid or distal

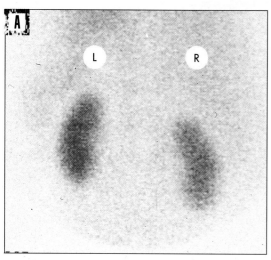

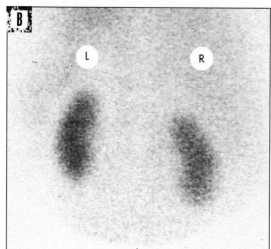

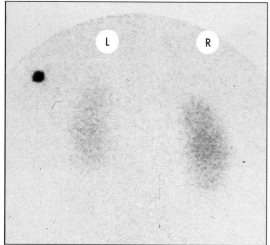

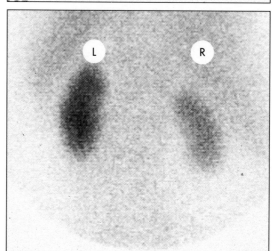

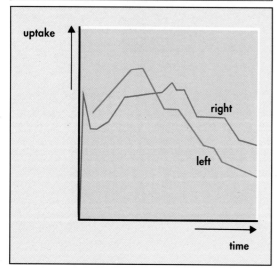

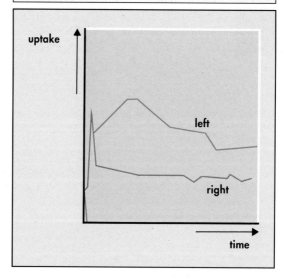

FIGURE 16.25 DTPA renal scans of patient with right renal artery stenosis. **(A)** The precaptopril study shows reduced and delayed uptake in the right kidney with delayed clearance of the isotope. **(B)** After 25 mg of captopril, marked reduction of function and failure to clear the isotope are seen. (Reproduced with permission; see Figure Credits)

pearance of any of the isotopes is proportional to the delivery of the agent via nal blood flow.

Since many parenchymal diseases may ultimately be accompanied by reduced nal perfusion, the reduction of renal blood flow to one or both kidneys is of sufficient specificity to identify renovascular disease. Since ACE inhibitors tenuate the autoregulation of GFR (as discussed above), isotopic scans are ow enhanced with the use of captopril.[20] In unilateral renal artery stenosis, oderate blood flow reduction to a single renal artery produces no apparent differences in isotope excretion in each kidney, as seen in the precaptopril study igs. 16.25, 16.26). One hour after the oral administration of captopril (25 mg), owever, a remarkable change occurs in the isotope excretion from the left kidney. Administration of the ACE inhibitor causes a sudden reduction in GFR in e affected kidney, resulting in a delayed "washout" of the isotope. Instead of a eep rise, followed by rapid disappearance of the isotope, the curve of the left dney now continues to rise and reaches a plateau. This is strongly indicative of emodynamically significant unilateral disease. In kidneys with long-standing enosis, presumably with profound ischemia, a flat curve may be seen in both e pre- and postcaptopril studies, indicative of very poor perfusion with no ptake of isotope. Bilateral renovascular disease, which may occur in 15% of patients, often presents difficulty in interpretation. False-positive results may occur in patients who suffer a profound fall in blood pressure following captopril.

Since activation of the RAS is central in the pathogenesis of renovascular hypertension, measurement of PRA might seem a logical means of screening for this condition. Many conditions that produce false-positive or false-negative results, however, hamper the reliability of this test.

Recently investigators have experimented with the PRA measurement after captopril administration, anticipating hyper-responsiveness of renin release in patients with renal artery stenosis. A standardized test that has been proposed by Muller et al[43] provides excellent sensitivity but less optimal specificity. The patient has all or most antihypertensive medications (particularly beta-blockers) withdrawn for 3 weeks and is placed on a normal salt intake with no diuretics. After 30 minutes of quiet sitting, a baseline venous PRA sample is drawn. Captopril (50 mg) is administered in 10 ml of water and, one hour later, a second venous PRA sample is drawn (Fig. 16.27).

Definitive radiographic diagnosis of renovascular disease is required if either angioplasty or surgical correction (see discussion below) is anticipated. Ideally, the study would consist of aortography combined with selective injections of the renal arteries. Selective renal angiography best depicts distal or segmental

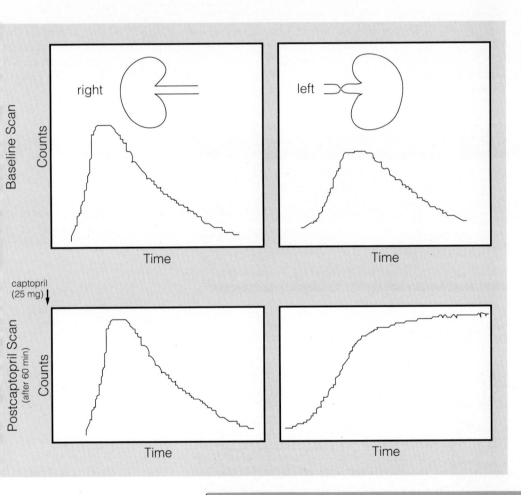

FIGURE 16.26   Representations of scan before (baseline) and after captopril administration in unilateral (left) renovascular hypertension.

FIGURE 16.27 CRITERIA FOR POSITIVE CAPTOPRIL PRA TEST

1. Stimulated PRA of ≥12 ng/ml/hr
2. Absolute increase in PRA of ≥10 ng/ml/hr
3. ≥150% increment in PRA over baseline, or ≥400% increment in PRA over baseline if unstimulated value is <3 ng/ml/hr.

lesions. Digital subtraction angiography with aortic injection provides small contrast volumes but sacrifices good images of peripheral vessels.

The capacity of angiography to predict curable hypertension is enhanced by sampling the renal veins for renin activity. Interpretation of renal venous renins can be accomplished by deriving a "ratio" or an "index" (Fig. 16.28). An index greater than 1.5 indicates that renin secretion is predominantly from the ipsilateral kidney while the contralateral kidney is suppressed. This can be confirmed by a ratio that should exceed 0.24 in the ipsilateral kidney. However, in bilateral disease, the absence of suppression with ratios of more than 0.24 may be observed in both kidneys.

Our approach to the diagnosis of renovascular hypertension is similar to that described by Kaplan (Fig. 16.29). If the patient has the typical clinical features of renovascular disease, renal arteriography should be performed unless there is a relative contraindication (pre-existing renal insufficiency, allergy to radiocontrast, etc.). In such cases, isotopic captopril renography can be used. Therapeutic angioplasty is not employed at the time of diagnostic arteriography unless hemodynamically significant unilateral stenosis is clearly identified. Instead, definitive therapy should await interpretation of renal vein renins, in conjunction with the arteriographic images.

ADRENOCORTICAL HYPERTENSION
MINERALOCORTICOID EXCESS

Mineralocorticoids are sodium-retaining hormones produced in the adrenal cortex. The principal mineralocorticoids are aldosterone, synthesized in the outermost zona glomerulosa (ZG), and deoxycorticosterone (DOC), produced in the

zona fasciculata (ZF). The biosynthetic pathways for both hormones stem from a common precursor, cholesterol (Fig. 16.30). In the ZG pathway, both DOC and aldosterone are produced. In the ZF, 18-OH-DOC and the principal glucocorticoid, cortisol, are synthesized. The late products of steroid synthesis, both of these mineralocorticoids participate in the genesis of hypertension and can be assayed for diagnosis.

As discussed above (see Fig. 16.5), mineralocorticoid excess and hyperaldosteronism account for a very small proportion of unreferred cases of hypertension. Nonetheless, the potential curability of these cases warrants early diagnosis. Mineralocorticoids are principally responsible for transporting epithelia, particularly in the kidney and gastrointestinal tract. In the distal nephron, both aldosterone and DOC bind to cytosolic receptors where they are transported to the cell nucleus and induce specific mRNAs and protein synthesis. The resultant effects are an increase in serosal Na–K-ATPase activity with augmented extrusion of sodium into the extracellular, peritubular space and secretion of both hydrogen and potassium ions into the tubular lumen (Fig. 16.31). Hypokalemia and metabolic alkalosis are typical clinical elements in mineralocorticoid-induced hypertension. Unprovoked hypokalemia in a patient with hypertension should alert the physician to the possibility of this diagnosis.

The mechanisms by which aldosterone and other mineralocorticoids produce hypertension are shown in Figure 16.32. The early phenomena of sodium retention and extracellular volume expansion lead to an increase in cardiac output. Aldosterone may exert a direct action (perhaps by activating Na–K-ATPase) on myocardial contractility, thereby increasing cardiac output. Later, probably through secondary elaboration of a natriuretic hormone, increased peripheral resistance provokes increased vascular smooth muscle contractility. In addition,

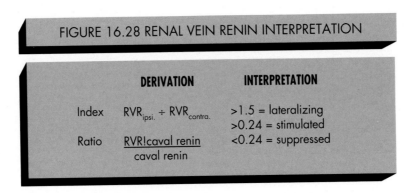

FIGURE 16.28 RENAL VEIN RENIN INTERPRETATION

	DERIVATION	INTERPRETATION
Index	$RVR_{ipsi.} \div RVR_{contra.}$	>1.5 = lateralizing >0.24 = stimulated
Ratio	$\dfrac{RVR!caval\ renin}{caval\ renin}$	<0.24 = suppressed

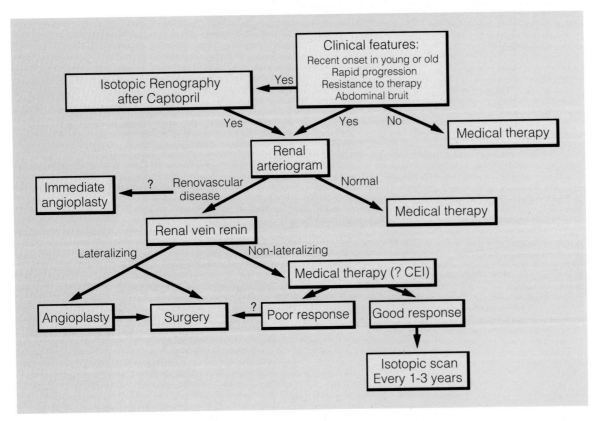

FIGURE 16.29 Algorithm for diagnosis and management of renovascular disease. (Redrawn with permission; see Figure Credits)

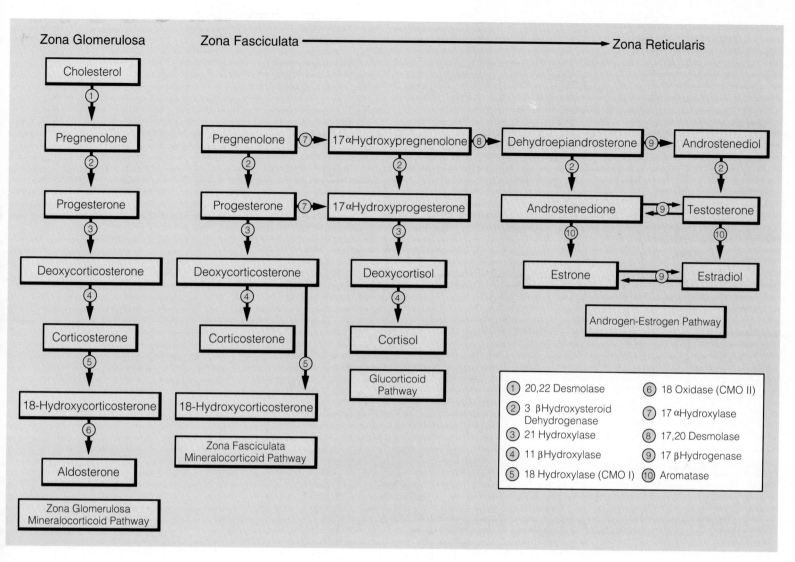

FIGURE 16.30 Biosynthetic pathways of steroid hormones. (Redrawn with permission; see Figure Credits)

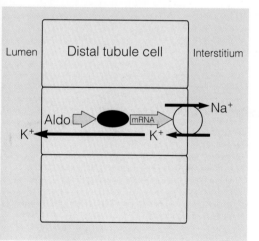

FIGURE 16.31 Mechanism of aldosterone (aldo) action in distal renal tubular cell.

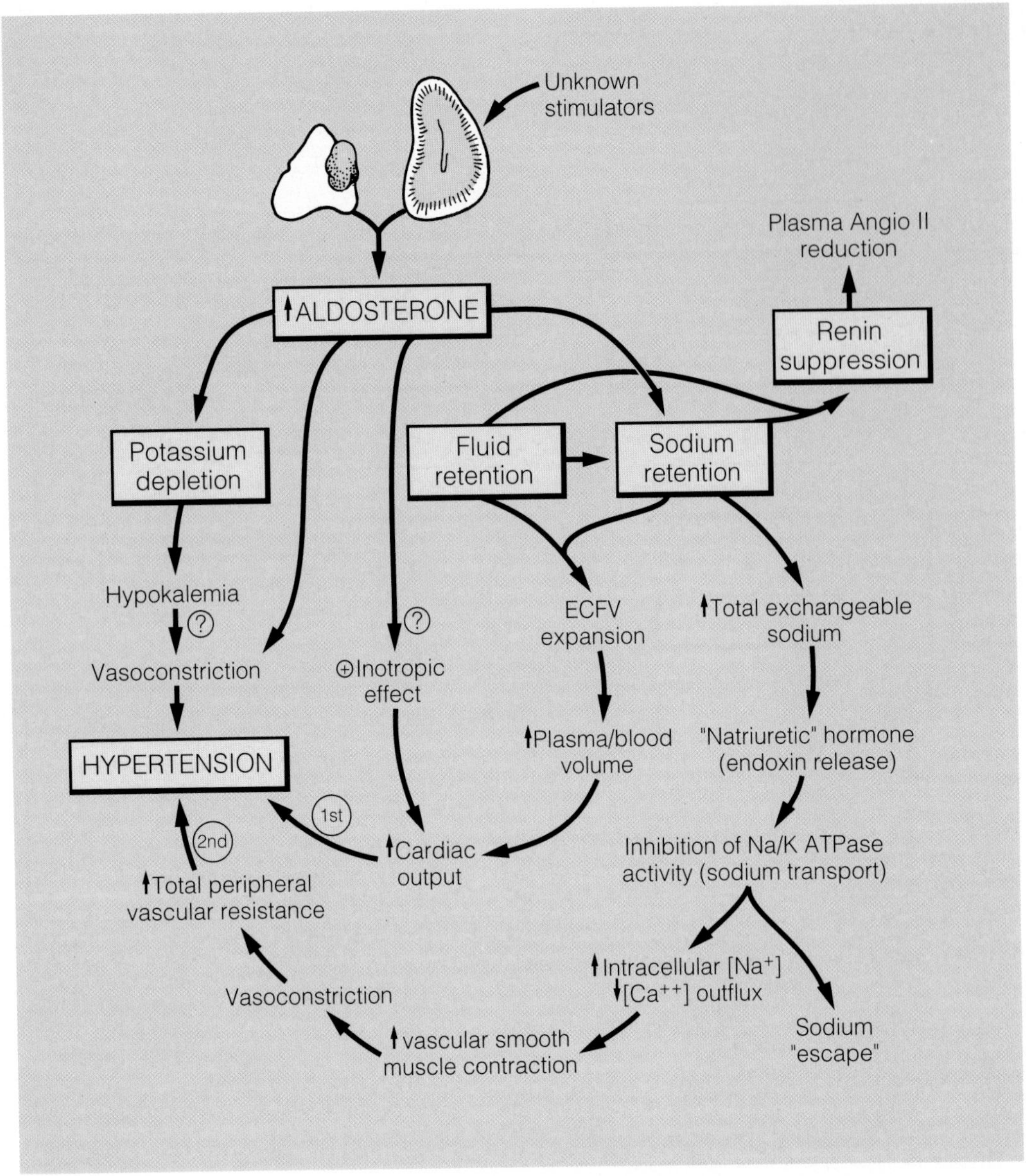

FIGURE 16.33 COMPARATIVE FEATURES OF
ADRENAL ADENOMAS AND IDIOPATHIC ADRENAL HYPERPLASIA IN
PRIMARY ALDOSTERONISM

CONDITION	ADENOMA	HYPERPLASIA
Plasma potassium	Low	Low-normal
Exchangeable sodium	High	Normal
Aldosterone response to exogenous angiostensin II	None	Augmented
Aldosterone response to upright posture	Decrease	Increase

ightened sensitivity to catecholamines may increase peripheral resistance. In addition to mineralocorticoids, glucocorticoid excess promotes hypertension. At least 80% of patients with Cushing's syndrome develop hypertension.[4] On the other hand, only 20% of individuals treated with glucocorticoids for other medical conditions become hypertensive. The weaker mineralocorticoid-like action of these synthetic agents may explain why they are less prone to raise elevated blood pressure.

In general, the mineralocorticoid syndromes can be divided into *primary aldosteronism* and conditions produced by excesses of other mineralocorticoids. Primary aldosteronism, presenting usually as hypertension with unprovoked hypokalemia, is further categorized into syndromes associated with either a benign *adrenal adenoma* (usually unilateral) or *idiopathic adrenal hyperplasia* (usually bilateral). Adrenal adenomas account for at least 85% to 90% of cases of primary aldosteronism.[7] Microscopically, they consist of cords of lipid-laden cells that ultrastructurally resemble aldosterone-producing ZG cells. In addition to hypertension and hypokalemia, the other manifestations of these tumors are elevation of plasma aldosterone accompanied by suppression of renin and angiotensin formation. Characteristically, aldosterone secretion by the tumors is unresponsive to exogenous angiotensin II or to maneuvers that activate the endogenous RAS.

Idiopathic adrenal hyperplasia usually appears with more subtle biochemical and hormonal abnormalities than those seen in patients with adrenal adenomas. Patients with adrenal tumors have more severe hypokalemia and higher exchangeable sodium than those with bilateral hyperplasia (Fig. 16.33). The greater severity of these abnormalities in the former group probably reflects higher ambient levels of aldosterone. Moreover, aldosterone secretion departs from the normal pattern in tumorous aldosteronism by failing to respond appropriately to administered angiotensin II or to upright posture.

There are other syndromes that produce hypertension and hypokalemia and are associated with non-aldosterone mineralocorticoids. In these cases, plasma aldosterone levels are low. Excessive secretion of DOC may occur in association with Cushing's syndrome (see discussion below) or as the result of enzymatic deficiencies (17- or 21-hydroxylase deficiency). Increased levels of DOC may also occur as the result of licorice ingestion. In these patients, the glycyrrhizinic acid contained in licorice produces *pseudoaldosteronism* by blocking the degradation of DOC and other mineralocorticoids.[17]

GLUCOCORTICOID EXCESS

The pathogenesis of hypertension in Cushing's syndrome (as occurs in adrenocortical carcinoma or ACTH-induced hypercortisolism) is complex. Although DOC and other mineralocorticoids may appear in excess, elevated free cortisol may also lead to hypertension (Fig. 16.34). Cortisol excess activates the RAS by increasing hepatic synthesis of renin substrate (angiotensinogen) with consequent angiotensin II-driven vasoconstriction. Inhibition of catecholamine uptake and degradation also augments vasoconstriction. In addition to an excess of vasoconstrictors, diminished vasodilator activity (kinins and prostaglandins) also occurs with elevated plasma cortisol levels. Blood volume may be expanded, either as the result of mineralocorticoid effects of cortisol or because of a shift of fluid from the intracellular to the extracellular compartment.

DIAGNOSIS

The diagnosis of hyperaldosteronism can usually be suspected by the appearance of hypertension, unprovoked (i.e., patient is not using kaliuretic agents) hypokalemia, and low PRA. Once the disease is clinically suspected, elevated

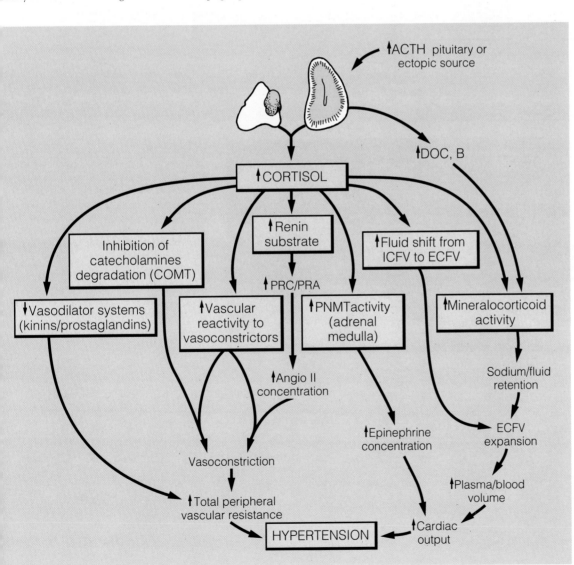

FIGURE 16.34 Pathogenesis of hypertension due to excess glucocorticoids. (Redrawn with permission; see Figure Credits)

plasma aldosterone will usually confirm the diagnosis. Distinguishing between bilateral hyperplasia and adrenal tumor may be difficult. Adenomas produce higher plasma aldosterone levels that may paradoxically fall when the patient assumes a standing posture (Fig. 16.35). Imaging procedures, however, are most helpful in differentiating tumor from bilateral hyperplasia. The CT scan can demonstrate either bilaterally enlarged adrenal glands or a single adenoma (Fig. 16.36). Radioisotopic imaging with ^{77}Se-cholesterol will localize either a single adenoma or bilateral enlargement (Fig. 16.37). A combination of biochemical and imaging parameters may provide the necessary differentiation (Fig. 16.38).

Evaluation of Cushing's syndrome usually requires measurement of cortisol levels. Patients with Cushing's syndrome fail to demonstrate the normal circadian dip in plasma cortisol levels at midnight (Fig. 16.39). Likewise, patients with glucocorticoid-induced hypertension fail to suppress ACTH and, hence, cortisol

levels with administration of dexamethasone. Once hypercortisolism is confirmed, differentiation between a pituitary tumor or adrenal overproduction may begin with a measurement of ACTH levels (Fig. 16.40). High ACTH levels usually point to a pituitary source and suggest radiologic work-up of the pituitary fossa. Contrariwise, low ACTH levels suggest feedback suppression by the adrenals, which should then be examined by imaging techniques.

PHEOCHROMOCYTOMA
PATHOPHYSIOLOGY

Chromaffin-cell tumors that secrete catecholamines are called pheochromocytomas. These tumors, usually of adrenal medullary origin (90%), arise from tissues derived from the neuroectoderm, which also include the sympathetic ganglia and the organs of Zuckerkandl. Tumors may be found in other sites in the

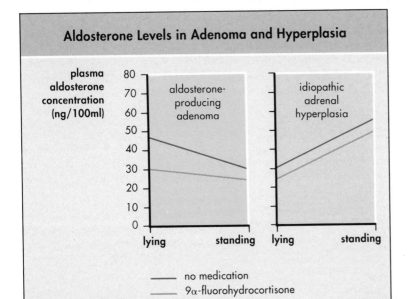

FIGURE 16.35   Contrasting responses of plasma aldosterone in adenoma and idiopathic hyperplasia. Patients with adenomas demonstrate a paradoxical fall in plasma aldosterone levels after 2 hours of upright posture. Those with adrenal hyperplasia demonstrate a physiologic increase in plasma aldosterone. Both conditions demonstrate suppression with 9-fluorohydrocortisone, although a larger decrement is observed in the patient with adenoma. (Reproduced with permission; see Figure Credits)

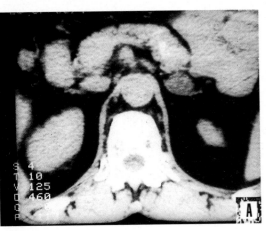

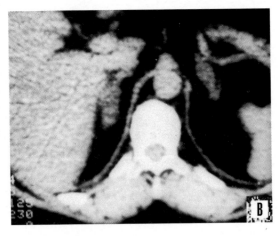

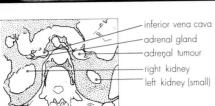

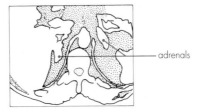

FIGURE 16.36   Computerized tomography in two patients with hyperaldosteronism. **(A)** Scan demonstrates a large adrenal mass above the right kidney. (The left kidney is incidentally small in this patient.) **(B)** Image shows bilaterally enlarged adrenals in a patient with idiopathic hyperplasia. (Reproduced with permission; see Figure Credits)

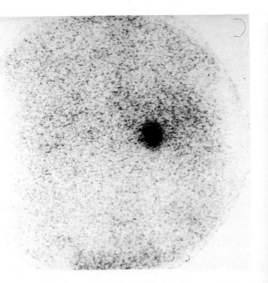

⁷⁵Se-cholesterol adrenal scan monstrating accumulation of isotope in an adrenal enoma. Image was obtained 7 days after the injec- n of isotope. (Reproduced with permission; see ure Credits)

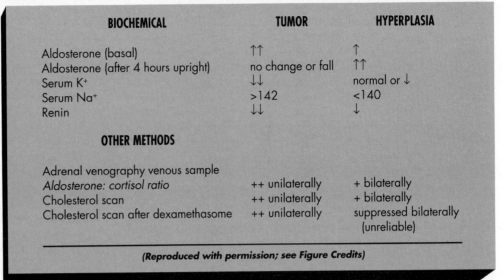

FIGURE 16.38 DIFFERENCES BETWEEN ADENOMA AND HYPERPLASIA

BIOCHEMICAL	TUMOR	HYPERPLASIA
Aldosterone (basal)	↑↑	↑
Aldosterone (after 4 hours upright)	no change or fall	↑↑
Serum K⁺	↓↓	normal or ↓
Serum Na⁺	>142	<140
Renin	↓↓	↓
OTHER METHODS		
Adrenal venography venous sample		
Aldosterone: cortisol ratio	++ unilaterally	+ bilaterally
Cholesterol scan	++ unilaterally	+ bilaterally
Cholesterol scan after dexamethasome	++ unilaterally	suppressed bilaterally (unreliable)

(Reproduced with permission; see Figure Credits)

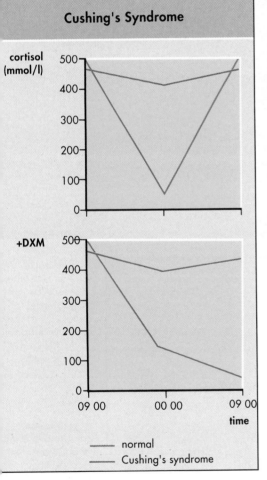

Cushing's Syndrome

cortisol (mmol/l)

+DXM

— normal
— Cushing's syndrome

FIGURE 16.39
Patterns of plasma cortisol in normal patients and those with Cushing's syndrome. The usual diurnal variation of plasma cortisol with midnight or early morning dip followed by a rise is absent in Cushing's. Likewise, dexamethasone fails to normally suppress cortisol in the patient with Cushing's. (Reproduced with permission; see Figure Credits)

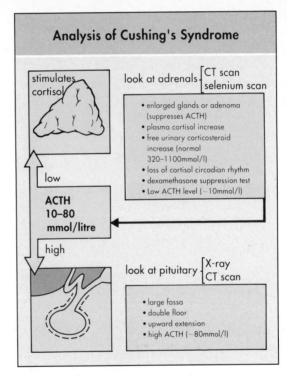

Analysis of Cushing's Syndrome

stimulates cortisol

look at adrenals — CT scan / selenium scan

- enlarged glands or adenoma (suppresses ACTH)
- plasma cortisol increase
- free urinary corticosteroid increase (normal 320–1100mmol/l)
- loss of cortisol circadian rhythm
- dexamethasone suppression test
- Low ACTH level (~10mmol/l)

low

ACTH 10–80 mmol/litre

high

look at pituitary — X-ray / CT scan

- large fossa
- double floor
- upward extension
- high ACTH (~80mmol/l)

FIGURE 16.40
Differentiation between pituitary and adrenal Cushing's syndrome. Analysis begins with ACTH levels, which are usually high in the former and suppressed in the latter. (Reproduced with permission; see Figure Credits)

abdominal or thoracic cavities. Although pheochromocytomas account for only 0.1% to 0.2% of cases of hypertension, recognition and diagnosis of the condition are important since deaths from stroke, myocardial infarction, and severe cardiomyopathy may occur and are preventable.

Hypertension, as well as the symptom–complex associated with pheochromocytomas (Fig. 16.41), correlates with the amount and rate of catecholamine secretion into the plasma. Often the symptoms are episodic; three fourths of patients suffer a symptomatic attack once or more weekly. Some have daily paroxysms, usually consisting of headache, diaphoresis, and palpitations. Attacks may be triggered by specific activities such as bending over, micturition, application of abdominal pressure, ingestion of tyramine-containing foods, exposure to certain drugs (tyramine, glucagon, histamine, phenothiazines), general anesthesia, or merely anxiety.

Although both epinephrine and norepinephrine are usually secreted, the clinical manifestations relate to the type of catecholamine receptor interaction that predominates. (In rare instances, dopamine may be secreted.) Vasoconstriction and hypertension result from the activation of alpha-receptors. Vasodilatory flushing, headache, and palpitations are due to beta-receptor stimulation. With some tumors the predominant symptom may be orthostatic hypotension, presumably from volume contraction coupled with desensitization of adrenergic receptors due to prolonged elevation of circulating catecholamine. Paradoxical hypertension following the administration of a beta-blocker, ganglionic blockers, or guanethidine should alert the physician to the possibility of pheochromocytoma.

Ten percent of pheochromocytomas occur in association with familial syndromes. Although 60% of familial pheochromocytomas occur without other

---

FIGURE 16.41 COMMON SIGNS AND SYMPTOMS OF PHEOCHROMOCYTOMAS

Hypertension—sustained, intermittent, or paroxysmal
Hypotension—usually orthostatic
Headache
Diaphoresis
Palpitations and tachycardia
Anxiety
Nausea and vomiting
Retinopathy

FIGURE 16.42 SYNDROMES AFFECTING MEN

TYPE I (WERMER'S SYNDROME)
Pituitary tumors
Pancreatic islet tumors (with Zollinger–Ellison)
Parathyroid tumors
Carcinoid tumors

TYPE II (SIPPLE'S SYNDROME)
Medullary carcinoma of the thyroid
Pheochromocytoma
Parathyroid hyperplasia or adenomas
Bilateral adrenocortical hyperplasia with Cushing's (uncommon)

TYPE III (OR IIB)
Medullary carcinoma of the thyroid
Pheochromocytoma
Mucosal neuromas
Bumpy lips
Thickened corneal nerves
Marfanoid habitus

Reliability of Urinary Catecholamine Tests

assays performed	patients with both assays normal	patients with both assays elevated	patients with one assay elevated		
			CA only	VMA only	MN only
CA & VMA	20%	60%	12%	8%	
MN & VMA	4%	70%		0%	25%
MN & CA	4%	75%			21%

FIGURE 16.43 Diagnostic reliability of urinary catecholamines and their metabolites in pheochromocytoma. (CA = free catecholamines, MN = metanephrine, VMA = vanillyllmandelic acid) (Reproduced with permission; see Figure Credits)

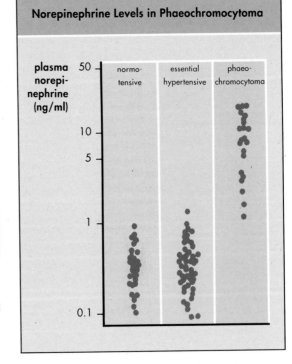

Norepinephrine Levels in Phaeochromocytoma

FIGURE 16.44
Plasma norepinephrine levels in normal subjects, patients with essential hypertension, and patients with pheochromocytoma. Although the values appear well-segregated, some patients with pheochromocytoma may present with values in the normal range, particularly if secretion of catecholamines is intermittent. (Reproduced with permission; see Figure Credits)

glandular dysfunctions, they may appear as part of a multiple endocrine neoplasia (MEN) syndrome (Fig. 16.42).[38] In MEN Type II, pheochromocytomas coexist with hyperplasia or medullary carcinoma of the thyroid and parathyroid hyperplasia. In Type III (or IIB) they occur with medullary thyroid carcinoma, mucosal neuromas, and unusual phenotypic signs, including bumpy lips and corneal nerve hyperplasia. In common with other familial neoplasia syndromes, hereditary pheochromocytomas appear at an earlier mean age and are more often bilateral tumors (45% to 80%). Sporadic tumors are more often unilateral and occur at a later age.

DIAGNOSIS

Pheochromocytoma should be suspected in any hypertensive patient who reports a certain symptom complex (see Fig. 16.41). However, because of the ubiquity of these symptoms such as headache and anxiety, the old adage, "many are called but few are chosen" clearly applies to this diagnosis. The use of a few reliable catecholamine assays, therefore, can confirm this condition. Urinary tests of free catecholamine, particularly metanephrines, provide the highest degree of sensitivity and specificity (Fig. 16.43).[9,41] In addition, plasma catecholamine, epinephrine, and norepinephrine are elevated to the highest levels in patients with pheochromocytoma (Fig. 16.44). However, the diagnostician should bear in mind that conditions such as anxiety, alcohol withdrawal, and hypothyroidism can produce moderate elevations in both plasma and urinary catecholamine.

In borderline cases, the clonidine suppression test can differentiate between these other conditions and pheochromocytoma.[8] Three hours after the centrally-acting sympatholytic agent clonidine (0.3 mg orally) is given, plasma catecholamines are reduced below normal in patients with essential hypertension but remain elevated in those with pheochromocytoma (Fig. 16.45).

Localization of the pheochromocytoma can prove difficult, but most tumors over 2 cm in diameter can be visualized by computerized tomography (Fig. 16.46). CT scan is also helpful in identifying bilateral tumors that occur frequently in MEN syndromes and metastases. The radiolabeled guanethidine analogue ^{131}I-MIBG, which is concentrated in adrenergic vesicles, has been found to be a sensitive imaging device for pheochromocytomas.

HYPERTENSION ASSOCIATED WITH PREGNANCY AND ORAL CONTRACEPTIVES

PREGNANCY-RELATED HYPERTENSION

Normal pregnancy is characterized by diminished blood pressure, with diastolic values often 10 mmHg lower than those taken before pregnancy. This phenomenon begins early in the first trimester, reaching its nadir by midtrimester. In the late third trimester, blood pressure levels usually return to normal. Lowered blood pressure is accompanied by a 30% to 50% increase in plasma volume and a similar increase in cardiac output, all of which indicate that the fall in blood pressure is due to peripheral vasodilation. Renal vasodilation results in a 50% increase in the GFR.

All of these phenomena occur despite marked stimulation of the RAS with elevations of both PRA and angiotensin II. Part of this augmentation may be related to estrogen-induced increases in renin substrate (angiotensinogen), although other factors (renal vasodilation, increased prostaglandin synthesis) are also at play. Circulatory vasorelaxation evidently stems from rises in vasodilatory prostaglandins, particularly prostacyclin, and insensitivity to angiotensin. The evidence supporting the role of vasodilatory prostaglandins in RAS stimulation is that cyclo-oxygenase inhibitors, such as indomethacin, markedly enhance vascular reactivity to angiotensin II.[19,32,58] Progesterone metabolites, such as 5 alpha-dihydroprogesterone, may also account for the vascular resistance to angiotensin II.[32]

Because of the lower than normal blood pressure observed during normal pregnancy, hypertension during gestation is defined as an increase in blood pressure of 30/15 mmHG or an absolute value of greater than 140/90 mmHg. Pregnancy-associated hypertension may be categorized as shown in Figure 16.47.

Pre-eclampsia (or toxemia of pregnancy) is a common disorder, developing in 5% to 10% of all pregnancies, with a preponderance among primigravidas.[32] Other associated risk factors for pre-eclampsia include diabetes, antecedent hypertension or renal disease, twin pregnancy, family history of toxemia, and age extremes. Pre-eclampsia is associated with excess morbidity for the mother and fetal loss.[32] If eclamptic seizures occur, maternal mortality rates are substantially higher, usually the result of intracerebral hemorrhage.

The pathogenesis of this disorder stems from hypoperfusion of the uteroplacental unit.[13,32,58] Inadequate placentation arises when the placental mass is too large, as might occur in a twin pregnancy, or the placental blood flow is attenuated, as might occur in disorders with vascular disease, such as diabetes or pre-existing hypertension. Inadequate placentation appears to be associated with a derangement in the balance of endothelial and circulating eicosanoids so that increased levels of vasoconstrictive thromboxane A2 and diminished levels of vasodilatory prostacyclin are found in pre-eclampsia. Both urinary measurements of excreted prostaglandin metabolites and studies of endothelial production of these products support this conclusion. However, whether this is a primary defect or a secondary response to a more generalized endothelial injury is unclear.

As might be anticipated with a decrease in prostacyclin, responsiveness to pressor substances is augmented in pre-eclamptic pregnancies. Hence, even though renal renin secretion is lower in pre-eclampsia than in normal pregnancy, sensitivity to angiotensin II is enhanced (Fig. 16.48).

A host of organ system abnormalities provides further evidence of endothelial injury in pre-eclampsia. These abnormalities appear to be the result of activation of the clotting system with intravascular fibrin deposition.

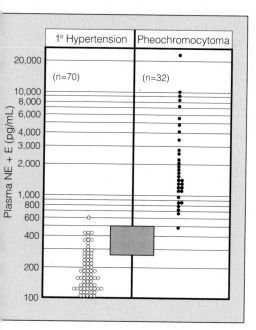

FIGURE 16.45
Clonidine suppression test results in 32 patients with pheochromocytoma and 70 with essential hypertension. Hatched area represents mean ± 2 SD of normal subjects. (Redrawn with permission; see Figure Credits)

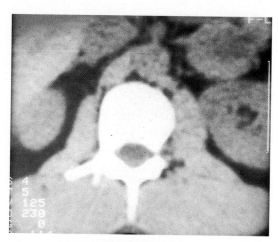

FIGURE 16.46
Abdominal CT of patient with pheochromocytoma visualized as a large mass anterior to the left kidney. (Reproduced with permission; see Figure Credits)

FIGURE 16.47 PREGNANCY-ASSOCIATED HYPERTENSION

SYNDROME	FEATURES
Pre-eclampsia/eclampsia Pre-eclampsia	Hypertension, proteinuria, edema, caogulopathy, or liver function abnormalities occurring after the 20th week of gestation.
Eclampsia	All of the above, plus convulsions
Chronic hypertension	Hypertension usually occurring before the 20th week of gestation uncomplicated by proteinuria or other systemic manifestations. This includes essential and all forms of secondary hypertension. May be complicated by superimposed pre-eclampsia.
Late/transient hypertension	Hypertension without proteinuria usually occurring in the last trimester of pregnancy. May be difficult to distinguish from pre-eclampsia.

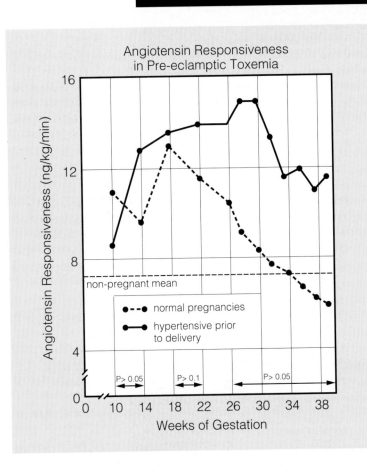

Angiotensin Responsiveness in Pre-eclamptic Toxemia

- ●---● normal pregnancies
- ●—● hypertensive prior to delivery

FIGURE 16.48
Responsiveness to angiotensin II (expressed as ng/kg/min of hormone required to raise blood pressure). The curve for patients with pre-eclampsia shows augmented sensitivity to the hormone by midtrimester when compared to pregnant subjects without hypertension. Late in the third trimester, angiotensin sensitivity in patients with pre-eclampsia exceeds that of non-pregnant individuals. (Redrawn with permission; see Figure Credits)

FIGURE 16.49 CAUSES OF DEATH IN ADULTS WITH AORTIC COARCTATION

CAUSE	% OF DEATHS
Congestive heart failure	25
Rupture of the aorta	21
Bacterial endocarditis	18
Intracranial hemorrhage	11

ral contraceptives are associated with an increased risk of death from cardiovascu-
r disease. This information, however, belies the observation that most of the car-
ovascular risk is seen in a relatively small proportion of pill users: those over the
e of 35 and those who smoke cigarettes. Likewise, only 5% of women who use oral
ntraceptives develop hypertension. Obesity and older age appear to be additional
k factors.[32] There is also some evidence that almost one half of women who are
pertensive and on the pill develop spontaneous hypertension after the contracep-
e is withdrawn, thereby suggesting some other predisposing factor.

The mechanism causing oral contraceptive-induced hypertension appears to
volve the RAS. Estrogens increase the hepatic production of renin substrate
th resultant increases in angiotensin II and aldosterone. PRA may actually be
w, owing to negative feedback from the increase in angiotensin II.

COARCTATION OF THE AORTA

oarctation of the aorta accounts for 1% or less of all hypertension.
ecognition and treatment, however, are mandatory because of the high rate of
ortality. More than one half of all infants with coarctated aortas die, the mor-
lity rate reaching almost 90% in untreated cases. Similarly, adults with unrec-
gnized coarctations reach a mean age of only 34 years. These deaths are all
lated to cardiovascular complications (Fig. 16.49).[33]

The pathogenesis of hypertension in coarctation is related to both increased
scular resistance and the obstruction of flow through the aortic conduit,
hich leads to vascular plethora of the upper extremities and head. The former
enomenon is related to activation of RAS, which is caused by relative hypop-
fusion to the renal circulation.

Diagnosis and Assessment of Hypertension

fore initiating any kind of treatment for high blood pressure, the physician
ould assess the reproducibility, severity, and associated target organ effects of
e syndrome. In particular, the finding of white coat or labile hypertension

might dictate a nonpharmacologic approach to the problem. Self-recording and
logging of blood pressures by the patient at home or at work provide important
supplementary evidence of the severity of the problem. Continuous ambulatory
monitoring of blood pressure is now possible with a variety of electronic devices
(see discussion below).

In addition, careful attention should be paid to the possibility of target organ
damage (see discussion below) and conditions, such as diabetes, that synergize
with hypertension in producing cardiovascular disease.

Diagnosis and Assessment of Hypertension
TARGET ORGAN COMPLICATIONS

The common thread in hypertensive complications is vascular disease. All cal-
ibers of vessels are potentially involved, from the microcirculation (e.g.,
glomerular capillaries) to the aorta. Small caliber vessels, particularly arterioles,
show signs of vascular hypertrophy with intimal smooth muscle proliferation
(Fig. 16.50). The mechanisms involved in this process are complex and not fully
understood (Figs. 16.51, 16.52). There is evidence suggesting that early baroin-
jury, signalled by endothelial damage, progresses with passage of circulating
white cells and macrophages across the denuded endothelium. Smooth muscle
proliferation develops in the next phase, possibly the result of stimulation of
intrinsic peptide growth factors or because of macrophage-stimulated cytokines
and growth factors. Angiotensin II, well-known for its vasoconstrictor activity,
has potent mitogenic and hypertrophying effects *in vitro*.[39] Thus, angiotensin-
mediated forms of hypertension might be characterized by more aggressive vascular disease.[1,10]

In addition to the changes described above, atherosclerosis with lipid deposition and plaque formation is frequently seen, particularly in the aorta and large
vessels at points where shear stress is high. Thrombus formation in the area of
plaques, particularly at points of intimal rupture, leads to ischemic infarction of
the brain and myocardium.

The specific types of organ system involvement in hypertension are listed in
Figure 16.53. Retinal changes include those associated with hypertension (hemorrhages, exudates, and papilledema), as well as those due to arteriosclerosis

FIGURE 16.50   Cross sections of small
arteries from hypertensive patients. **(A)**
Duplication of the internal elastic lamina.
(B) Micrograph demonstrating intimal
hyperplasia. (Reproduced with permission;
see Figure Credits)

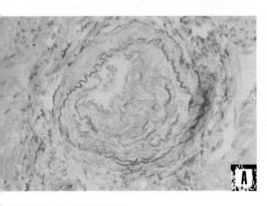
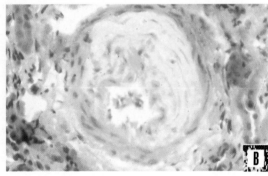

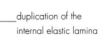
duplication of the
internal elastic lamina

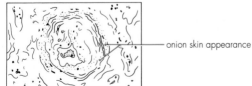
onion skin appearance

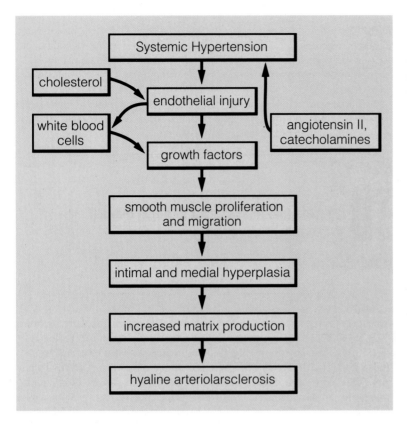

FIGURE 16.51 Pathogenesis of small vessel injury in systemic hypertension.

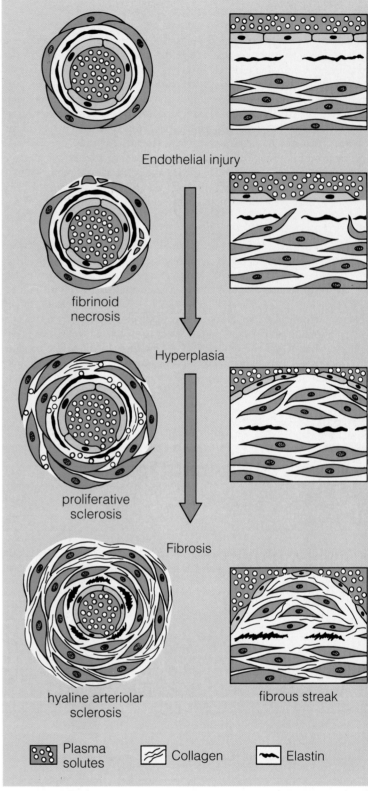

FIGURE 16.52 Comparison of small vessel arteriolar sclerosis (left) with large vessel atherosclerosis (right). Both processes begin with endothelial injury, leading to smooth muscle proliferation. Growth factors either from serum, migratory white cells, or smooth muscle itself contribute to these processes. (Redrawn with permission; see Figure Credits)

narrowed caliber, crossing changes, and silver wiring). Classification of hypertensive retinopathy has been useful in defining the severity and chronicity of hypertension. The Keith–Wagener–Barker classification combines changes associated with hypertension and arteriosclerosis (Fig. 16.54). Figures 16.55 and 16.56 demonstrate retinal changes observed in hypertension. Grading of retinopathy serves as a guide to the severity and duration of hypertension. Grade III or IV changes may be seen with accelerated or malignant hypertension and therefore connote urgent treatment.

The neurologic manifestations in hypertension range from the subtle to the severe. Small lacunar infarcts may present with insidious neurologic signs, such as dementia (Fig. 16.57). Larger thrombotic events are more easily identified. However, in a hypertensive patient, the therapeutic distinction between hemorrhagic (Fig. 16.58) and nonhemorrhagic stroke must be made. Full discussion of this complication is beyond the scope of this chapter. However, use of magnetic resonance imaging (MRI) (Fig. 16.59) or CT scanning devices augments the neurologic examination. A serious but reversible consequence of malignant hypertension is hypertensive encephalopathy. Characterized by generalized depression of the sensorium, hypertensive encephalopathy may represent diffuse

FIGURE 16.53 TARGET ORGAN INVOLVEMENT IN HYPERTENSION

ORGAN SYSTEM	TYPE OF INVOLVEMENT
Ocular	Retinopathy (Grades III or IV with malignant hypertension)
CNS	Encephalopathy
	Cerebral hemorrhage
	Cerebral thrombosis
Myocardium	Congestive heart failure
	Left ventricular hypertrophy
	Myocardial infarction
Renal	Benign or malignant nephrosclerosis
	Accelerated loss of renal mass (e.g., in diabetic nephropathy)
Vascular	Aortic dissection
	Atherosclerosis
	Peripheral vascular disease and claudication syndromes

FIGURE 16.54 CLASSIFICATION OF HYPERTENSIVE RETINOPATHY (KEITH–WAGENER–BARKER)

GRADE	DESCRIPTION
0	Normal optic fundi
I	Arteriolar spasm (copper or silver wiring)
II	Above symptoms, plus evidence of arteriolar sclerosis with increased light reflex and arteriovenous "nicking"
III	All the above symptoms, plus hemorrhages and soft or hard exudates
IV	All of the above symptoms, plus papilledema with circumferential blurring of the optic disc margin and/or elevation of the optic nerve

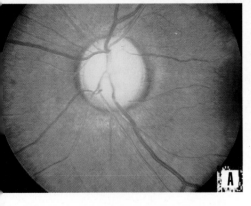
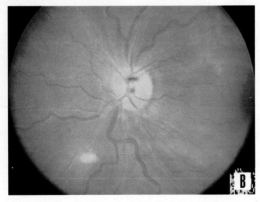
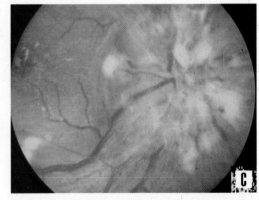
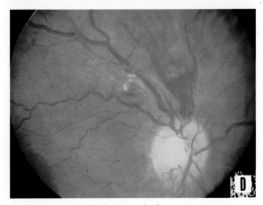

FIGURE 16.55   Retinal changes associated with systemic hypertension. **(A)** The retina of a 49-year-old black woman with asymptomatic essential hypertension of at least 10 years' duration displays arteriolar narrowing and straightening, increased light reflex, irregular caliber, loss of small arteriolar branches, and early arteriovenous crossing changes. **(B)** A 42-year-old black woman with essential hypertension and blood pressure levels averaging 260/130 was asymptomatic except for headaches. Retinal examination revealed severe vascular sclerosis, seen as marked irregularity of arteriolar caliber, "sheathing," and nearly complete loss of the arterioles. A "cotton wool" exudate is seen at seven o'clock. The nasal disk margin is blurred, which may occur normally. **(C)** A 38-year-old black man with malignant hypertension, bilateral papilledema, and azotemia had no visual disturbance. Retinal examination revealed massive edema, hemorrhages, and exudates completely obscuring the disk and burying the blood vessels. The veins are congested, and the arterioles show diffuse thickening ("copper wire"). There are hard exudates (edema residues) forming in the nerve bundle grooves in the macular region at ten o'clock. **(D)** The retina of a 50-year-old black woman with severe hypertension of 25 years' duration shows evidence of arteriosclerosis: marked narrowing, irregular caliber, increased light reflex, and arteriovenous crossing changes. Atherosclerosis is also suggested by the large fan-shaped superficial hemorrhage, due to occlusion of a branch of the superior temporal vein as it enters the disk region. (Reproduced with permission; see Figure Credits)

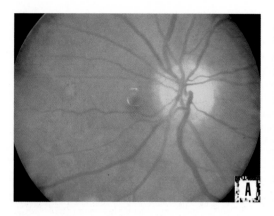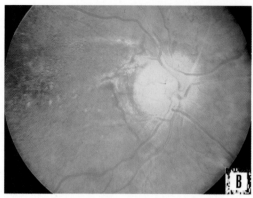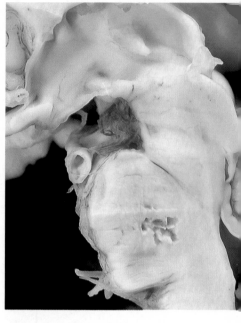

FIGURE 16.56   Retinal changes associated with systemic hypertension. **(A)** The retina of a 68-year-old white man with hypertension and mild diabetes mellitus shows very small red dots, or capillary aneurysms, scattered between the disk and the macular region. There is also a faint "cotton wool" exudate at seven o'clock. **(B)** A 36-year-old white woman with pseudoxanthoma elasticum presented with severe hypertension, marked visual disturbance, and renal insufficiency. Retinal examination revealed characteristic brownish angioid streaks around the disk, extending toward the macula. Also seen are marked retinal arteriosclerotic changes, sheathing, irregular caliber, occluded vessels, and hard exudates with a "smudge" hemorrhage at seven o'clock. (Reproduced with permission; see Figure Credits)

FIGURE 16.57   Median section through the pons reveals a clustering of multiple lacunar infarcts due to hypertension. (Reproduced with permission; see Figure Credits)

FIGURE 16.59
Magnetic resonance image demonstrating large intracerebral hemorrhage in a patient with hypertension.

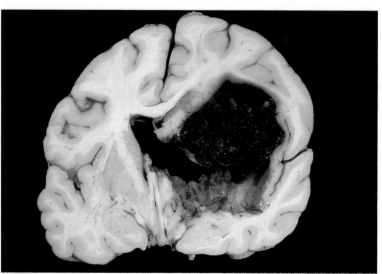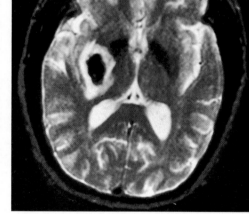

FIGURE 16.58   A massive intracerebral hemorrhage ruptured into the ventricular system. (Reproduced with permission; see Figure Credits)

ortical vasospasm and is therefore a functional equivalent to vascular constriction seen in other circulations, such as the eye.

Hypertensive myocardial disease most often presents as left ventricular hypertrophy (LVH), a direct result of the high impedance to chamber outflow (Fig. 16.60). LVH may present on physical examination as a more prominent and sustained apical impulse. More often, though, it is found by electrocardiography (Fig. 16.61). However, the ECG may demonstrate false–positive results, particularly in young adults. Echocardiography now provides definitive evidence of left ventricular wall thickening (Fig. 16.62), and is more sensitive than the ECG.[15]

Congestive heart failure may result directly from prolonged or severe hypertension, again due to severe outflow impedance. However, myocardial disease directly associated with hypertrophy (hypertensive cardiomyopathy) or the result of myocardial ischemia or infarction may present the typical findings of left ventricular or biventricular failure. Data from the Framingham study indicate that hypertensive patients have a sixfold greater likelihood than normal subjects of developing congestive heart failure. Moreover, the appearance of congestive heart failure in a hypertensive patient confers a much higher mortality rate: only 50% survived 5 years in the Framingham cohort.[27] A complete discussion of heart failure is presented in Chapter 3.

Renal insufficiency almost inevitably complements long-standing hypertension. As described above, hypertension is a common consequence of renal parenchymal disease. However, primary hypertension often leads to renal damage. In a recent study, 15% of patients with an initially normal serum creatinine, followed for an average of approximately 5 years, suffered a fall in GFR.[51] A rise in serum creatinine in this study was more likely to occur in older subjects, those who missed follow-up appointments, and those who were laborers. African-American subjects had twice the likelihood of developing renal insufficiency, compared with whites. Unfortunately, even pharmacologic control of blood pressure, as demonstrated in the aforementioned study, confers no certain protection against renal damage. After diabetes, hypertension is the most common etiology of end-stage renal failure necessitating dialysis in the United States (Fig. 16.63).

Figure 16.64 depicts the current theory[16,59] linking hypertension and progressive renal insufficiency. A common pathway is intraglomerular hypertension, which can develop as a result of other forms of renal disease, diabetes, or systemic hypertension. Increased intracapillary hydraulic pressure leads to mesangial (and possibly other glomerular cell) injury, glomerulosclerosis, and eventual loss of renal mass. Loss of renal tissue feeds back and accelerates the processes of intraglomerular hypertension and further loss of nephrons. A recent modification of this theory places equal emphasis on factors leading to renal (and glomerular) hypertrophy. Many of these factors, such as dietary protein and sodium as well as diabetes, share properties causing both capillary hypertension and glomerular hypertrophy.

Glomerular sclerosis is probably the common pathway by which renal mass is lost in a host of renal diseases. Glomerular injury in these cases is often heralded by increased urinary protein excretion of up to 2 g per day. The nephrotic range for proteinuria (>3.5 g per day) is seldom seen in primary hypertension and should raise suspicion of a primary glomerular disease.

Arteriolar nephrosclerosis is common to both diabetes and hypertension and is generally associated with slowly progressing renal loss. *Malignant nephrosclerosis*, however, is a distinct lesion, seen in conjunction with malignant or accelerated hypertension and consisting of fibrinoid necrosis of arterioles and, often, of glomerular tufts (Fig. 16.65). Loss or "pruning" of small peripheral vessels is the equivalent arteriographic picture (Fig. 16.66).

Just as microvascular disease occurs in renal and retinal vessels, large vessel disease, particularly atherosclerosis, may complicate hypertension. The relationship is particularly close in the cerebral and coronary vasculature. In both man

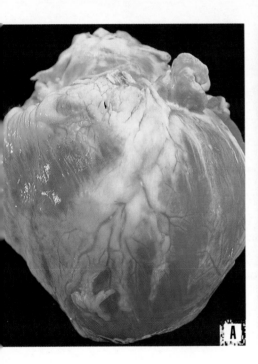 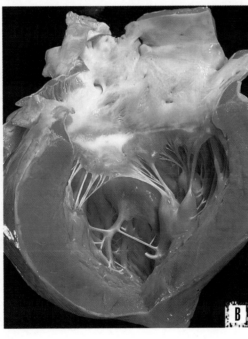

FIGURE 16.60 Globose heart (**A**). The specimen is opened (**B**) to reveal left ventricular wall hypertrophy, an adaptive phenomenon to long-standing systemic hypertension. (Reproduced with permission; see Figure Credits)

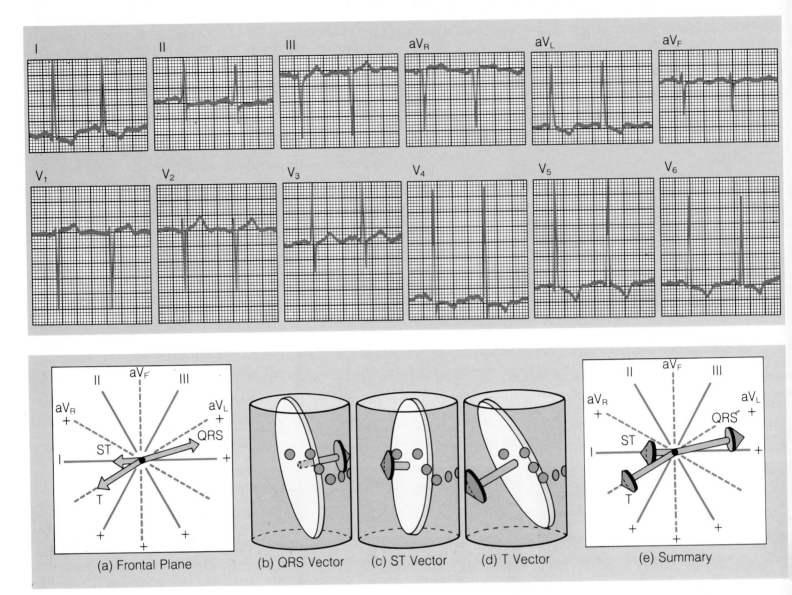

FIGURE 16.61   ECG from a 61-year-old patient with essential hypertension and left ventricular hypertrophy. The QRS complex is large and positive in lead I, resultantly positive in lead II, and resultantly negative in lead aV$_F$. The mean QRS vector is therefore directed relatively parallel to the positive limb of lead I, but it must be directed slightly cephalad in order to project a slightly negative quantity on lead aV$_F$. The T wave is large and negative in lead I and flat in lead II. The mean T vector is therefore directed perpendicular to lead II. The ST segment displacement is greatest in lead I and least in lead aV$_F$. Accordingly, the mean ST vector is directed parallel to the negative limb of lead I. The spatial orientation of the mean QRS, ST,

and T vectors is illustrated. The mean QRS vector is directed 20° posteriorly, because the transitional pathway passes between V$_2$ and V$_3$. The mean ST vector is directed 30° anteriorly, because the transitional pathway passes between V$_3$ and V$_4$. The mean spatial ST vector is relatively parallel to the mean spatial T vector. Final summary reveals the spatial arrangement of the vectors. The mean QRS vector is directed to the left and posteriorly, and the mean T vector is directed to the right and anteriorly. The QRS voltage is increased, and the spatial QRS–T angle is 175°. The mean ST vector is relatively parallel to the mean T vector and represents forces of repolarization. (Redrawn with permission; see Figure Credits)

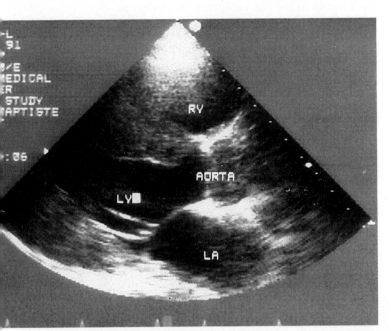

FIGURE 16.62   Two-dimensional echocardiogram demonstrating left ventricular hypertrophy in a patient with hypertension.

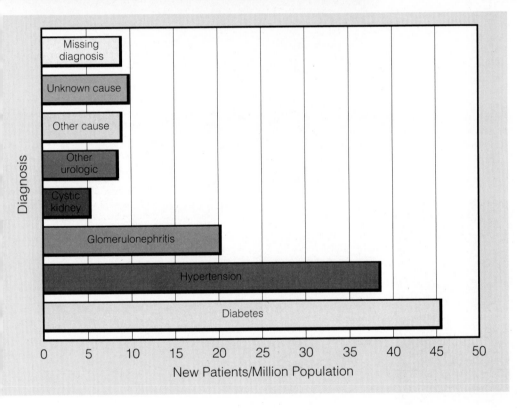

FIGURE 16.63   Causation of end-stage kidney failure by diagnosis in 1989. Hypertensive renal disease was the second most common underlying diagnosis. (Data compiled; see Figure Credits)

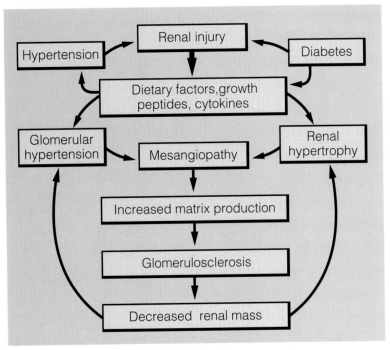

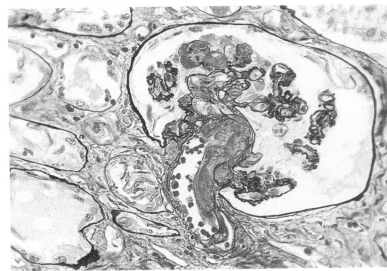

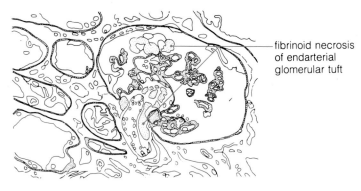

fibrinoid necrosis of endarterial glomerular tuft

FIGURE 16.64 Role of hypertension in the pathogenesis of progressive renal failure. Renal injury, produced initially by hypertension, diabetes, or inflammatory conditions (such as glomerulonephritis), eventuates in nephron loss. The resultant compensation includes the elaboration of growth factors and other peptides, which contribute both to intraglomerular hypertension and glomerular hypertrophy. These processes lead to changes in the growth characteristics of the glomerular mesangial cell (and perhaps other glomerular cells) with mesangial hypertrophy and overproduction of matrix products. The resultant glomerulosclerosis engenders further loss of renal mass and a vicious cycle ensues. (Data used with permission; see Figure Credits)

FIGURE 16.66 Cortical nephrogram of a patient with malignant nephrosclerosis. Distended main branches show "pruning" of small arteries and minimal opacification despite preservation of the renal mass. (Reproduced with permission; see Figure Credits)

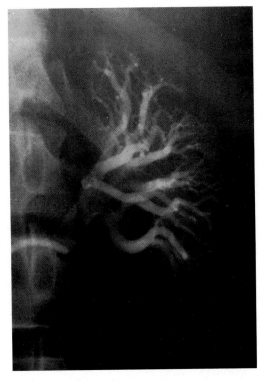

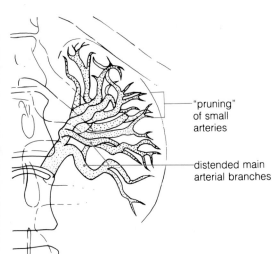

"pruning" of small arteries

distended main arterial branches

nd animals with experimental hypertension, however, atherosclerotic lesions re seen in the aorta, particularly at branch points or ostia of smaller vessels Fig. 16.67). Atherosclerotic lesions are particularly severe with combinations of yperlipidemia and hypertension, presumably stemming from the synergy of hese factors in the development of the vascular lesion (Fig. 16.68; compare ith Fig. 16.63).

Forms of vascular disease associated with hypertension include abdominal aor- ic and dissecting thoracic aneurysms, both of which occur predominantly in hypertensive subjects. Dissection often develops as an intimal tear in the ascending or descending thoracic aorta. However, a false lumen often extends well into the abdominal aorta (Figs. 16.69, 16.70).

ACCELERATED OR MALIGNANT HYPERTENSION

Accelerated or malignant hypertension is caused by extreme elevation of blood pressure (diastolic blood pressure greater than 120 to 140 mmHg) with multisys- tem involvement (Fig. 16.71). It is often a severe manifestation of primary or

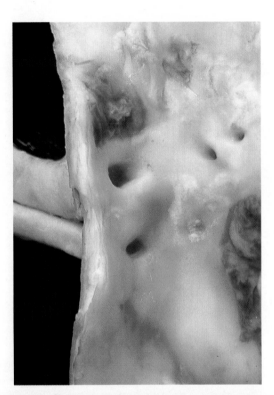

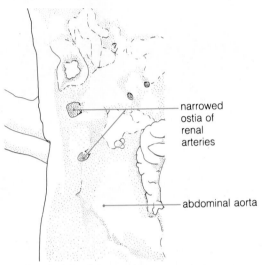

FIGURE 16.67   Abdominal atherosclerosis leading to narrowing of the orifices of the renal arteries. In this case there are two separate arter- ies for the right kidney. This condition may under- lie renovascular hypertension. (Reproduced with permission; see Figure Credits)

narrowed ostia of renal arteries

abdominal aorta

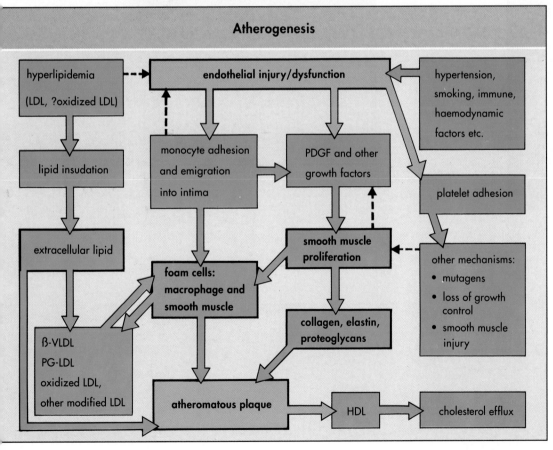

FIGURE 16.68   Pathogenesis of ather- osclerosis. (PG-LDL = proteoglycan–low- density lipoprotein; HDL = high-density lipoprotein) (Reproduced with permis- sion; see Figure Credits)

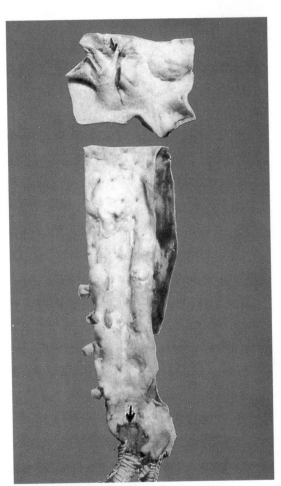

FIGURE 16.69 Dissecting aortic aneurysm with point of re-entry of blood flow into the lumen. (Reproduced with permission; see Figure Credits)

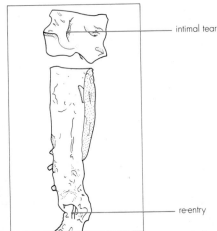

intimal tear

re-entry

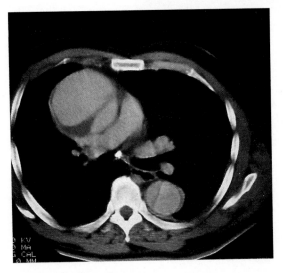

FIGURE 16.70
CT of aortic dissection demonstrating extravasation of blood into the media. Intimal tear often occurs in the ascending aorta. (Reproduced with permission; see Figure Credits)

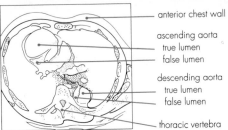

anterior chest wall

ascending aorta
true lumen
false lumen

descending aorta
true lumen
false lumen

thoracic vertebra

FIGURE 16.71 CLINICAL CHARACTERISTICS OF MALIGNANT HYPERTENSION

ORGAN SYSTEM	SYMPTOMS
CNS	Headache, encephalopathy
Ocular	Papilledema, blurring of vision
Cardiac	Congestive heart failure, angina
Renal	Azotemia, microscopic hematuria and proteinuria, oliguria
Hematologic	Microangiopathic hemolytic anemia

essential hypertension but may also accompany any secondary form of hypertension.

In addition to an alarmingly high blood pressure reading, a patient with malignant hypertension might present with a host of other clinical signs or symptoms (see Fig. 16.71). Encephalopathy generally appears as lethargy or confusion. Papilledema is common. Patients often present with pulmonary edema and sometimes angina pectoris, particularly in patients with coronary disease. Renal manifestations include azotemia, usually with urinary findings including microscopic hematuria (occasionally with red blood cell casts) and proteinuria. The urinary findings manifest the necrotic glomerular injury that accompanies malignant nephrosclerosis (see discussion above). Oliguria and acute renal failure are less common findings and might suggest a primary renal disease.

The hypothetical pathogenesis of malignant hypertension is depicted in Figure 16.72. Severe hypertension induces endothelial injury and subsequent vasculopathy, which, primarily through activation of RAS, aggravates the hypertension and accelerates the vascular injury.

LOOKING FOR SECONDARY CAUSATION OF HYPERTENSION
In an office practice, essential hypertension will be the basis for an overwhelming proportion of patients with high blood pressure. Nonselective application of screening tests for secondary causes of hypertension is unwise and costly in such a setting. The low prevalence of secondary hypertension increases the likelihood of false-positive screening tests,[37] which inevitably leads to the performance of more procedures. In most patients with mild-to-moderate hypertension, a prudent work-up should consist of the steps listed in Figure 16.73. These steps assess the severity of hypertension and the degree of target organ damage and serve to alert the physician to certain secondary forms of hypertension.

Atypical hypertension should provoke further inquiry into specific secondary causes (Fig. 16.74). If secondary hypertension is suggested by these findings, initial screening procedures can be performed[37] (Fig. 16.75).

HOME AND AMBULATORY BLOOD PRESSURE MONITORING
As mentioned earlier in the chapter, blood pressure recordings fluctuate dramatically with stress and other emotional factors, which are collectively known as white coat hypertension. The effects of these factors were impressively examined by Mancia et al.[40] Continuous 24-hour intra-arterial blood pressure monitoring was done in patients for 5 to 7 days until stable, steady-state recordings were obtained. After forewarning the subjects, either a male physician or a female nurse entered the room and recorded three successive blood pressure readings in the opposite arm with a conventional sphygmomanometer. When

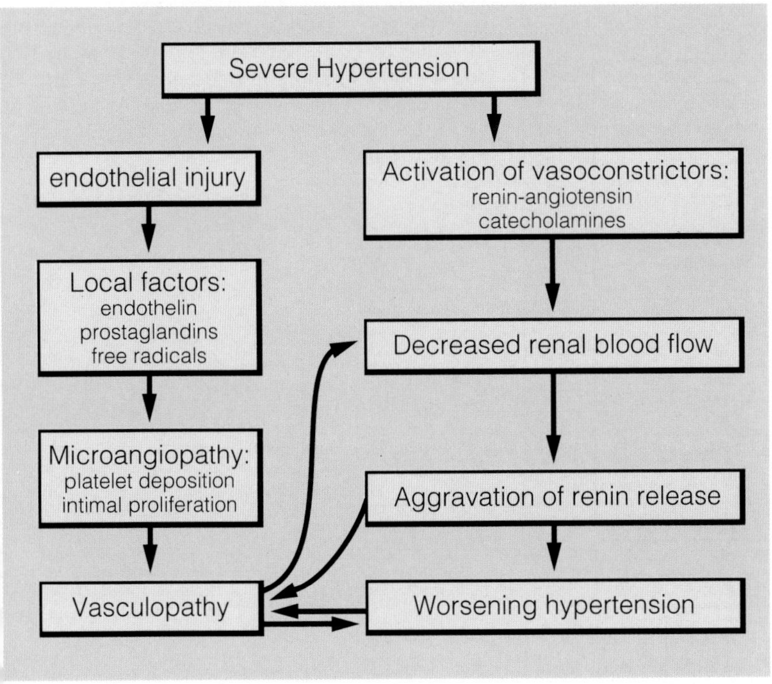

FIGURE 16.72 Hypothetical pathogenesis of malignant hypertension.

FIGURE 16.73 LIMITED EVALUATION FOR PATIENTS WITH MILD-TO-MODERATE HYPERTENSION

History
Physical examination
Urine analysis
Serum creatinine and electrolytes
Two-hour postprandial blood sugar
Lipid profile—total cholesterol, HDL, LDL, triglyceride
Electrocardiogram (or echocardiogram?)

FIGURE 16.74 FEATURES OF "INAPPROPRIATE" HYPERTENSION

1. Age of onset: before 20 or after 50
2. Level of blood pressure >180/110 mmHg
3. Organ damage
   Funduscopy grade II or beyond
   Serum creatinine >1.5 mg%
   Cardiomegaly or LVH by ECG
4. Presence of features indicative of secondary causes
   Unprovoked hypokalemia
   Abdominal bruit
   Variable pressures with tachycardia, sweating tremor
   Family history of renal disease
5. Poor response to effective therapy

(Reproduced with permission; see Figure Credits)

FIGURE 16.75 OVERALL GUIDE TO WORKUP OF HYPERTENSION

DIAGNOSTIC PROCEDURE

DIAGNOSIS	INITIAL	ADDITIONAL
Chronic renal disease	Urinalysis, serum creatinine, sonography	Isotopic renogram, renal biopsy
Renovascular disease	Bruit, plasma renin before and 1 hr after captopril	Aortogram, isotopic renogram 1 hr after captopril
Coarctation	Blood pressure in legs	Aortogram
Primary aldosteronism	Plasma potassium, plasma renin and aldosterone (ratio)	Urinary potassium, plasma or urinary aldosterone after saline load
Cushing's syndrome	AM plasma cortisol after 1 mg dexamethasone at bedtime	Urinary cortisol after variable doses of dexamethasone
Pheochromocytoma	Spot urine for metanephrine	Urinary catechols; plasma catechols, basal and after 0.3 mg clonidine

(Reproduced with permission; see Figure Credits)

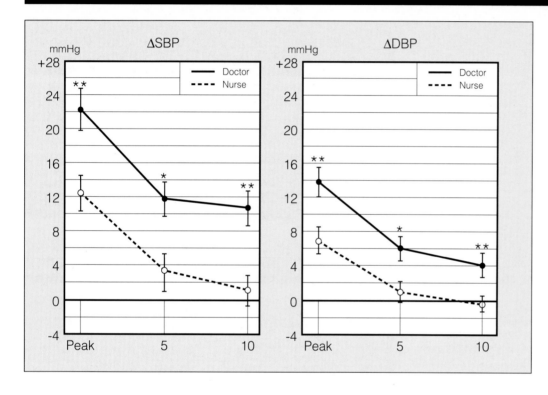

FIGURE 16.76   Comparison of blood pressure measurements taken by physicians and nurses in 30 subjects, expressed as increments in systolic and diastolic readings from baseline (intra-arterial) values 4 minutes earlier. Data are expressed as mean ± S.E.M. (Redrawn with permission; see Figure Credits)

physicians took the initial recordings, blood pressure increased by more than 22 mmHg and declined toward baseline during subsequent readings over the next 0 minutes (Fig. 16.76). Nurses provoked a similar but less severe response. These data support the hypothesis that office recordings of blood pressure, particularly those taken by physicians, may be spuriously high.

To circumvent this problem, home recordings of blood pressure have been advocated. Intermittent self-measurements, performed at home or work with automated sphygmomanometers, can provide reliable data for confirming diagnosis, gauging severity, and assessing the response to therapy. Patients should be encouraged to perform measurements in a quiet place at the same times each day. Recordings should be logged with notations about concurrent activities, such as exercise or eating.

Twenty-four hour ambulatory blood pressure monitoring (ABPM) provides information similar to intermittent home recordings, with the added benefit of nocturnal recordings while the subject sleeps. New noninvasive devices utilize standard cuffs that automatically inflate every 15 or 30 minutes (longer intervals may be used over night.) Automated recordings are accomplished by electronic auscultation or by oscillometric readings of cuff pressures. Indications for ABPM are listed in Figure 16.77.

ASSESSMENT OF CARDIOVASCULAR RISK

Since the mortality and morbidity of cardiovascular disease represent the greatest threat to a patient with hypertension, appraisal of concurrent risk factors, including hyperlipidemia, cigarette smoking, and glucose intolerance, is warranted. At every level of systolic blood pressure, the effects of additional risk factors are cumulative (Fig. 16.78).

Laragh and others have long championed the theory that RAS activity correlates with cardiovascular risk. They prospectively examined the relationship between cardiovascular disease and the renin–sodium profile (i.e., the index of PRA and 24-hour urinary sodium excretion).[37] In 1717 subjects with hyperten-

---

FIG.16.77 INDICATIONS FOR AMBULATORY BLOOD PRESSURE MONITORING

UNCERTAIN HYPERTENSION

"White coat," labile, or borderline hypertension
Normal blood pressure readings at home
Absence of evident target organ damage and other
  cardiovascular risk factors

UNCERTAIN NORMOTENSION

Suggestion of target organ damage (e.g., left ventricular
  hypertrophy)
Additional cardiovascular risk factors

MANAGEMENT OF HYPERTENSION

Appraisal of blood pressure control on therapy
Orthostatic hypotension or other possible adverse side effects

---

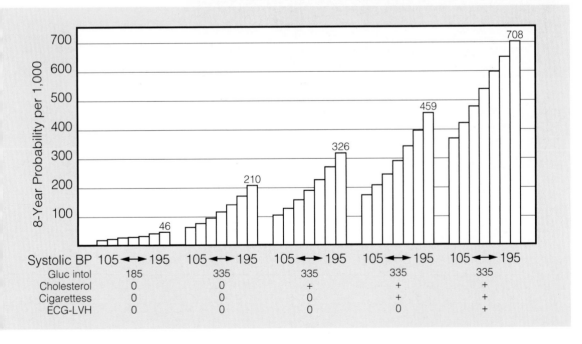

FIGURE 16.78 Eight-year risk of cardiovascular events in a cohort of 40-year-old men in Framingham with graded levels of systolic blood pressure with additional risk factors. (Redrawn with permission; see Figure Credits)

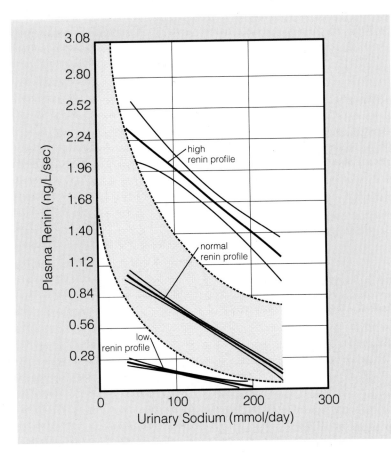

FIGURE 16.79 Relation between plasma renin activity and urinary sodium excretion in patients with hypertension. The renin–sodium profile for normal subjects is indicated by the shaded area. The profiles for high, low, and normal patients with hypertension are indicated by regression lines and 95% confidence intervals. (Redrawn with permission; see Figure Credits)

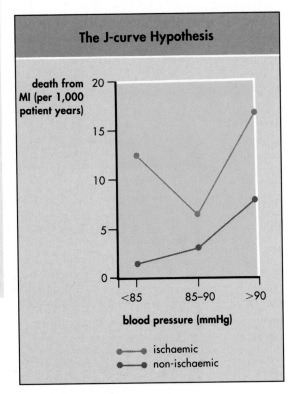

FIGURE 16.81 J-shaped curve demonstrating the relationship between mortality and a lowered blood pressure in patients with (top) and without (lower) ischemic heart disease. (Reproduced with permission; see Figure Credits)

FIGURE 16.80 Incidence of myocardial infarction, adjusted for age, sex, and race, in relation to renin profile and smoking status, cholesterol level, or fasting blood glucose level. (Redrawn with permission; see Figure Credits)

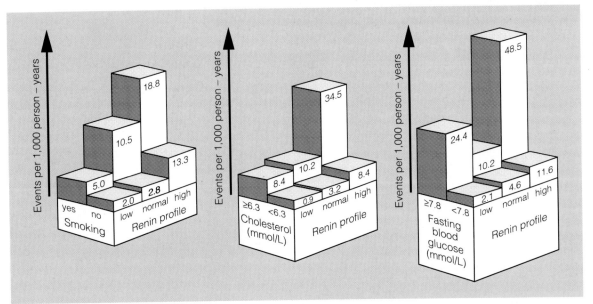

on and no known cardiovascular disease, distinct high, normal, and low renin profile groups were found (Fig. 16.79). A high renin–sodium profile correlated with substantially greater risk of subsequent cardiovascular events, independent of other risk factors (Fig. 16.80).

A full interpretation of these data suggests that either a RAS component accelerates cardiovascular disease or that silent vascular disease is manifest by a high renin profile. Models of hypertension that produce elevations of angiotensin II and the peptide itself cause vascular damage. However, subtle vascular damage in the kidney, as evidenced by microalbuminuria, may contribute to elevated renin levels and also correlates with cardiovascular morbidity.[29]

The results of hundreds of drug-intervention studies provide evidence that low-ering of blood pressure prevents cardiovascular mortality and morbidity. The overwhelmingly favorable outcomes, however, are confined to patients with *severe* hypertension. The evidence that blood pressure control benefits those with *mild* hypertension is far more limited.

The Veterans Administration Cooperative Studies in 1967 and 1970[56,57] were the first controlled trials to show that pharmacologic control of blood pressure reduced mortality. However, the mortality reduction was chiefly limited to those patients whose initial diastolic pressures were 105 to 114 mmHg. In mild hypertension, a meta-analysis of seven trials with placebo controls and two with treated controls demonstrated a substantial reduction in morbidity from strokes in the intervention groups. The antihypertensive therapy, however, afforded no

FIGURE 16.82 EXAMPLES OF ORAL ANTIHYPERTENSIVE AGENTS

DRUG TYPE OR CLASS	DOSAGE RANGE (MG/D)	DOSES/DAY	COMMON SIDE EFFECTS
DIURETICS			
Thiazide			Volume depletion, hypokalemia, hyperuricemia and gout, hyperlipidemia, glucose intolerance, hypomagnesemia, water retention and hyponatremia
Hydrochlorothiazide	12.5–50	1	
Indapamide	2.5–5	1	
Metolazone	0.5–10	1	
Chlorthalidone	12.5–50	1	
Loop			Volume depletion and prerenal azotemia, hypokalemia, hyperuricemia and gout, hyperlipidemia, glucose intolerance, hypomagnesemia, water retention and hyponatremia
Furosemide	20–500	2	
Ethacrynic acid	25–100	2	
Bumetanide	0.5–5	2	
Potassium Sparing			Hyperkalemia, metabolic acidosis, GI disturbance
Amiloride	5–10	1	
Spironolactone	25–100	1–2	Also menstrual abnormalities and gynecomastia
Triamterene	50–150	1	Also nephrolithiasis
SYMPATHOLYTIC AGENTS			
Centrally Acting			Sedation, dry mouth, rebound hypertension upon withdrawal, headache
Clonidine (TTS Patch)	0.1–1.2	2	
	0.1–0.3	1 q wk	
Guanabenz	4–64	2	
Methyldopa	250–2000	2	Above and immune hepatitis, dermatitis, Coombs-positive hemolytic anemia, thrombocytopenia, drug-induced lupus
Peripherally Acting		1	
Guanethidine	10–150		Orthostatic hypotension, edema, diarrhea, retrograde ejaculation
Reserpine	0.05–0.25	1	Mental depression, fatigue, bradycardia

such protection against coronary disease. Examination of the effects of antihypertensive treatment on the course of renal disease also yields discouraging results. A recent study has shown that despite good blood pressure control, renal function may deteriorate in at least 15% of subjects.[51] Factors that appeared to contribute to progressive loss of renal function were advanced age, African-American race, missed office visits, and occupation as laborer.

The J-curve concept demonstrates how lowered blood pressure and reduced risk of mortality are correlated (Fig. 16.81). At a definable point, however, risk increases again, perhaps the result of adverse effects such as reduced coronary perfusion. Many researchers dispute the latter idea, however, suggesting that the higher mortality rate at lower blood pressures may be due to pre-existing disease, particularly coronary disease.

THERAPY OPTIONS

Exercise and dietary measures have proven to lower blood pressure. Obesity, particularly in the truncal area, is associated with insulin resistance, glucose intolerance, and hypertension. In addition to weight reduction, a modest reduction in sodium intake (2 g per day), potassium and calcium supplementation, and relax-

ation therapy appear to assist in lowering blood pressure.

The development of new and potent antihypertensive drugs, such as the ACE inhibitors, calcium channel blockers, newer alpha$_1$-blockers, and vasodilators, enables the clinician to normalize blood pressure in almost every patient. Although a detailed description of available antihypertensive drugs is beyond the mission of this chapter, a summary of oral agents from all classes is presented in Figure 16.82. Previous JNC reports recommended a "stepped care" approach to hypertensive management in which a second or third agent was added if blood pressure normalization did not occur with the primary drug. Injudicious use of multiple drug therapy involved several problems, however, including additive side effects and confusing dosing regimens. The JNC currently recommends use of a single agent, tailored to the individual patient's demographic background (age, race) and underlying disease (diabetes, coronary disease, etc.).

THE SPECIAL PATIENT

Treatment of patients with malignant hypertension requires urgent (hours) or emergent (minutes) blood pressure control. Concomitant CNS (stroke or encephalopathy) or cardiac (ischemia, heart failure) manifestations dictate

FIGURE 16.82 EXAMPLES OF ORAL ANTIHYPERTENSIVE AGENTS continued

DRUG TYPE OR CLASS	DOSAGE RANGE (MG/D)	DOSES/DAY	COMMON SIDE EFFECTS
α1-blockers			First-dose syncope, orthostasis, headache, priapism, palpitations
Prazosin	1–20	2	
Terazosin	1–20	1	
β-blockers			Fatigue, depression, impotence, bradycardia, exacerbation of CHF, hyperlipidemia, bronchospasm, exacerbation of vascular insufficiency, blunted symptoms of hypoglycemia, withdrawal-exacerbated angina
Atenolol	25–150	1–2	Cardioselective
Metoprolol	50–200	1	Cardioselective
Nadalol	40–320	1–2	
Pinodol	10–60	2	Intrinsic sympatheomimetic; less apt to cause bradycardia
Timolol	20–80	2	
Combined α-and β-blocker			Similar to βblockers
Labetolol	200–1600	2	
Vasodilators			
DIRECT VASODILATORS			
Hydralazine	25–300	2–3	Headache, tachycardia, edema, exacerbation of angina, drug-induced lupus
Minoxidil	2.5–80	1–2	Edema, hair growth, tachycardia, exacerbation of angina
ACE INHIBITORS			Skin rash, cough, metallic taste and anorexia, hyperkalemia, autoregulatory failure with acute azotemia in bilateral renal artery stenosis or pre-existing renal disease, anemia, agrunolocytosis (particularly in patient with pre-existing azotemia)
Captopril	6.25–450	2–3	
Enalapril	2.5–40	1–2	
Fosinopril	10–40	1	
Lisinopril	5–40	1	
CALCIUM CHANNEL BLOCKERS			GI complaints (reflux, nausea, constipation), flushing, edema, tachycardia
Diltiazem SR	60–360	2	
Nicardipine	30–180	3	
Nifedipine	30–180	3 (1 with XL)	
Nitrendipine	5–40	1–2	
Verapamil SR	120–480	1–2	Also bradyarrhythmias and AV block

ergent care. Hypertensive emergencies require parenteral drug treatment (Fig. .83). Less severe hypertensive "urgencies" could alternatively be treated with l agents. For example, malignant hypertension occurring without cardiac or JS findings could be treated more slowly.

Iypertension in patients with cardiac disease requires tailored management. ongestive heart failure in the setting of hypertension may require urgent man-ement. In general, the use of diuretics and vasodilator therapy is recommend-, the latter for afterload reduction. Acute myocardial ischemia with hyperten-n (either evolving myocardial infarction or unstable angina) is most suitably ated with nitroglycerin or other nitrate therapy, both for blood pressure low-ng (and afterload reduction) as well as for preload reduction and coronary sodilation.

Treatment of hypertension in the elderly presents major challenges to the clin-an and to society. Systolic hypertension may represent arterial rigidity in ich case intra-arterial blood pressure readings may be much lower. This may d to overtreatment. In general, the clinician should aim for a systolic pressure 160 to 170 mmHg, below which the risk of stroke is considerably diminished. addition, the choice of medication should be simplified to avoid the unwant-effects of polypharmacy. Also to be noted is that medications are more likely accumulate, given diminished hepatic and renal function in the elderly.

Management of hypertension during pregnancy is complicated by several prob-lems, including fetal toxicity and risk. Recognition of hypertension is confound-ed by the normal lowering of blood pressure by midtrimester. Hence, blood pres-sures of greater than 130 to 140/90 should be considered suspect and retested. The physician must also differentiate between the various types of pregnancy-related hypertension and pre-eclampsia. The latter may be suspected in patients who are particularly young or old, who are primigravidas, or who have large weight gains or edema. Contrariwise, those with hypertension onset before 20 weeks or with a previous history of hypertension or renal disease are more likely to have chronic pre-existing disease. Antihypertensive drug treatment in preg-nancy must be tempered by the recognition that lowering of perfusion to the uteroplacental unit may pose hazards to the fetus and worsen a pre-eclamptic condition.

Treatment of patients with renovascular hypertension is a complex and often contentious subject. The clinician must choose among medical, surgical, or angioplastic approaches. Medical therapy, particularly with the newer agents available such as ACE inhibitors and calcium channel blockers, may be quite successful but more definitive treatment is often sought. Medical therapy should therefore be reserved for elderly patients or those patients with conditions pre-cluding surgery or angioplasty.

FIGURE 16.83 PARENTERAL DRUGS FOR HYPERTENSIVE EMERGENCIES

DRUG OR CLASS	DOSAGE RANGE	ONSET OF ACTION (MIN)	PREFERRED USE	ADVERSE EFFECTS
VASODILATORS **Direct**				
Nitroprusside	0.25–10 µ/kg/min IV infusion	Instant	Malignant hypertension, stroke, myocardial ischemia, heart failure	Nausea, vomiting, diaphoresis, thiocyanate toxicity
Nitroglycerine	5–100 µ/min IV infusion	2–5	Myocardial ischemia, heart failure	Headache, tachycardia, flushing, nausea, vomiting
Diazoxide	50–100 mg IV bolus or 15–30 mg/min IV infusion	2–4	Malignant hypertension	Nausea, hypotension, exacerba-tion of angina, ? exacerbation of aortic dissection
Hydralazine	10–20 mg IV bolus	10–20	Malignant hypertension, other agents preferred	Exacerbation of angina, tachy-cardia, flushing, unpredictable response
ACE inhibitor Enalaprilat	1.26–5 mg IV q 6hr	15		Marked hypotension in renin-dependent conditions
Ca Channel Blocker Nicardipine	5–10 mg/hr IV	10	Malignant hypertension, myocardial ischemia	Tachycardia, headache, flushing
ADRENERGIC INHIBITORS **Ganglionic Blocker**				
Trimethophan	0.5–5 mg/min IV infusion	1–5	Malignant hypertension, stroke	Orthostatic hypotension and syn-cope, flushing, tachycardia, exacerbation of angina, dry mouth, urinary retention
α-blocker Phentholamine	5–15 mg IV	1–2	Aortic dissection, stroke	Flushing, tachycardia
β-blockers Esmolol	500 µg/kg/min IV x 4 min, then 150–300 µg/kg/min	1–2	Aortic dissection, stroke, myocardial ischemia	Brochospasm, exacerbation of heart failure, vascular insufficiency
Propranolol	1–5 mg IV bolus, then 3 ng/hr	1–2	Other β-blockers preferred	Same as above
Labetolol	20–80 mg IV bolus q 10 min, then 2 mg/min IV	5–10	Malignant hypertension, stroke, aortic dissection	Same as above and nausea, vomiting, orthostasis

⚡ FIGURE CREDITS:

Figs. 16.1, and 16.2 compiled from data in Joint National Committee: The 1988 report of Joint National Committee on detection, evaluation, and treatment of high blood pressure. Arch Intern Med 148:1023, 1988.

Figs. 16.3, 16.4, 16.66 from Hurst JW (ed): The Heart, 6th ed. McGraw-Hill, New York, 1986.

Figs. 16.6, 16.7, 16.11–16.13, 16.15–16.19, 16.22, 16.23, 16.25, 16.35–16.40, 16.43, 16.44, 16.46, 16.50, 16.68–16.70 from Swales JD, Sever PS, Peart S: Clinical Atlas of Hypertension. Gower, London, 1991.

Fig. 16.18 modified and redrawn from Bing RF, Russell GI, Swales, JD, et al: Effect of 12 hours of saralasin or captopril on blood pressure of hypertension conscious rats. Relationship to plasma renin, hypertension, and effect of unclipping. J Lab Clin Med 98:302, 1981.

Figs 16.29, 16.74, 16.75 from Kaplan NM (ed): Clinical Hypertension, 5th ed. Williams & Wilkins, Baltimore, 1990. Fig. 16.29 is redrawn.

Figs. 16.30, 16.32, 16.34 redrawn from Biglieri EG: Adrenocortical forms of hypertension. In Laragh JH, Brenner BM (eds): Hypertension: Pathophysiology, Diagnosis, and Management. Raven Press, New York. 1990.

Fig. 16.45 redrawn from Bravo EL, Gifford RW Jr: Current concepts. Pheochromocytoma: diagnosis, localization and management. N Engl J Med 311:1298, 1984.

Fig. 16.48 redrawn from Gant NF, Daley GL, Chand S, et al: A study of angiotensin II pressor response throughout primigravid pregnancy. J Clin Invest 52:2682, 1973.

Fig. 16.52 redrawn from Schwartz SM, Ross R: Cellular proliferation in atherosclerosis and hypertension. Prog Cardiovasc Dis 26:355, 1984.

Figs. 16.55, 16.56 from Hurst JW (ed): The Heart, 1st ed. McGraw-Hill, New York, 1966. Courtesy of Joseph A. Wilber, MD, Atlanta, GA.

Figs. 16.57, 16.58, 16.60, 16.65, 16.67 from Hurst JW: Atlas of the Heart. Gower, New York, 1988.

Fig. 16.61 redrawn from Hurst JW, Woodson GC: Atlas of Spatial Vector Electrocardiography. The Blakiston Co., New York, 1952.

Fig. 16.63 data from United States Renal Data Systems. Am J Kid Dis, 18:Supp 2, 1991.

Fig. 16.64 data from United States Renal Data Systems. Am J Kid Dis, 1989.

Fig. 16.69 modified and redrawn from Cotran RS, Munro JM: Pathogenesis of atherosclerosis: Recent concepts. In Grundy SM, Bearn AG (eds): The Role of Cholesterol in Atherosclerosis: New Therapeutic Opportunities. Hanley and Belfus, Philadelphia, 1988.

Fig. 16.76 redrawn from Mancia G, Parati G, Pomidossi G, et al: Alerting reaction and rise in blood pressure during measurement by physician and nurse. Hypertension 9:209, 1987.

Fig. 16.78 redrawn from Kannel WB: In Kaplan NM, Stamler J (eds): Prevention of Coronary Heart Disease. WB Saunders, Philadelphia, 1983.

Figs. 16.79, 16.80 redrawn from Alderman MH, et al: Association of the renin–sodium profile with the risk of myocardial infarction in patients with hypertension. N Engl J Med 324:1098, 1991.

Fig. 16.81 modified and redrawn from Cruikshank JM, et al: Lancet 1:581, 1987.

⚡ REFERENCES:

1. Alderman MH, Madhavan S, Ooi WL, et al: Association of the renin-sodium profile with the risk of myocardial infarction in patients with hypertension. N Engl J Med 324:1098, 1991.

2. Babka JC, Cohn MS, Sode J: Solitary intrarenal cyst causing hypertension. N Engl J Med 291:343, 1974.

3. Berk BC, Vallega G, Muslin AJ, et al: Spontaneously hypertensive rat vascular smooth muscle cells in culture exhibit increased growth and Na+/H+ exchange. J Clin Invest 83:822, 1989.

4. Biglieri EG, Irony I, Kater CE: Adrenocortical forms of human hypertension. In Laragh JH, Brenner BM (eds): Hypertension: Pathophysiology, Diagnosis, and Management. Raven Press, New York, 1990.

5. Blaustein MP, Hamlyn JM: Sodium transport inhibition, cell calcium, and hypertension. Am J Med 77:45, 1984.

6. Brands MW, Hildebrandt DA, Mizelle HL, et al: Sustained hyperinsulinemia increases arterial pressure in conscious rats. Am J Physiol Regul Integr Comp Physiol 260:R764, 1991.

7. Bravo EL, Tarazi RC, Dustan HP, et al: The changing clinical spectrum of primary aldosteronism. Am J Med 74:641, 1983.

8. Bravo EL, Tarazi RC, Fouad FM, et al: Clonidine-suppression test. A useful aid in the diagnosis of pheochromocytoma. N Engl J Med 305:623, 1981.

9. Bravo EL, Tarazi RC, Gifford RW, et al: Circulating and urinary catecholamines pheochromocytoma. Diagnostic and pathophysiologic implications. N Engl J M 301:682, 1979.

10. Brunner HR, Gavras H: Vascular damage in hypertension. Hosp Pract: 97, 1975.

11. Christlieb AR, Krolewski AS, Warram JH, et al: Is insulin the link between hypertension and obesity? Hypertension 7:1154, 1985.

12. Cohen AJ, McCarthy DM, Stoff JS: Direct hemodynamic effect of insulin in the isolated perfused kidney. Am J Physiol 257:F580, 1989.

13. Cunningham FG, Lindheimer MD: Hypertension in pregnancy. N Engl J M 326:927, 1992.

14. De Wardener HE: Kidney, salt intake, and Na +,K+ ATPase inhibitors in hypertension: 1990 Corcoran Lecture. Hypertension 17:830, 1991.

15. Devereux RB: Evaluation of cardiac structure and function by echocardiography and other noninvasive techniques. In Laragh JH, Brenner BM (eds): Hypertension Pathophysiology, Diagnosis, and Management. Raven Press, New York, 1990.

16. Dunn BR, Zatz R, Rennke HG, et al: Prevention of glomerular capillary hypertension in experimental diabetes mellitus obviates functional and structural glomerular injury. J Hypertens 4:S251, 1986.

17. Farese RV Jr, Biglieri EG, Shackleton CH, et al: Licorice-induced hypermineralocorticoidism. N Engl J Med 325:1223, 1991.

18. Ferrannini E, Buzzigoli G, Bonadonna R, et al: Insulin resistance in essential hypertension. N Engl J Med 317:350, 1987.

19. Fitzgerald DJ, Fitzgerald GA: Eicosanoids in the pathogenesis of preeclampsia. Laragh JH, Brenner BM (eds): Hypertension: Pathophysiology, Diagnosis, and Management. Raven Press, New York, 1990.

20. Fommei E, Ghione S, Palla L, et al: Renal scintigraphic captopril test in the diagnosis of renovascular hypertension. Hypertension 10:212, 1987.

21. Goldblatt H: Studies on experimental hypertension V. The pathogenesis of experimental hypertension due to renal ischemia. Ann Intern Med 11:69, 1937.

22. Goldblatt H, Lynch J, Hanzal RF, et al: Studies on hypertension 1. The production persistent elevation of systolic blood pressure by means of renal ischemia. J Exp M 59:347, 1934.

23. Guyton AC: Arterial Pressure and Hypertension. W.B. Saunders, Philadelphia, 198

24. Hollenberg NK, Moore T, Shoback D, et al: Abnormal renal sodium handling essential hypertension. Relation to failure of renal and adrenal modulation responses to angiotensin II. Am J Med 81:412, 1986.

25. Hommel E, Mathiesen ER, Giese J, et al: On the pathogenesis of arterial blood pressure elevation early in the course of diabetic nephropathy. Scand J Clin Lab Inve 49:537, 1989.

26. Joint National Committee: The 1988 report of the Joint National Committee detection, evaluation, and treatment of high blood pressure. Arch Intern M 148:1023, 1988.

27. Kannel WB, Castelli WP, McNamara PM, et al: Role of blood pressure in the development of congestive heart failure. The Framingham Study. N Engl J Med 287:782, 1972.

28. Kannel WB, Gordon T, Schwartz MJ: Systolic versus diastolic blood pressure and risk of coronary heart disease. The Framingham study. Am J Cardiol 27:335, 1971.

29. Kannel WB, Stampfer MJ, Castelli WP, et al: The prognostic significance of proteinuria: The Framingham study. Am Heart J 108:1347, 1984.

30. Kaplan NM: The deadly quartet. Upper-body obesity, glucose intolerance, hypertriglyceridemia, and hypertension. Arch Intern Med 149:1514, 1989.

31. Kaplan NM: Hypertension in the individual patient. In Kaplan NM (ed.): Clinical Hypertension. Williams & Wilkins, Baltimore, 1990.

32. Kaplan NM: Hypertension with pregancy and the pill. In Kaplan NM (ed.): Clinical Hypertension. Williams & Wilkins, Baltimore, 1990.

33. Kaplan NM: Other forms of secondary hypertension. In Kaplan NM (ed.): Clinical Hypertension. Williams & Wilkins, Baltimore, 1990.

34. Kaplan NM: Renal vascular hypertension. In Kaplan NM (ed.): Clinical Hypertension. Williams & Wilkins, Baltimore, 1990.

35. King AJ, Marsden PA, Brenner BM: Endothelin. A potent vasoactive peptide endothelial origin. In Laragh JH, Brenner BM (eds): Hypertension: Pathophysiology, Diagnosis, and Management. Raven Press, New York, 1990.

36. Kopp E, Aurell M, Nilsson I-M, et al: The role of beta-1-adrenoreceptors in the renin release response to graded renal sympathetic nerve stimulation. Pfleugers Ar 387:107, 1980.

37. Laragh JH, Sealey JE: Renin-sodium profiling: Why, how, and when in clinical practice. Cardiovasc Med 2:1053, 1977.

38. Lips KJM, Der Sluys Veer JV, Struyvenberg A, et al: Bilateral occurrence of pheochromocytoma in patients with the multiple endocrine neoplasia syndrome type 2A (Sipple's syndrome). Am J Med 70:1051, 1981.

39. Lyall F, Morton JJ, Lever AF, et al: Angiotensin II activates Na+-H+ exchange and stimulates growth in cultured vascular smooth muscle cells. J Hypertens 6:S438, 1988.

40. Mancia G, Casadei R, Groppelli A, et al: Effect of stress on diagnosis of hypertension. Hypertension 17:III56, 1991.

41. Manger WM, Gifford RW: Pheochromocytoma. In Laragh JH, Brenner BM (eds): Hypertension: Pathophysiology, Diagnosis, and Management. Raven Press, New York, 1990.

42. Mbanya JC, Thomas TH, Taylor R, et al: Increased proximal tubular sodium reabsorption in hypertensive patients with type 2 diabetes. Diab Med 6:614, 1989.

43. Muller FB, Sealey JE, Case CB, et al: The captopril test for identifying renovascular disease in hypertensive patients. Am J Med 80:633, 1986.

44. Naftilan AJ, Zuo WM, Inglefinger J, et al: Localization and differential regulation of angiotensinogen mRNA expression in the vessel wall. J Clin Invest 87:1300, 1991.

45. Palmer RMJ, Ferrige AG, Moncada S: Nitric oxide release accounts for the biological activity of endothelium-derived relaxing factor. Nature 327:524, 1987.

46. Panza JA, Quyyumi AA, Brush JE Jr, et al: Abnormal endothelium-dependent vascular relaxation in patients with essential hypertension. N Engl J Med 323:22, 1990.

47. Reaven GM: Banting lecture 1988. Role of insulin resistance in human disease. Diabetes 37:1595, 1988.

48. Reisin E: Sodium and obesity in the pathogenesis of hypertension. Am J Hypertens 3:164, 1990.

49. Rocchini AP: Insulin resistance and blood pressure regulation in obese and nonobese subjects: Special lecture. Hypertension 17:837, 1991.

50. Rocchini AP, Moorehead C, Deremer S, et al: Hyperinsulinemia and the aldosterone and pressor responses to angiotensin II. Hypertension 15:861, 1990.

51. Rostand SG, Brown G, Kirk KA, et al: Renal insufficiency in treated essential hypertension. N Engl J Med 320:684, 1989.

52. Siegel WC, Blumenthal JA, Divine GW: Physiological, psychological, and behavioral factors and white coat hypertension. Hypertension 16:140, 1991.

53. Simonson DC: Insulin sensitivity and the effects of antihypertensive agents: Implications for the treatment of hypertension in the patient with diabetes mellitus. Postgrad Med J 64:39, 1988.

54. Simonson MS, Dunn MJ: Cellular signaling by peptides of the endothelin gene family. Faseb J 4:2989, 1990.

55. Vaughan ED, Sosa RE: Hypertension and hydronephrosis. In Laragh JH, Brenner BM (eds): Hypertension: Pathophysiology, Diagnosis, and Management. Raven Press, New York, 1990.

56. Veterans Administration Cooperative Study Group on Antihypertensive Agents: Effects of treatment on morbidity in hypertension. Results in patients with diastolic blood pressures averaging 115-129 mmHg. JAMA 202:1028, 1967.

57. Veterans Administration Cooperative Study Group on Antihypertensive Agents: Effects of treatment on morbidity in hypertension II. Results in patients with diastolic blood pressure averaging 90-114 mmHg. JAMA 213:1143, 1970.

58. Walsh SW: Preeclampsia: An imbalance in placental prostacyclin and thromboxane production. Am J Obstet Gynecol 152:335, 1985.

59. Zatz, R, Anderson S, Meyer TW, et al: Lowering of arterial blood pressure limits glomerular sclerosis in rats with renal ablation and in experimental diabetes. Kidney Int 20:S123, 1987.

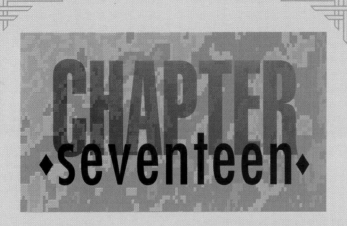

CHAPTER ◆seventeen◆

LIPOPROTEIN METABOLISM AND CORONARY ARTERY DISEASE

STUART R. CHIPKIN, MD

Physiologic mechanisms have evolved in humans to meet cellular needs for cholesterol and its derivatives. However, diet, aging, genetic abnormalities, and various diseases can affect these pathways, causing them to facilitate atherosclerosis. Cholesterol is a necessary component of cell membranes and is the precursor for bile acids, sex hormones, and adrenal steroid synthesis. It is either absorbed from the intestines or synthesized in the liver. Since lipids are not water soluble, cholesterol and triglycerides must be transported in the bloodstream within discrete particles as *lipoproteins*. The proteins within these lipoproteins, which may signal receptors, enhance membrane transport, or activate enzymes, are termed *apoproteins* or *apolipoproteins*. Although human physiology is efficient at absorbing, synthesizing, and transporting cholesterol, similarly effective mechanisms for degrading cholesterol do not normally exist. With increased dietary fat, cells will maintain intracellular cholesterol concentrations even if circulating levels increase. Clinical problems in lipid metabolism can frequently be traced to an imbalance between the rate of entry of cholesterol into serum and the rate of degradation.

The Relation Between Lipids and Coronary Heart Disease

To understand the medical studies that have been done to help define the relation between lipids and heart disease, it is important to consider study design, time course, population characteristics, lipid fractions being analyzed, end points being measured, and means of expressing risk. Beside differences in retrospective versus prospective design, studies may vary in length of patient follow-up and whether an intervention was continued throughout the follow-up.

Investigators may compare different stable populations or changes within a single population. Different studies have attempted to relate coronary disease to total cholesterol; very low density, low density, and high density lipoproteins; triglycerides; specific apoproteins; and ratios of the above factors (Fig. 17.1). Whereas some studies have used nonfatal myocardial infarction as an end point, others have used angiographic evidence of coronary artery disease, and still others have evaluated the effects of lipids on mortality from heart disease. Coronary heart disease can be expressed as an absolute rate or as a relative risk reflecting the increase conferred by a given parameter. The risk ratio can be calculated using the risk for any given cholesterol concentration as a numerator and the risk for coronary heart disease at a "normal" cholesterol as a denominator. However, this risk ratio does not take into account duration of the abnormality or age-related increases in disease. Despite variations in all these parameters, the correlation between serum cholesterol and coronary disease remains strong.

Total cholesterol correlates linearly with coronary death rates in different countries (Fig. 17.2). As Japanese have migrated from Japan to Hawaii and then to San Francisco, an increase in coronary disease has paralleled an increase in cholesterol (Fig. 17.3). The Framingham study and the Multiple Risk Factor Intervention Trial (MRFIT) are large prospective epidemiologic surveys that documented a strong curvilinear relationship between cholesterol and coronary disease (Fig. 17.4).[1,28]

Although several studies have now documented an increase in coronary heart disease and mortality with elevated cholesterol, separate studies have been needed to prove that decreases in cholesterol levels improve survival (Fig. 17.5). Decreases in coronary heart disease incidence have been demonstrated with reduction of serum cholesterol achieved by altering diet.[9,23]

In summary, through the use of different epidemiologic approaches, serum cholesterol has been linked to coronary heart disease and cardiac mortality. Populations of individuals with elevated cholesterol are at higher risk than those with lower cholesterol . In addition, interventions that successfully lower serum cholesterol result in a decreased risk for coronary artery disease.

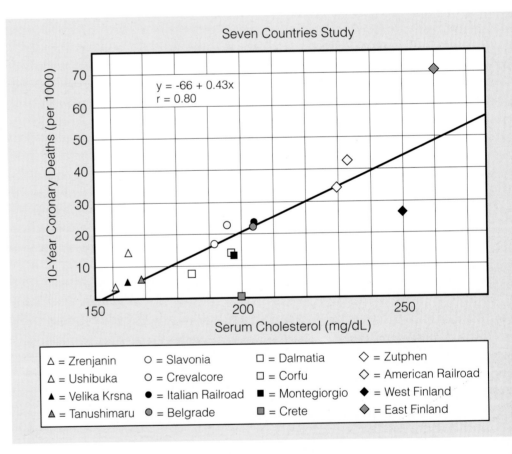

FIGURE 17.1 PREDICTORS OF CORONARY ARTERY DISEASE

LIPIDS	APOPROTEINS
Increased total cholesterol	—
Increased LDL cholesterol	Increased APO B
Decreased HDL (HDL₂)	Decreased APO A-I
Increased Lp(a)	—

Seven Countries Study

y = -66 + 0.43x
r = 0.80

10-Year Coronary Deaths (per 1000)

Serum Cholesterol (mg/dL)

△ = Zrenjanin	○ = Slavonia	▢ = Dalmatia	◇ = Zutphen
△ = Ushibuka	○ = Crevalcore	▢ = Corfu	◇ = American Railroad
▲ = Velika Krsna	● = Italian Railroad	■ = Montegiorgio	◆ = West Finland
▲ = Tanushimaru	● = Belgrade	■ = Crete	◆ = East Finland

FIGURE 17.2   Epidemiologic evidence from seven countries establishing high levels of serum cholesterol as a major risk factor for coronary heart disease (Modified with permission; see Figure Credits).

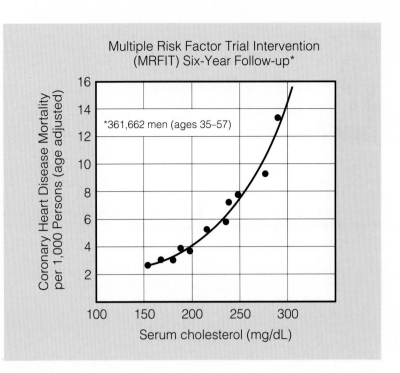

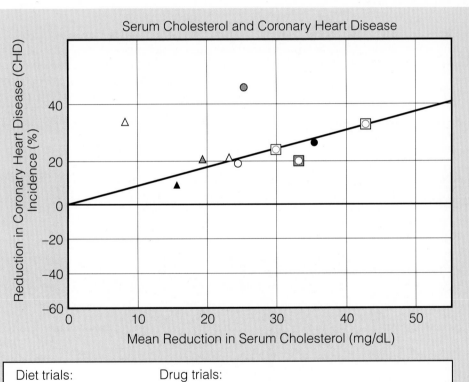

FIGURE 17.3 COMPARISON OF CHOLESTEROL LEVELS AND CHD RATES IN JAPANESE LIVING IN JAPAN, HAWAII, AND SAN FRANCISCO

	JAPAN	HAWAII	SAN FRANCISCO
Serum cholesterol (mg/dL)	181	218	228
CHD Rate	25.4	34.7	44.6

(Reproduced with permission; see Figure Credits)

FIGURE 17.4 Follow-up survey of 360,000 men with high total cholesterol. Further evidence that high cholesterol levels are a risk factor for coronary heart disease. (Modified with permission; see Figure Credits).

FIGURE 17.5 Clinical trial evidence indicating a connection between serum cholesterol and the development of coronary heart disease. Therapeutic lowering of cholesterol levels in hypercholesterolemic patients reduced the risk. (Modified with permission; see Figure Credits).

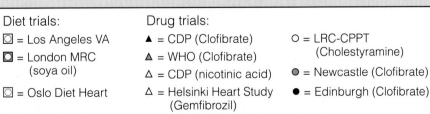

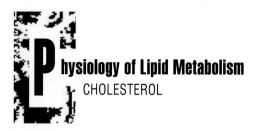

Physiology of Lipid Metabolism
CHOLESTEROL

To appreciate how cholesterol increases the risk for coronary disease, it is necessary to understand how cholesterol is synthesized, absorbed, transported, taken up, and excreted by cells.[11,13] A defect in any one of these processes may augment the risk for atherosclerotic changes. Conversely, therapeutic options in the future will be directed toward each of these areas.

Cholesterol synthesis begins with the condensation of three molecules of acetate which form 3-hydroxy-3-methylglutaryl co-enzyme A (HMG CoA). The step converting HMG CoA to mevalonic acid is rate limiting and controlled by HMG CoA reductase. If this enzyme is inhibited, cellular synthesis of cholesterol decreases.

Cholesterol is a steroid that has structural and functional roles in cell biology (Fig. 17.6). It is a major component of cell membranes, serving to anchor specialized proteins and facilitate transport into cells. Cholesterol is also used for the production of bile acids, which enhance intestinal fat absorption. In addition, it is used to synthesize hydrocortisone and aldosterone in adrenal glands, as well as androgens and estrogens in reproductive organs. Cholesterol, therefore, is necessary for normal cellular function.

Cholesterol enters the circulation following either intestinal absorption or hepatic synthesis. Intestinal cholesterol is derived from diet (250 to 500 mg/day) or from bile (600 to 1000 mg/day) (Fig. 17.7). Dietary cholesterol comes from animal products; plants (and therefore fruits, vegetables, and grains) do not contain cholesterol. Biliary cholesterol is derived from hepatic synthesis. Fifty percent of intestinal cholesterol (diet and bile) is absorbed after being solubilized by bile acids and other polar lipids; the rest is excreted.

Cholesterol produced in the liver can be released into the circulation, converted into bile acids (to facilitate intestinal fat absorption), or excreted into the intestines via bile. Increased cholesterol feeds back to the liver, decreasing hepatic cholesterol synthesis (see below discussion) and increasing intestinal

excretion. However, cholesterol is efficiently reabsorbed from the intestine i... the portal circulation, creating an enterohepatic cycle and minimizing amount of cholesterol excreted from the body. Ninety-seven percent of b acids and 50% of biliary cholesterol are reabsorbed from the intestine. The ab... ty to reabsorb cholesterol maximally probably evolved in response to a dietary intake, but as "civilized" diets increased in cholesterol, this physiolo... mechanism became potentially detrimental.

Cholesterol released from the liver is transported in the circulation in com... nation with apoproteins (or apolipoproteins). Cholesterol esters and triglyceri... are nonpolar lipids and tend to be located within the center of the lipoprot... particle. Free cholesterol and phospholipids, which are more polar, are located the periphery. The relative contribution of lipids and apoproteins alters lipop... tein density, thus creating distinct categories of lipoproteins (Fig. 17.8).

CHYLOMICRONS

Chylomicrons transport dietary fat from intestine to liver. Epithelial cells of t... small intestine are stimulated postprandially to synthesize chylomicrons by bile a... micelles containing intestinal lipids. Although chylomicrons are the largest lipop... teins, they are also the least dense because of the large component of triglycer... (98%–99%). From the intestine, chylomicrons are absorbed into mesenteric lym... and enter the circulation via the thoracic duct. Triglyceride is hydrolyzed from c... lomicrons via the enzyme lipoprotein lipase, which is synthesized in adipose tiss... muscle, breast, and lung and is located along capillary endothelial surfaces. The l... erated fatty acids may be used for fuel (e.g., muscle), storage (e.g., fat), or synthe... of nonpolar compounds (e.g., breast or liver). The resulting triglyceride-poor pa... cles are termed *chylomicron remnants*. The importance of triglyceride as a cardiov... cular risk factor has not been uniformly agreed upon.[38,39]

VERY LOW DENSITY LIPOPROTEINS

Very low density lipoproteins (VLDL) are somewhat analogous to chylomicro... because these particles also transport triglyceride. However, instead of bringi... dietary fat to the liver, VLDL transports triglyceride from the liver where it... synthesized to peripheral tissues. Lipoprotein lipase also acts on VLDL particl... releasing triglyceride and forming intermediate density lipoproteins (IDL). II... is taken up in the liver, most likely by the same receptor that takes up low de... sity lipoproteins (LDL). VLDL can also be metabolized directly to LDL ... hepatic triglyceride lipase (Fig. 17.9).

FIGURE 17.6 FUNCTIONS OF CHOLESTEROL

ESSENTIAL COMPONENT OF	PRECURSOR OF
Cell membranes (required for transmembrane transport) Serum lipoproteins (required for transport of triglycerides)	Bile acids (required for fat absorption) Adrenal steroid (hydrocortisone, aldosterone) Sex hormones (estrogens, androgens)

(Reproduced with permission; see Figure Credits)

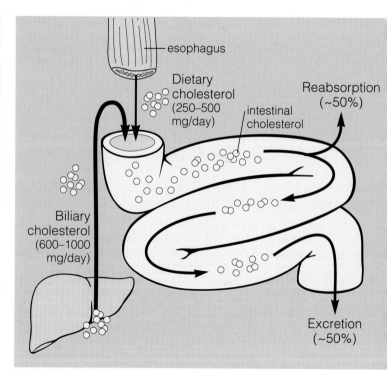

FIGURE 17.7   Origins and fates of intestinal cholesterol. (Reproduced with permission; see Figure Credits)

FIGURE 17.8 LIPOPROTEINS AND THEIR ATTRIBUTES

LIPOPROTEIN	DIAMETER (Å) RELATIVE SIZE	MAJOR COMPONENT	APOPROTEIN	ORIGIN	FUNCTION
Chylomicron	800–5000	Triglyceride	B-48 A-I A-II	Intestine	Transport Tg & Chol from intestine
VLDL	300–800	Triglyceride	B-100 E C	Liver	Transport Tg from liver
IDL	150–350	Triglyceride / Cholesterol	B-100 E	Hydrolysis of VLDL	Precursor of LDL Partial uptake by liver
LDL	180–280	Cholesterol	B-100	VLDL IDL	Transport chol Uptake by apo B, E receptor; Correlate with CHD
HDL	50–120	Cholesterol Phospholipid	A-I A-II C	Liver	Transport cholesterol from periphery to liver for removal; Inverse correlation with CHD
Lipoprotein (a)	—	Cholesterol	B-100 apo (a)	Liver	Correlates directly with CHD

(Modified with permission; see Figure Credits)

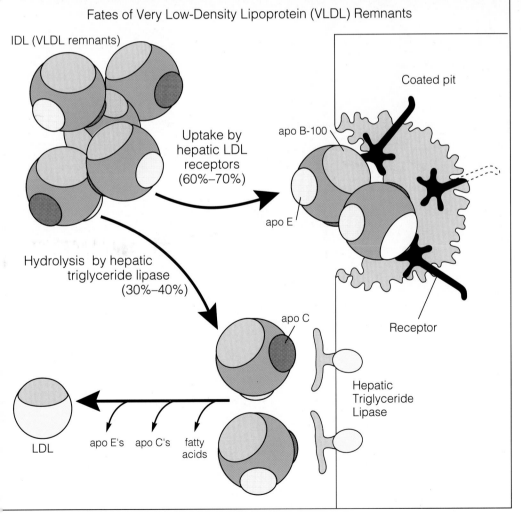

Fates of Very Low-Density Lipoprotein (VLDL) Remnants

IDL (VLDL remnants)

Uptake by hepatic LDL receptors (60%–70%)

Coated pit

apo B-100

apo E

Hydrolysis by hepatic triglyceride lipase (30%–40%)

Receptor

apo C

Hepatic Triglyceride Lipase

LDL

apo E's   apo C's   fatty acids

FIGURE 17.9   VLDL remnants can be taken up by the liver or transformed into low density lipoproteins (Modified with permission; see Figure Credits).

Under certain circumstances, the relative amount of cholesterol in VLDL increases and its electrophoretic mobility is similar to LDL. These lipoproteins, called *beta-VLDL*, are relatively more atherogenic, and disorders producing increased *beta-VLDL* are associated with premature coronary disease.

▒▒▒ LOW DENSITY LIPOPROTEINS

Low density lipoproteins (LDL) transport 70% of the total plasma cholesterol and have been recognized as atherogenic. The liver takes up the majority of LDL (75%); the remaining 25% is taken up by all other tissues. LDL is largely taken up via specific receptors that recognize specialized apoproteins (Fig. 17.10). After undergoing endocytosis, the LDL-receptor complex dissociates; the receptor recycles to the cell surface and, LDL is broken down in lysosomes. The free cholesterol liberated from LDL particles it may be used to meet cellular demands (cell membrane or steroid synthesis) or may be stored as cholesterol ester. In the liver, cholesterol can also be secreted into bile for excretion.

LOW DENSITY LIPOPROTEIN RECEPTOR

The LDL receptor (also called apo-B,E receptor) (Fig. 17.11) plays a critical role in lipoprotein metabolism because of its interaction with LDL, IDL, and VLDL. There are five distinct domains within its 839 amino acid structure. The first domain, at the amino terminal third, binds specific apoproteins on circulating lipoproteins (see below discussion). Within this domain, the repetitions of a 40

amino acid sequence has reinforced the concept of multiple ligand-binding sites.[17] The next portion of the receptor has sequence homology to epidermal growth factor, and other sequences are homologous to factors IX and X and to protein C. The third domain is extensively glycosylated, and the fourth spans the plasma membrane. The fifth domain, located at the carboxy terminal, projects into the cytoplasm and appears to play a role in clustering receptors in coated pits and internalizing the lipoprotein-receptor complex.

The number of LDL receptors are one means of regulating the concentration of intracellular cholesterol (Fig. 17.12). Receptor synthesis is inversely correlated with intracellular cholesterol; as the amount of cholesterol within the cell increases, LDL-receptor production is regulated downward. Conversely, receptor synthesis increases with decreased cellular cholesterol (see Fig. 17.10). This mechanism appears to apply in vivo since high fat and cholesterol diets, which would initially increase intracellular cholesterol levels, cause a reduction in hepatic LDL-receptor expression, and this reverses with cholestyramine.[6] Thus, in high fat and cholesterol diets, the regulation of LDL receptors may maintain intracellular cholesterol at the expense of increased plasma levels of cholesterol.

Mutated LDL (apo-B,E) receptors have been identified in humans and can be classified by sites of functional impairment (Fig. 17.13). The most basic anomaly is abnormal or absent LDL-receptor precursor synthesis in the endoplasmic reticulum (Fig. 17.13a). Another mutation involves a normal precursor that is not processed in the Golgi normally (Fig. 17.13b). A third class of genetic aberrations includes normal precursors that are processed correctly but are unable to

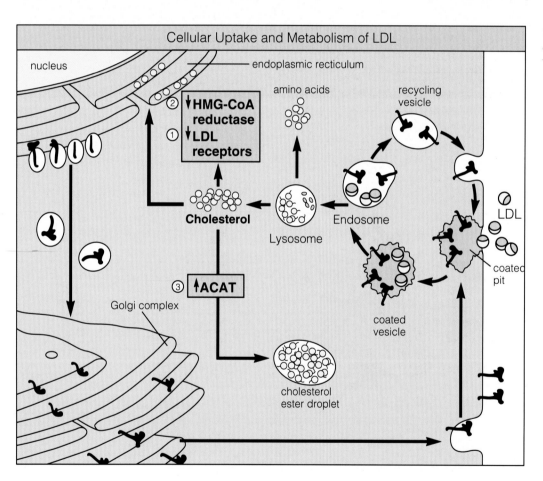

FIGURE 17.10   Pathways for uptake and degradation of LDL at the cellular level (Modified with permission; see Figure Credits).

nd LDL (Fig. 17.13c). Finally, normal precursors may be processed correctly and bind LDL but they may be unable to cluster in coated pits (Fig 17.13d). All these inborn errors result in increased circulating LDL and increased risk of coronary artery disease.[27]

In addition to LDL-receptor feedback regulation, there are two other mechanisms by which intracellular cholesterol is maintained within a narrow range (see Fig. 17.10). As intracellular cholesterol increases, cellular synthesis of cholesterol decreases by inhibition of the rate-limiting enzyme HMG-CoA reductase. In addition, excess intracellular cholesterol can be decreased by converting it to a form for storage (cholesteryl ester) via the enzyme acyl-CoA:cholesterol acyltransferase (ACAT). Thus, there are three distinct mechanisms by which intracellular cholesterol is tightly regulated (see Fig. 17.12).

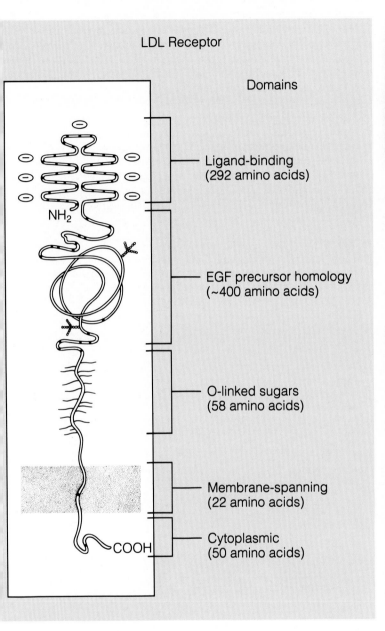

IGURE 17.11   Structure of the LDL receptor with its functional domains. Reproduced with permission; see Figure Credits)

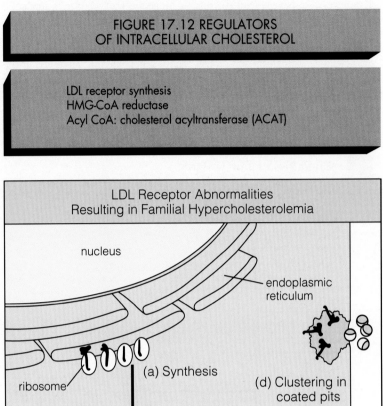

FIGURE 17.12 REGULATORS OF INTRACELLULAR CHOLESTEROL

LDL receptor synthesis
HMG-CoA reductase
Acyl CoA: cholesterol acyltransferase (ACAT)

FIGURE 17.13   Genetic defects underlying familial hypercholesterolemia. Abnormalities are found in LDL-receptor synthesis in the endoplasmic reticulum, the transport of receptors to the Golgi complex, the binding of receptors to LDL, and the clustering of receptors in coated pits (Modified with permission; see Figure Credits).

Increased circulating LDL heightens the risk for atherosclerosis because of changes that occur beneath the endothelial and smooth muscle cells of arterial walls (Fig. 17.14). LDL is thought to traverse endothelial cells and, if in excess, it may accumulate beneath the arterial lining. Endothelial cells and smooth muscle cells have the ability to modify LDL via oxidation. Oxidized LDL has been observed to have several atherogenic properties (Fig. 17.15).[18] Circulating monocytes appear to be attracted to the oxidized LDL and take it up via alternative receptors, termed *scavenger receptors*.[20,33] These cells then become transformed into lipid-filled macrophages. If the amount of LDL is small, this process could facilitate its removal and protect against atherosclerosis. However, in the presence of continued excess LDL, macrophages themselves oxidize LDL and increase the expression of scavenger receptors.[8] The continued accumulation of oxidized LDL inhibits macrophage movement[8] and, additionally, may inhibit endothelium-derived relaxing factors.[22] As the process continues, foam cells develop and the first clinical lesion in atherosclerosis, the fatty streak, appears.

HIGH DENSITY LIPOPROTEINS

High density lipoproteins (HDL), although the smallest of the lipoproteins, are the densest in volume because of the relatively small amount of lipid (50%) and large amount of protein (50%) per lipoprotein particle (see Fig. 17.8). HDL subclassified into three categories: HDL_1, which is enriched in cholester HDL_2, which correlates best with protection against coronary disease, a HDL_3, the most abundant HDL.

When initially synthesized in the liver or intestine, nascent HDL is thought be primarily composed of apoproteins and a phospholipid bilayer. As free chol terol is taken up and esterified by the enzyme lecithin; cholesterol acyltrar ferase (LCAT), a mature, spherical HDL particle is created.

HDL has been found in several studies to correlate inversely with corona artery disease.[29,30] Although reverse cholesterol transport from the periphery the liver is most often sited as the mechanism, HDL has other actions that m be protective. HDL inhibits binding of LDL to matrix proteins, oxidation LDL, and receptor uptake of oxidized LDL.

LIPOPROTEIN(a) [LP(a)]

Intermediate in density between LDL and HDL, Lp(a) is becoming increasing important in understanding lipoproteins and atherosclerosis. This particle is co posed of apoprotein B and the glycoprotein apo (a), which has strong homology plasminogen. Although it does not vary with age, sex, total cholesterol, or trigly eride, Lp(a) appears to correlate closely with coronary artery disease.[2] Thus f. Lp(a) has not been amenable to dietary or pharmacologic therapy.

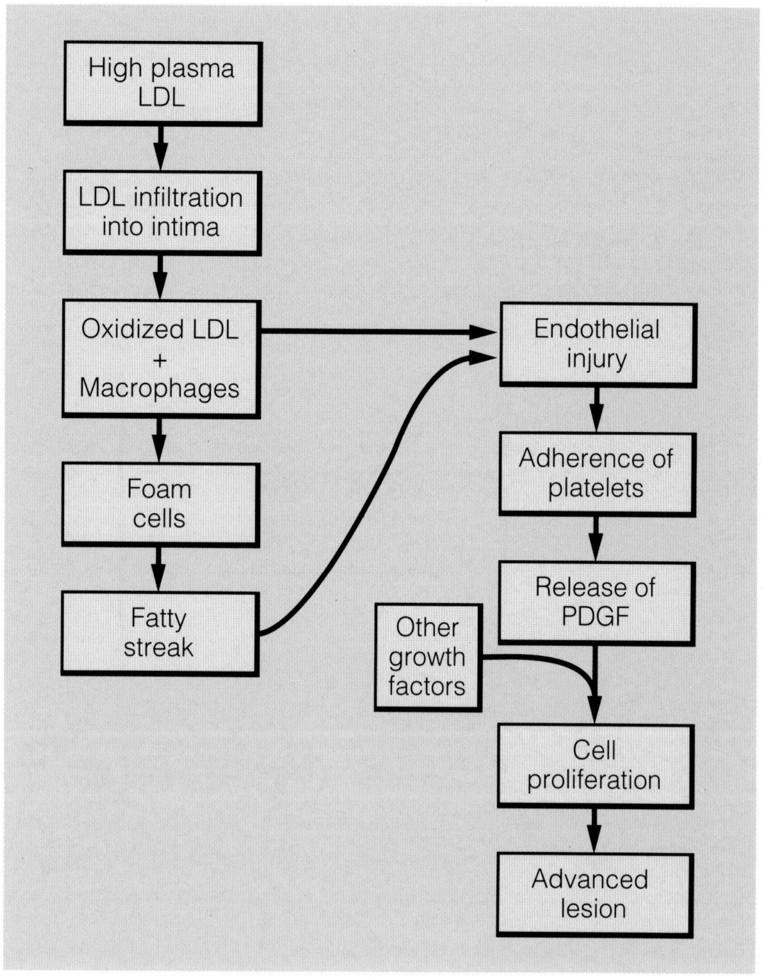

FIGURE 17.14 Possible linkage between the hypotheses for lipid infiltra tion and endothelial injury. Lipid infiltration (right column) may be sufficier to account for fatty streaks, and endothelial injury may account for progres sion of the fatty streaks to more advanced lesions. (PDGF = platelet-derived growth factor) (Reproduced with permission; see Figure Credits)

APOPROTEINS

Apoproteins (apo), which are generally located on the outer surface of lipoproteins, serve key roles in lipoprotein production, structure, metabolism, and cellular uptake (Fig. 17.16). These proteins may enhance membrane transport, act as ligands for receptors, or serve as cofactors for enzymes. They are typically classified into the following four groups (Fig. 17.17).

APOPROTEIN B

Apoproteins B-48 and B-100 are located in triglyceride-rich lipoproteins and are among the largest of the circulating proteins. Apo B-48 is synthesized in the intestine where it is used in the formation of chylomicrons. Similarly, apo B-100 is produced in the liver and used in the production of VLDL. Apo B-100 serves as a ligand for binding to the LDL (apo-B,E) receptor. As VLDL is metabolized to IDL and LDL, apo B-100 is the only apoprotein remaining within the lipoprotein.

If apo B is absent or abnormally produced, triglyceride levels are low; the decreases in LDL and chylomicrons can also produce vitamins E and A deficiency, respectively. Genetic excess of apo B-100 results in increased VLDL and produces a familial combined hyperlipidemia, with an increased risk for cardiovascular disease.[40] It is the most frequently inherited lipid abnormality among survivors of myocardial infarction.

APOPROTEIN A

There are three types of apoprotein A, which are synthesized in the intestines and the liver and are found on chylomicrons and HDL. Apo A is transferred from chylomicrons to HDL in exchange for apo C-II. As part of HDL, Apo A-I appears to avidly take up cholesterol from cells and esterify it by activating LCAT; the cholesterol is then transported to the liver where it undergoes further metabolism. Thus apo A plays a major role in transporting cholesterol from peripheral sites back to the liver. Abnormal apo A is found in Tangier disease and produces hypertriglyceridemia with very low concentrations of HDL.

APOPROTEIN C

Apoprotein C is manufactured in the liver and is located on HDL, and triglyceride-containing particles such as chylomicrons, VLDL, and IDL. Apo C is transferred to chylomicrons from HDL in the lymph, in exchange for apo A. Apo C-II is necessary for the activation of lipoprotein lipase, which hydrolyzes the triglycerides from lipoproteins. Apo C-II abnormalities present similarly to lipoprotein lipase deficiencies with severe hypertriglyceridemia.

APOPROTEIN E

Apoprotein E, similar to Apo C, is present on chylomicrons, VLDL, IDL and HDL. These proteins serve as ligands for apo E and LDL (apo B,E) receptors and thus play an important role in cellular uptake of cholesterol from all lipoproteins except LDL.[25] Apo E has a greater affinity than apo B for the LDL (apo B, E) receptor; this helps to explain the more rapid clearance of apo E–containing lipoproteins (minutes) compared with that of apo B–containing LDL (days). Apo E appears to also play a role in the uptake of chylomicron remnants.

There are three isoforms of apo E (E-2, E-3, E-4), and one isoform is inherited from each parent; thus, there are six different possible genotypic expressions. The affinity of each isoform for the apo E receptor varies; apo E-4 has the greatest and E-2 has the least. As a result, homozygotes for apo E-2 have elevated VLDL and IDL and can develop premature coronary disease[5] (genetic abnormalities, beta-VLDL).

FIGURE 17.15 PROPERTIES OF OXIDIZED LDL

Chemotactic for monocytes/macrophages
Greater uptake by scavenger receptors on
    monocytes/macrophages
Inhibits tissue macrophage motility
Directly cytotoxic

FIGURE 17.16 FUNCTIONS OF APOPROTEINS

Necessary for the synthesis and secretion of lipoproteins
Stabilize lipoprotein structure
Cofactors in enzyme activation
Ligands for specific cell-surface receptors

FIGURE 17.17 CLASSIFICATION OF APOPROTEINS

APOPROTEINS	FUNCTION
B-100	VLDL synthesis
	Ligand for LDL(apo-B/E) receptor
B-48	Chylomicron synthesis
E	Ligand for LDL (apo-B,E) receptor
	Facilitates uptake of chylomicron remnants and portions of VLDL, IDL, and HDL
A-I	LCAT activation in HDL
A-II	Structural protein of HDL
A-IV	LCAT activation in chylomicrons
C-I	LCAT activation
C-II	Lipoproteins lipase activation
C-III	Uptake of VLDL and chylomicrons (triglyceride-rich lipoproteins)

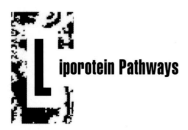

Liporotein Pathways

Cholesterol and triglyceride must be transported from points of origin to various destinations throughout the body and ultimately to a site of degradation. If the source is external (dietary), cholesterol and triglyceride are taken up in the intestine and the pathway is termed *exogenous*. When synthesized in the liver, cholesterol and triglyceride travel via VLDL through the *endogenous* pathway. *Reverse cholesterol transport* occurs when HDL brings cholesterol from the periphery back to the liver.

EXOGENOUS PATHWAY

As long as dietary fat is present and absorbed from the intestine, chylomicrons with apos B-48 and A will form (Fig. 17.18). After acquiring apo E and C, lipoprotein lipase can be stimulated by insulin and liberated fatty acids can be taken up by muscle, adipose tissue, or liver. Apos A and C are released and the residual chylomicron remnant, containing cholesteryl esters, is taken up by the liver.

There is no feedback in the exogenous pathway; increased dietary fat consumption will produce higher plasma triglyceride levels. Impairment or absence of lipoprotein lipase, which is the rate-limiting step for exogenous triglyceride metabolism, will also produce hypertriglyceridemia[37]; impaired insulin stimulation of LPL is thought to be the cause of hypertriglyceridemia in diabetes. Apo C-II deficiency has also been identified as a cause of elevated circulating triglyceride.[4]

ENDOGENOUS PATHWAY

Unlike the exogenous pathway, this pathway is cyclic and has feedback mechanisms through the hepatic LDL (apo B,E) receptor. It begins with hepatic synthesis of VLDL (see Fig. 17.18A) containing apo C, E, and B-100. As with chylomicrons, hydrolysis of VLDL triglyceride by LPL liberates fatty acids for use in muscle and adipose tissue (see Fig. 17.18B). The resulting IDL can either be taken up by the liver (apo E receptors) or be further metabolized to LDL (see Fig. 17.18C,D). LDL delivers cholesterol to the periphery and to the liver (see Fig. 17.18E,F) where uptake occurs via the LDL receptor. As the liver takes up increasing amounts of LDL-derived cholesterol, intracellular cholesterol normally provides feedback by inhibiting HMG-CoA reductase (thereby limiting VLDL synthesis), increasing ACAT activity (thereby increasing intracellular cholesterol storage), and decreasing LDL receptor synthesis (thereby decreasing cholesterol uptake). Since this feedback only affects hepatic cholesterol metabolism, its impact on circulating concentrations is decreased in the presence of a high cholesterol diet.

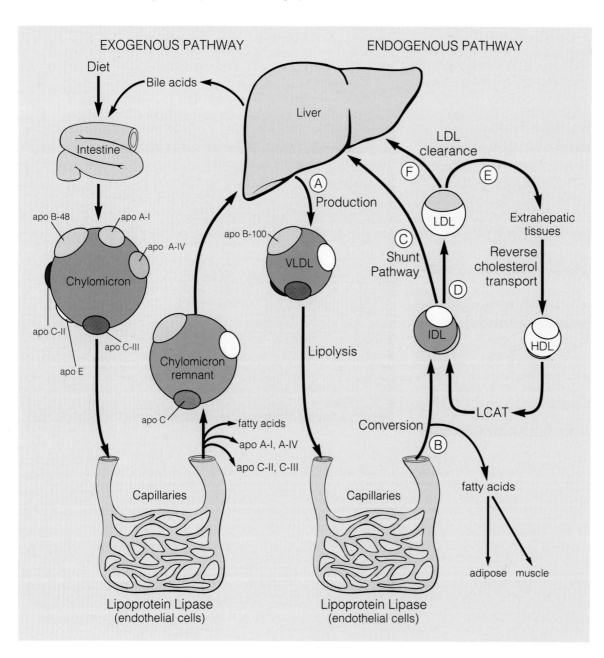

FIGURE 17.18 Pathways for metabolism of lipoproteins carrying endogenous and exogenous cholesterol. (Modified with permission; see Figure Credits)

REVERSE CHOLESTEROL TRANSPORT

HDL plays a key role in transporting cholesterol from the periphery to the liver where it can be degraded and excreted; this process is known as reverse cholesterol transport (Fig. 17.19). Excess free cholesterol is taken up by nascent HDL (see Fig.17.19A) and esterified by LCAT. Cholesteryl–ester transfer proteins appear to moderate an exchange of cholesterol for triglyceride between HDL and the lipoproteins VLDL, IDL, or LDL (B). These particles, which contain apo E, can now be taken up by the liver (C) and their cholesterol load can be excreted. An additional pathway in which cholesterol containing HDL is taken up directly by the liver (D) has also been proposed.

Although this process delivers cholesterol to the liver, it does not guarantee its degradation. After converting cholesterol into bile acids or excreting it into bile, enterohepatic circulation results in reabsorption of over 50% of intestinal cholesterol. All of these pathways have evolved in order to maximally retain and distribute cholesterol; prehistoric humans did not consume sufficiently large amounts of cholesterol to benefit from developing degradative pathways.

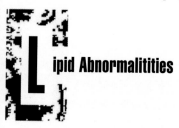

Lipid Abnormalitities

The homeostasis maintained by the above mechanisms can be adversely affect-ed by several processes. In the most general sense, cholesterol or triglyceride levels become elevated if too much lipid enters the bloodstream or too little is metabolized or excreted. Since cholesterol enters the circulation from the intestine and the liver, both of these are potential sources for increasing serum cholesterol. Impaired degradation of cholesterol can occur because of alterations in reverse transport, receptor number, or receptor signalling (via apoproteins). Serum triglycerides can increase because of excess dietary intake or because of impaired degradation from deficient or absent enzymes (LPL) or cofactors (apoproteins).

There are several factors that can increase cholesterol's entry into the bloodstream or decrease its removal; these include diet, age, genetic abnormalities, and diseases that produce secondary hypercholesterolemia.

DIET

Elevations in serum cholesterol have been correlated with the ingestion of foods containing cholesterol, diets high in saturated fatty acids, and obesity-related caloric intake.[13] Dietary sources of cholesterol can be divided into meats, eggs, and animal fats (including milk products) (Fig. 17.20). Eggs and organ meat contain the greatest amount of cholesterol. Increased dietary cholesterol raises LDL levels. The negative feedback on the LDL (apo B,E) receptor then further decreases uptake of LDL and VLDL.

Saturated fatty acids are those without double bonds; coconut oil, butter fat, palm oil, and cocoa butter contain over 50% saturated fatty acids. Although the precise way in which saturated fatty acids increase serum cholesterol is not known, they are believed to suppress LDL receptors, thereby decreasing hepatic cholesterol uptake.

FIGURE 17.19
Mechanisms for reverse cholesterol transport (Modified with permission; see Figure Credits).

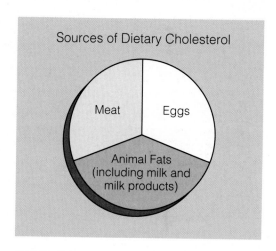

FIGURE 17.20   Typical sources of dietary cholesterol (Modified with permission; see Figure Credits).

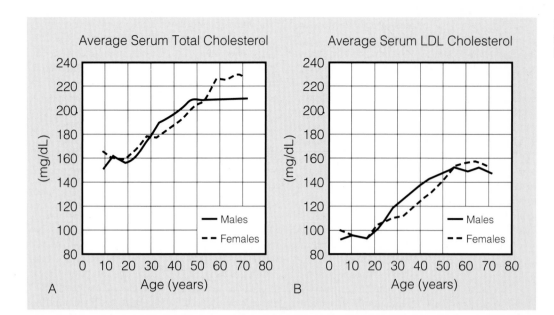

FIGURE 17.21   Increases with age in serum total cholesterol **(A)** and LDL-cholesterol **(B)**. (Reproduced with permission; see Figure Credits)

FIGURE 17.22 GENETIC DISORDERS OF LIPID METABOLISM

DEFICIENCY	XANTHOMAS	ASSOCIATED DISEASE	AVG. CHOLESTEROL	AVG. TRIGYLCERIDE
INCREASED TRIGLYCERIDES—TYPE V HYPERLIPOPROTEINEMIA				
Lipoprotein lipase	Eruptive	Pancreatitis lipemia	300–400	>2000
Apo C-II		Retinalis		
Type V HLP				
Familial combined hyperlipidemia	see below			
Familial hypertriglyceridemia	see below			
INCREASED VLDL—TYPE III HYPERLIPOPROTEINEMIA				
Dysbetalipoproteinemia	Tuberoeruptive		400–500	600–800
Apo E-2 homozygote				
Apo E deficiency				
Hepatic lipase, hyperuricemia		Diabetes deficiency		
INCREASED VLDL–TYPE IV HYPERLIPOPROTEINEMIA				
Familial combined hyperlipidemia	None usually	Obesity, diabetes, hyper-uricemia	225–275	400–500
Familial hypertriglyceridemia			<240	300–800
INCREASED LDL				
Familial combined hyperlipidemia	Tendinous	Corneal arcus	350–400	100–150
Familial hypercholesterolemia			Heterozygotes = 350–500 Homozygotes = 700–1000	
DECREASED HDL				
Tangier disease	None	Orange tonsils, normal tonsils	HDL <30	Vary
HDL deficiency				
Apo A-I/C-III deficiency	Palmar			
LCAT deficiency				
Hypoalphalipoproteinemia				

Obesity and excess caloric intake must be coupled in order to increase [ser]um cholesterol; people who ingest high amounts of calories and exercise [do] not demonstrate hypercholesterolemia. Obese individuals appear to over-[pro]duce VLDL containing apo-B.[14] In addition, obesity is associated with [de]creased HDL.

AGE

[In] both men and women between the ages of 20 and 60, total cholesterol and [LD]L increases between the ages of 20 and 60 (Fig. 17.21). These changes in lev-[els] appear to be due to an increase in production and a decrease in clearance of [ch]olesterol containing lipoproteins.[10,15]

GENETIC ABNORMALITIES

[On]ce the normal pathways of lipid metabolism are understood, the effects of a [spe]cific genetic abnormality can be easily predicted. Figure 17.22 lists some of [th]e known genetic diseases and their characteristics, grouped according to the [cli]nical abnormality. Figure 17.23 portrays the spectrum of lipoprotein abnor-[ma]lities for these inherited disorders and their underlying defects.

[Hy]pertriglyceridemia, resulting from accumulation of chylomicrons, usually [oc]curs because of either a lack of lipoprotein lipase or its cofactor apo C-II.[4] [Bo]th of these are inherited in an autosomal recessive pattern and patients typi-cally present with abdominal pain and pancreatitis. Debate persists as to whether these patients are at increased risk for coronary artery disease.

Increased beta-VLDL (from type III hyperlipoproteinemia or dysbetalipoproteine-mia) represents impaired conversion of VLDL to LDL. As a result, levels of VLDL and IDL are elevated and the VLDL/TG ratio is greater than 0.3 (normal greater than 0.25). Apo E that either is deficient or binds poorly to its receptor may explain the impaired clearance of VLDL.[5,47] Physical examination typically demonstrates tuberoeruptive xanthomas on palms, elbows, knees, buttocks (Figs. 17.24, 17.25).

While beta-VLDL is not considered to be a primary atherogenic lipoprotein, there is evidence that it plays a role in atherogenesis.[26,43] Animals that develop athero-sclerotic lesions after being fed high fat diets typically have increased beta-VLDL. High cholesterol and fat diets may increase beta-VLDL because of a regulation downward of LDL (apo B,E) receptors.[6] Macrophages, which play a critical role in foam cell development, contain beta-VLDL receptors and can also take up VLDL remnants via LDL (apo B,E) receptors. In addition, cholesteryl esters increase in cultured macrophages incubated with VLDL and chylomicrons but not with LDL.

Increased VLDL is a common presentation in two different inherited disorders: familial hypertriglyceridemia and familal combined hyperlipidemia. Familial hyper-triglyceridemia is an autosomal dominant condition whose precise defect is unknown. Although LDL and apo B/cholesterol are normal, VLDL and triglyc-erides are increased and HDL is low. This disorder has been identified in 5% of

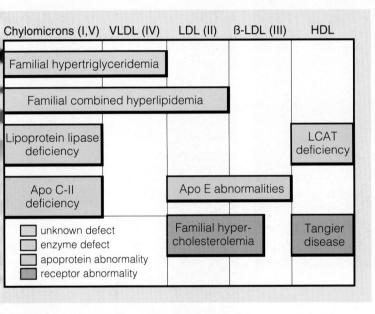

FIGURE 17.23 Spectrum of lipoprotein abnormalities for inherited disorders. (Modified with permission; see Figure Credits)

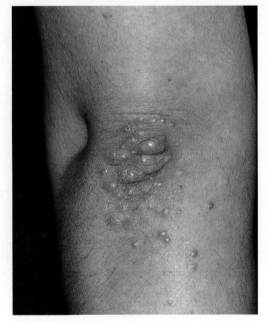

FIGURE 17.24
Tuberous and tuberoeruptive xan-thomas of the elbow secondary to type III hyperlipoproteinemia (Reproduced with per-mission; see Figure Credits).

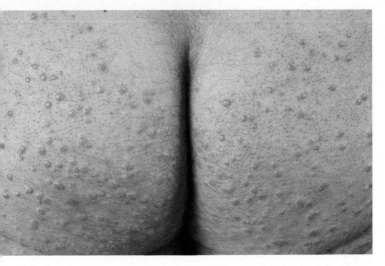

FIGURE 17.25 Eruptive skin xanthomas of the buttocks secondary to type V hyperlipoproteinemia (Reproduced with permission; see Figure Credits).

patients with myocardial infarctions who are less than 60 years of age. Familial combined hyperlipidemia, which is also associated with elevated VLDL, presents with *elevated* LDL levels.

Inherited disorders that produce increased LDL cholesterol are associated with increased risk for premature coronary artery disease. Familial combined hyperlipidemia, an autosomal dominant abnormality, can be diagnosed in 1 to 2% of the American population and 10 to 15% of patients with myocardial infarctions before the age of 60.[12] Lipid profiles vary with increases in cholesterol, triglycerides, or both.[12] VLDL, LDL, and apo B production are usually increased. Physical examination does not usually reveal xanthomas; obesity is common.

Another autosomal dominant disease, familial hypercholesterolemia, is found in 5% of patients with myocardial infarctions who are under age 60.[12] These patients have a defect either in one (heterozygous) or both (homozygous) genes for the LDL receptor.[46] Heterozygotes occur with a frequency of 1 in 500, but homozygotes are quite rare. Since the defective LDL (apo B,E) receptor cannot take up LDL and IDL, the clinical manifestations are decreased clearance of

VLDL and IDL and increased conversion of VLDL to LDL. In the physical examination, corneal arcus and xanthomas on dorsal hands and Achilles tendons are found (Fig. 17.26). Defects in apo B-100 also produce elevations of LDL, but VLDL is not affected because normal apo E can bind to the LDL (apo B,E) receptor. These patients have lower cholesterol levels than patients with familial hypercholesterolemia because of the normal VLDL metabolism.

Decreased concentrations of HDL impair reverse cholesterol transport and result in cholesterol deposits. In Tangier disease, an autosomal recessive disorder, cholesterol esters are deposited in the reticuloendothelial system, giving rise to the characteristic orange tonsils, lymphadenopathy, and hepatosplenomegaly. The lipid profile shows hypertriglyceridemia, which is due to increased chylomicrons and VLDL, and hypocholesterolemia, due to decreased LDL and markedly low HDL (<5 mg/dl). In pure HDL deficiency, tonsils are normal, but palmar xanthomas develop. LCAT deficiency prevents cholesteryl ester formation. As the amount of free cholesterol increases in this autosomal recessive disorder, anemia, corneal opacification, and proteinuria with renal failure can result.

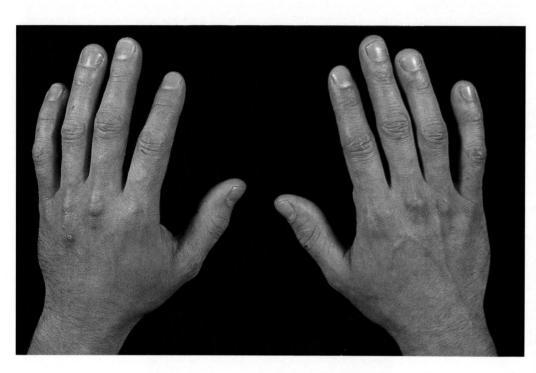

FIGURE 17.26 Tendon xanthomas secondary to familial hypercholesterolemia (Reproduced with permission; see Figure Credits).

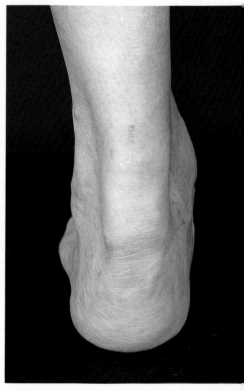

SECONDARY LIPID ABNORMALITIES

[L]ipid metabolism can be altered by diseases affecting hormonal balance, the [li]ver, and the kidney (Figs. 17.27). Hypothyroid patients have been observed to [h]ave hypercholesterolemia.[24,32] and hypertriglyceridemia.[31] although it is not [c]lear whether this specifically increases their risk for cardiovascular disease. [E]levated circulating levels of both LDL and HDL are thought to be due to [im]paired lipoprotein clearance.[24,46]

Patients with diabetes mellitus typically have hypertriglyceridemia with [in]creased VLDL; an increase in remnant particles (IDL) has also been report-[e]d.[16] Elevated triglyceride concentrations occur in diabetes because of increased [sy]nthesis and decreased degradation. Triglyceride synthesis is stimulated by [in]creased concentrations of glucose and fatty acids. Decreased hydrolysis of [tr]iglycerides in diabetes occurs because of impaired insulin-stimulated lipopro-[te]in lipase activity. For diabetic patients, elevated triglyercides are a strong pre-[d]ictor of cardiovascular disease.[36,41] However, this may also reflect the contribu-[ti]on of diabetes to cardiovascular disease since, with improved glucose control,

triglyceride levels tend to normalize.[34,42] In addition to triglyceride abnormalities, HDL levels are frequently low in type II (non-insulin–dependent) diabetes, even after they are corrected for obesity.[3,44]

Pharmacologic use of hormones can also affect lipid profiles. Estrogens increase HDL and lower total cholesterol; use of progestins is associated with decreased HDL levels.[19,21] Anabolic steroids also appear to raise LDL concentrations.

Obstructive liver disease blocks the only path of cholesterol excretion and results in hypercholesterolemia. Impaired secretion of bile and bile acids will decrease their synthesis and cause downward regulation of LDL (apo B,E) receptors.

The nephrotic syndrome is frequently associated with hypercholesterolemia. Hypoalbuminemia stimulates lipoprotein synthesis and increases LDL. An increase in VLDL is periodically observed and is mostly due to impaired metabolism. In more chronic cases, hypertriglyceridemia is also observed. With the development of renal failure, VLDL predominates because of impaired LPL activity. The increase in VLDL and IDL produces the common finding of hypertriglyceridemia.[7,35]

FIGURE 17.27 CAUSES OF SECONDARY HYPERLIPIDEMIAS

Hypothyroidism
Noninsulin-dependent diabetes mellitus
Drugs that raise LDL-cholesterol levels
  Progestins
  Anabolic steroids
Obstructive liver disease
Nephrotic syndrome
Chronic renal failure

(Reproduced with permission; see Figure Credits)

FIGURE CREDITS

Figs. 17.2–17.7, 17.9–17.11, 17.13, 17.14, 17.19, 17.20 redrawn from Grundy SM: Cholesterol and Atherosclerosis: Diagnosis and Treatment. Gower, New York, 1990.

Fig. 17.2 from Keys A: Coronary heart disease in seven countries. Circulation 41(suppl 1): 1–211, 1970.

Fig. 17.4 modified from Martin MJ, Hulley SB, Browner WS, et al: Serum cholesterol, blood pressure, and mortality: implications from a cohort of 361,662 men. Lancet 2: 933–936, 1986.

Fig. 17.5 adapted from Lipid Research Clinics Program. The Lipid Research Clinics Coronary Primary Prevention Trial results. I. Reduction in incidence of coronary heart disease. JAMA 251: 351–364, 1984; and Trial results II. The relationship of reduction in incidence of coronary heart disease to cholesterol lowering. JAMA 251: 365–374, 1984.

Fig. 17.8 modified from Mahley RW: Biochemistry and physiology of lipid and lipoprotein metabolism. In Becker AE, et al (ed): Principles and Practice of Endocrinology. JB Lippincott, Philadelphia, 1990.

Figs. 17.10, 17.11, 17.13 modified from Brown MS, Goldstein JL:Receptor-mediated pathway for cholesterol homeostasis. Science 232: 34–47, Copyright 1986 by the AAAS.

Fig. 17.14 redrawn from Steinberg D: Metabolism of lipoproteins and their role in the pathogenesis of atherosclerosis. In Stokes J III, Mancini M (eds): Hypercholesterolemia: Clinical and therapeutic implications. Atheroscler Rev 18:13, 1988.

Fig. 17.18 modified from Grundy SM: Cholesterol and Atherosclerosis: Diagnosis and Treatment. Gower, New York, 1990.

Fig. 17.21 adapted from the Lipid Research Clinics Population Studies Data Book. Vol 1, The Prevalence Study. NIH Publication No. 79–1527. Bethesda, MD, July 1979.

Fig. 17.23 modified from Schaeffer EJ: Hyperlipoproteinemias and other lipoprotein disorders. In Becker AE, et al (ed): Principles and Practice of Endocrinology. JB Lippincott, Philadelphia, 1990.

Figs. 17.24–17.27 courtesy of Jean Davignon, MD, Montreal, Canada.

REFERENCES

1. Anderson KM, Castelli WP, Levy D: Cholesterol and mortality: 30 years of follow-up from the Framingham study. JAMA 257:2176, 1987.
2. Berg K, Dahlen G, Frick MH: Lp(a) lipoprotein and pre-b₁-lipoprotein in patients with coronary heart disease. Clin Genet 6:230, 1974.
3. Biesbroeck RC, Albers JJ, Wahl PW, et al: Abnormal composition of high density lipoproteins in non-insulin dependent diabetics. Diabetes, 31:126, 1982.
4. Breckinridge WC, Little A, Steiner G, et al: Hypertriglyceridemia associated with a deficiency of apolipoprotein C-II. N Engl J Med 298:1265, 1978.
5. Brewer HB Jr, Zech LA, Gregg RE, et al: Type III hyperlipoproteinemia diagnosis, molecular defects, pathology, and treatment. Ann Intern Med 98:623, 1983.
6. Brown MS, Goldstein JL: Lipoprotein receptors in the liver. Control signals for plasma cholesterol traffic. J Clin Invest 72:743, 1983.
7. Camejo F, Riera G, Lee M, et al: Lipoprotein structural abnormalities in chronic renal failure with and without hemodialysis. Biomed Biochem Acta, 47:239, 1988.
8. Fogelman AM, Haberland ME, Seager J, et al: Factors regulating the activities of the low-density lipoprotein receptor and the scavenger receptor on human monocyte-macrophages. J Lipid Res 22:1131, 1981.
9. Frick MH, Elo O, Haapa K, et al: Helsinki heart study: Primary-prevention trial with gemfibrozil in middle-aged men with dyslipidemia. Safety of treatment, changes in risk factors and incidence of coronary heart disease. N Engl J Med 20:317, 1987.
10. Fulwood R, Kalsbeck W, Rifkind B, et al: Total serum cholesterol levels of adults 20-74 years of age: United States 1976-1980. National Center for Health Statistics. Ser. II, No. 236. DHHS Pub No. (PHS) 86-1686. Public Health Service United States Gov't. Printing Office. Washington DC, May 1986.
11. Ginsberg HN: Lipoprotein physiology and its relation to atherogenesis. Endo Metab Clin No Amer, 19:211, 1990.
12. Goldstein JL, Schrott HG, Hazzard WR, et al: Hyperlipidemia in coronary heart disease. II. Genetic analysis of lipid levels in 176 families and delineation of a new inherent disorder, combined hyperlipidemia. J Clin Invest 52:1544, 1973.

13. Grundy SM: Cholesterol and Atherosclerosis: Diagnosis and Treatment. Gower, New York 1990.

14. Grundy SM, Mok HYI, Zech LA, et al: Transport of very low density lipoprotein triglyceride in varying degrees of obesity and hypertriglyceridemia. J Clin Invest 63:1274, 1979.

15. Grundy SM, Vega GL, Bilheimer DW: Kinetic mechanisms determining variability in low density lipoprotein levels and their rise with age. Arteriosclerosis 5:623, 1985.

16. Hughes TA, Clements RS, Fairclough PR, et al: Effects of insulin therapy on lipoproteins in non-insulin dependent diabetes mellitus (NIDDM). Atherosclerosis 67:105, 1987.

17. Innerarity TL, Kempner ES, Hui DY, et al: Functional unit of the low density lipoprotein receptor of fibroblasts: A 100,000 dalton structure with multiple binding sites. Proc Nat Acad Sci 78:4378, 1981.

18. Kita T, Ishii K, Yokode M, et al: The role of oxidized low-density lipoprotein in the pathogenesis of atherosclerosis. Eur Heart J 11 (suppl):122, 1990.

19. Knopp RH, Walden CE, Wahl PW, et al: Oral contraception and postmenopausal estrogen effects on lipoprotein triglyceride and cholesterol in an adult female population. J Clin Endocrinol Metab 53:1123, 1981.

20. Kodama T, Freeman M, Rohrer L, et al: Type I macrophage scavenger receptor contains a helical and collagen-like coiled coils. Nature 343:531, 1990.

21. Kugiyama K, Kerns SA, Morrisett JD, et al: Impairment of endothelium-dependent arterial relaxation by lysolecithin in modified low-density lipoproteins. Nature 344:160 1990.

22. Leren P: The Oslo diet-heart study. Eleven-year report. Circulation 76:515, 1987.

23. Lithell H, Boberg J, Hellsing K, et al: Serum lipoprotein and apolipoprotein concentrations and tissue lipoproteins lipase activity in overt and subclinical hypothyroidism: The effects of substitution therapy. Eur J Clin Invest 11:3, 1981.

24. Mahley RW: Apolipoprotein E: Cholesterol transport protein with expanding role in cell biology. Science 240:622, 1988.

25. Mahley RW: Atherogenic lipoproteins and coronary artery disease: Concepts derived from recent advances in cellular and molecular biology. Circulation 72:943, 1985.

26. Mahley RW, Innerarity TL, Rall SC Jr, et al: Lipoproteins of special significance in atherosclerosis: Insights provided by studies of type III hyperlipoproteinmia. Ann NY Acad Sci 454:209, 1985.

27. Martin JH, Hulley SB, Browner WS, et al: Serum cholesterol, blood pressure, and mortality: Implications from a cohort of 361,662 men. Lancet 2:933, 1986.

28. Miller NE, Thelle DS, Forde OH, et al: The Tromso heart study. High-density lipoproteins as a protective factor against coronary heart disease: A prospective case-control study. Lancet I:965, 1977.

29. Miller M, Kwiterovich PO Jr.: Isolated low HDL-cholesterol as an important risk factor for coronary heart disease. Eur Heart J 11(suppl):9, 1990.

30. Nikkila E, Kekki M: Plasma triglyceride metabolism in thyroid disease. J Clin Inve: 51:2103, 1973.

31. O'Hara DD, Porte D Jr, Williams RH: The effect of diet and thyroxine on plasm lipids in myxedema. Metabolism 15:123, 1966.

32. Quinn MT, Parthasarathy S , Fong LG, et al: Oxidatively modified low-densit lipoproteins: A potential role in recruitment and retention of monocyte/macrophag: during atherogenesis. Proc Nat Acad Sci 84:2995, 1987.

33. Rabkin SW, Boyko E, Streja DA: Change in high density lipoprotein cholester after initiation of insulin therapy in non-insulin dependent diabetes mellitu Relationship to changes in body weight. Am J Med Sci 285:14, 1983.

34. Ron D, Aviram M, Better OS, et al: Accumulation of lipoprotein remnants i patients with chronic renal failure. Atherosclerosis 46:67, 1983.

35. Santen RJ, Willis PJ, Fajans SS: Atherosclerosis in diabetes mellitus. Correlations wit serum lipid levels, adiposity, and serum insulin levels. Arch Intern Med 130:833, 1972.

36. Schaefer EJ, Levy RI: The pathogenesis and management of lipoprotein disorders. Engl J Med 312:1300, 1985.

37. Schwandt P: The TG controversy: A review of the data. Eur Heart J 11(suppl):3 1990.

38. Sirtoli CR, Mancini M, Paoletti R: Consensus: Hypertriply ceridensa as a vascula risk factor. Eur Heart J 11(suppl):44, 1990.

39. Sniderman AD, Wolfson C, Teng B, et al: Association of hyperapobetalipoprotein mia with endogenous hypertriglyceridemia and atherosclerosis. Ann Intern Me 97:833, 1982.

40. Solerte SB, Carnevale-Schiana GP, Adamo S, et al: Lipid and lipoprotein changes i diabetes mellitus in relation to metabolic control and vascular degenerative compli cations. Med Biol Environ 13:755, 1985.

41. Sosenki JM, Breslow J, Miettinen OS, et al: Hyperglycemia and plasma lipid level Covariation in insulin-dependent diabetes. Diab Care 5:40, 1982.

42. Steinberg D, Corew TE, Fielding C, et al: Lipoproteins and the pathogenesis of athe osclerosis. Circulation. 80:719, 1989.

43. Taskinen MR, Nikkila EA, Kuusi T, et al : Lipoprotein lipase activity and serur lipoproteins in untreated type 2 (insulin-independent) diabetes associated with obesi ty. Diabetologia 22:46, 1982.

44. Thompson GR, Soutar AK, Spengel FA, et al: Defects of receptor mediated low den sity lipoprotein catabolism in homozygous familial hypercholesterolemia an hypothyroidism. Proc Soc Nat Acad Sci 78:2591, 1981.

45. Tolleshaug J, Hobgood KK, Brown MS, et al: The LDL receptor locus in familia hypercholesterolemia: Multiple mutations disrupt transport and processing of a mem brane receptor. Cell 32:941, 1983.

46. Utermann GM, Jaescke J, Menzel J: Familial hyperlipoproteinemia type III deficienc of a specific apolioprotein (apo E-III) in the very low density lipoproteins. FEBS Let 56:352, 1985.

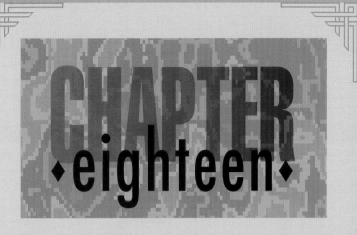

CHAPTER ·eighteen·

OBESITY AND THE HEART

ANN WARD, PhD

JAMES M. RIPPE, MD

J. WILLIS HURST, MD

JAMES K. ALEXANDER, MD

ANTON E. BECKER, MD

Obesity is a major public health problem because of its prevalence and association with morbidity and mortality. About 25% of adults in the United States are overweight, which is defined as 20% above ideal weight.[14] Obesity in children is increasing and, in a high percentage of cases, obesity in childhood leads to obesity in the adult.

Obesity is related to diabetes, hyperlipidemia, hypertension, coronary artery disease, sudden death, respiratory problems, gallbladder disease, and some cancers.[14] The health risks are curvilinear, increasing progressively and disproportionately with the increasing degree of overweight. The purpose of this chapter is to define obesity and emphasize the relationship between obesity and coronary artery disease, hypertension, and cardiomyopathy.

Height–weight charts such as the Metropolitan Life Insurance tables[13] and body mass index (BMI) (weight in kg/height[2] in m) have been used to evaluate obesity in population studies since these measures are simpler to make. The BMI shows the highest correlation with independent measures of body fat. A simple nomogram to calculate BMI is given in Figure 18.1.[7] A BMI above 25 is associated with increased morbidity and mortality.

Coronary Heart Disease and Obesity

Prospective studies of cardiovascular morbidity and mortality have shown an association with obesity. Whether obesity is an independent risk factor for coro-

nary heart disease (CHD) is still a matter of debate. Hubert et al.[8] have presented evidence from the Framingham Heart Study that it is; Alexander,[1] on the other hand, has reviewed the evidence accrued from other epidemiologic studies, as well as angiographic and pathologic studies, and has concluded that obesity is not an independent risk factor. Barrett-Connor[6] reached the same conclusion. However, recent results from the Nurse's Health Study[12] indicate that even mild-to-moderate overweight measurements increased the risk of coronary disease in middle-aged women.

Whether or not obesity presents an independent risk for CHD, it is unquestionably associated with other established risk factors of heart disease. The relative risk for hypertension for overweight adults aged 20 to 75 years is three times greater than that for non-overweight adults; the relative risk of elevated cholesterol is 1.5 and the relative risk of diabetes is 2.9 (Fig. 18.2).[17] When the data were analyzed by age, overweight adults aged 20 to 44 years were at greater risk of developing hypertension, elevated cholesterol, or diabetes. Obesity is also related to low levels of high-density lipoprotein (HDL) cholesterol and hypertriglyceredemia.

Hypertension and Obesity

As body mass increases, the incidence of hypertension is greater. Hemodynamic studies have shown that obesity is associated with an expanded blood volume

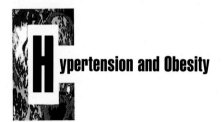

FIGURE 18.1 Nomogram for determining body mass index. A straight edge is placed from patient's weight to height to indicate the body mass index, which is measured in metric units. (Redrawn with permission; see Figure Credits)

d elevated cardiac output. Normotensive obese persons have reduced periph-al vascular resistance, while in obese hypertensive people peripheral vascular sistance is normal or elevated.

Not only is hypertension more frequent in obese people than in those of nor-al weight, but weight gain in young adults is a potent risk factor for subsequent velopment of hypertension. In addition, recent studies have suggested an sociation between distribution of body fat and blood pressure. Centrally locat-or upper body fat (high waist-to-hip ratio) is positively related to levels of th systolic and diastolic blood pressure.

A mechanism associating upper body fat distribution to hyperinsulinemia and pertension has been suggested (Fig. 18.3).[9] According to this mechanism, creased androgenic activity (as seen in males in general and in some women) the presence of a positive energy balance leads to deposition of fat in the domen and upper body. Obesity is accompanied by an increase in pancreatic insulin secretion and hyperinsulinemia reflecting peripheral insulin resistance. Abdominal fat is more responsive to adrenergic agonists that stimulate lipolysis, resulting in greater release of free fatty acids into the portal circulation. These fatty acids cause hypertriglyceridemia and appear to interfere with insulin clear-ance by the liver. The hyperinsulinemia may elevate blood pressure by (1) reducing urinary sodium excretion, which results in volume expansion; and (2) increasing plasma norepinephrine which also increases sodium reabsorption. This mechanism may explain why some, but not all, obese individuals develop hypertension.

Other suggested mechanisms for hypertension accompanying obesity include abnormal aldosterone–renin relationships and increased noradrenergic activity due to overfeeding. As body weight increases, the aldosterone/renin activity ratio rises due to a progressive fall in plasma renin activity. In addition, studies have shown that fasting and refeeding influence catecholamine metabolism.

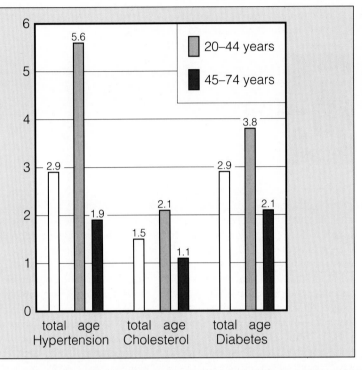

FIGURE 18.2 Relative risk for hypertension, cholesterol, and elevated serum cholesterol in overweight American adults. (Reproduced with permis-sion; see Figure Credits)

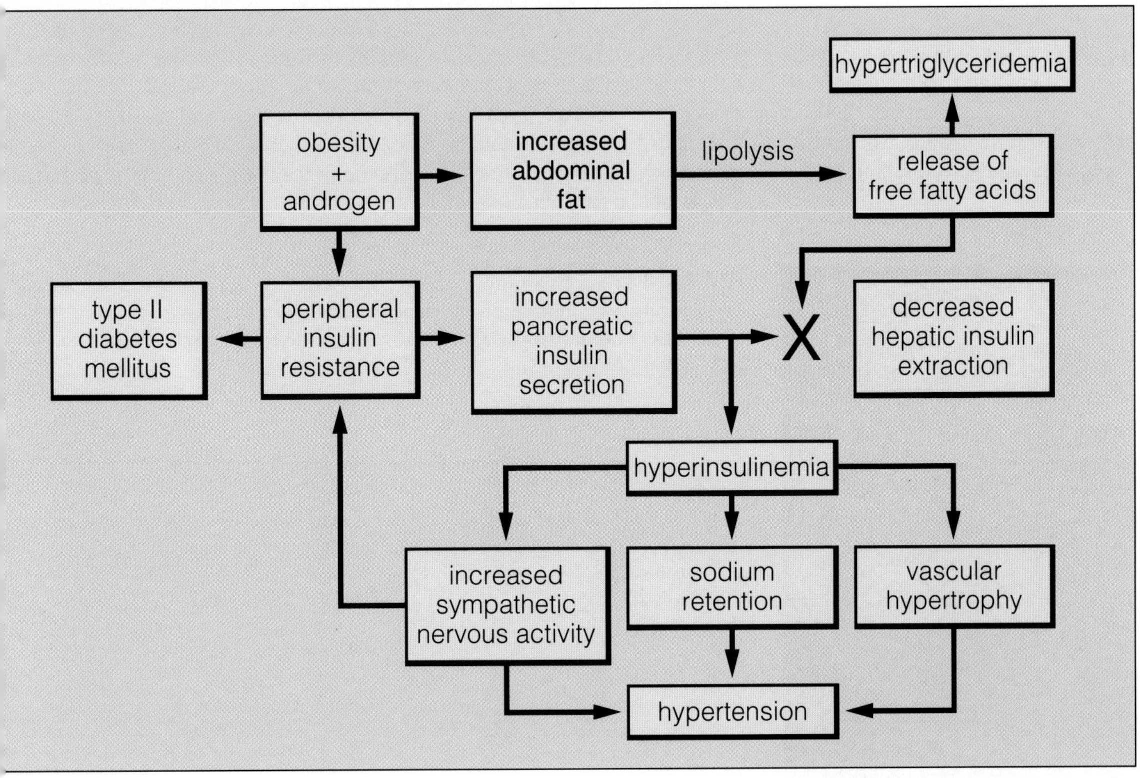

FIGURE 18.3 Proposed mecha-nism for the development of hyper-insulinemia. (Redrawn with permis-sion; see Figure Credits)

Cardiomyopathy of Obesity

Very obese patients have left ventricular hypertrophy and, at times, right ventricular hypertrophy. Heart failure is often seen. Fatty infiltration of the heart muscle, including the conduction system, may be seen, but this abnormality rarely causes any difficulty (Fig. 18.4).

Patients who are extremely obese have altered hemodynamics. Notably there is an increase in circulating blood volume, a normal or slightly increased hematocrit, an increase in cardiac output, an increase in stroke volume, and a slight increase in the arteriovenous oxygen difference, as compared to subjects of normal weight. Cerebral blood flow is normal; renal blood flow may be slightly less than it is in normal subjects. The splanchnic blood flow, in contrast, may be increased as compared with subjects who are not obese.

The majority of extremely obese patients have pulmonary hypertension and systemic hypertension with high cardiac output. The left ventricular end-diastolic pressure is elevated both at rest and during exercise.[2] Recent studies indicate that the heart failure seen in extremely obese patients may be due to one of two mechanisms. Some patients develop "diastolic" heart failure because of volume overload in the setting of decreased ventricular compliance.[4] Other patients develop heart failure associated with myocardial systolic dysfunction. The prognosis appears to be better in patients with diastolic dysfunction of the myocardium. The two types of heart failure can be distinguished by echocardiography, nuclear scanning, or angiography. These patients may have recurrent bouts of worsening heart failure or sudden death, the latter perhaps as a consequence of atrial arrhythmias and conduction defects.[5]

Sleep Apnea

About 50% of patients with sleep apnea are obese. The condition occurs more often in middle-aged men than women. The systemic and pulmonary blood pressures rise during apnea; at the same time the Po_2 decreases and the Pco_2 rises. Cardiac arrhythmias, such as sinus arrest, asystole, high-grade atrioventricular block, and ventricular tachycardia, also occur, possibly precipitating sudden death.[10,15,16]

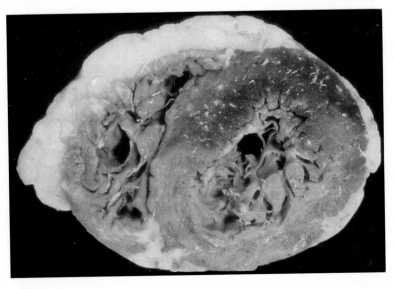

Obesity Hypoventilation Syndrome

A small percent of obese patients have hypoventilation, hypoxemia, hypercardia, respiratory acidosis, and erythrocytosis. This chronic syndrome often begins with sleep apnea, which dulls the hypoxic drive for ventilation. There is also decreased chest wall compliance, an increase in the work of breathing, and a decrease in the ventilatory response to CO_2. Chronic hypoxemia induces pulmonary arteriolar constriction, which, when added to the hemodynamic effects of obesity, imposes an increase in pulmonary and arterial venous pressures. This all leads to biventricular hypertrophy and failure; rarely these are associated with predominant right ventricular dysfunction.

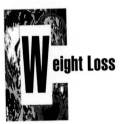

Weight Loss

Treatment of obesity may reduce cardiovascular mortality by decreasing blood pressure, cholesterol, triglycerides, and glucose intolerance and by increasing HDL cholesterol. The obese patient with angina pectoris due to coronary atherosclerosis is likely to experience fewer episodes of angina when extra weight is significantly diminished. Weight reduction is also a treatment component for obesity hypoventilation syndrome (OHS).

In addition, weight loss has been shown to decrease left ventricular hypertrophy and improve depressed systolic and diastolic cardiac function.[18] Because weight loss reduces the elevated preload and afterload typical of the severely obese patient, it may be beneficial in the prevention and control of congestive cardiac failure.

Many strategies for losing weight have been tried. However, patients often find keeping weight off extremely difficult. Of patients who lose weight, 80% to 100% regain it. Recent data from the Framingham Heart Study[11] indicate that men and women who repeatedly gained and lost weight had increased mortality from CHD and morbidity due to CHD. Consequently, strategies are needed to help patients lose weight and keep it off. Combining a weight loss diet with a moderate exercise program that includes both aerobic and resistance activities may help patients maintain weight loss. Not only does this type of exercise increase energy expenditure, but it also helps maintain lean body mass and resting metabolic rate, which normally decrease with a caloric-restricted diet.

FIGURE 18.4   Heart of an obese patient displaying excessive epicardial fat deposits with infiltration of myocardium. With the macro-enzyme staining technique, viable myocardium stains purple. (Reproduced with permission; see Figure Credits)

ACKNOWLEDGMENT

This chapter is based in part on Alexander JK: The heart and obesity. In Hurst JW (ed): The Heart, 6th ed. McGraw-Hill, New York, 1986.

FIGURE CREDITS

Fig. 18.1 redrawn from Bray GA: Definitions, measurements and classifications of the syndromes of obesity. Int J Obes 2:99, 1978.

Fig. 18.2 data from Van Itallie TB: Health implications of overweight and obesity in the United States. Ann Int Med 103:983–988, 1985.

Fig. 18.3 modified and redrawn from Kaplan NM: The Deadly Quartet: Upper-body obesity, glucose intolerance, hypertriglyceridemia, and hypertension. Arch Intern Med 149:1514, 1989.

Fig. 18.4 from Hurst JW (ed): Atlas of the Heart. Gower, New York, 1988.

REFERENCES

Alexander JK: Obesity and coronary heart disease. In Conner WE, Bristow JD (eds): Coronary Heart Disease, Prevention, Complications and Treatment. JB Lippincott, Philadelphia, 1985.

Alexander JK, Peterson KL: Cardiovascular effects of weight reduction. Circulation 45:310, 1972.

Alexander JK, Pettigrove JR: Obesity and congestive heart failure. Geriatrics 22:101, 1967.

Alexander JK, Woodard CB, Quinones MA, et al: Heart failure from obesity. In Mancini M, Lewis B, Cantaldo F (eds): Medical Complications of Obesity. Academic Press, London, 1978.

Balsaver M, Morales AR, Whitehouse FW: Fat infiltration of myocardium as a cause of cardiac conduction defect. Am J Cardiol 19:216, 1967.

6. Barrett-Connor EL: Obesity, atherosclerosis and coronary artery disease. Ann Intern Med 101:1010, 1985.

7. Bray GA: Definitions and classifications of the syndromes of obesity. Int J Obes 2:99, 1978.

8. Hubert HB, Feinleib M, McNamara PM, et al: Obesity as an independent risk factor for cardiovascular disease: A 26-year follow-up of participants in the Framingham Heart Study. Circulation 67:968, 1983.

9. Kaplan NM: The deadly quartet: Upper-body obesity, glucose intolerance, hypertriglyceridemia, and hypertension. Arch Intern Med 149:1514, 1989.

10. Kryger M, Quesney LP, Holder D, et al: The sleep deprivation syndrome of the obese patient. Am J Med 56:531, 1974.

11. Lissner L, Odell PM, D'Agostino RB, et al: Variability of body weight and health outcomes in the Framingham population. N Engl J Med 324:1839, 1991.

12. Manson JE, Graham AC, Stampfer MJ, et al: A prospective study of obesity and risk of coronary heart disease in women. N Engl J Med 322:882, 1990.

13. Metropolitan Life Insurance Company. Metropolitan height and weight tables. Stat Bull 64:2, 1983.

14. Pi-Sunyer FX: Obesity. In Shils ME, Young VR (eds): Modern Nutrition in Health and Disease, 16th ed. Lea & Febiger, Philadelphia, 1988.

15. Schroeder JS, Motta J, Guilleminault C: Hemodynamic studies in sleep apnea. In Guilleminault C, Dement WC (eds): Sleep Syndromes. Alan R. Liss, New York, 1978.

16. Tilkian A, Motta J, Guilleminault C: Cardiac arrhythmias. In Guilleminault C, Dement WC (eds): Sleep Syndromes. Alan R. Liss, New York, 1978.

17. Van Itallie T: Health implications of overweight and obesity in the United States. Ann Intern Med 103:983, 1985.

18. Webb JG, Birmingham CL: Cardiac effects of dieting. Prac Cardiol 14:104, 1987.

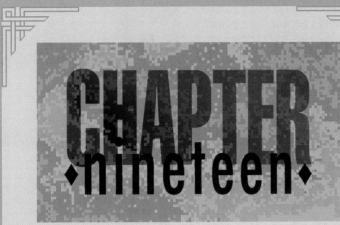

CHAPTER
nineteen

AGING OF THE CARDIOVASCULAR SYSTEM

J. V. NIXON, MD

CAROLYN A. BURNS, MD

It is generally accepted that aging accompanied by a more sedentary lifestyle produces a linear decline in the functional capabilities of the human body. This decline is represented physiologically by a reduction in the cardiovascular and pulmonary reserves and a decrease in strength and endurance of the musculoskeletal system.[4,44] From a cardiovascular perspective, changes in the structure and function of the heart and the peripheral vasculature are seen.[50] In particular, left ventricular function becomes the ultimate determinant for the assessment of aging changes in myocardial tissue structure and functional capability, together with its response to hormonal and other physiologic interventions.[50]

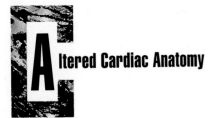

ltered Cardiac Anatomy

Relatively recently, autopsy review has documented a gradual increase in cardiac weight with age (Fig. 19.1).[31] The advent of noninvasive cardiac imaging techniques has permitted the documentation of increasing left ventricular mass and wall thickness with age.[15,17,39,46] A series of endomyocardial biopsies in older patients has shown that this age-related increase in left ventricular mass is due principally to a cellular hypertrophy, rather than hyperplasia, similar to that classically associated with valvular disease or hypertension.[49] These findings do not necessarily contrast with experimental reports of age-related loss of cardiac myocytes associated with an increase in fibrous tissue, both associated with clinical hypertrophy.[24]

The Baltimore Longitudinal Study on Aging has provided further evidence of altered cardiac anatomy with aging. Aortic root dilatation and left atrial enlargement are both associated with increasing age.[17] All these changes appear to be adaptive in response to the increased systolic pressure and the altered diastolic compliance associated with the normal process of aging.

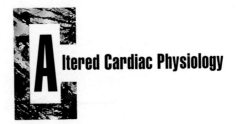

ltered Cardiac Physiology

Several age-related changes have been demonstrated in a series of experimental studies of cardiac function (Fig. 19.2). In vitro studies have shown that relaxation of cardiac muscle is prolonged by aging, due to age-related changes in the sarcoplasmic reticulum of cardiac muscle, and manifested by prolonged contraction duration and myocardial relaxation time without altering time to peak tension.[28] These findings are consistent with studies documenting an age-related increase in dynamic stiffness in the aged myocardium.[47] Other studies have shown a diminished intrinsic inotropic response to norepinephrine and to ouabain, as well as to sympathetic stimulation by isoproterenol.[18,29]

Further in vitro studies have shown that a number of myocardial cellular functional characteristics remain unchanged. Active tension, maximal rate of tension development (dt/dt), and time to peak tension are not age-dependent.[29] The inotropic response to mediators, such as calcium or postsystolic potentiation, that do not require cell-membrane receptors is also not age-dependent.[18,29] Furthermore, the time course of electrical depolarization and repolarization is not influenced by the aging process.[9,28]

Some of the age-related changes in the myocardium, such as prolonged contraction duration and changes in the sarcoplasmic reticulum, are remarkably

FIGURE 19.1 ALTERED ANATOMY OF PRESBYCARDIA

Increased cardiac weight
Increased left ventricular
  wall mass
Cardiac hypertrophy
Decreased myocytes
Dilated aortic root
Left atrial enlargement

FIGURE 19.2 ALTERED PHYSIOLOGY OF PRESBYCARDIA:

1. Changes
Prolonged contraction duration
Prolonged relaxation time
Diminished responses to ouabain, norepinephrine,
  and isoproterenol

2. No Changes
Active tension
Time to peak tension
Maximal rate of tension development

nilar to those associated with the increases in left ventricular mass.[21,26] It has en suggested that inactivity and gradual deconditioning may be responsible for ese age-related changes. Increased calcium transportation and faster myocar- al relaxation are both the results of physical training in animals.[5,35]

In vivo experimental studies have shown that the cardiac performance of older arts augmented by preloading with a dextran infusion remains unchanged (Fig. .3).[30] The addition of superimposed pressure loading by angiotensin II showed altered increase in stroke volume in older animals, suggesting an age-associ- ed decrease in the ventricular response to increased pressure afterload, despite augmentation of end-diastolic fiber length.[30] Other studies have shown an e-associated increase in diastolic stiffness in intact hearts.[48] Furthermore, an e-related increase in wall mass occurs in the absence of increased arterial pres- re, leading to the suggestion that age-related, increased left ventricular wall ass has a higher output impedance than that found in younger cardiovascular stems at all levels of dynamic exercise.[47,53]

With noninvasive imaging techniques, an accurate evaluation of cardiovascu- r structure and function can be made in a healthy elderly population.[20] While has been well established that the heart rate response to dynamic exercise and e heart rate and blood pressure responses to phenylephrine and isoprotenenol e attenuated in an elderly population,[19,36,42] the central cardiac effects of these anges were not known until recently. In normotensive elderly subjects, there an increase in stroke work and left ventricular wall thickness.[17,39] This latter nding appears to manifest physiologically as a reduction in diastolic filling, rticularly early diastolic filling.[15,16] Furthermore, it has been shown that, dur- g exercise, the older heart compensates for the attenuated heart rate response increasing end-diastolic and stroke volumes to preserve cardiac output.[39] hus, the increase in left ventricular wall mass in these older subjects serves to aintain a normal wall stress in the presence of increased left ventricular vol- nes during exercise.[27]

Maintenance of normal wall stress during other physiologic and pharmacologic terventions due to the adaptive changes associated with aging has been found.

Increases and decreases in volume preload by as much as 20% of the end-diastolic volume, while resulting in an attenuated end-diastolic and stroke volume response in older subjects, fails to significantly alter left ventricular wall stress.[34] Further- more, the administration of intravenous isoproterenol and phenylephrine to older subjects in doses sufficient to produce 25% increases in heart rate and mean blood pressure also failed to significantly alter left ventricular wall stress.[41] These find- ings are consistent with observations made in experimental studies.[30]

Recently, it has been shown that while diastolic stiffness estimated by direct measurements of end-diastolic volumes and pressures is increased in older normal people, this increase is very variable.[38] Furthermore, estimations of dynamic exercise performance in the same subjects and other similar stud- ies suggest that the experimental observations of change in left ventricular stiffness may be the result of gradual deconditioning.[6]

Altered Systemic Vascular Anatomy and Reflex Responses

Morphologically, there is a decrease in peripheral vascular distensibility or com- pliance with increasing age.[51] This alteration may be attributed to a decrease in vascular connective tissue elasticity or an increase in the prevalence of athero- sclerosis, or both.[23,51] In fact, there is a close inverse correlation between large vessel compliance and systolic blood pressure in older individuals.[45]

More information is readily available in humans regarding vascular reflex responses in the elderly (Fig. 19.4). It appears that the age-related alterations in peripheral vascular resistance found in the elderly are due to a combination of

---

FIGURE 19.3 ALTERED PHYSIOLOGY OF PRESBYCARDIA:

1. Changes
Increased LV wall thickness
Increased LV stroke work
Increased LV stroke volume during exercise
Increased LV diastolic stiffness
Decreased LV diastolic filling

2. No Changes
Normal LV wall stress at rest, during exercise, and during different physiological and pharmacological interventions

---

FIGURE 19.4 ALTERED PERIPHERAL VASCULATURE

STRUCTURE
Decreased distensibility
Increased prevalence of atherosclerosis

FUNCTION
Maintained alpha-adrenergic responsiveness
Decreased beta-adrenergic responsiveness
Altered dependence on calcium

vascular structural and functional changes. Studies of the alpha-adrenergic responsiveness in older individuals have produced variable results, but the data appear to suggest that it is unchanged with age.[2,13] Conversely, substantial data, both direct and indirect, exist to show that beta-adrenergic responsiveness is attenuated by age.[14,19,52] These changes appear to be confined to the sympathetic nervous system, as the responses to other vasodilators such as nitroglycerin are unaffected by age.[2,14] Furthermore, they effectively attenuate the cardiovascular response to stress with increasing age.[23,25] It has been suggested that the increasing peripheral vascular resistance in the elderly is due, at least in part, to the imbalance of alpha- and beta-adrenergic tone created by the gradual diminution of beta-adrenergic responsiveness, while alpha responsiveness remains unchanged.[3]

Serum calcium levels and the calcium ion appear to play a role in the increasing peripheral vascular resistance associated with age.[7,25] This was confirmed in both animals and humans by the dependence on extracellular calcium of the degree of norepinephrine-induced vascular contraction, and the favorable response of elderly patients to calcium antagonist therapy.[1,8,11,37]

Other Significant Alterations

Renal blood flow diminishes with age (Fig. 19.5).[33] The most likely cause for this is the gradual increase in renal vascular resistance, which is undoubtedly multifactorial (see discussion above). Glomerular filtration rate also appears to gradually fall off with increasing age.[32,40]

Plasma renin activity clearly decreases with age.[43] In the presence of congestive heart failure, however, the renin-angiotensin system becomes reactivated to maintain arterial perfusion pressures.[12] In contrast, norepinephrine levels rise with increasing age, particularly in normotensive subjects.[33] It has been suggested that these increases in plasma norepinephrine levels are due to the gradual reduction in beta-adrenergic responsiveness associated with aging.[32]

Intravascular volume appears to be maintained in the normal older individual.[10] However, the older normal subject appears to be sensitive to relatively small changes in intravascular volume compared to younger subjects.[34] In hypertensive elderly patients, there is a significant reduction in intravascular volume.

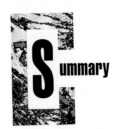

Summary

The anticipated decline in the structure and functional capabilities of the aging cardiovascular system has been described in some detail (Fig. 19.6). Significant increases in cardiac weight and left ventricular hypertrophy, together with dilatation of the aortic root and the left atrium, have been recorded with the histologic wastage of myocytes and the laydown of collagen fibrous tissue. Cellular changes include a prolonged contraction duration and relaxation time, together with a diminished response to digitalis glycosides, norepinephrine, and isoproterenol. Studies in humans have documented increased stroke volume during exercise, diastolic stiffness, and decreased diastolic filling. Vascular changes incorporate alterations in distensibility and impedance, with a decreased beta-adrenergic responsiveness and an altered dependence on calcium. Other significant age-related changes involving the cardiovascular system are a decrease in renal blood flow and glomerular filtration rate, an increase in renal vascular resistance (together with an increase in plasma norepinephrine levels), and a decrease in plasmic renin activity.

FIGURE 19.5 OTHER SIGNIFICANT CHANGES

Decrease in renal
   blood flow
Increase in renal
   vascular resistance
Decrease in glomerular filtration rate
Decrease in plasma renin activity
Increase in plasma
   norepinephrine
Intravascular volume maintained

FIGURE 19.6 ALTERATIONS IN THE AGING CARDIOVASCULAR SYSTEM

CENTRAL EFFECTS

Preload	Attenuated
Contractility	Not attenuated
Heart rate	Attenuated at all levels of exercise
Afterload	No attenuation

PERIPHERAL EFFECTS

Decreased distensibility
Decreased beta-adrenergic responsiveness
Altered dependence on calcium

◪ ACKNOWLEDGMENT

The authors wish to acknowledge Valerie Roy, RN, for her help with the literature search, and Jeanie Toombs for her assistance in preparing the manuscript.

◪ REFERENCES

1. Abernathy DR, Swartz JB, Todd EL, et al: Verapamil pharmacodynamics and disposition in young and elderly hypertensive patients: Altered electrocardiographic and hypotensive responses. Ann Intern Med 105:329, 1986.
2. Abrass IB: Catecholamine levels and vascular responsiveness in aging. In Horan MJ, Steinberg GM, Dunbar JB, et al (eds): Blood Pressure Regulation and Aging: An NIH Symposium. Biomedical Information, New York, 1986.
3. Applegate WB: Hypertension in elderly patients. Ann Intern Med 110:901, 1989.
4. Befitis H, Sargent F: Human physiological adaptibility through the life sequence. J Gerontol. 32:402, 1977.
5. Bersolm MM, Scheuer J: Effects of physical training on end-diastolic volumes and myocardial performance of isolated rat hearts. Circ Res 40:510, 1977.
6. Blumenthal JA, Emery CF, Madden DJ, et al: Effects of exercise training on cardiorespiratory function in men and women over 60 years of age. Am J Cardiol 67:633, 1991.
7. Bohr DF: Vascular smooth muscle: Dual effect of calcium. Science 139:597, 1963.
8. Bravo EL, Krakoff LR, Friedman CP: Antihypertensive effectiveness of nifedipine GITS in the elderly. Am J Hypertens 3:3265, 1990.
9. Caverto FV, Kelliher GJ, Roberts J: Electrophysiological changes in the rat atrium with age. Am J Physiol 225:1293, 1974.
10. Chien S, Usaim S, Simmons RL, et al: Blood volume and age: Repeated measurements on normal men after 17 years. J Appl Physiol 21:583, 1966.
11. Cohen ML, Berkowitz BA: Vascular contraction: Effective age and extracellular calcium. Blood Vess 13:139, 1976.
12. Dzau VJ, Colucci WS, Hollenberg NK, et al: Relation of the renin-angiotensin-aldosterone system to clinical state in congestive heart failure. Circulation 63:645, 1981.
13. Elliott HL, Sumner BJ, McLein K: Effect of age on vascular alpha responsiveness in man. Clin Sci 63:305S, 1982.
14. Fleisch JH, Hooker CS: The relationship between age and relaxation of vascular smooth muscle in the rabbit and rat. Circ Res 38:243, 1976.
15. Gardin JM, Henry WL, Savage DD, et al: Echocardiographic measurements in normal subjects: Evaluation of an adult population without clinically apparent heart disease. J Clin Ultra 7:439, 1979.
16. Gerstenblith G, Fleg JL, Becker LC: Maximum left ventricular filling rate in healthy individuals measured by gated blood pool scans: Effects of age. Circulation 68 (Suppl III):III-101, 1983.
17. Gerstenblith G, Fredrickson J, Yin FCP, et al: Echocardiographic assessment of a normal adult aging population. Circulation 56:273, 1977.
18. Gerstenblith G, Spurgeon HA, Froehlich JP, et al: Diminished inotropic responsiveness to ouabain in aged rat myocardium. Circ Res 54:517, 1979.
19. Gribbin B, Pickering TG, Sleight P, et al: Effect of age and high blood pressure on baroreflex sensitivity in man. Circ Res 29:424, 1971.
20. Harrison FR, Dixon K, Russell RO, et al: The relation of age to the duration of contraction, ejection and relaxation of the normal heart. Am Heart J 67:189, 1964.
21. Jordahl LA, McCollum WB, Wood WG, et al: Mitochondric and sarcoplasmic reticulum function in cardiac hypertrophy and failure. Am J Physiol 224:497, 1973.
22. Julius S, Antoon A, Whitlock LS, et al: Influence of age on the hemodynamic response to exercise. Circulation 36:222, 1967.
23. Kannel WB, Wolf PA, McGee DL, et al: Systolic blood pressure, arterial rigidity and risks of stroke: The Framingham Study. JAMA 245:1225, 1981.
24. Lakatta EG: Alterations in the cardiovascular system that occur with advanced age. Fed Proc 38:163, 1979.
25. Lakatta EG: Age-related alterations in the cardiovascular response to adrenergic-mediated stress. Fed Proc 39:3173, 1980.
26. Lakatta EG: Do hypertension and aging have a similar effect on the myocardium? Circulation 75 (Suppl I):I-69, 1987.
27. Lakatta EG: Is normotensive aging of the cardiovascular system a muted form of hypertensive cardiovascular disease? In Masserli FH (ed): The Heart and Hypertension. York Medical Books, New York, 1987.
28. Lakatta EG, Gerstenblith G, Angell CS, et al: Prolonged contraction duration in aged myocardium. J Clin Invest 55:61, 1975.
29. Lakatta EG, Gerstenblith G, Angell CS, et al: Diminished inotropic response of aged myocardium to catecholamines. Circ Res 44:517, 1979.
30. Lee JC, Karpeles LM, Downing SE: Age-related changes of cardiac performance in male rats. Am J Physiol 222:432, 1972.
31. Linzbach AJ, Aknamoa-Boateng E: Die Alernsversanderungen des wenschlichen Verzens. 1. Das Verzgenwicht in Alter. Klin Wochensk 51:156, 1973.
32. Masserli FH: Essential hypertension in the elderly. Nephron 24:35, 1985.
33. Masserli FH, Sundguard-Riise K, Ventina HO, et al: Essential hypertension in the elderly: Hemodynamics, intravascular volume, plasma renin activity and circulating catecholamine levels. Lancet 2:983, 1983.
34. Nixon JV, Hallmark H, Page P, et al: Ventricular performance in human hearts aged 61 to 73 years. Am J Cardiol 56:932, 1985.
35. Penpargkul S, Repke DI, Katz AM, et al: Effect of physical training on calcium transport by rat cardiac sarcoplasmic reticulum. Circ Res 40:134, 1977.
36. Pickering TG, Gribbin B, Petersen ES, et al: Effects of autonomic blockade on the baroreflex in man at rest and during exercise. Circ Res 30:177, 1972.
37. Pool PE, Massie BM, Venkatarat AN: Diltiazem as a model therapy for systemic hypertension: A multicenter, randomized, placebo-controlled trial. Am J Cardiol 57:212, 1982.
38. Porter TR, Arrowood JA, Roy V, et al: Effect of preload changes on altered left ventricular function characteristics of older normal subjects. Clin Res 38:4, 1990.
39. Rodeheffer RJ, Gerstenblith G, Becker LC, et al: Exercise cardiac output is maintained with advancing age in healthy human subjects: Cardiac dilatation and increased stroke volume compensate for diminished heart rate. Circulation 69:203, 1984.
40. Rowe JW, Chock NW, DeFronzo RA: The influence of age on the renal response to water deprivation in man. Nephron 17:270, 1976.
41. Sanchez E, Sweeney M, Nixon JV: Effects of isoproterenol and phenylephrine on cardiac function in the older normal heart. Clin Res 34:174, 1986.
42. Schlant RC, Blomquist CG, Brandenburg RO, et al: Guidelines for exercise testing. JACC 8:725, 1986.
43. Scott P, Giese J: Age and the renin-angiotensin system. Acta Med Scand (Suppl) 676:45, 1983.
44. Shock NW: Physiological aspects of aging in man. Ann Rev Physiol 23:97, 1961.
45. Simor AC, Safar MA, Levenson JA, et al: Systolic hypertension: Hemodynamic mechanism and choice of antihypertensive treatment. Am J Cardiol 44:505, 1979.
46. Sjogren AL: Left ventricular wall thickness in patients with circulatory overload of the left ventricle. Ann Clin Res 4:310, 1972.
47. Spurgeon HA, Thorne P, Yin FCP, et al: Changes in dynamic stiffness of aged rat myocardium. Am J Physiol 232:373, 1977.
48. Templeton GH, Platt MR, Willerson JT, et al: Influence of aging on left ventricular hemodynamics and stiffness in beagles. Circ Res 44:189, 1979.
49. Unverforth DV, Fetter JK, Unverforth BJ, et al: Human myocardial histologic characteristics in congestive heart failure. Circulation 68:1194, 1983.
50. Weisfeldt ML: Left ventricular function. In Weisfeldt ML (ed): The Aging Heart. Raven Press, New York, 1980.
51. Yin FCP: The aging vasculature and its effect on the heart. In Weisfeldt ML (ed): The Aging Heart. Raven Press, New York, 1980.
52. Yin FCP, Spurgeon HA, Greene HL, et al: Age-associated decrease in heart rate response to isoproterenol in dogs. Mech Aging Dev 10:15, 1979.
53. Yin FCP, Weisfeldt ML, Milnor WR: Role of aortic input impedance in the decreased cardiovascular response to exercise with aging in dogs. J Clin Invest 68:28, 1981.

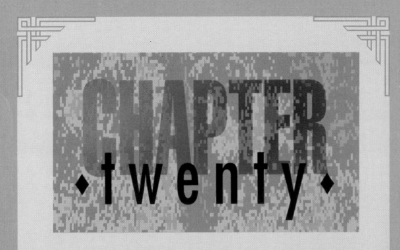

CHAPTER
◆ twenty ◆

ALCOHOL
AND THE HEART

J. WILLIS HURST, MD

TIMOTHY J. REGAN, MD

ANTON E. BECKER, MD

JOSEPH S. ALPERT, MD

Paul Dudley White[7] was among the first to call attention to the relationship of alcohol and cardiac dysfunction, arrhythmias, and angina. The advent of modern technology has permitted the identification of certain cardiac abnormalities that may be related to overconsumption of alcohol of any type. Experimental studies in normal animals and humans have generally documented that acute and chronic alcohol ingestion leads to myocardial and thus ventricular systolic and diastolic dysfunction. Alcohol also produces changes in preload and afterload that complicate the analysis of its effects on circulatory function. Ventricular dysfunction following alcohol administration is almost universally observed in patients with pre-existing heart disease (Figs. 20.1–20.4).[3,6]

FIGURE 20.1 HEMODYNAMIC RESPONSES TO WHISKEY (2 OZ) IN NORMAL SUBJECTS AND IN PATIENTS WITH CARDIAC DISEASE

TYPE	NORMALS	CARDIAC DISEASE
Heart rate	—	—
Cardiac index	⬆	⬇
Stroke index	⬆	⬇
Systolic vascular resistance??	⬇	⬆
Blood pressure	—	—
LV work	⬆	⬇
LV end-diastolic pressure	—	—

— = no change (Data from Gould L, et al: Cardiac effects of a cocktail. JAMA 218:1799, 1971)

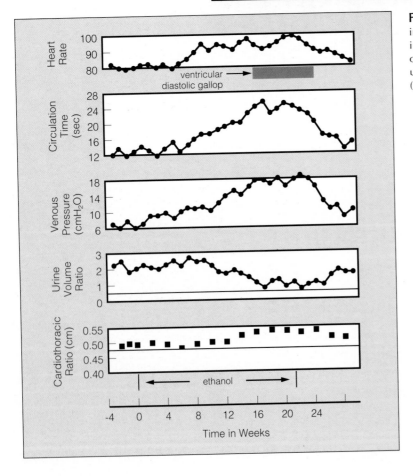

FIGURE 20.2   Ethanol and the well-fed patient. Observations were made in a single patient who received 12 to 16 oz of Scotch daily, which resulted in evidence of heart failure. Note the rise in resting heart rate, prolongation of circulation time, and elevation of venous pressure after 6 weeks. The failure regressed without medical treatment after alcohol intake was stopped. (Redrawn with permission; see Figure Credits)

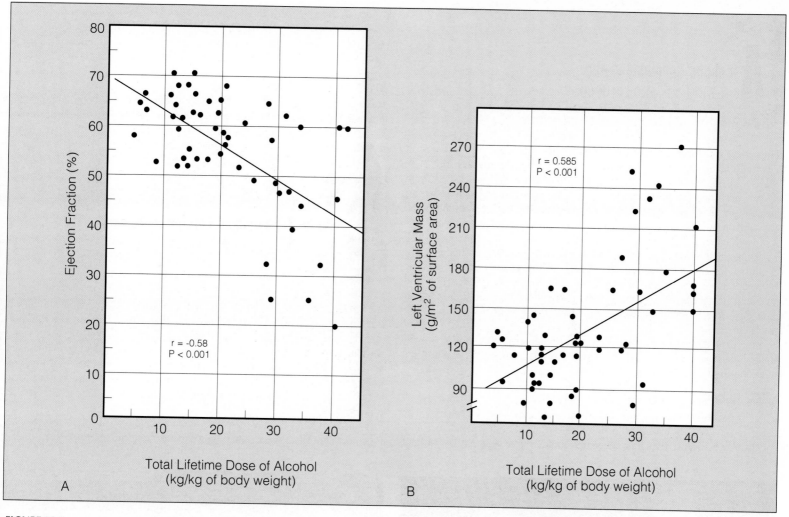

FIGURE 20.3   Correlation between the total lifetime consumption of ethanol and the left ventricular ejection fraction
(A) and left ventricular mass **(B)** in 52 alcoholic patients. (Redrawn with permission; see Figure Credits)

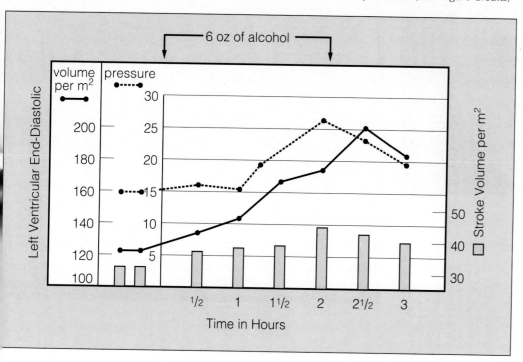

FIGURE 20.4   Ethanol in the cardiac patient.
Observations made during the ingestion of 6 oz
of Scotch by an alcoholic patient with cardiac
decompensation. A depressant effect on the left
ventricle is seen at a dose that has no effect in
the noncardiac alcoholic. (Redrawn with permission; see Figure Credits)

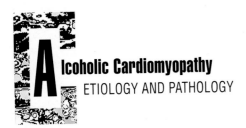

Alcoholic Cardiomyopathy
ETIOLOGY AND PATHOLOGY

The patient with alcoholic cardiomyopathy has ingested alcohol for many years. It is not possible to state that all patients who have cardiomyopathy and drink alcohol have alcoholic cardiomyopathy, because such patients often have hypertension or they may have had unrecognized viral myocarditis. There is, however, an increasing body of circumstantial evidence indicating that alcohol is harmful to the myocardium in certain susceptible patients. The biochemical derangement produced by alcohol within the myocardial cell is discussed by Sarma and colleagues.[5]

Prior to the development of heart failure, the asymptomatic alcoholic patient exhibits reduced cardiac contractility.[4] Early in the course of the illness the echocardiogram reveals a normal internal diameter of the left ventricle and increased ventricular wall thickness. Later in the illness there is evidence of an increase in the internal diameter of the heart with a normal ventricular wall thickness.[2]

The gross and microscopic pathology of the cardiomyopathy associated with alcohol abuse is nonspecific. In advanced stages the heart usually exhibits features of dilated cardiomyopathy (Fig. 20.5).

CLINICAL MANIFESTATIONS

The clinical features are those of dilated cardiomyopathy (see Chapter 8). The heart is enlarged with no diagnostic murmurs; atrial and ventricular gallop sounds may be heard. The chest radiograph shows a large heart with or without pulmonary congestion. The electrocardiogram (ECG) may show atrial fibrillation, other arrhythmias, or bundle branch block, while the echocardiogram displays a decrease in cardiac contractility. Heart failure ensues, gradually worsening over a period of months and years. Sudden death is common.

NATURAL HISTORY

The outcome for patients with alcoholic cardiomyopathy is poor. Patients may improve if abstinence from alcohol can be achieved and if heart damage is not too advanced. However, alcoholic patients often have damage to other organs, and there are no assurances that abstinence will be permanent.

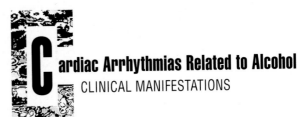

Cardiac Arrhythmias Related to Alcohol
CLINICAL MANIFESTATIONS

A cardiac arrhythmia may be the first sign of alcoholic heart disease although it is not usually appreciated as such at the time (Fig. 20.6). Patients with the "holiday heart" syndrome may not have clinical signs of cardiomyopathy.[1] These patients are often chronic users of alcohol who have cardiac arrhythmias in association with an acute binge. Supraventricular arrhythmias predominate, most commonly atrial fibrillation. Other arrhythmias and sudden death may occur. The exact chemical derangement that is responsible for the arrhythmias is not known.

A variety of ECG changes have been observed in chronic alcoholics; particularly common are ST–T wave changes and conduction disturbances (see Fig. 20.6).

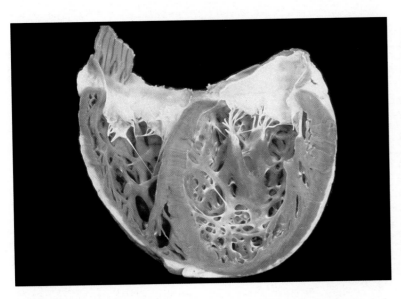

FIGURE 20.5   Cross section of the heart of a patient with chronic alcohol abuse shows dilation of both ventricular chambers, which is also seen in other types of dilated cardiomyopathy. (Reproduced with permission; see Figure Credits)

FIGURE 20.6 ECG FINDINGS IN PATIENTS WITH ALCOHOLIC CARDIOMYOPATHY (SUMMARY OF THE LITERATURE)

Rhythm disturbance
Sinus tachycardia
Premature ventricular contractions
Ventricular tachycardia
Ventricular fibrillation
Premature atrial contractions
Atrial fibrillation or flutter
Atrial tachycardia

Conduction disturbance
First-degree atrioventricular block
Left anterior hemiblock
Left posterior hemiblock
Left bundle-branch block

Right bundle-branch block
Intraventricular conduction defect

Atrial abnormality
Left atrial enlargement
Right atrial enlargement
Biatrial enlargement

Ventricular abnormality
Left ventricular hypertrophy
Right ventricular hypertrophy
Biventricular hypertrophy

Other abnormality
ST–T changes

(Adapted from Moushmoush B, and Abi-Monsour P: Alcohol and the heart. Arch Intern Med 151:38, 1991)

ACKNOWLEDGMENT

This chapter is based in part on Regan TJ: The heart, alcoholism, and nutritional disease. In Hurst JW (ed): The Heart, 6th ed. McGraw-Hill, New York, 1986.

FIGURE CREDITS

Fig. 20.1 data from Gould L, et al: Cardiac effects of a cocktail. JAMA 218:1799, 1971. Reproduced with permission.

Fig. 20.2 redrawn from Regan TJ, Levinson GE, Oldewurtel HA, et al: Ventricular function in noncardiacs with fatty liver: Role of ethanol in the production of cardiomyopathy. Reproduced from J Clin Invest 48:397, 1969 by copyright permission of the American Society for Clinical Investigation.

Fig. 20.3 redrawn from Urbano-Marquez A, Estruch R, Navarro-Lopez F, et al: The effects of alcoholism on skeletal and cardiac muscle. N Engl J Med 320:409, 1989.

Fig. 20.4 redrawn from Regan TJ, Haider B, Ahmed SS: Whiskey and the heart. Cardiovasc Med 165, Feb 1977.

Fig. 20.5 from Hurst JW (ed): Atlas of the Heart. Gower, New York, 1988.

Fig. 20.6 adapted from Moushmoush B, Abi-Monsour P: Alcohol and the heart. Arch Intern Med 151:38, 1991.

REFERENCES

1. Ettinger PO, Wu CF, de La Cruz C Jr, et al: Arrhythmias and the "holiday heart": Alcohol-associated cardiac rhythm disorders. Am Heart J 95:555, 1978.
2. Matthews EC Jr, Gardin JM, Henry WL, et al: Echocardiographic abnormalities in chronic alcoholics with and without overt congestive heart failure. Am J Cardiol 47:570, 1981.
3. Moushmoush B, Abi-Mansour P: Alcohol and the heart—The long-term effects of alcohol on the cardiovascular system. Arch Int Med 151:36, 1991.
4. Regan TJ, Levinson GE, Oldewurtel HA, et al: Ventricular function in noncardiacs with alcoholic fatty liver: Role of ethanol in the production of cardiomyopathy. J Clin Invest 48:397, 1969.
5. Sarma JSM, Shigeaki I, Eischer R, et al: Biochemical and contractile properties of heart muscle after prolonged alcohol administration. J Mol Cell Cardiol 8:951, 1976.
6. Urbano-Marquez A, Estruch R, Navarro-Lopez F, et al: The effects of alcoholism on skeletal and cardiac muscle. N Engl J Med 320:409, 1989.
7. White PD: Heart Disease. Macmillan, New York, 1951.

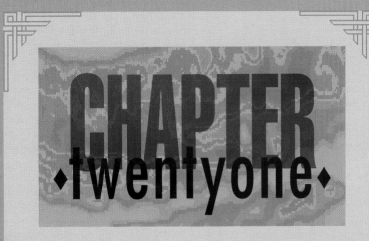

CHAPTER
◆twentyone◆

COCAINE AND THE HEART

JEFFREY M. ISNER, MD

Acute Myocardial Infarction

Among the alleged cardiac consequences of cocaine abuse, the one that has been reported most frequently is acute myocardial infarction.[4,6,7,9,12-15] At least 58 cases of acute myocardial infarction temporally related to cocaine abuse have been reported in the English language medical literature. All 58 reports were of young individuals, with a mean age of 32.6 years and an age range between 19 and 44 years. Of these 58 patients, 49 were male and 9 were female, a reflection, perhaps, of the demographics of cocaine use. Only 3 of these 58 individuals were first-time cocaine users; the remainder used cocaine on a chronic basis. Various routes of cocaine administration related to acute infarction were identified: intranasal in 38, intravenous in 17, inhalation by smoking in 1 and free-base/mixed form in 2. A history of pre-existing angina or prior myocardial infarction unrelated to cocaine use was positive in 18 of the 58 individuals; the 40 remaining persons had no antecedent cardiac history. Seven of the 58 (12%) individuals died as a complication of acute infarction.

The results of selective coronary angiography have been reported for 45 of the 58 above-mentioned patients in whom myocardial infarction was temporally related to cocaine use. Filling defects involving the infarct-related major epicardial coronary arteries were observed in 31 cases. These defects included occlusive lesions as well as focal stenoses. Intraluminal filling defects inferred to represent intracoronary thrombi were documented in 10 of 31 patients who received thrombolytic therapy (either streptokinase or tissue plasminogen activator) within 6 hours of onset of symptoms of acute infarction. Thrombolytic therapy was successful in lysing the clot and re-establishing patency of the "culprit" artery in all of these cases. In contrast, 14 of 45 (31%) patients were found to have angiographically normal epicardial coronary arteries; although 8 of these 14 patients underwent ergonovine provocative testing, all 8 failed to develop angiographic evidence of focal coronary narrowing.

The finding of intracoronary thrombus in cases of myocardial infarction related to cocaine abuse has been confirmed in multiple cases studied at necropsy. We previously reported on a 37-year-old man in whom cocaine-related acute infarction was associated with thrombotic occlusion of the left anterior descending coronary artery at the site of 90% cross-sectional area narrowing by atherosclerotic plaque.[7] Simpson and Edwards[12] observed platelet thrombi in one or more major coronary arteries of a 21-year-old cocaine user who died suddenly and at necropsy was found to have "microfocal" areas of fibrosis or granulation tissue that were interpreted to be ischemic in origin. Each of the major epicardial coronary arteries was severely narrowed by 50% to 95% in the cross-sectional area. Mittleman and Wetli reported 24 cases of sudden death associated with cocaine abuse and attributed the etiology in 15 of these to ischemic heart disease.[9] Two victims had evidence of acute infarction, while 10 others had gross or histologic findings of myocardial fibrosis. Complete thrombotic occlusion of one epicardial coronary artery was observed in three cases, while hemorrhage into an atherosclerotic plaque was observed in two. All cases were notable for the presence of severe focal arterial narrowing by atherosclerotic plaque in at least one major epicardial coronary artery.

Virmani et al.[15] studied two individuals at necropsy, one in whom there was "severe coronary atherosclerosis" and another in whom an occlusive platelet thrombus in the left anterior descending coronary artery was superimposed upon atherosclerotic plaque that had the native lumen by 40% in the cross-sectional area. Likewise, Stenberg et al.[13] observed underlying atherosclerotic plaque that narrowed the left anterior descending and right coronary arteries by 70% and 50%, respectively, in a 38-year-old man who died 13 hours after the onset of clinically documented acute myocardial infarction.

Finally, Dressler et al.[4] reported quantitative analysis of coronary arterial narrowing by atherosclerotic plaque among 22 chronic cocaine users studied at necropsy over a 10-year period. Of the 12 individuals in whom death was believed to be related to cocaine, at least one major epicardial coronary artery was narrowed by >96%, while in 6 cases, at least one artery was narrowed by 76% to 95%; 51% to 75% cross-sectional area narrowing was observed in all but cases. In 1 of these 12 cases, intracoronary thrombus was superimposed upon underlying atherosclerotic plaque; in this and 2 other of the 12 cases, examination of the myocardium disclosed microscopic foci of necrosis.

It is interesting to note that *qualitative assessment of the site of the thrombotic occlusion in these individuals at necropsy has failed to disclose evidence of plaque rupture, plaque fissure, or plaque hemorrhage.*[15] These findings have been routinely observed in noncocaine-related thrombotic coronary arterial occlusion. The absence of these features in cocaine-related infarction has been interpreted as evidence that cocaine-induced spasm, rather than plaque rupture, may constitute the primary event in the pathogenesis of infarction in cocaine users.

A second pathologic finding that has been cited to support the role of spasm in cocaine-related infarction is the finding of increased foci of contraction band necrosis in cases of cocaine-related deaths studied at necropsy.[14] This finding is also consistent with the concept that myocardial damage resulting from cocaine abuse may represent the consequence of cocaine-induced catecholamine excess, since contraction bands have been previously observed in association with pheochromocytoma and exogenous catecholamine administration.

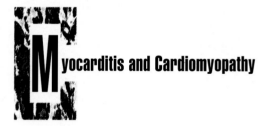

Myocarditis and Cardiomyopathy

Myocarditis temporally related to cocaine has been documented in vivo in a 25-year-old frequent cocaine user who used free-base cocaine twice on the day of hospital admission.[7] On arrival in the emergency room the patient was found to have complete heart block, which was treated with a transvenous temporary pacemaker. An endomyocardial biopsy performed one day after admission showed foci of myocyte necrosis and a diffuse inflammatory cell infiltrate, including eosinophils (Fig. 21.1). The patient was treated with prednisone and azothiaprine. Three days later, the patient's conduction disturbance resolved. Two weeks following admission, a second biopsy showed rare isolated foci of myocarditis. A biopsy obtained 6 months after admission, while the patient was believed to be abstaining from cocaine, was normal.

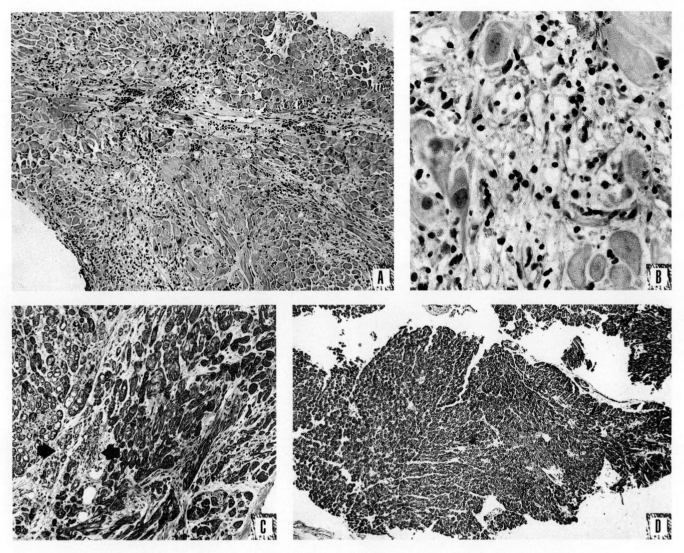

FIGURE 21.1　　Light photomicrographs of endomyocardial biopsy specimens in cocaine user with myocarditis. **(A)** Myocarditis is demonstrated (x90). **(B)** At higher magnification, a focus of mononuclear inflammatory cell infiltrate and myocyte necrosis is seen (x225). **(C)** A second specimen demonstates a persistent focus of myocarditis (x38). **(D)** The final specimen shows normal myocardium. (A–C, H&E stain; D, Masson trichrome stain) (Reproduced with permission; see Figure Credits)

In necropsy studies, evidence of myocarditis has been observed in as many as 17.5% of patients who died a natural or homicide-related death and had cocaine detected in their blood.[15] Several of the patients studied at necropsy were also observed to have a prominent eosinophilic component. The finding of eosinophils in patients with myocarditis, while by no means specific for cocaine, nevertheless raises the question of whether cocaine and/or accompanying contaminants could cause a drug-induced vasculitis/myocarditis.

Weiner et al.[16] reported on two patients in whom dilated cardiomyopathy was documented in association with cocaine abuse. In one, a 42-year-old male cocaine user with normal coronary arteries, recurrent myocardial infarctions appeared responsible for the development of a dilated, globally hypocontractile left ventricle. In the second patient, a 28-year-old woman who presented with signs and symptoms of biventricular dilation and failure, evidence of atherosclerotic coronary arterial narrowing was absent.

In at least one well-documented case, acute dilated cardiomyopathy temporally related to the use of free-base crack cocaine led to cardiogenic shock, unassociated with signs of acute infarction or biopsy evidence of myocarditis.[3] Two weeks later, however, serial echocardiograms showed reversal of the patient's cardiomyopathy with a marked improvement in left ventricular systolic function (Fig. 21.2). The patient's clinical course was similar to previously reported patients, with pheochromocytoma associated with the development of catecholamine cardiomyopathy. Biventricular dilation and reduced left ventricular ejection fraction proved reversible in these patients after surgical excision of the adrenal tumor. Such reversible depression of myocardial systolic function has been attributed to a direct "toxic" effect of high levels of circulating catecholamines on cardiac myocytes. Histologic examination of myocytes from these patients has typically shown "contraction-band necrosis." The argument that this disorder is analogous to cocaine-induced left ventricular dysfunction is compelling, both because of the profound sympathomimetic augmentation typical of cocaine and the previously noted finding of contraction-band necrosis at necropsy.

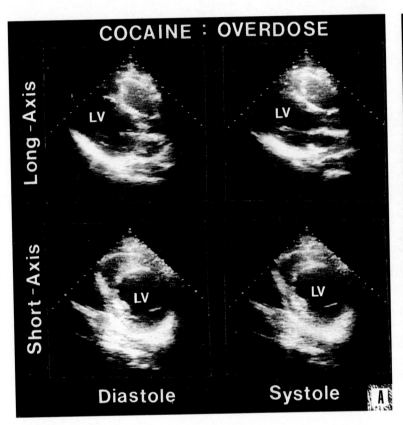

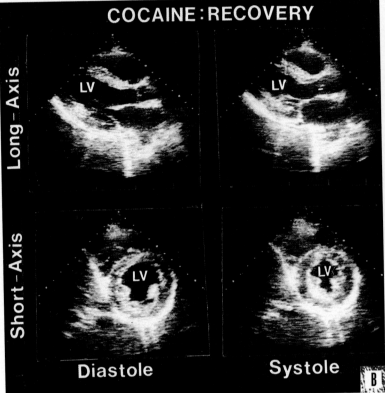

FIGURE 21.2 Two-dimensional echocardiograms recorded in long- and short-axis views during diastole and systole. **(A)** Recording taken shortly after cocaine overdose shows a dilated, globally hypocontractile left ventricle (LV). **(B)** Recording taken during the recovery period shows nondilated left ventricle with markedly improved left ventricular ejection fraction. (Reproduced with permission; see Figure Credits)

Arrhythmias and Conduction Disturbances

The concept that cocaine may have primary arrhythmogenic properties is supported by both clinical[1,2,5,10,11] and experimental[8] findings. Cocaine used as a local anesthetic agent during laryngoscopy has been observed to increase the frequency of premature ventricular complexes.[11] Benchimol et al. described a 37-year-old man who presented with a wide QRS-complex dysrhythmia at a rate of 94 beats per minute after 2 days of intravenous cocaine abuse.[1] The ectopic rhythm had a left bundle branch block configuration and was occasionally ushered in by fusion beats, suggesting its ventricular origin. Nanji and Filipenko reported asystole and ventricular fibrillation as the presenting signs of cocaine intoxication.[10] We previously described a 37-year-old man who, following intranasal use of cocaine, developed ventricular tachycardia that degenerated into ventricular fibrillation requiring DC cardioversion[7] (Fig. 21.3). Geggel et al. described a ventricular arrhythmia temporally associated with cocaine abuse involving a 2.41-kg infant girl delivered at 36 weeks' gestation to a 30-year-old woman who had used approximately 1.5 g of cocaine intranasally during the 48 hours preceding delivery.[5] Cocaine metabolites were detected qualitatively in the infant's urine sample. Resolution of the ventricular tachycardia corresponded to disappearance of cocaine metabolites from the urine.

Finally, in two previously reported patients with Wolff–Parkinson–White syndrome, intranasal administration of cocaine appeared to unmask electrophysiologically silent accessory pathways, precipitating life-threatening arrhythmias.[2]

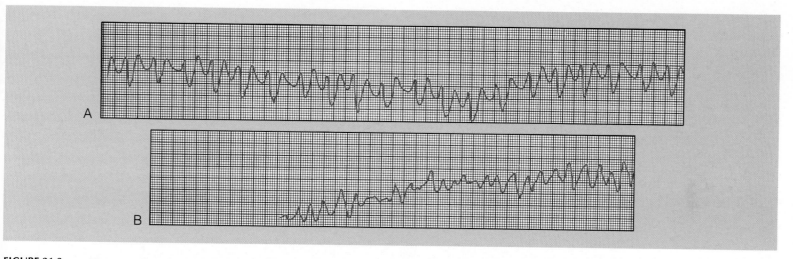

FIGURE 21.3   Electrocardiogram of a cocaine user recorded on admission to emergency department. Strip shows ventricular tachycardia **(A)** followed by ventricular fibrillation **(B).** (Reproduced with permission; see Figure Credits)

FIGURE CREDITS

Figs. 21.1, 21.3 from Isner JM, et al: Acute cardiac events temporally related to cocaine abuse. N Engl J Med 315:1458, 1985.

Fig. 21.2 from Chokshi SK, et al: Reversible cardiomyopathy associated with cocaine intoxication. Ann Intern Med 111:1039, 1989.

REFERENCES

1. Benchimol A, Bartall H, Dresser KB: Accelerated ventricular rhythm and cocaine abuse. Ann Intern Med 88:519, 1978.
2. Chokshi SK, Miller G, Rongione A, et al: Cocaine and cardiovascular diseases. The Leading Edge: Cardiology III:1, 1989.
3. Chokshi SJ, Moore R, Pandian NG, et al: Reversible cardiomyopathy associated with cocaine intoxication. Ann Intern Med 111:1039, 1989.
4. Dressler FA, Malekzadeh S, Roberts WC: Quantitative analysis of amounts of coronary arterial narrowing in cocaine addicts. Am J Cardiol 65:303, 1990.
5. Geggel RL, McInerny J, Estes NAM: Transient neonatal ventricular tachycardia associated with maternal cocaine use. Am J Cardiol 63:383, 1989.
6. Isner JM, Chokshi SK: Cocaine and vasospasm. N Engl J Med 321:1604, 1989.
7. Isner JM, Estes NAM, Thompson PD, et al: Acute cardiac events temporally related to cocaine abuse. N Engl J Med 315:1438, 1985.
8. Kabas JS, Blanchard SM, Matsuyama Y, et al: Cocaine-mediated impairment of cardiac conduction in the dog: A potential mechanism for sudden death following cocaine. J Pharmacol Exp Ther 252:185, 1990.
9. Mittleman RE, Wetli CV: Cocaine and sudden "natural" death. J Foren Sci 32:11, 1987.
10. Nanji AA, Filipenko JD: Asystole and ventricular fibrillation associated with cocaine intoxication. Chest 85:132, 1984.
11. Orr D, Jones I: Anesthesia for laryngoscopy. A comparison of the cardiovascular effects of cocaine and lignocaine. Anaesthesia 23:194, 1968.
12. Simpson RW, Edwards WD: Pathogenesis of cocaine-induced ischemic heart disease. Autopsy findings in a 21-year-old man. Arch Pathol Lab Med 110:479, 1986.
13. Stenberg RG, Winniford MD, Hillis LD, et al: Simultaneous acute thrombosis of two major coronary arteries following intravenous cocaine use. Arch Pathol Lab Med 113: 521, 1989.
14. Tazelaar HD, Karch SB, Stephens BG, et al. Cocaine and the heart. Hum Pathol 18:195, 1987.
15. Virmani R, Robinowitz M, Smialek JE, et al: Cardiovascular effect of cocaine: An autopsy study of 40 patients. Am Heart J 115:1068, 1988.
16. Weiner RS, Lockhart JT, Schwartz RG: Dilated cardiomyopathy and cocaine abuse. Am J Med 81:699, 1986.

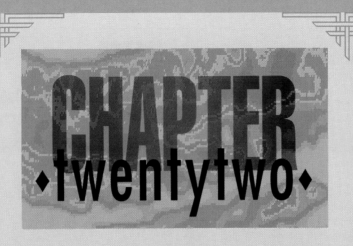

CHAPTER twentytwo

NEOPLASTIC AND HEMATOLOGIC DISEASES OF THE HEART

MARY ELLEN M. RYBAK, MD

THOMAS W. GRIFFIN, MD

J. WILLIS HURST, MD

ROBERT J. HALL, MD

ANTON E. BECKER, MD

The heart may be the site of primary neoplastic disease, secondary neoplastic processes extending from adjacent structures, or metastatic disease from a distant primary tumor.[22] In addition, the heart may be affected as a consequence of chemotherapy or radiation therapy for neoplastic disease at other sites. It may be involved in a paraneoplastic syndrome, or it may be a target of a product secreted by a tumor.

The clinical manifestations of neoplastic cardiac disease include pericarditis, myocardial disease, congestive heart failure, obstructive disease simulating valvular disease, arrhythmias, emboli, and systemic symptoms (Fig. 22.1). Neoplasms must always be included in the differential diagnosis of the etiology of these clinical symptoms. It should be noted, however, that many tumors involving the heart may be totally asymptomatic.

Primary nonmalignant tumors of the heart are uncommon, found in only 0.01% to 0.28% of all autopsies. The type and frequency of primary cardiac tumors and cysts recorded in the classic study of McAllister and Fenogolio[23] are shown in Figure 22.2. A review of all primary cardiac tumors at the University of Minnesota between 1959 and 1989 revealed 83% benign lesions and 17% malignant lesions.[25] The vast majority of primary malignant lesions were sarcomas. A similar trend was observed in a recent French study,[5] which also noted a marked increase in the frequency of preoperative diagnosis of these lesions.

Metastatic disease to the heart occurs more commonly (Fig. 22.3) than do primary cardiac tumors. A review of 8,571 sequential autopsies by the Gade Institute from 1975 to 1984 found 2,833 patients with malignant tumors. Cardiac involvement was found in 130 cases (4.5%).[16] The diagnosis of cardiac tumors requires clinical suspicion, followed by strategic laboratory testing (Fig. 22.4).[20,26,34]

Benign Primary Tumors of the Heart
CARDIAC MYXOMAS

Myxomas comprise 50% of benign tumors of the heart. Twenty-five percent of myxomas are located in the left atrium, 18% in the right atrium, 4% in the right ventricle, and 4% in the left ventricle. Cardiac myxomas usually present as a pedunculated mass.[20] Left atrial myxomas may obstruct the mitral orifice (Fig. 22.5) or the pulmonary venous orifice. Histologically, they are composed of polygonal myxoma cells embedded with a mucoid ground substance (Fig. 22.6).

FIGURE 22.1 MANIFESTATIONS OF NEOPLASTIC HEART DISEASE

PERICARDIAL INVOLVEMENT
Pericarditis—pain
Pericardial effusion
Radiographic evidence of enlargement
Arrhythmia—predominantly atrial
Tamponade
Constriction

MYOCARDIAL INVOLVEMENT
Arrhythmias—ventricular and atrial
Electrocardiographic changes
Radiographic evidence of enlargement
Generalized
Localized
Conduction disturbances and heart block
Congestive heart failure
Coronary involvement
Angina—infarction

INTRACAVITARY TUMOR
Cavity obliteration
Valve obstruction and valve damage
Embolic phenomena—systemic, neurologic, coronary
Constitutional manifestations

(Reproduced with permission; see Figure Credits)

FIGURE 22.2 TUMORS AND CYSTS OF THE HEART AND PERICARDIUM

TYPE	NUMBER	PERCENT
Benign		
Myxoma	130	24.4
Lipoma	45	8.4
Papillary fibroelastoma	42	7.9
Rhabdomyoma	36	6.8
Fibroma	17	3.2
Hemangioma	15	2.8
Teratoma	14	2.6
Mesothelioma of atrioventricular node	12	2.3
Granular cell tumor	3	
Neurofibroma	3	
Lymphangioma	2	
Subtotal	319	59.8
Pericardial cyst	82	15.4
Bronchogenic cyst	7	1.3
Subtotal	89	16.7
Malignant		
Angiosarcoma	39	7.3
Rhabdomyosarcoma	26	4.9
Mesothelioma	19	3.6
Fibrosarcoma	14	2.6
Malignant lymphoma	7	1.3
Extraskeletal osteosarcoma	5	
Neurogenic sarcoma	4	
Malignant teratoma	4	
Thymoma	4	
Leiomyosarcoma	1	
Liposarcoma	1	
Synovial sarcoma	1	
Subtotal	125	23.5
Total	533	100.0

(Reproduced with permission; see Figure Credits)

CLINICAL MANIFESTATIONS

Patients with cardiac myxomas may be asymptomatic. When symptoms are present, they may be systemic, embolic, obstructive, or a combination of these.[27]

Systemic Manifestations The majority of patients with cardiac myxomas have systemic symptomatology, including fever, weight loss, fatigue, anemia (including hemolytic anemia), an elevated sedimentation rate, elevated polyclonal immunoglobulin levels, an elevated white count, thrombocytopenia, clubbing, Raynaud's phenomenon, breast fibroadenomas, and erythrocytosis. When a constellation of these symptoms occurs simultaneously, the disorder may mistakenly be diagnosed as collagen vascular disease.[14] In some patients with myxoma, elevated levels of interleukin-6 have been cited as a mechanism for the systemic symptomatology.[13] In addition to direct effects, the tumor may become infected with a variety of micro-organisms, resulting in positive blood cultures and a clinical picture simulating endocarditis even more closely.

FIGURE 22.3 SOURCE OF METASTATIC TUMORS OF THE HEART

Lung
Melanoma
Mesothelioma
Breast
Sarcoma
Lymphoma
Renal cell carcinoma (direct extension)
Leukemia
Uterine

FIGURE 22.4 DIAGNOSTIC EVALUATION OF CARDIAC TUMORS

1. Blood work including sedimentation rate, red and white blood cell count, and serum protein electrophoresis
2. Electrocardiogram (ECG)
3. Chest radiograph
4. *Two-dimensional echocardiogram*
5. Radionuclide studies
6. *Computerized tomography*
7. Magnetic resonance imaging*
8. *Cardiac catheterization* (pressure measurements, cineangiography, coronary angiography)
9. Endomyocardial biopsy
10. Pericardiocentesis (pericardial fluid analysis)

Highest diagnostic yield in italics.
* May assume greater utility
(Reproduced with permission; see Figure Credits)

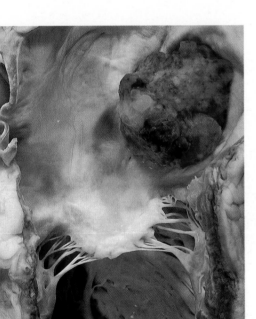

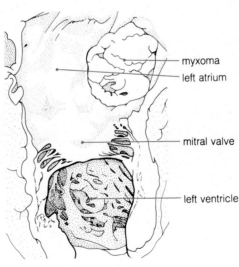

- myxoma
- left atrium
- mitral valve
- left ventricle

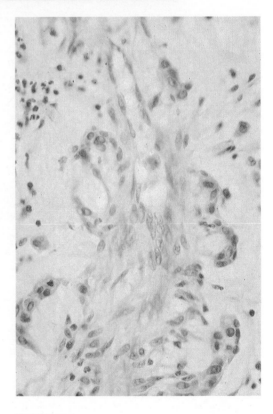

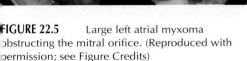

FIGURE 22.5 Large left atrial myxoma obstructing the mitral orifice. (Reproduced with permission; see Figure Credits)

FIGURE 22.6 Histologic section of a myxoma with polygonal cell strands within a mucoid stroma (H &E). (Reproduced with permission; see Figure Credits)

Systemic emboli are common when the myxoma is left atrial in location. The first clinical suspicion of a myxoma may arise from microscopic examination of a skin biopsy of a necrotic area or other systemic embolus. Emboli may affect brain, retina, skin, coronary arteries, kidneys, extremities, or aortic bifurcation. When the coronary arteries are involved, an episode of myocardial infarction may be produced in the absence of any other manifestations of myxoma.

SPECIFIC SYMPTOMS AND SIGNS RELATED TO THE LESION SITE

Left Atrial Myxoma   When the lesion is located in the left atrium, the mitral valve orifice or pulmonary vein may be obstructed, producing pulmonary venous hypertension, secondary pulmonary arterial hypertension,

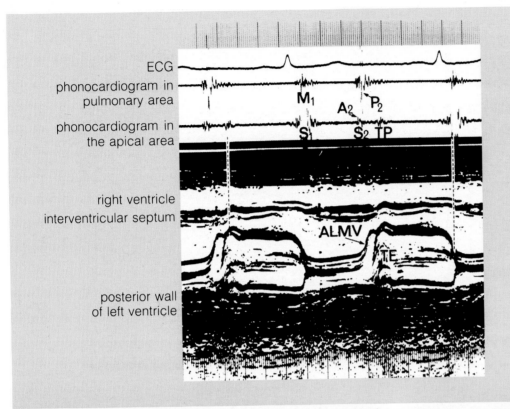

FIGURE 22.7   Recordings from a patient with a cystic left atrial myxoma: ECG, phonocardiograms from the pulmonary and apical areas at medium frequency, and M-mode echocardiogram at the level of the mitral valve are seen. Time lines indicate 0.01-sec intervals The right ventricle, the interventricular septum, and the posterior wall of the left ventricle are identified. The loud component of the first sound (M_1) is delayed (Q–M_1 = 0.09 sec). The pulmonary second sound (P_2) is accentuated. Multiple linear tumor echoes (TE) are seen behind the anterior leaflet of the mitral valve (ALMV), first appearing at the mitral level 0.04 sec after the onset of mitral opening. The forward movement is completed 0.09 sec after the onset of mitral opening, at which point the tumor plop (TP) is recorded The A_2–TP interval measures 0.10 sec. (Reproduced with permission; see Figure Credits)

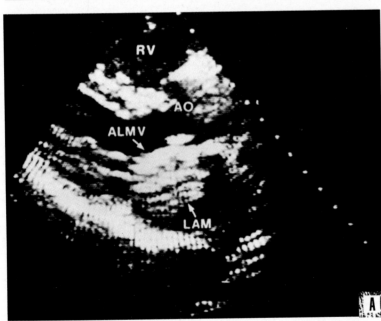
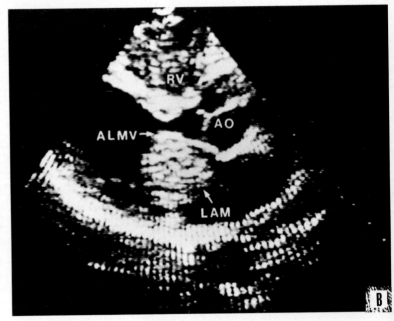

FIGURE 22.8   Cross-sectional echocardiograms in the long-axis parasternal view recorded during systole **(A)** and diastole **(B)** in a 56-year-old woman. A large left atrial myxoma (LAM) is seen in the left atrium behind the anterior leaflet of the mitral valve (ALMV). The myxoma prolapses and fills the mitral orifice during diastole. This tumor was attached to the posterior leaflet of the mitral valve and the adjacent posterior wall of the left atrium. (RV = right ventricle; Ao = aorta) (Reproduced with permission; see Figure Credits)

ulmonary congestion, dyspnea on effort, pulmonary edema, cough, hemoptysis, atigue, syncope, or sudden death. The symptoms may occasionally be either pro-oked or relieved by a change in body position. For example, assumption of a ecumbent position may relieve the symptoms in some patients.

The physical examination is suggestive of mitral stenosis. There may be a oud first heart sound, a diastolic rumble at the apex, and a systolic murmur. A umor "plop" simulating the opening snap of the mitral valve may be heard and he pulmonary valve closure sound may be loud. The tumor, which is often mobile in the left atrium, may damage the mitral valve producing severe mitral regurgitation. The M-mode echocardiogram may simulate the abnormalities associated with mitral stenosis (Fig. 22.7). Cross-sectional echocardiography may enhance visualization of the tumor (Fig. 22.8) and usually precludes the need for cardiac catheterization and angiography to make the diagnosis. Magnetic resonance imaging may also reveal evidence of the tumor. Transesophageal echocardiography (Fig. 22.9) and computerized tomography may also be diagnostic (Fig. 22.10).[26,28]

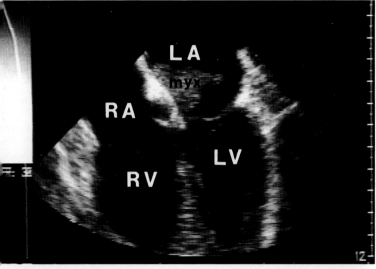
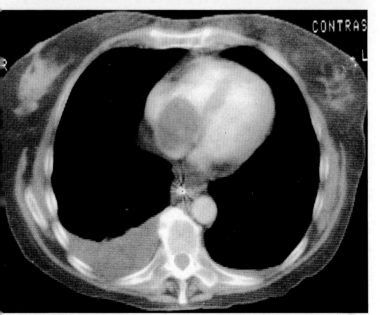
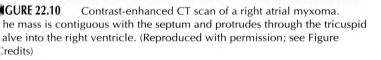

FIGURE 22.10 Contrast-enhanced CT scan of a right atrial myxoma. The mass is contiguous with the septum and protrudes through the tricuspid valve into the right ventricle. (Reproduced with permission; see Figure Credits)

FIGURE 22.9 Transesophageal echocardiogram of a left atrial myxoma (myx). This myxoma is triangular and sessile, with a wide-based attachment to the interatrial septum. (LA = left atrium; LV = left ventricle; RA = right atrium; RV= right ventricle) (Reproduced with permission; see Figure Credits)

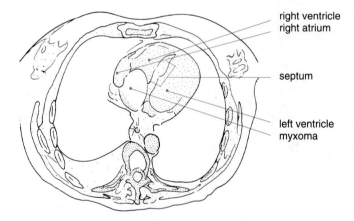

right ventricle
right atrium

septum

left ventricle
myxoma

Cardiac catheterization reveals pulmonary hypertension, a notch on the ascending limb of the left ventricular pressure curve, a rapid Y descent in the left atrial or the wedge pressure curve, and a large V wave in the wedge pressure curve. The angiogram reveals the myxoma. Coronary arteriography may reveal a tumor blush from small arteries that supply the myxoma. Because echocardiography is so reliable in identifying myxomas, a coronary arteriogram is usually performed before surgery only to identify coronary atherosclerosis; it is not employed to make the diagnosis of myxoma.

In summary, *left* atrial myxomas simulate mitral valve disease, endocarditis, and collagen vascular disease.

Right Atrial Myxomas

Systemic symptoms are less common in patients with right than with left atrial myxoma. Polycythemia and cyanosis may occur because of a right-to-left shunt through the foramen ovale. Erythrocytosis may be the result of elevated erythropoietin produced by the tumor.

The patient may exhibit a large A wave in the deep jugular venous pulse, ascites, edema, an enlarged liver, cyanosis, syncope, and episodes of dyspnea. The action of the mobile tumor may damage the tricuspid valve, producing tricuspid regurgitation. Pulmonary emboli may occur and myxomatous material may infiltrate the pulmonary arteries, producing aneurysms. Paradoxical emboli may also occur.

A loud sound may be heard in systole after the first sound and it may be preceded by a murmur. These auscultatory abnormalities are due to the rapid movement of the tumor from the right ventricle to the right atrium. There is a loud diastolic rumble heard best at the lower left sternal border and a loud systolic murmur due to tricuspid regurgitation caused by the damaged tricuspid valve. A tumor plop is sometimes heard. These sounds may be altered by repositioning the patient.

The electrocardiogram may be normal or may reveal a right atrial abnormality, a right axis deviation of the mean QRS vector, and right bundle branch block. The chest radiograph may show right atrial enlargement, right ventricular enlargement, or calcification of the tumor (Fig. 22.11). Echocardiography reveals the presence of the tumor (Fig. 22.12). Cardiac catheterization reveals prominent A wave in the right atrium and a pressure gradient across the tricuspid valve. There may be a conspicuous notch in the upstroke of the right ventricular pressure curve. A rapid Y descent can be seen. The right atrial myxoma can be visualized by angiography (Fig. 22.13).

In summary, *right* atrial myxoma must be differentiated from rheumatic tricuspid stenosis, Epstein's anomaly, pulmonary emboli and carcinoid syndrome.

Left Ventricular Myxomas

Left ventricular myxomas are rare and more likely to occur in young women than in young men. Emboli are frequent and syncope is common; however, systemic symptoms are uncommon.

The symptoms and physical signs are suggestive of aortic valve stenosis, subaortic obstruction,[6] or mitral valve stenosis or insufficiency (Fig. 22.14). The echocardiogram reveals a mobile tumor during systole, moving into the open aortic valve area. Left ventricular thrombus may simulate a left ventricular myxoma, but usually the thrombus is located in the left ventricular apex. Angiography is usually diagnostic.

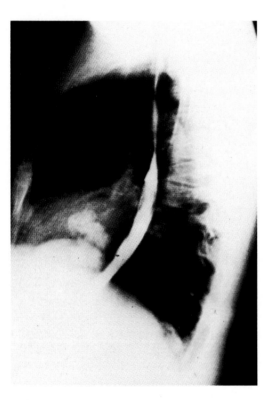

FIGURE 22.11 Lateral chest radiograph demonstrating the dense calcification of a right atrial myxoma. (Reproduced with permission; see Figure Credits)

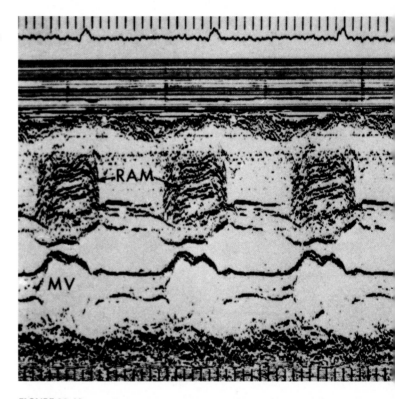

FIGURE 22.12 M-mode echocardiogram obtained through the ventricular chambers. It demonstrates a mass of echoes, filling the tricuspid funnel (RAM, *arrows*). At surgery this patient had a large right atrial myxoma. (MV = mitral valve) (ECG at top of tracing is for reference.) (Reproduced with permission; see Figure Credits)

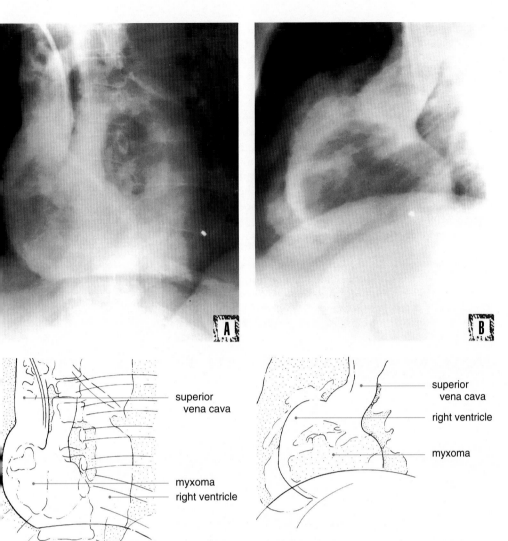

FIGURE 22.13   Frontal **(A)** and lateral **(B)** projections of right atriogram of a right atrial myxoma. The views were obtained after injection of contrast material into the superior vena cava and show a large filling defect that represents the myxoma. The mass occupies approximately 50% of the atrial chamber and extends through the tricuspid orifice into the right ventricle. (Reproduced with permission; see Figure Credits)

superior
vena cava

myxoma
right ventricle

superior
vena cava

right ventricle

myxoma

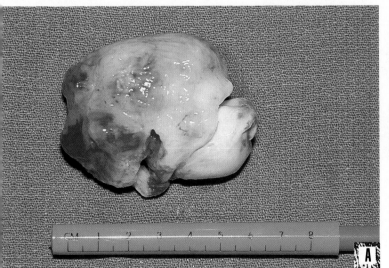

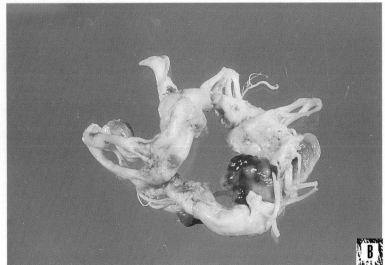

FIGURE 22.14   **(A)** Resected specimen of a left ventricular myxoma found to arise from the posterior papillary muscle. The mass caused mitral stenosis and insufficicieny and necessitated a resection of the mitral valve **(B)**. (Reproduced with permission; see Figure Credits)

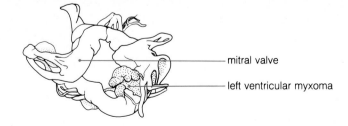

mitral valve

left ventricular myxoma

Right Ventricular Myxomas   Right ventricular myxomas produce right-sided heart failure, syncope, fever, and a murmur suggesting pulmonary valve stenosis. Pulmonary emboli may occur. A tumor "plop" may be heard in diastole, an ejection sound may be detected, and the pulmonary soft closure sound may be delayed. A calcified myxoma may be seen on chest radiography. An echocardiogram usually reveals the tumor, and the angiogram is diagnostic.

MRI is assuming an increasingly important role in the diagnosis of myxomas, including atrial and ventricular myxomas (Fig. 22.15).

RHABDOMYOMA

Rhabdomyomas are the most common cardiac tumors found in infants and children. The clinical significance is largely determined by the size and location of the lesion within the myocardium. Intracavitary extension is particularly prominent in patients with functional impairment (Fig. 22.16A). The demonstration of an intracardiac mass in a symptomatic child under 5 years of age is strongly suggestive of this diagnosis. Histologically, the tumor is composed of grotesquely swollen myocytes with an almost empty cytoplasm traversed by strands of cellular matrix (Fig. 22.16B).

The tumor usually presents with obstructive symptomatology, such as syncope and hypoxic spells that result from occlusion of the pulmonary, aortic, or mitral valve. Cardiac arrhythmias such as atrioventricular block, pericardial effusion, and sudden death are common. The tumor can be identified by chest radiography, echocardiographic examination, radionuclear angiography, cardiac angiography, and cardiac catheterization (Figs. 22.17, 22.18).

FIBROMA

Cardiac fibromas are often circumscribed and slow-growing but are potentially aggressive lesions, with a distinct tendency to occur in the ventricular septum (Fig. 22.19A). Histologically, the lesion is composed of interweaving bundles of collagen fibers, elastin fibers, and smooth muscle cells (Fig. 22.19B). These benign cardiac tumors occur most often in infants and children. They may produce sudden death, cardiac arrhythmias, and ventricular outflow obstruction. These tumors are usually identified by echocardiography and angiography.

PAPILLARY FIBROELASTOMA

Fibroelastomas arise from cardiac valves or the endocardium (Fig. 22.20). Villous tumors may also arise from the aortic valve and obstruct the coronary ostia, producing angina pectoris and sudden death. Tumors of the tricuspid valve may obstruct the outflow tract of the right ventricle. Fibroelastomas may be recognized by echocardiography and angiography.

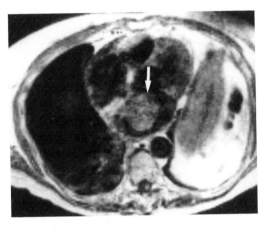

FIGURE 22.15   Transverse MR image of an atrial myxoma (arrow). The solid tissue in the left hemithorax is liver and subdiaphragmatic fat, occupying this position due to eventuation of the left hemidiaphragm. (Reproduced with permission; see Figure Credits)

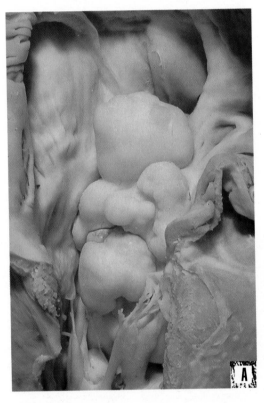

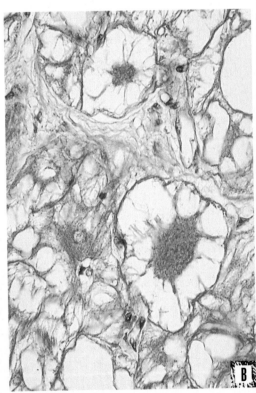

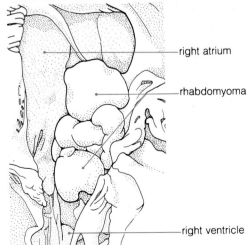

right atrium

rhabdomyoma

right ventricle

FIGURE 22.16   (A) Rhabdomyoma of the heart with intracavitary extension through the tricuspid orifice. (B) Histologic section of rhabdomyoma demonstrating bizarrely vacuolated cells with centrally placed nuclei suspended by thin cytoplasmic strands (H&E). (Reproduced with permission; see Figure Credits)

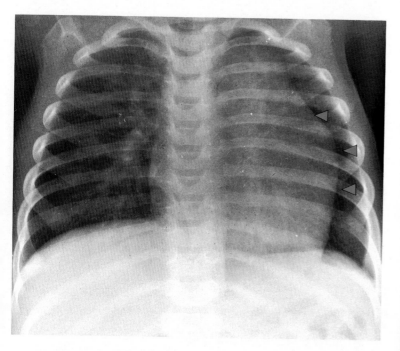

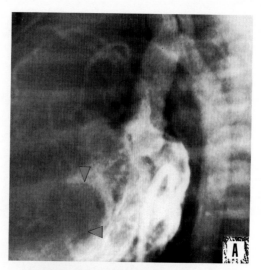

FIGURE 22.18 Early (A) and late (B) phases of a left ventriculogram demonstrating an oval-shaped rhabdomyoma (arrows) deforming the apical (trabecular) portion of the left ventricle. The mass encroaches on the ventricle lumen, causing cavitary obstruction. (Reproduced with permission; see Figure Credits)

FIGURE 22.17 Frontal chest x-ray demonstrating a deformity of the left cardiac contour (arrows) caused by a rhabdomyoma involving the antero-lateral wall of the left ventricle. (Reproduced with permission; see Figure Credits)

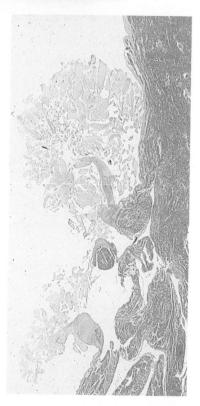

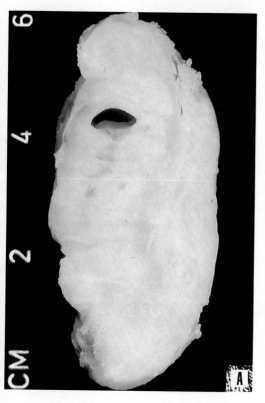

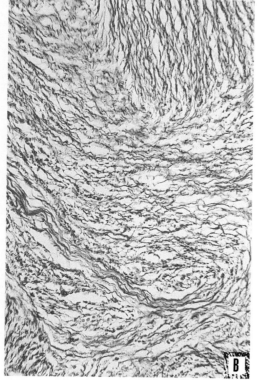

FIGURE 22.19 (A) Cut surface of an excised cardiac fibroma with typical features of fibromatous lesion. (B) Histologic section of the tumor demonstrating a bundled arrangement of collagen and elastin fibers sparsely intermingled with smooth muscle cells. (Reproduced with permission; see Figure Credits)

FIGURE 22.20 Fibroelastoma seen to arise from the mural endocardium (H&E). (Reproduced with permission; see Figure Credits)

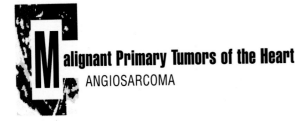

LIPOMA

Lipomas are small or large benign tumors that may occur in the pericardium, atrial septum, or ventricular myocardium. They may be asymptomatic or produce pericardial effusions, cardiac arrhythmias, or sudden death. The tumor may be identified by echocardiography and angiography.

MESOTHELIOMA OF THE ATRIOVENTRICULAR NODE

Mesotheliomas involve the atrioventricular node, producing complete heart block and Stokes–Adams attacks. Even a small tumor in this area can produce sudden death. The tumors, which occur predominantly in females, are recognized at autopsy, but they should be suspected in any child or young adult with sudden death.

HEMANGIOMA

Hemangiomas are rare benign tumors but should be suspected whenever coronary angiography reveals a tumor blush. Hemangiomas are usually discovered at autopsy (Fig. 22.21).

Malignant Primary Tumors of the Heart
ANGIOSARCOMA

Angiosarcomas are more common in males than in females and usually arise from the right atrium or the pericardium (Fig. 22.22). A continuous murmur may be heard because of the extreme vascularity of the tumor. A pericardial

tumor may produce hemorrhagic pericardial effusion and cardiac tamponade. Intracavitary tumors may produce valvular obstruction and congestive heart failure. The diagnosis may be suggested by evidence on the echocardiogram or angiogram. Coronary arteriography may reveal abnormal vessels over the tumor area. This malignant tumor may metastasize to other areas.

RHABDOMYOSARCOMA

Rhabdomyosarcomas are more commonly found in males than in females and may involve multiple sites of the heart. Valvular obstruction is present in one half of the patients with this disease. Chest radiography, echocardiography, and cardiac angiography may aid in identifying the location of the neoplasm.

OTHER MALIGNANT NEOPLASMS

Fibrosarcoma, liposarcoma, primary malignant lymphoma, and sarcomas of other varieties comprise the remaining malignant tumors of the heart. These tumors may fill the cardiac chambers, causing obstruction of the cardiac valves and congestive heart failure.

Tumors of the Pericardium
PERICARDIAL CYST

As noted on chest radiography, a benign pericardial cyst is usually located in the right costophrenic angle. The cyst rarely connects with the pericardial space. The patient with a pericardial cyst is usually asymptomatic, but may complain of

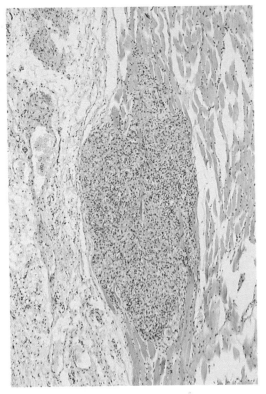

FIGURE 22.21
Histologic section of a capillary hemangioma of the heart (H&E). (Reproduced with permission; see Figure Credits)

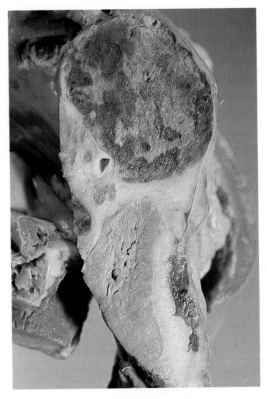

FIGURE 22.22
Angiosarcoma of the heart localized in the atrioventricular groove. (Reproduced with permission; see Figure Credits)

chest pain, dyspnea, cough, or paroxysmal heart action. Pericardial echocardiography and computerized tomography assist in making the diagnosis.

TERATOMA OF THE PERICARDIUM

Teratomas, which are rarely malignant, occur most commonly in female infants. The tumor arises and receives its blood supply from the root of the aorta of the pulmonary artery. Most of these tumors are extracardiac and lie within the pericardial space. Rarely, intracardiac tumors are identified. The intrapericardial teratoma should be considered in a child who has recurrent nonhemorrhagic effusion. Cardiac function can be compromised when the tumor attains a large size. Echocardiography and computerized tomography assist in the identification of these tumors.

MESOTHELIOMA OF THE PERICARDIUM

Mesothelioma, which are malignant neoplasms, involve the pericardium and myocardium (Fig. 22.23). The tumor occurs more commonly in males than in females. The patient may experience pericarditis, constrictive pericardial disease, or obstruction of the superior vena cava. The pericardial fluid is bloody, and malignant cells may be found in the fluid.

Secondary Neoplasms of the Heart

Neoplasms originating in other organs may metastasize to the heart. Secondary tumors of the heart and pericardium are 20 to 40 times more common than primary tumors of the heart. Several authors have found cardiac metastases in 20% of all routine autopsies of patients with metastatic neoplasms, and this number increased by another 12% when the heart specifically was investigated more thoroughly.[36] Cardiac involvement may be the result of contiguous growth from an adjacent structure in the mediastinum (Figs. 22.24, 22.25), hematogenous or lymphatic spread (Figs. 22.26–22.28), or direct contiguous growth of the primary tumor into the pulmonary veins or vena cava (Fig. 22.29).

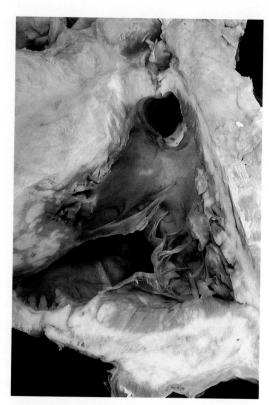

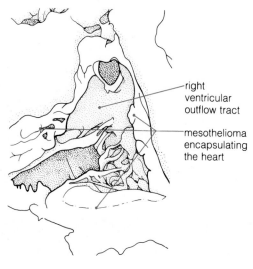

right ventricular outflow tract

mesothelioma encapsulating the heart

FIGURE 22.23   Primary mesothelioma of the pericardium. The tumor presents as a thick pericardial layer covering the heart, with local invasion into the myocardium. (Reproduced with permission; see Figure Credits)

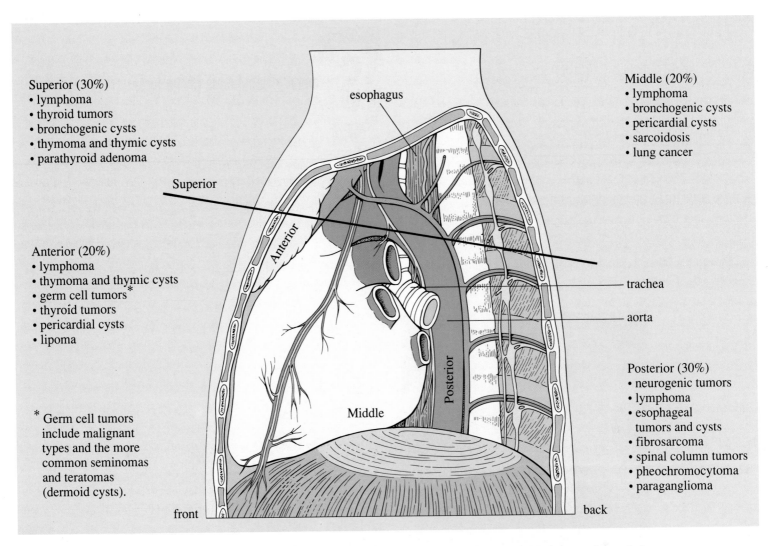

Superior (30%)
• lymphoma
• thyroid tumors
• bronchogenic cysts
• thymoma and thymic cysts
• parathyroid adenoma

Anterior (20%)
• lymphoma
• thymoma and thymic cysts
• germ cell tumors*
• thyroid tumors
• pericardial cysts
• lipoma

* Germ cell tumors
include malignant
types and the more
common seminomas
and teratomas
(dermoid cysts).

esophagus

Superior

Anterior

Posterior

Middle

front

Middle (20%)
• lymphoma
• bronchogenic cysts
• pericardial cysts
• sarcoidosis
• lung cancer

trachea

aorta

Posterior (30%)
• neurogenic tumors
• lymphoma
• esophageal
  tumors and cysts
• fibrosarcoma
• spinal column tumors
• pheochromocytoma
• paraganglioma

back

FIGURE 22.24   Tumors of the mediastinum. Included are a partial listing of the tumors found in the mediastinum and the relative frequency of their occurrence in the various mediastinal divisions. (Reproduced with permission; see Figure Credits)

FIGURE 22.25   Cross sections through the heart and lungs of a patient with a central bronchial carcinoma revealing directed spread of the tumor into the heart. (Reproduced with permission; see Figure Credits)

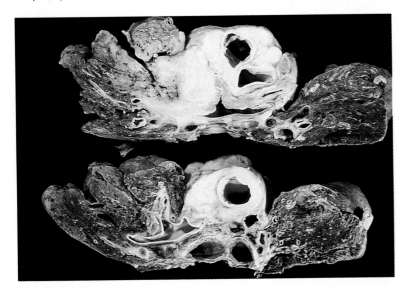

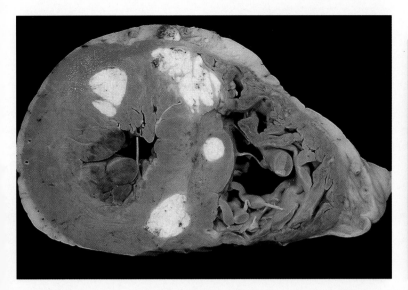

FIGURE 22.26 Hematogenous metastases in the myocardium of a patient with primary renal carcinoma. (Reproduced with permission; see Figure Credits)

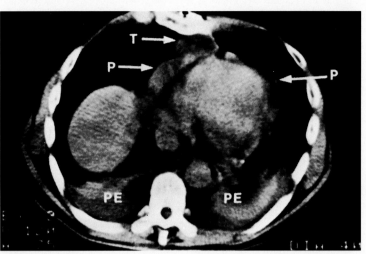

FIGURE 22.27 CT scan of the heart in a patient with renal cell carcinoma. Metatases to the anterior mediastinum (T) and pericardium (P) are revealed. Bilateral pleural effusions (PE) are also evident. (Reproduced with permission; see Figure Credits)

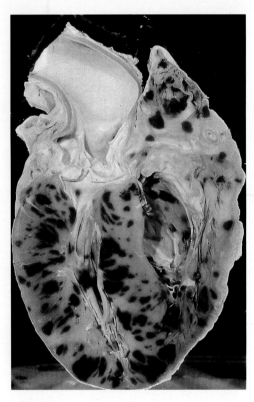

FIGURE 22.28 Section through the heart depicting numerous pigmented deposits of metastatic melanoma throughout the myocardium. (Reproduced with permission; see Figure Credits)

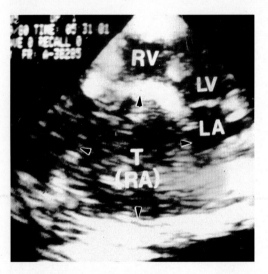

FIGURE 22.29 Very large mass deforming and distorting the right atrium primarily, but involving the other three chambers as well. The tumor, a malignant thymoma, propagated down from the superior vena cava. (Reproduced with permission; see Figure Credits)

DeLoach and Haynes[9] recorded the results of 2,547 consecutive autopsies performed at Walter Reed Army Hospital. They found malignant disease of the heart in 980 of these cases, 13.9% with metastatic disease of the heart and pericardium. Cancer of the lung involved the heart and pericardium more often than any other process (21% of 105 cases). Lymphatic leukemia also invaded the heart and pericardium in about the same number of cases. The Gade Institute series[14] from Norway also found lung cancer to be the most frequent of metastatic cardiac tumors, followed by melanoma, mesothelioma, breast cancer, and sarcoma. Chronic myelogenous leukemia and acute myelogenous leukemia may also directly invade the heart.[7,29] Lymphomas[1,8] and, rarely, chronic lymphocytic leukemia may involve the pericardium and myocardium in immunocompetent patients and, in increasing numbers, in patients with HIV infection. In breast cancer, cardiac involvement has been reported in 12% to 30% of cases.[35] Cardiac metastases occur in 15% to 35% of lung cancer patients.[15] One retrospective review showed that most of these patients were symptomatic. In fact, only 4% of patients who were pathologically proven to have cardiac metastases from lung cancer had no clinical signs or symptoms, often due to the signs and symptoms being missed clinically.[33] At autopsy, pericardial involvement (88%) was more common than myocardial involvement (45% often by extension) for all types of lung cancer. An elevated venous pressure, arrhythmias, change in cardiac silhouette, or congestive heart failure can all antecede cardiac tamponade in the patient with lung cancer, and such symptoms warrant prompt investigation of the possibility of cardiac metastases. The physician should not wait for the development of classic findings of cardiac tamponade to begin an investigation; in particular, echocardiography should be undertaken.

PERICARDIAL INVOLVEMENT

The patient with metastatic disease of the pericardium may have the signs and symptoms of pericarditis, cardiac tamponade, and cardiac arrhythmias. The echocardiogram (Fig. 22.30) and CT scan (Figs. 22.27, 22.31) may reveal fluid and the mass, while in some cases thickening of the pericardium may be the only finding. In addition, the pericardium may be abnormally dense due to tumor infiltration (imaging may also demonstrate encapsulated pericardial fluid). The pericardial fluid is usually but not always bloody. Pericardial sequelae, such as constrictive pericarditis, may also be the result of radiation therapy.

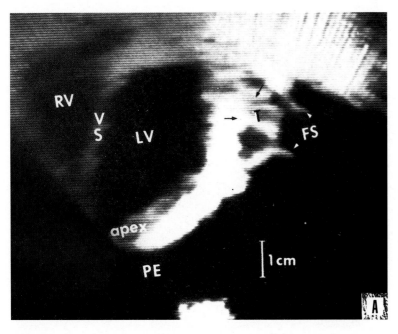

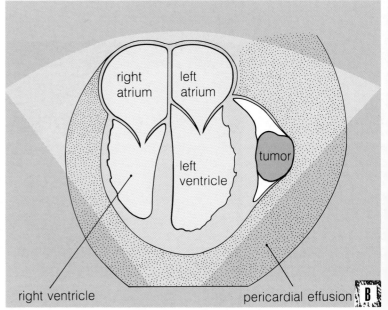

FIGURE 22.30 **(A)** Still frame, modified four-chamber view of cross-sectional echocardiogram obtained in a patient with a large pericardial effusion. A large tumor mass within the pericardial space is attached to the epicardium (T, arrows), and fibrinous strands (FS) extend from the tumor. This patient had had a mastectomy several years previously for adenocarcinoma; the diagnosis was a metastatic tumor to the pericardium. **(B)** Representation of the position of the tumor, as well as the view obtained on echocardiography. (RV = right ventricle; VS = ventricular septum; LV = left ventricle; PE = pericardial effusion). (Reproduced with permission; see Figure Credits)

MYOCARDIAL INVOLVEMENT

Neoplastic infiltration of the atria may result in atrial fibrillation and atrial flutter. Serious ventricular arrhythmias or heart failure may occur when the ventricle is inundated by metastatic growth. The ECG may show nonspecific ST–T wave changes and may mimic myocardial infarction due to persistent elevation of the ST segment. In cases of osteogenic sarcoma, bone fragments may be seen in the myocardium on chest radiography.

CORONARY ARTERY INVOLVEMENT

Coronary artery disease manifested as angina pectoris or myocardial infarction in patients with malignant neoplasm may be due to coronary atherosclerosis unrelated to the neoplasm, tumor emboli to a coronary artery, and compression or occlusion of the coronary arteries.[17] In addition, there is evidence to support the theory that cardiac radiation may accelerate atherosclerosis; this is further discussed below.

INTRACAVITARY TUMOR GROWTH

Cardiac chambers may become occluded by tumor when the myocardial mass increases in size or when certain neoplasms extend directly into the atrium.

This latter occurrence may be seen with renal cell carcinoma, hepatoma, or uterine leiomyosarcoma extending into the vena cava and subsequently into the atrial cavity. The clinical syndrome produced by intracavitary lesions simulates obstructive valvular disease and constrictive pericarditis. Echocardiography, computerized tomography, and cardiac angiography may assist in the diagnosis.[26]

LEUKEMIA

At autopsy, the heart has been found to be involved in 69% of patients with leukemia.[29] In most of these patients, the pericardium is also involved. The cardiac involvement is not usually recognized prior to the autopsy although a variety of symptoms and signs may occur, which include mitral valve involvement and congestive heart failure.[2] Cardiac rupture has been reported in the literature. Cardiac tamponade due to hemorrhagic pericardial effusion from chronic myelogenous leukemia and chronic lymphocytic leukemia have been described.[4,7] Infiltration of the conduction system is also seen (Fig. 22.32). Susceptibility to infection in these patients, including fungal endocarditis, can also lead to cardiac sequelae.

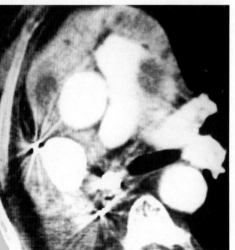

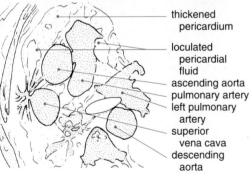

thickened pericardium

loculated pericardial fluid

ascending aorta

pulmonary artery

left pulmonary artery

superior vena cava

descending aorta

FIGURE 22.31 Contrast-enhanced CT scan at the level of the great arteries in a patient with pericardial metastasis. The heart is displaced to the right as a result of a pneumonectomy that was done for carcinoma of the lung. The aorta and pulmonary arteries are surrounded by thickened pericardium, which is abnormally dense due to tumor infiltration. (Reproduced with permission; see Figure Credits)

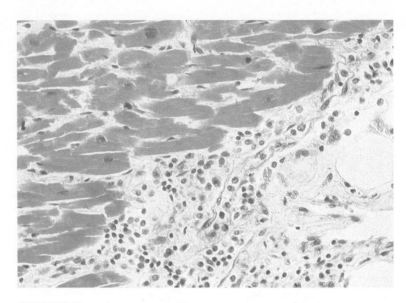

FIGURE 22.32 Histologic section showing leukemic infiltration of the myocardium.

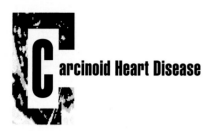

Carcinoid Heart Disease

Carcinoid heart disease is produced by substances released by the carcinoid tumor. Serotonin is one of the best characterized substances involved, which also include bradykinin. Carcinoid tumors originate from the organs in the gastrointestinal tract—the small intestine, stomach, appendix, and rectum. They may also arise from a variety of other sites, including the bronchus, biliary tract, pancreas, ovaries,[12] testes, and thyroid. Carcinoid tumor in the appendix rarely produces the carcinoid syndrome. Most cases of carcinoid tumor associated with the carcinoid syndrome will have liver metastasis. For the most part, these tumors contain 5-hydroxytryptamine that is excreted in the urine as 5-hydroxyindoleacetic acid. Carcinoid tumors of the bronchus, pancreas, and stomach produce different substances, differ morphologically, and metastasize more widely than carcinoid of the ileum. These tumors also produce 5-hydroxytryptamine and excrete 5-hydroxyindoleacetic acid in the urine, but the clinical syndrome may be different from that found with the ileal carcinoid. Carcinoid tumors in the rectum do not produce 5-hydroxytryptamine.

The liver usually deactivates substances produced by the ileal carcinoid, but metastatic lesions produce the substances that are delivered into the hepatic and renal veins, which may damage the heart and produce the clinical syndrome. Ovarian carcinoid tumors and tumors arising from other extraportal venous structures can deliver the mediators into the ovarian vein and inferior vena cava without metastases to the liver. These agents produce cardiac damage and others (e.g., vasoactive amines) produce flushing of the skin, bronchospasm, and hypermotility of the intestine and edema.

CARDIAC LESIONS

The left side of the heart is the usual site involved by lesions produced by the ileal carcinoid. The lesions known as *carcinoid plaques*, occur in the pulmonary valve, the tricuspid valve, and the endocardium. These lesions may be present on the left side of the heart in patients who have extensive right-sided involvement or who have an interatrial communication. Bronchial carcinoids tend to produce lesions in the mitral valve and the left side of the heart.

Clinical manifestations include characteristic episodes of flushing and cardiac lesions. There may be evidence of severe right-sided heart disease and heart failure, pulmonary valve stenosis or regurgitation, and tricuspid regurgitation. Mitral stenosis and regurgitation seldom occur. The clinical diagnosis is usually suspected because of the uniqueness of the syndrome. Unusual flushing portends pulmonary and tricuspid valve disease and should always alert the physician to consider the possibility of carcinoid syndrome. Pellagra may also be present because tryptophan is diverted into the metabolic pathway that leads to the production of 5-hydroxyindoleacetic acid.

Echocardiography and cardiac catheterization provide evidence of tricuspid valve abnormalities (Fig. 22.33). Computerized tomography reveals metastatic alterations in the liver and carcinoid tumors of the ovaries.

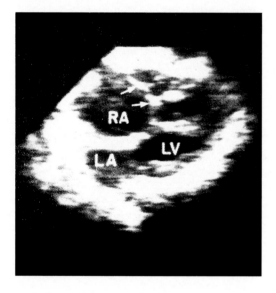

FIGURE 22.33
Subcostal cross-sectional long-axis echocardiogram of the tricuspid valve recorded in a patient with the carcinoid syndrome. The valve leaflets *(arrows)* and cords are thickened. In this diastolic frame there is no evidence of valve opening. In real time, the valve appeared completely fixed and stenotic, with no observable motion from diastole to systole. The right atrium (RA) is dilated. (LV = left ventricle = LA, left atrium) (Reproduced with permission; see Figure Credits)

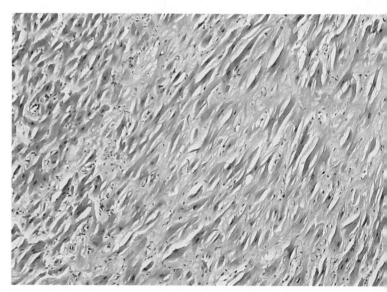

FIGURE 22.34 Histologic section demonstrating cardiac amyloidosis.

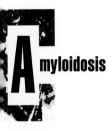

Amyloidosis

Amyloidosis is a pathologic process in which there is deposition of a unique protein in a twisted, pleated sheet fibril. The amyloidogenic protein may be a monoclonal light chain (AL) or another protein (AA), and may even contain part of the calcitonin molecule in special cases of medullary carcinoma of the thyroid. Amyloidosis is seen in 6% to 15% of cases of multiple myeloma, 4% of cases of Hodgkin's disease, and 1% of cases of other lymphomas. Carcinomas associated with amyloidosis include medullary carcinoma of the thyroid, and tumors of the bladder, kidneys, pelvis, cervix, and biliary tract.

Signs and symptoms include "inch purpura," cutaneous papules, peripheral neuropathy, autonomic neuropathy, and restrictive cardiomyopathy (Fig. 22.34). The latter may be manifested by right-sided heart failure, low voltage on the ECG, and digitalis sensitivity.

Diagnosis is made by demonstration of characteristic emerald green dye reagents of tissue biopsy (from bone marrow, gingiva, skin, or the rectum). A characteristic echocardiogram (Fig. 22.35) may be helpful in raising a diagnostic suspicion.

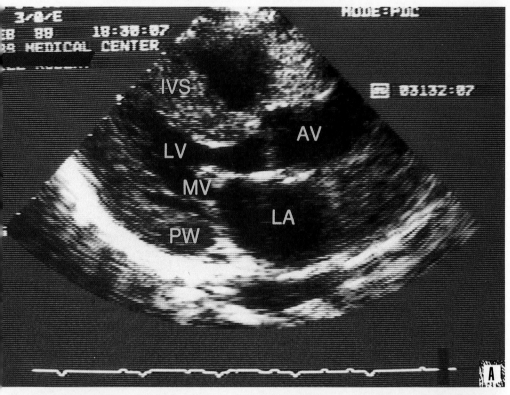

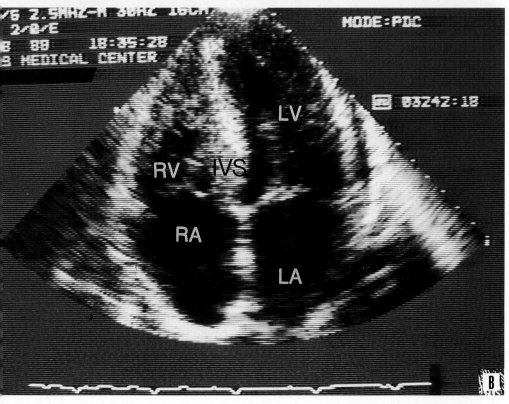

FIGURE 22.35 Two-dimensional echocardiogram from patient with biopsy-proven amyloidosis. **(A)** Parasternal long-axis view of the left ventricle (LV), left atrium (LA), and aortic valve (AV). The interventricular septum (IVS) and posterior wall (PW) of the left ventricle are thickened and have a specific appearance, characteristic of infiltrative cardiomyopathy. The mitral valve (MV) is also thickened. **(B)** Apical four-chamber view. There is enlargement of both the right atrium (RA) and LA and marked thickening of the IVS. (RV = right ventricle).

Cardiac Complications of Chemotherapy and Radiation Therapy

Several widely used chemotherapeutic agents—most prominently anthracyclines, mitomycin-C, and mitoxantrone—may produce cardiac toxicity. Free radical formation has been implicated as a major mechanism, although several other mechanisms have been proposed (Fig. 22.36). Clinical manifestations include acute arrhythmias, myocarditis–pericarditis syndrome, and a chronic cardiomyopathy that is related primarily to cumulative doses of drugs.[10] Risk factors for cardiac toxicity include age, mediastinal radiation, hypertension, individual dose size, and co-administration of other drugs such as cyclophosphamide.

A major characteristic of the pathologic picture is the development of focal lesions in which both dilation of the sarcoplasmic reticulum and destruction of myofibrils are prominent. There is a correlation between biopsies and clinical congestive heart failure; however, myocardial changes may be seen in patients who are totally asymptomatic and have no clinical evidence of cardiac dysfunction.

Monitoring for cardiac toxicity includes radionuclide cineangiography, echocardiography, and recording of systolic time intervals; less commonly, cardiac catherization and endomyocardial biopsy are employed. A proposed sequence of evaluation and monitoring of the clinical cardiac toxicity of chemotherapy is shown in Figure 22.37.[32] Late cardiac toxicity is also of concern. Analysis of children who had been treated for acute lymphoblastic leukemia with anthracycline containing chemotherapy regimens revealed that more than 50% of patients had abnormal ventricular wall thickness or contractility a median of 6.4 years after completion of therapy, despite cumulative doses of doxorubicin less than 500 mg/M^2.[19]

Cardiac complications can also occur following radiation therapy. Such problems were first reported in the treatment of Hodgkin's disease. Their occurrence has become relatively uncommon with awareness of the problem and with limitations in the volume of pericardium radiated and restriction of radiation fraction to less than 2.5 Gy. When the entire heart is radiated to doses of greater than 30 Gy, as many as 50% of patients develop pericardial complications. The symptoms seen are usually pericarditis and, rarely, cardiac tamponade and pericardial fibrosis. There also may be an increased risk of asthma or acceleration of atherosclerosis, with premature myocardial infarction. In addition, immunotherapy of cancer with interleukin-2 has been associated with a syndrome of lymphocytic myocarditis.[18]

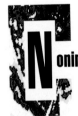

Noninfective Thrombotic Endocarditis

Noninfective endocarditis can develop in the cancer patient with or without clinical manifestations of disseminated intravascular coagulation (DIC). In fact, these two disorders may be related aspects of the same pathophysiologic process.[31] Thromboembolic or hemorrhagic complications (Fig. 22.38) may result. Patients most often present with embolic phenomenon to the brain and other organs, such as the heart, kidneys, spleen, and extremities. Both small and large vessels can be involved. These patients, in contrast to those with infective endocarditis, are usually afebrile, and only one third or fewer have a detectable heart murmur. Paraneoplastic endocarditis can present early as well as later in malignancy.[21]

Noninfective endocarditis can be seen in a variety of malignancies. As reported by Rosen, the autopsy incidence of NBTE in patients with adenocarcinoma of the lung (7.5%) was twice that seen with adenocarcinoma of the prostate or pancreas (3%–4%) and more than seven times that seen with other solid tumors, lymphomas, and leukemias.[30] In related analyses, an increased frequency of adenocarcinomas of the lung, gastrointestinal tract, and pancreatic cancer was found in patients with endocarditis and cerebral infarcts.[3,11,16] The differential diagnosis includes infectious endocarditis, DIC of malignancy without endocarditis, microangiopathic hemolytic anemia of malignancy, and embolic lesions from other sites.

FIGURE 22.36 MECHANISMS OF CHEMOTHERAPY-INDUCED CARDIAC TOXICITY

1. Free radical, superoxide, and hydrogen peroxide membrane damage
2. Alteration in calcium metabolism
3. Inhibition of Na–K-ATPase
4. Direct membrane effects

FIGURE 22.37 SUGGESTED MONITORING GUIDELINES FOR PATIENTS RECEIVING ANTHRACYCLINE THERAPY

1. Baseline LVEF (left ventricular ejection fraction)
2. Second LVEF at 250–300 mg/M^2
3. Third LVEF at 400 mg/M^2 (risk factors) and 450 mg/M^2 (no risk factors)
4. Then sequential studies prior to each dose
5. STOP drug if absolute decline in LVEF is 10% or more, on a decline to 50% or more

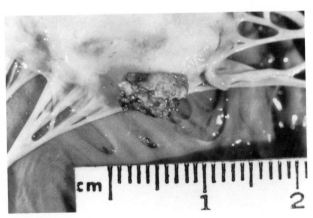

FIGURE 22.38 Mitral anterior leaflet in a patient with Hodgkin's disease exhibiting a large vegetation adherent to the leaflet surface. (Reproduced with permission; see Figure Credits)

ACKNOWLEDGMENT

This chapter is partially derived from Hall RJ, Cooley DA: Neoplastic heart disease. In Hurst JW (ed): The Heart, 6th ed. McGraw-Hill, New York, 1986; Hurst JW (ed): Atlas of the Heart. Gower, New York, 1988.

FIGURE CREDITS

Figs. 22.1, 22.7, 22.8, 22.11, 22.27, from Hurst JW: The Heart, 6th ed. McGraw-Hill, New York, 1986. Fig. 22.27 courtesy of F. Parker Gregg, MD, Houston, TX.

Fig. 22.2 from McAllister HA Jr, Fenoglio JJ Jr: Tumors of the Cardiovascular System. Armed Forces Institute of Pathology, Washington, D.C., 1978.

Fig. 22.4 modified from Tillmanns H: Clinical aspects of cardiac tumors. Thorac Cardiovasc Surg 38:152, 1990.

Figs. 22.5–22.8, 22.14, 22.19B, 22.21–22.23, 22.25, 22.26, from Hurst JW: Atlas of the Heart. Gower, New York, 1988.

Figs. 22.6, 22.16, 22.19A, 22.20 from Becker AE, Anderson RH: Cardiac Pathology. Raven, New York, 1983.

Figs. 22.9, 22.15, 22.29, 22.38 from Chatterjee K, et al: Cardiology: An Illustrated Text Reference. Gower, New York, 1992. Fig. 22.39 courtesy of Margaret Billingham, MD, Stanford, CA.

Figs. 22.10, 22.13, 22.17, 22.18, 22.31 from Kassner EG: Atlas of Radiologic Imaging. Gower, New York, 1989.

Fig. 22.12 from Brest AN: Cardiovascular Clinics. FA Davis, Philadelphia, 1980.

Figs. 22.24, 22.28 from Skarin AT: Atlas of Diagnostic Oncology. Gower, New York, 1991.

Fig. 22.30 from Nasser FN, Giuliani ER: Clinical Two-dimensional Echocardiography. Year Book Medical Publishers, Chicago, 1983.

Fig. 22.33 from Weyman AE: Cross-sectional Echocardiography. Lea & Febiger, Philadelphia, 1982.

REFERENCES

1. Acierno LJ: Cardiac complications in acquired immune deficiency syndrome (AIDS): A review. J Am Coll Cardiol 13:1141, 1989.

2. Applefeld MM, Milner SD, Vigorito RD, et al: Congestive heart failure and endocardial fibroelastosis caused by chronic lymphocytic leukemia. Cancer 46:1479, 1980.

3. Biller J, Challa VR, Toole JF, Howard VJ: Nonbacterial thrombotic endocarditis. Arch Neurol 33:95, 1982.

4. Bjorkholm M, Ost A, Biberfeld P: Myocardial rupture with cardiac tamponade as a lethal early manifestation of acute myeloblastic leukemia. Cancer 50:1967, 1982.

5. Blondeau PH: Primary cardiac tumors—French studies of 533 cases. Thorac Cardiovasc Surg 38:192, 1990.

6. Bradham RR, Gregorie HB Jr, Howell JS Jr, et al: Aortic obstruction from embolizing cardiac myxoma. J SC Med Assoc 75:7, 1982.

7. Cassis N Jr, Porterfield J: Massive hemopericardium as the initial manifestation of chronic myelogenous leukemia. Arch Intern Med 142:2193, 1982.

8. Dalli E, Quesada A, Paya R: Cardiac involvement by non-Hodgkin's lymphoma in acquired immune deficiency syndrome. Intern J Cardiol 26:223, 1990.

9. DeLoach JF, Haynes JW: Secondary tumors of heart and pericardium: Review of the subject and report of one hundred thirty-seven cases. Arch Intern Med 91:224, 1953.

10. Doroshow JH: Doxorubicin-induced cardiotoxicity. N Engl J Med 324:843, 1991.

11. Graus F, Rogers LR, Posner JB: Cerebrovascular complications in patients with cancer. Medicine 64:16, 1985.

12. Hurst JW, Whitworth HB, O'Donoghue S, et al: Heart disease due to ovarian carcinoid: Successful replacement of the pulmonary and tricuspid valves with porcine heterografts and removal of the tumor. In Hurst JW (ed): Clinical Essays on the Heart, vol 5. McGraw-Hill, New York, 1985.

13. Jourdan M, Bataille R, Seguin J, et al: Constitutive production of interleukin-6 and immunologic features in cardiac myxomas. J Arthr Rheumat 33:398, 1990.

14. Kaminsky ME, Ehlers K, Engle ME, et al: Atrial myxoma mimicking a collagen disorder. Chest 75:93, 1979.

15. Karwinski B, Svendsen E: Trends in cardiac metastasis. Acta Pathol Microbiol Immunol Scand 7:1018, 1989.

16. Kookier JC, MacLean JM, Sumi SM: Cerebral embolism, marantic endocarditis and cancer. Arch Neurol 32:260, 1976.

17. Kopelson G, Herwig KJ: The etiologies of coronary artery disease in cancer patients. Int J Rad Oncol Biol Phys 4:895, 1978.

18. Kragel AH, Travis WD, Steis RG, et al: Myocarditis or acute myocardial infarction associated with interleukin-2 therapy for cancer. Cancer 66:1513, 1990.

19. Lipshultz SE, Colan SD, Gelber RD, et al: Late cardiac effects of doxorubicin therapy for acute lymphoblastic leukemia in childhood. N Engl J Med 324:808, 1991.

20. Liu HY, Panadis I, Soffer J, et al: Echocardiographic diagnosis of intracardiac myxomas. Chest 84:63, 1984.

21. MacDonald RA, Robbins SL: The significance of non-bacterial thrombotic endocarditis: Autopsy and clinical study of 78 patients. Ann Intern Med 46:255, 1957.

22. McAllister HA Jr: Primary tumors and cysts of the heart and pericardium. In Harvey WP (ed): Current Problems in Cardiology, vol IV, no. 2. Year Book, Chicago, 1979.

23. McAllister HA Jr, Fenoglio JJ Jr: Tumors of the Cardiovascular System. Armed Forces Institute of Pathology, Washington, D.C., 1978.

24. Meltzer V, Korompai FL, Mathur VS, et al: Surgical treatment of leukemic involvement of the mitral valve. Chest 67:119, 1975.

25. Molina JE, Edward JE, Ward HB: Primary cardiac tumors: Experience at the University of Minnesota. Thorac Cardiovasc Surg 38:183, 1990.

26. Mugge A, Daniel WG, Haverich A, et al: Diagnosis of noninfective cardiac mass lesions by two-dimensional echocardiography. Comparison of transthoracic and transesophageal approaches. Circulation 83:70, 1991.

27. Peters MN, Hall RJ, Cooley DA, et al: The clinical syndrome of atrial myxoma. JAMA 230:694, 1974.

28. Rienmuller R, Tiling R: MR and CT for detection of cardiac tumors. Thorac Cardiovasc Surg 38 (Suppl 2):168, 1990.

29. Roberts WC, Bodey GC, Wertlake PT: The heart in acute leukemia: A study of 420 autopsy cases. Am J Cardiol 21:388, 1968.

30. Rosen P, Armstrong D: Nonbacterial thrombotic endocarditis in patients with malignant neoplastic disease. Am J Med 54:23, 1975.

31. Sack GH, Levin J, Bell WR: Trousseau's syndrome and other manifestations of chronic disseminated intravascular coagulation and neoplasms. Medicine 56:1, 1977.

32. Schwartz RG, McKenzie WB, Alexander J, et al: Congestive heart failure and left ventricular dysfunction complicating doxorubicin therapy: Seven year experience using radionuclide angiography. Am J Med 82:1109, 1987.

33. Strauss BL, Matthews MJ, Cohen MH, et al: Cardiac metastases in lung cancer. Chest 71:607, 1977.

34. Tillmanns H: Clinical aspects of cardiac tumors. Thorac Cardiovasc Surg 38:152, 1990.

35. Volk MJ, Carbone PP, Pozniak MA, et al: Cardiac involvement in metastatic breast cancer. Wisc Med J 89(2):56, 1990.

36. Young JM, Goldman IR: Tumor metastasis to the heart. Circulation 19:220, 1954.

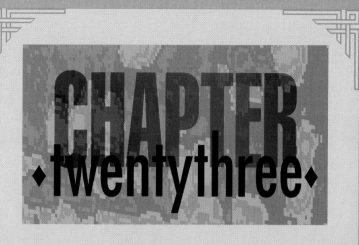

CHAPTER
•twentythree•

CEREBROVASCULAR
DISORDERS

MARC FISHER, MD
KAZUO MINEMATSU, MD

The generic term *stroke* is frequently used for patients who suffer acute cerebrovascular events. Stroke is a broad term which refers to a group of similar, but diverse, clinical syndromes, which affect the brain in relationship to its vascular supply.[5] Approximately 450,000 new strokes per year occur in the United States, and 150,000 deaths are related to these acute strokes.[4] Many stroke patients do not die as a direct consequence of their cerebrovascular event; they expire because of medical complications such as sepsis, pulmonary embolus, cardiac arrhythmias, and aspiration pneumonia.

Stroke is more common in the elderly than in middle-aged or younger adults. Therefore, despite the decline in stroke incidence over the past two decades (Fig. 23.1), which may now be ebbing, we can anticipate an increased incidence of stroke as the population continues to age. Stroke-related neurologic dysfunction is a major cause of disability in the United States and is also a substantial financial burden. Accurate diagnosis, appropriate management, and prevention of stroke remain an important challenge for primary care physicians and neurologists alike.

Vascular and Functional Anatomy

The vascular supply to the brain is divided into two major sources (Fig. 23.2), the carotid artery (anterior circulation) and the vertebral–basilar system (posterior circulation).[5] The carotid artery territory encompasses approximately 80% of the brain and the vertebral–basilar system supplies the remainder. A wide variety of symptoms may occur as a result of carotid system stroke (Fig. 23.3),

and the particular signs and symptoms will relate to the areas of the brain involved that are supplied by a particular branch of the carotid artery. The most commonly encountered neurologic signs in patients with carotid territory stroke include contralateral weakness, sensory loss, visual field loss, and language disturbance, if the stroke is in the dominant hemisphere. Nondominant hemisphere strokes cause a variety of behavioral abnormalities, such as denial of deficit and neglect of the hemiparetic limbs or space. Vertebral basilar strokes are associated with such signs as double vision, vertigo, cerebellar limb and/or gait disturbance, and contralateral weakness and/or numbness (see Fig. 23.3). The hallmark of posterior circulation stroke is the presence of cranial nerve deficits ipsilateral to the lesion and somatic deficits contralateral to the lesion. This typically relates to the decussation of motor and sensory fibers below the area of involvement in the brainstem. The initial step in evaluating stroke patients should be an accurate history and physical examination, which will allow for accurate localization of the site of the lesion within the brain.

Stroke Subtypes

Stroke is readily divisible into four major subcategories (Fig. 23.4), and the prognosis, evaluation and management of each category differ.[5] The four categories are (1) large vessel atherothrombotic stroke (40% of the total), (2) small vessel lacunar stroke (20%), (3) cardiogenic brain embolism (20%), and (4) intracerebral hemorrhage (15%). A small group of patients, approximately 5%, do

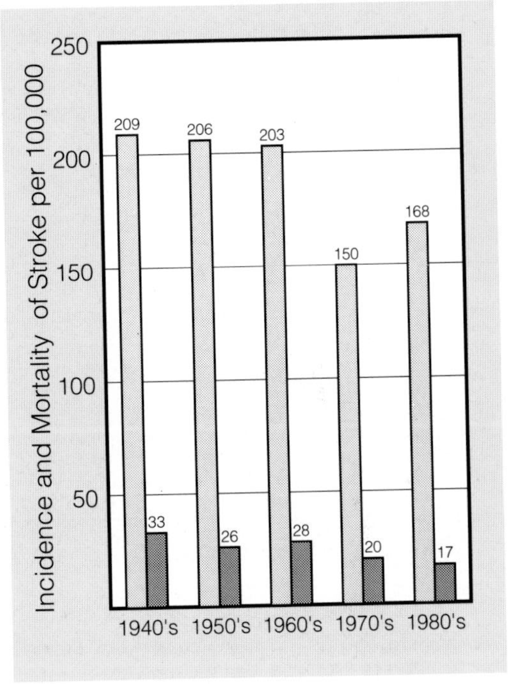

FIGURE 23.1   Stroke incidence (light gray bar) and mortality (dark gray bar) over five decades. (Data compiled with permission; see Figure Credits)

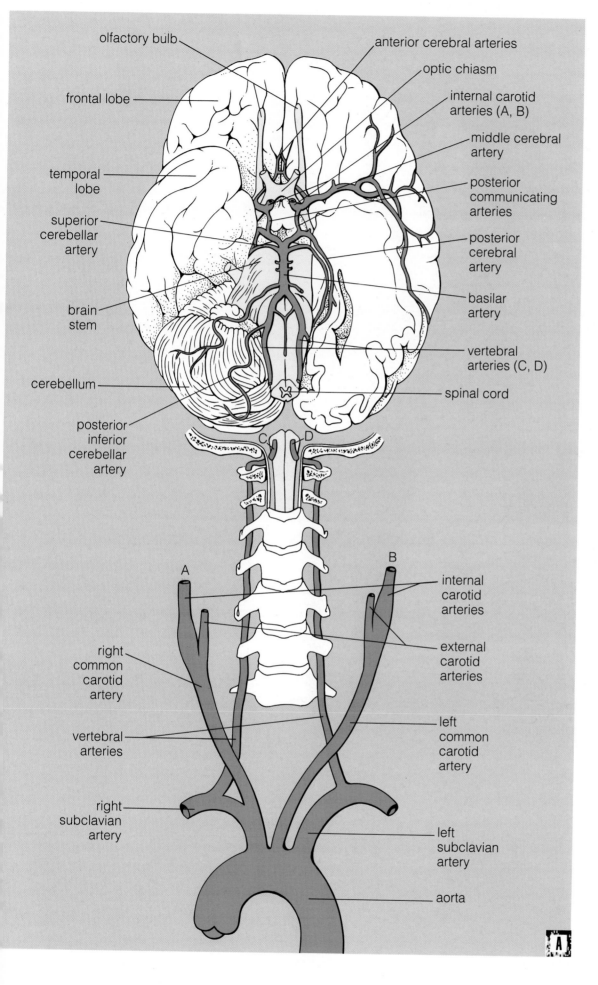

olfactory bulb

frontal lobe

temporal lobe

superior cerebellar artery

brain stem

cerebellum

posterior inferior cerebellar artery

right common carotid artery

vertebral arteries

right subclavian artery

anterior cerebral arteries

optic chiasm

internal carotid arteries (A, B)

middle cerebral artery

posterior communicating arteries

posterior cerebral artery

basilar artery

vertebral arteries (C, D)

spinal cord

internal carotid arteries

external carotid arteries

left common carotid artery

left subclavian artery

aorta

FIGURE 23.2 **(A)** Major blood vessels supplying the brain.

FIGURE 23.2 (B) Functional vascular territories.

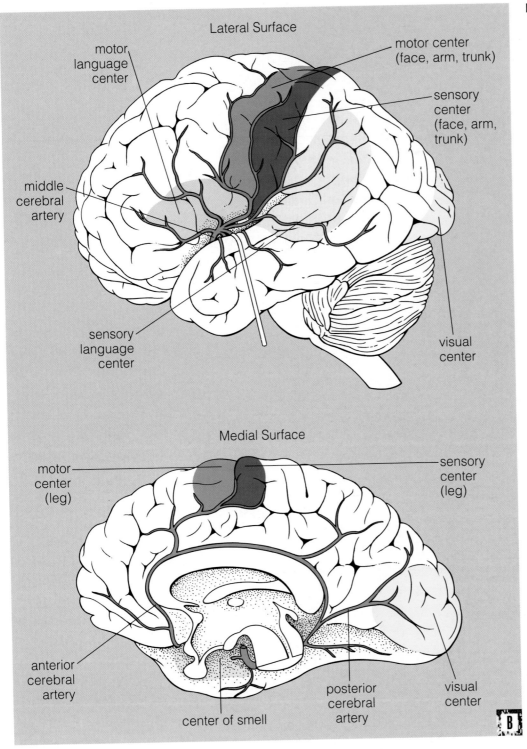

Lateral Surface

motor
language
center

motor center
(face, arm, trunk)

sensory
center
(face, arm,
trunk)

middle
cerebral
artery

sensory
language
center

visual
center

Medial Surface

motor
center
(leg)

sensory
center
(leg)

anterior
cerebral
artery

center of smell

posterior
cerebral
artery

visual
center

FIGURE 23.3 MOST COMMONLY ENCOUNTERED NEUROLOGIC SIGNS IN CAROTID AND VERTEBRAL–BASILAR STROKE

Carotid Territory

A. Hemiparesis
B. Hemisensory loss: cortical sensory modalities
C. Homonymous hemianopsia or quadrantanopsia
D. Aphasia: global, receptive or expressive, if dominant hemisphere involved
E. Neglect syndromes if non-dominant hemisphere involved

Vertebral–Basilar Territory

A. Ipsilateral cranial nerve deficits with contralateral weakness or sensory loss
B. Diplopia
C. Vertigo
D. Visual field loss, may cause cortical blindness
E. Gait and/or limb ataxia

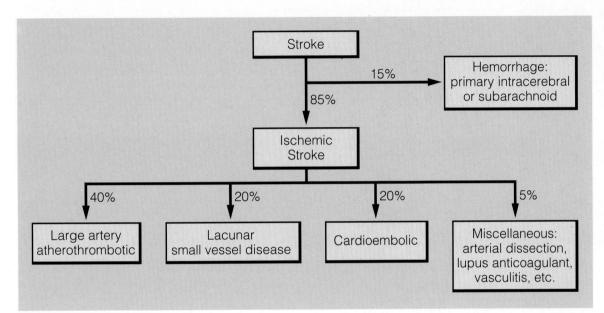

FIGURE 23.4   Major subcategories of stroke and their relative frequency. (Data compiled; see Figure Credits)

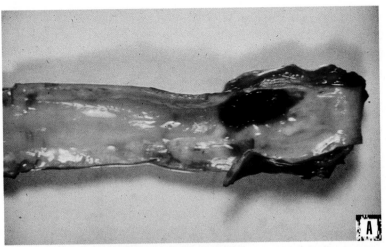

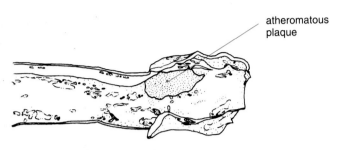

atheromatous plaque

FIGURE 23.5   **(A)** Pathologic specimen of a carotid athero-sclerotic lesion. **(B)** Angiogram of carotid atherosclerosis. **(C)** Noninvasive image of the same lesion, causing complete occlusion.

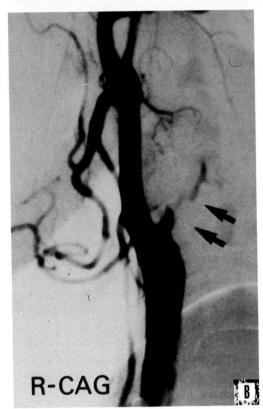

R-CAG

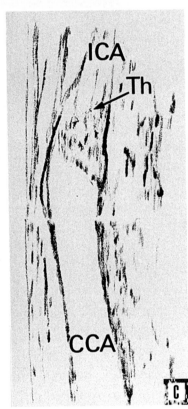

ICA

Th

CCA

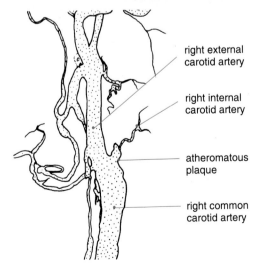

right external carotid artery

right internal carotid artery

atheromatous plaque

right common carotid artery

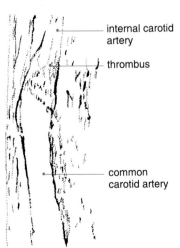

internal carotid artery

thrombus

common carotid artery

THE HEART AND OTHER CONDITIONS

not fall into one of these categories; these patients represent a group with other potential etiologies for their stroke. Each of the major subcategories of stroke has distinctive clinical, radiologic and pathophysiologic characteristics, which allow for their differentiation. Most stroke patients can be assigned to one of these four major categories after initial clinical and laboratory evaluations have been obtained. The characteristics of each major stroke subcategory are outlined in this chapter to help the clinician diagnose the patient's stroke accurately.

LARGE VESSEL ATHEROTHROMBOTIC STROKE

Atherothrombotic stroke represents the largest etiologic category for stroke and shares many pathophysiologic features with atherosclerotic disorders in other vascular territories, such as the heart.[3] These stroke patients have atherosclerotic lesions that occur at the carotid bifurcation (Fig. 23.5) or, occasionally, more distally within the intracranial carotid artery. In the vertebral-basilar system, atherosclerotic lesions are commonly noted at the origin of the vertebral arteries or, more distally, within the basilar artery. Large artery atherothrombotic stroke may begin abruptly, but in many patients it follows a stuttering, or step-wise, progressive course. Many large artery atherothrombotic strokes develop while the patient is asleep and the symptoms are initially noted upon awakening. The symptoms and signs in these patients reflect the area of ischemia, as previously outlined. Large artery atherothrombotic strokes may develop either secondary to distal embolization of thrombi, which form upon proximal atheromata, or secondary to hemodynamic compromise, as a large vessel narrows or becomes occluded. A prior history of transient ischemic attack within the same vascular territory is most common in patients with large artery atherothrombotic stroke and supports this diagnosis. Risk factors for atherosclerosis, such as hypertension, diabetes mellitus, hyperlipidemia, and cigarette smoking, are also risks for the

development of this stoke subtype.

LACUNAR STROKE

Small vessel degenerative changes can lead to vascular compromise in such vital arteries as the lenticulostriate branches of the middle cerebral artery (Fig. 23.6) and penetrators into the brainstem from the basilar artery.[5] In these vascular territories and others, a small infarction can cause substantial neurologic deficits because vital structures are compromised. The term *lacunar syndrome* is typically used for such small infarctions, but other vascular lesions can cause similar symptoms and the diagnosis of a lacunar syndrome should not be entirely equated with a small infarction in all cases.

The most common lacunar syndrome observed in clinical practice is pure motor hemiplegia. In this disorder, weakness of the face, arm, and leg are typically observed with relatively equal severity. However, in some cases there may be greater involvement in some of these areas than in others. While other neurologic findings should be present, on occasion mild sensory loss can be seen. Pure motor hemiplegia usually occurs secondary to a small infarction within the internal capsule or basis pontis. Pure sensory stroke is observed much less commonly and usually represents a similar infarction within the thalamus. A large variety of other lacunar syndromes have been described; the two most likely to be encountered are clumsy hand dysarthria syndrome and ipsilateral ataxia in an arm or leg with weakness as well. The diagnosis of a lacunar syndrome is important, because the prognosis when these vascular events are secondary to small infarctions is much better than that associated with atherothrombotic and cardioembolic stroke.

Approximately 75% of lacunar patients have no or little neurologic residual after 1 to 2 months. Many, but not all of these patients, have a history of hyper-

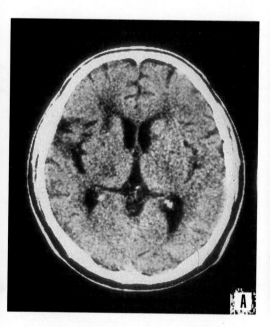

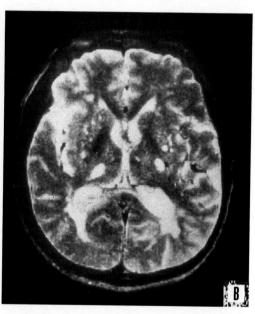

FIGURE 23.6   Lacunar infarctions demonstrated by CT (**A**) and MRI (**B**) scans in the same patient.

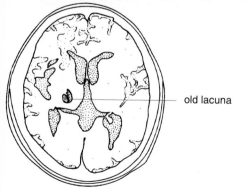

old lacuna

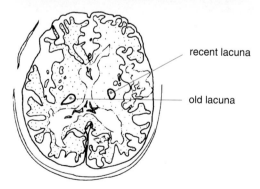

recent lacuna

old lacuna

tension and/or diabetes mellitus. The vascular pathology associated with small vessel occlusion is lipohylanosis or microatheromatous change of the vessel. These changes differ from the typical atherosclerotic plaque observed in larger arteries.

INTRACEREBRAL HEMORRHAGE

The third major subtype of acute stroke is primary intracerebral hemorrhage, and this subtype includes strokes with substantial differences in pathophysiology, prognosis, and management from those associated with ischemic stroke (Fig. 23.7).[5] Primary intracerebral hemorrhages usually occur within the basal ganglia, thalamus, brainstem, cerebellum, or cerebral hemispheres. Primary intracerebral hemorrhage in deeper structures is typically associated with a history of hypertension; cortical hemorrhages have this association less commonly. The neurologic deficit in primary intracerebral hemorrhage usually progresses in a relatively smooth fashion over hours. Obtundation or coma may be seen relatively early in the course of primary intracerebral hemorrhage, while such clouding of consciousness is very unusual early in the course of ischemic stroke. Headache, nausea, and vomiting are also more commonly seen with primary intracerebral hemorrhage than with ischemic stroke. The prognosis for primary intracerebral hemorrhage is much worse than with the ischemic stroke subtypes, as the rate of mortality in these patients ranges from 20% to 40%, substantially higher than that seen with ischemic stroke.

Primary intracerebral hemorrhage should be suspected in patients complaining of headache who become obtunded in association with a progressive focal neu-

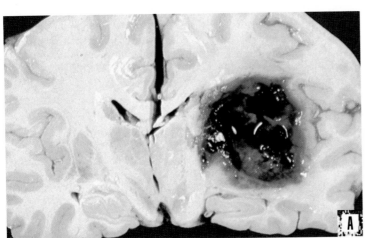

FIGURE 23.7 **(A)** Large basal ganglial hemorrhage with mass effect. **(B)** CT and MRI examples of an acute intracerebral hemorrhage and its course. (Reproduced with permission; see Figure Credits)

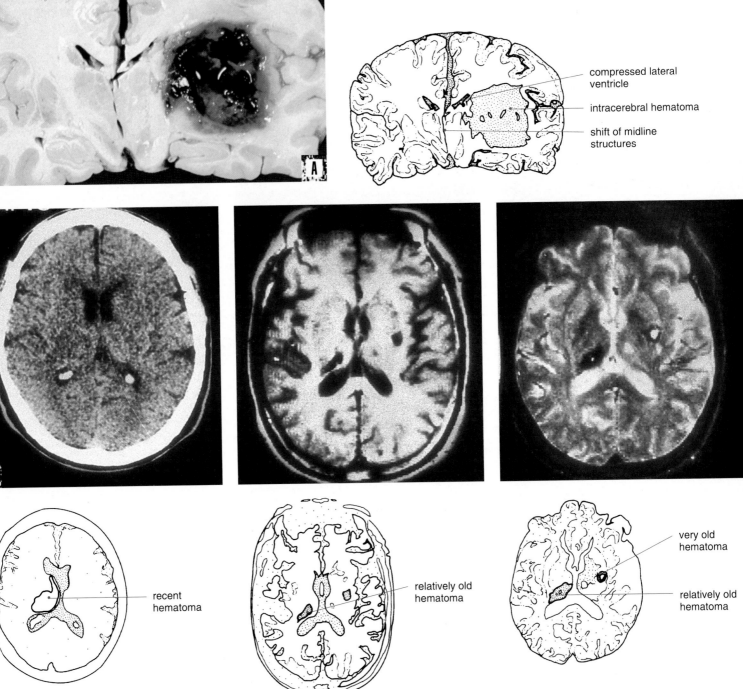

THE HEART AND OTHER CONDITIONS

rologic deficit. Imaging studies should be performed early to differentiate this stroke subtype. Such studies as computerized tomography (CT) and magnetic resonance imaging (MRI) are very sensitive and specific for establishing an accurate diagnosis.

Subarachnoid hemorrhage (SAH) is an intracerebral hemorrhage that primarily involves the subarachnoid space, and not the brain parenchyma.[5] Patients with SAH typically seek medical evaluation because of an acutely developing, violent headache associated with nausea and vomiting. Focal neurologic signs occur in a minority of patients. Rupture of an intracranial arterial aneurysm (Fig. 23.8) or arteriovenous malformation (Fig. 23.9) causes SAH in most patients, although blood dyscrasias and anticoagulants occasionally may be the etiology. SAH should be easy to differentiate from ischemic stroke or primary intracerebral hemorrhage by clinical criteria. In some SAH patients, the blood may dissect into the brain tissue, causing a hematoma and focal neurologic signs. Diagnostic confusion may ensue, although imaging studies usually clarify the anatomic source of intracranial bleeding. Early performance of a CT or MRI scan is mandatory for diagnosis. If these studies are unremarkable, a lumbar puncture should be performed to look for the presence of bloody cerebrospinal fluid. The mortality rate for acute SAH approaches 50%. Its management should include early aneurysm clipping, if an aneurysm is the bleeding source and the patient is clinically stable. SAH is commonly associated with a variety of electrocardiographic abnormalities and, rarely, with cardiac arrest.

CARDIOGENIC BRAIN EMBOLISM

Cardiogenic brain embolism (CBE) is the last stroke subtype to be discussed and is the major focus of this chapter.[6] The clinical diagnosis of CBE and its distinction from other stroke subtypes may be difficult, but several clinical features should engender suspicion. CBE should be considered in all patients who have potential cardiac sources for emboli (Fig. 23.10). However, the presence of a potential cardiac source for emboli does not establish with certainty that a CBE has caused the patient's stroke. Approximately one third of patients with a potential cardiac source for emboli will be found to have large and/or small vessel atherosclerosis, when they are appropriately studied. Abrupt onset of maximal neurologic deficit should lead to the suspicion of CBE, but such maximal deficit at onset may also be seen in patients with large artery atherothrombotic stroke and small vessel–related stroke on occasion. Transient ischemic attacks precede CBE much less commonly than large vessel atherothrombotic stroke. The presence of systemic emboli in association with stroke and a potential cardiac source would be supportive evidence for CBE, but this scenario is relatively uncommon. At present, CBE should be strongly considered in stroke patients with a potential cardiac source for emboli in the absence of large vessel cerebrovascular disease and lacunar syndrome.

The most common cardiac sources for CBE are nonvalvular atrial fibrillation, sick sinus syndrome, acute myocardial infarction (MI) with dyskinetic segments, ventricular aneurysms remote from MI, valvular heart disease, bacterial endo-

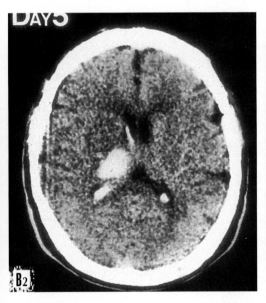
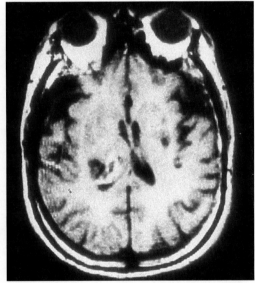
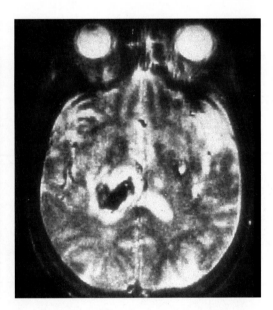

FIGURE 23.7   Continued.

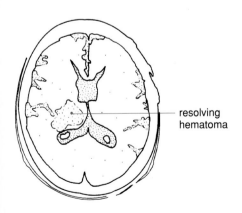
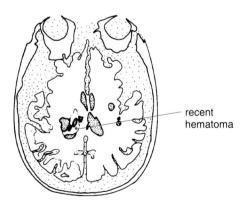
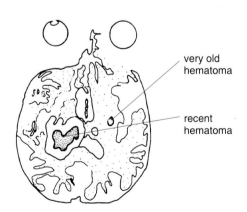

resolving hematoma

recent hematoma

very old hematoma

recent hematoma

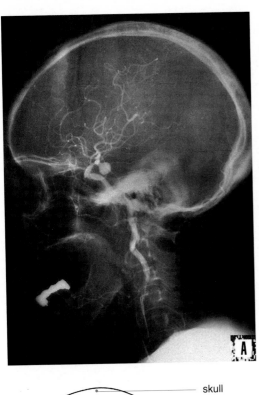

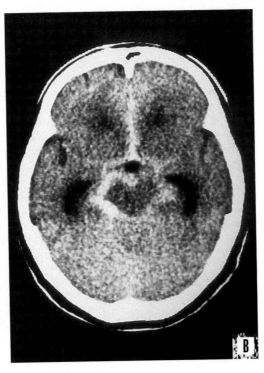

FIGURE 23.8   (A) Lateral cerebral angiogram of a large aneurysm at the internal carotid artery–posterior communicating artery junction. (B) CT evidence of blood in the subarachnoid space.

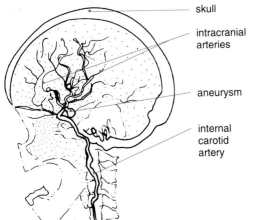

skull

intracranial arteries

aneurysm

internal carotid artery

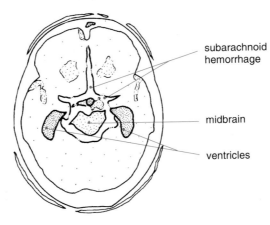

subarachnoid hemorrhage

midbrain

ventricles

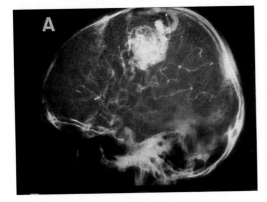

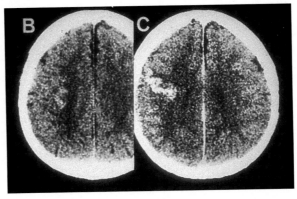

FIGURE 23.9   (A) Angiographic and (B,C) CT studies of a patient with an arteriovenous malformation (AVM).

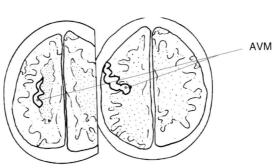

draining vein

AVM

AVM

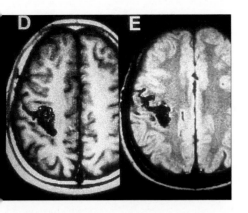
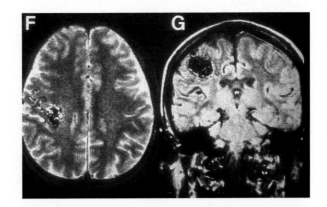

FIGURE 23.9 Continued. **(D–G)** MRI studies in a patient with an arteriovenous malformation (AVM).

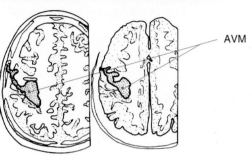
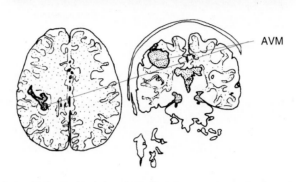

AVM

AVM

FIGURE 23.10 COMMON AND UNCOMMON CARDIAC SOURCES FOR EMBOLIC STROKE

Common Cardiac Sources

A. Nonvalvular atrial fibrillation
B. Ventricular segment dysfunction: acute MI or ventricular aneurysm
C. Infective endocarditis
D. Prosthetic cardiac valves, especially mitral
E. Patent foramen ovale, atrial septal defect leading to paradoxical emboli

Uncommon Sources

A. Atrial myxoma
B. Atrial septal aneurysm
C. Cardiomyopathy
D. Mitral valve prolapse
E. Sick sinus syndrome
F. Mitral annulus calcification
G. Valvular vegetations associated with lupus or prothrombotic states

carditis, and prosthetic cardiac valves.[1] Paradoxical emboli related to patent foramen ovale are being increasingly recognized in younger stroke patients.[7] A large variety of other less common cardiac conditions may be associated with CBE (see Fig. 23.10). The clinical features of the more common cardiac sources for CBE will be discussed in detail in later sections, and less common sources for CBE will also be outlined.

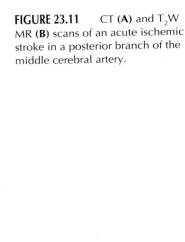

Diagnostic Testing

The history and general physical and neurologic examinations are very important for localization and subtyping of patients with acute stroke. The presence of a potential source for CBE should be readily apparent after the performance of the initial clinical evaluation of the patient. A standard 12-lead electrocardiogram should be performed in all patients with acute stroke, not only to look for potential sources of CBE but also to identify dysrhythmias and morphologic changes of the electrocardiogram that may occur secondary to the cerebrovascular event. An imaging study, either CT or MRI (Fig. 23.11), should be obtained in all stroke patients as soon as possible. These studies will help to differentiate between ischemic and hemorrhagic strokes, as well as give information concerning the size and location of the cerebrovascular event.[9] MRI scanning is the recommended procedure, because the yield for demonstrating early changes in ischemic stroke is better than that obtained with CT scanning. However, cost considerations may have an impact upon the choice for imaging studies. MRI scanning is also more sensitive for patients with vertebral-basilar strokes, as the posterior fossa structures are more accurately seen on MR than CT scanning. Early performance of an imaging study, within the first 24 hours after ischemic stroke onset, may in many cases not demonstrate the area of ischemia and will also miss potential hemorrhagic transformation of the ischemic lesion.[8] Therefore, in some cases, repeat imaging studies may be necessary several days after stroke onset, especially if deterioration is noted clinically.

Echocardiography is frequently used in suspected CBE patients.[5] In most older stroke patients, echocardiography should not be performed unless cardiac disease is appreciated by physical examination, standard electrocardiography, or chest x-ray. In younger patients, echocardiography is recommended routinely, as the yield of this procedure will be higher than in older patients for the demonstration of a cardiac source for stroke. Two-dimensional echocardiography may demonstrate a cardiac source for stroke in 10% to 15% of all patients with ischemic stroke. Transesophageal echocardiography may demonstrate a potential source for cardiac stroke in a larger number of patients, as this new technique appears to be more sensitive than two-dimensional echocardiography. Contrast echocardiography, employing the injection of air bubbles, should be

FIGURE 23.11   CT (**A**) and T$_2$W MR (**B**) scans of an acute ischemic stroke in a posterior branch of the middle cerebral artery.

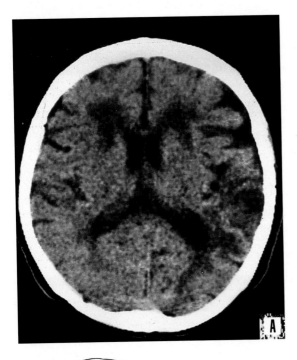
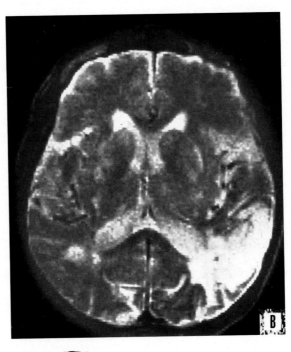

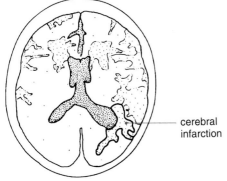
cerebral infarction

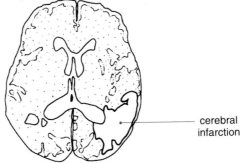
cerebral infarction

considered in most younger stroke patients, as the presence of a potential right-to-left cardiac shunt is common in this setting. Other cardiac imaging modalities, such as ultra-fast CT, MRI (Fig. 23.12), and isotope-labelled platelet scintigraphy are interesting but of unproven value at this time. Prolonged electrocardiographic monitoring, either by ambulatory means or by telemetry for in-patients, should be reserved for special situations. The yield concerning a potential cardioembolic arrhythmia, such as atrial fibrillation or sick sinus syndrome, is only about 2% in unselected ischemic stroke patients. However, in patients in whom such a dysrhythmia is suspected or in younger stroke patients, the yield may be substantially higher and therefore electrocardiographic testing should be considered.

Cerebral angiography should only be performed in selected patients with ischemic stroke, particularly if CBE is suspected. There are angiographic features, such as proximal occlusion of an intracranial artery, intraluminal filling defects, and rapid disappearance of an arterial occlusion, that support the diagnosis of embolus and, therefore, may influence diagnosis and therapy. Angiography should be used, however, in patients in whom the performance of this invasive technique will influence patient management. It is now possible with MRI techniques to visualize the extracranial and intracranial vasculature (Fig. 23.13). The technology for MRI angiography is rapidly evolving and this technique should be widely available in the near future. MRI angiography may

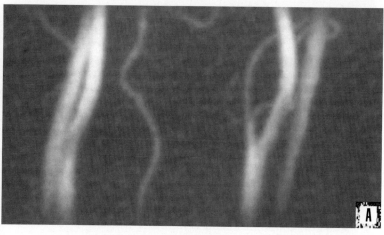

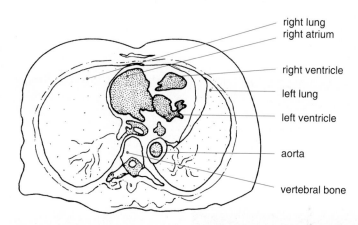

FIGURE 23.12   Cardiac MRI study clearly outlining cardiac structures.

right lung
right atrium

right ventricle

left lung

left ventricle

aorta

vertebral bone

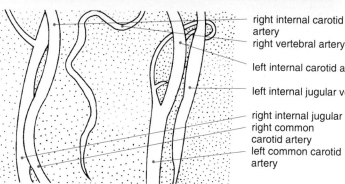

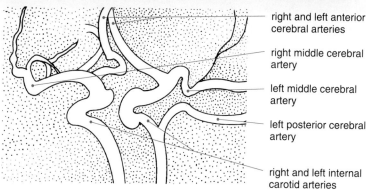

right internal carotid artery
right vertebral artery

left internal carotid artery

left internal jugular vein

right internal jugular vein
right common carotid artery
left common carotid artery

right and left anterior cerebral arteries

right middle cerebral artery

left middle cerebral artery

left posterior cerebral artery

right and left internal carotid arteries

FIGURE 23.13   **(A)** Normal MRI angiogram of the carotid bifurcation. **(B)** Circle of Willis well visualized on MRI angiogram.

afford a noninvasive mechanism to evaluate the vasculature of patients with acute stroke and contribute to our knowledge about stroke mechanism and its management.

A variety of noninvasive arterial imaging techniques are also available to evaluate the extracranial and intracranial cerebrovasculature. These techniques include B-mode ultrasound and Doppler. The evaluation of extracranial carotid atherosclerosis is well documented, and transcranial Doppler ultrasound (Fig. 23.14) is now being standardized for the evaluation of both carotid territory vascular lesions and vertebral–basilar disease.

ommon Sources for Cardiogenic Brain Embolism

NONVALVULAR ATRIAL FIBRILLATION AND SICK SINUS SYNDROME
Nonvalvular atrial fibrillation (NVAF) is a relatively common cardiac arrhythmia in the elderly (Fig. 23.15A). This arrhythmia is associated with a substantial risk for stroke, approximately five to six times that of an age-matched population without atrial fibrillation. Patients with NVAF also have a substantial risk for "silent" or asymptomatic strokes, as demonstrated by imaging studies. NVAF is associated with hypertensive heart disease, ischemic heart disease, and thyro-

toxic heart disease and, in some cases, may be of idiopathic origin. The stroke risk may be greater in NVAF patients who are elderly and have evidence of cardiac dilatation and/or congestive heart failure. Patients with idiopathic NVAF appear to be at lower risk.

Sick sinus syndrome (SSS) represents another arrhythmia with a substantial stroke risk (Fig. 23.15B). The risk for stroke may approach 8% to 10% per year in SSS patients. Those patients who have both tachyrhythmias and bradyrhythmias appear to be at higher risk for stroke in comparison to patients who have only bradyrhythmias. Atrial fibrillation is commonly associated with SSS and the distinction may be somewhat artificial.

MYOCARDIAL INFARCTION
Stroke within 2 to 3 weeks after acute MI occurs in 2% to 3% of patients. Patients with transmural anterior MIs are at much higher risk than patients with inferior MIs. MI patients who have a demonstrable ventricular thrombus on echocardiography appear to be a subgroup at particularly high risk for CBE. Additionally, patients with substantial ventricular wall motion abnormalities may also represent a subgroup at higher risk. The stroke risk in acute MI is greatest during the first week and diminishes over the following 2 to 3 weeks. A patient who suffers an MI may develop a chronic dyskinetic ventricular wall area or a ventricular aneurysm. Such ventricular wall abnormalities may be associated with the development of ventricular thrombi (Fig. 23.16) and, therefore, an increased risk for CBE. The risk for stroke in patients with left ventricular thrombi who are untreated may approach 5% per year.

Patients who develop a stroke acutely after an MI or who have a remote history of MI, should undergo echocardiographic studies to look for the presence of ventricular wall dyskinesia, aneurysms, or thrombi. The observation of one of

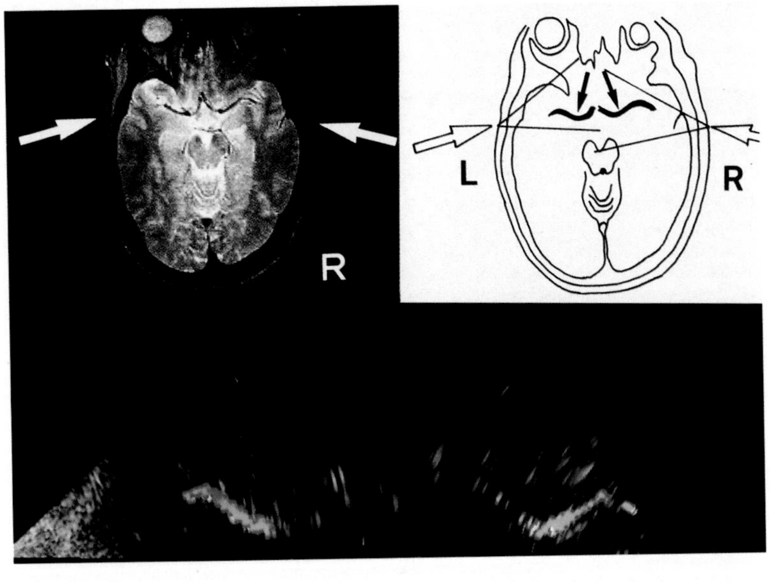

FIGURE 23.14   Transcranial Doppler studies of the horizontal portion of the middle cerebral artery and MRI of the artery. (Reproduced with permission; see Figure Credits)

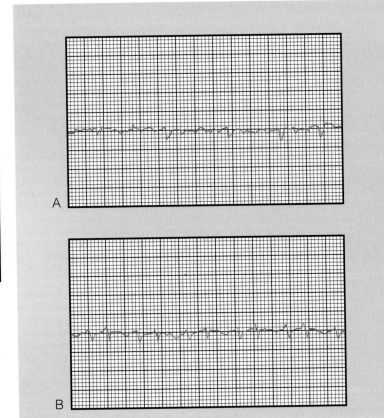

FIGURE 23.15   ECGs of atrial fibrillation **(A)** and tachycardia **(B)** associated with sick sinus syndrome.

these abnormalities may have an impact upon acute and chronic management. However, the potential presence of a cerebrovascular source for stroke should not be overlooked in this population.

VALVULAR HEART DISEASE

CBE is a common complication of rheumatic valvular heart disease—up to 20% of patients with rheumatic mitral stenoses experience stroke. The relative contribution of rheumatic heart disease to ischemic stroke has waned as the incidence of rheumatic heart disease has declined. Patients with rheumatic mitral stenoses and coexistent atrial fibrillations are at substantial risk for stroke in comparison to patients with mitral stenoses but no atrial fibrillation. The presence of atrial thrombi or enlargement on echocardiography (Fig. 23.17) may identify other risk factors for stroke in patients with rheumatic mitral stenoses. Patients with this valvular disorder who have an initial stroke are at substantial risk for recurrence, and therefore, appropriate therapy to reduce the risk of stroke is indicated.

PROSTHETIC CARDIAC VALVES

Although the total number of patients who have prosthetic cardiac valves is relatively small in comparison to the population at large, patients with such valves appear to have an inordinate risk for stroke (Fig. 23.18). Approximately 10% of

CBE patients have a prosthetic cardiac valve in place. A mechanical prosthetic valve appears to confer greater risk for stroke than does a bioprosthetic valve. Mitral prostheses are associated with greater risk of producing CBE than are aortic valves, and the presence of coexistent atrial fibrillation with prosthetic valves at either site adds to the risk for CBE. Many patients with CBE and an associated prosthetic valve are on anticoagulation therapy when their stroke occurs. Such patients should probably have their anticoagulants discontinued for a short period of time if the size of their stroke is substantial. The possibility of an infected prosthetic valve should also be considered in patients with CBE and a valve replacement.

MITRAL VALVE PROLAPSE

Mitral valve prolapse is a common disorder that on occasion may be associated with CBE (Fig. 23.19).[2] Mitral valve prolapse should be considered a source for CBE in the absence of other identifiable sources. It may be commonly associated with a patent foramen ovale, and therefore the contribution of the valvular disorder may be obscured. The association of mitral valve prolapse with CBE is easier to identify in younger patients than in older patients because other stroke sources are not as readily identifiable. Mitral valve prolapse may be associated with persistent or intermittent atrial fibrillation, and this arrhythmia should be

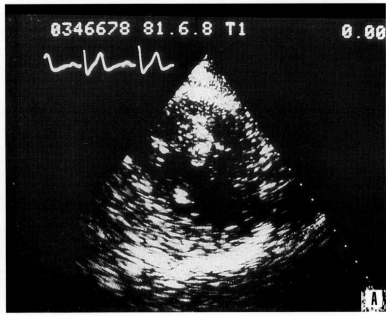

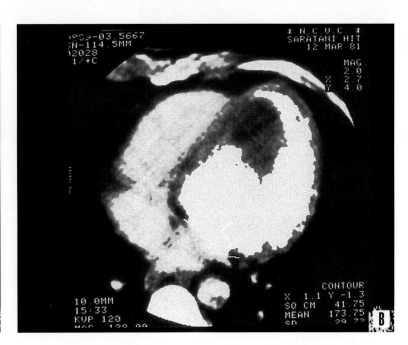

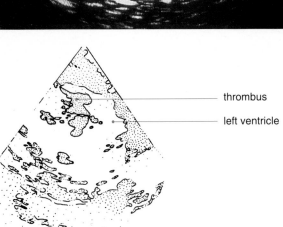

thrombus

left ventricle

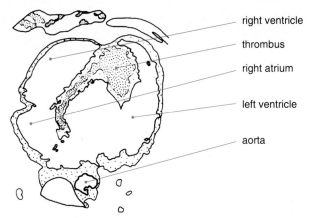

right ventricle

thrombus

right atrium

left ventricle

aorta

FIGURE 23.16   (A) Echocardiogram of an intraventricular thrombus. (B) Cardiac CT scan of the thrombus. (Reproduced with permission; see Figure Credits)

sought in patients with stroke and mitral valve prolapse. The risk for CBE in asymptomatic mitral valve prolapse is minute, and prophylactic therapy is therefore not indicated. However, patients with mitral valve prolapse who suffer CBE may be at substantial risk for recurrence, and therapeutic intervention in such patients should be considered.

BACTERIAL ENDOCARDITIS

Stroke complicates bacterial endocarditis in 10% to 20% of cases and is not an unusual initial manifestation of this disorder (Fig. 23.20).[10] Stroke in bacterial endocarditis typically occurs early in the course, and the risk is reduced as the infection is treated. Stroke may be seen with endocarditis associated with either mitral or aortic valvular infection and is more common in patients with *Staphylococcus aureus*. Infection of a mechanical prosthetic valve may put patients at an even higher risk for stroke than infection of a native valve. The detection of valvular vegetations by echocardiography may identify patients

with bacterial endocarditis who are at higher risk for embolic complications. Bacterial endocarditis may lead to the development of mycotic aneurysms within the cerebral vasculature and an associated risk for subarachnoid hemorrhage.

PARADOXICAL EMBOLI

The widespread employment of echocardiographic techniques in younger stroke patients has lead to the identification of a potential pathway for paradoxical emboli in 40% to 50% of stroke patients under the age of 45 who have no other obvious source for their stroke.[7] The prevalence of a potential right-to-left shunt is four to five times that of a control population without stroke. A patent foramen ovale can be readily demonstrated by contrast echocardiography and may be seen both at rest or with Valsalva maneuver (Fig. 23.21). Patients with a shunt at rest may be at higher risk for emboli. An atrial septal defect is another commonly identifiable abnormality that may cause stroke. The sources of thrombi for paradoxical emboli include venous thrombi or thrombi within the

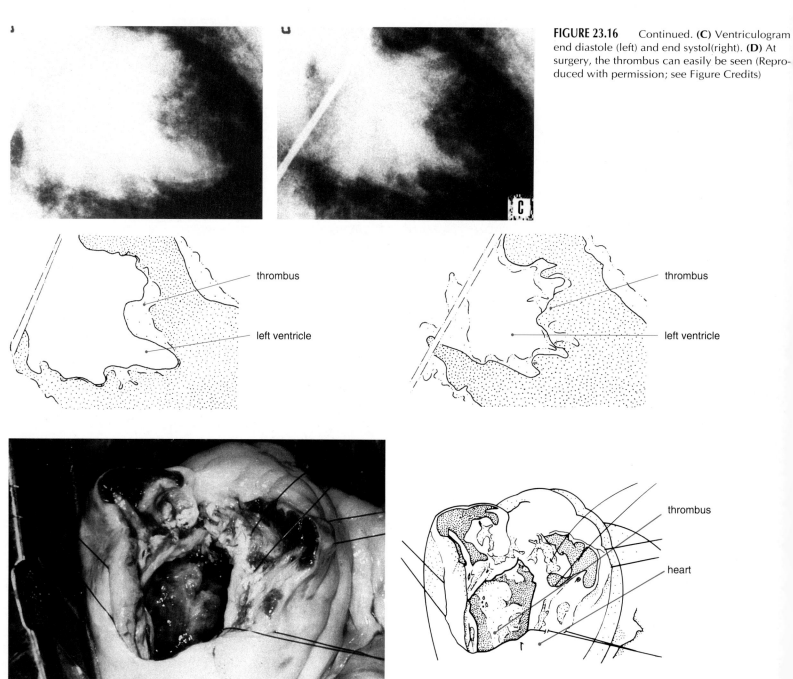

FIGURE 23.16 Continued. **(C)** Ventriculogram end diastole (left) and end systol(right). **(D)** At surgery, the thrombus can easily be seen (Reproduced with permission; see Figure Credits)

ghtside of the heart that can then bypass the pulmonary circulation by going through the intracardiac shunt. In many patients, no obvious source for the thrombus can be identified; therefore, it is only presumptive that the right-to-left shunt identifiable by echocardiography is the source of stroke in patients who have no other obvious source. The primary risk or the risk for recurrence of this disorder has not been established.

LESS COMMON SOURCES FOR CBE

As outlined in Fig. 23.10, a wide variety of other cardiac disorders are associated with an increased risk for stroke, although they are less commonly implicated.[1] Mitral annulus calcification may be seen with rheumatic mitral stenosis and atrial fibrillation, but is unclear whether the disorder by itself is associated with

an increased risk for stroke. Mitral annulus calcification is also associated with hypertension and diffuse atherosclerosis, and therefore stroke in these patients may be secondary to large vessel or small vessel cerebrovascular disease.

Nonbacterial thrombotic endocarditis (NBTE) is associated with collagen vascular disorders and underlying malignancies. Many of these patients are relatively hypercoagulable, and this state may be associated with the development of valvular thrombi (Fig. 23.22). The diagnosis of NBTE should be considered in patients with appropriate underlying disease who develop ischemic stroke. The diagnosis may be suspected by physical examination and confirmed occasionally by echocardiography.

Cardiomyopathies, both ischemic and idiopathic, are another group of cardiac disorders that may be associated with an increased risk for CBE. However, with-

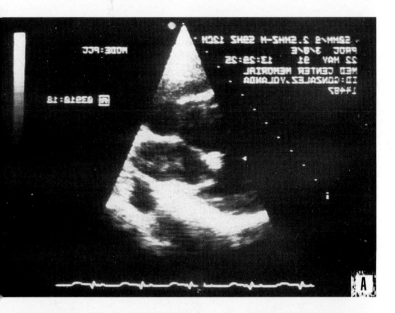

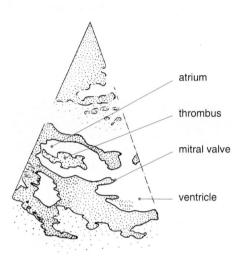

atrium

thrombus

mitral valve

ventricle

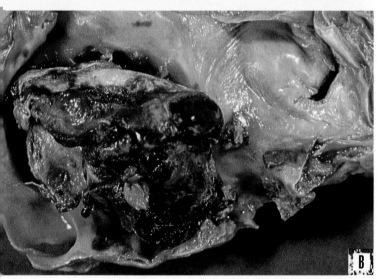

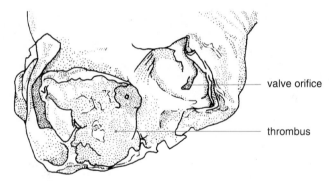

valve orifice

thrombus

FIGURE 23.17   (A) Echocardiogram demonstrating an atrial thrombus. (B) Large atrial thrombus in a patient with mitral stenosis. (Reproduced with permission; see Figure Credits)

out atrial fibrillation, cardiomyopathy is only rarely associated with CBE. Calcific aortic stenosis is not rare on routine echocardiographic studies. However, CBE is rarely associated with aortic valvular disease in the absence of arrhythmias or invasive procedures such as cardiac catheterization or percutaneous balloon valvuloplasty. Atrial septal aneurysms represent a congenital redundancy of the atrial septum identifiable by echocardiography. This is a rare cardiac disorder, but it has been associated with CBE. Therefore, if an atrial septal aneurysm is seen in a patient with ischemic stroke undergoing echocardiography, the aneurysm may be the source of the stroke.

While atrial myxomas are unusual, they are the most common primary intracardiac tumor (Fig. 23.23). Stroke may be the presenting clinical manifestation of atrial myxoma, and this tumor should be a considered diagnosis in younger stroke patients, especially when they manifest systemic symptoms, such as weight loss, fever, and joint pain, as well as abnormal findings on cardiac examination. Atrial myxomas can lead to stroke either by embolization of tumor material or associated thrombi. The disorder can be readily identified by appropriate echocardiographic techniques and confirmed by CT or MR imaging of the heart.

Complications of Cardiac Catheterization

Transient focal cerebral ischemic attacks or completed stroke occur infrequent as a complication of cardiac catheterization (0.1% to 0.4%). When associate with cardiac catheterization, cerebral ischemic symptoms occur most common in the posterior circulation. The most frequent symptoms relate to visual fie loss and, typically, these symptoms resolve within hours to a few days after th episode. Completed infarctions in the occipital lobe have been reported occ sionally. Other signs and symptoms associated with posterior circulation ischem may be seen in association with the visual field abnormalities. In only a sma

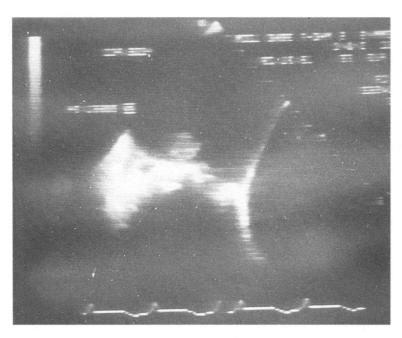

FIGURE 23.18   Large valve vegetation well visualized on transesophageal echocardiogram in a patient with a prosthetic cardiac valve.

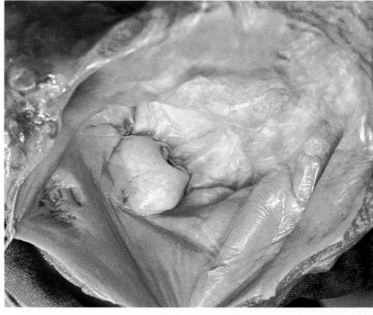

FIGURE 23.19   Prolapsed mitral valve observed from the left ventricle. (Reproduced with permission; see Figure Credits)

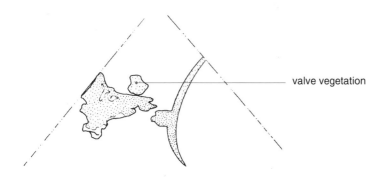

valve vegetation

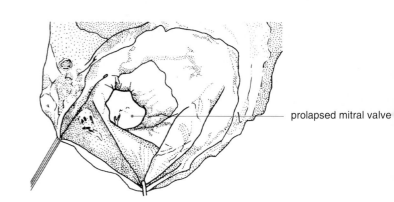

prolapsed mitral valve

minority of cases are symptoms and signs referable to the carotid circulation identified when a complication of cardiac catheterization occurs. Cerebral ischemic complications of cardiac catheterization are probably related to emboli in most cases, as thrombi or atheromatous material may be dislodged by the catheter (Fig. 23.24). Additionally, vasospasm associated with the catheterization, hypotensive events, or contrast media toxicity are alternative explanations in some cases. Most patients who suffer cerebral ischemic symptoms associated with cardiac catheterization resolve rapidly and are left with no long-term sequelae.

Complications of Electrical Cardioversion

Cardioversion is frequently performed in patients with new onset atrial fibrillation, atrial flutter, and supraventricular tachycardia. Embolism appears to be an infrequent complication of cardioversion done for the latter two arrhythmias; therefore, atrial fibrillation is the major concern. Up to 5% of patients undergo-

ing cardioversion for atrial fibrillation suffer embolic complications, if they are not treated. Formation of an atrial clot in patients with atrial fibrillation probably takes several days and, therefore, if the arrhythmia has begun within 1 to 2 days, anticoagulation may not be necessary prior to elective cardioversion. Beyond that time frame, elective cardioversion should be preceded by adequate anticoagulation therapy for several weeks to reduce embolic complications. Anticoagulants should probably be continued for several weeks after elective cardioversion, as emboli may occur during this period.

Cardiac Effects of Acute Stroke

Acute stroke, particularly an intracranial hemorrhage, may be associated with a variety of arrhythmias, morphologic electrocardiographic changes, and focal myocardial damage (Fig. 23.25).[10] Morphologic electrocardiographic changes, such as enlarged or inverted T waves and a prolonged QT interval, are common-

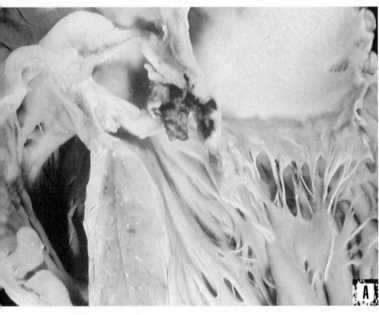

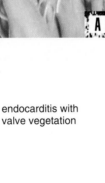

endocarditis with valve vegetation

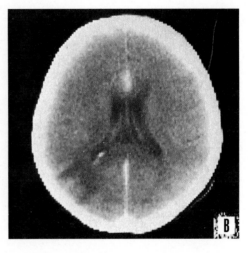

FIGURE 23.20
(A) Aortic valve associated with bacterial endocarditis and a thrombus. **(B)** Left posterior infarct visualized by CTscan. (Reproduced with permission; see Figure Credits)

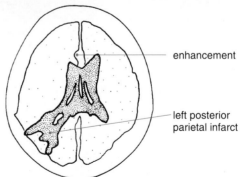

enhancement

left posterior parietal infarct

ly encountered in patients with acute intracerebral hemorrhage and, occasionally, in patients with ischemic stroke. Other morphologic electrocardiographic changes seen with acute stroke include depressed or elevated ST segments, high amplitude T waves, Q waves, increased QRS voltage, and U waves. These morphologic abnormalities may evolve over several days after the onset of the stroke.

Cardiac arrhythmias are also commonly encountered after acute stroke, espe-cially after intracerebral hemorrhage. Commonly observed arrhythmias include supraventricular tachycardia, ectopic ventricular contractions, multifocal ventricular tachycardia, ventricular flutter or fibrillation, and chronic or paroxysmal atrial fibrillation. Malignant arrhythmias, such as ventricular fibrillation, may cause acute cardiovascular collapse in patients with primary intracerebral or subarachnoid hemorrhage leading to sudden death. Approximately 1% of patients with sudden death have an associated intracerebral hemorrhage, and this should

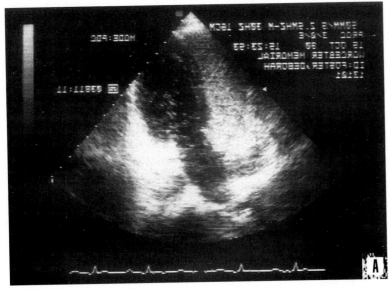

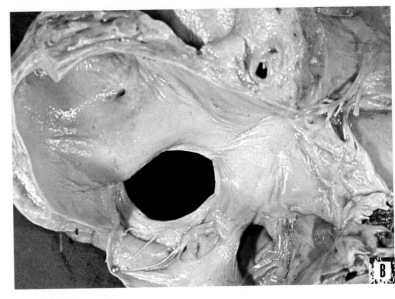

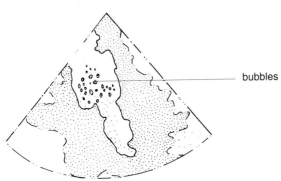

bubbles

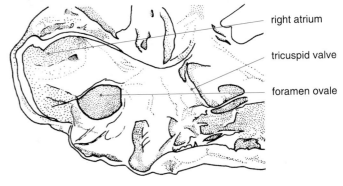

right atrium

tricuspid valve

foramen ovale

FIGURE 23.21 **(A)** Contrast echocardiogram (bubble study) demonstrating bubbles in both atria in a patient with a patent foramen ovale who had a brainstem infarction. **(B)** Pathologic specimen with a patent foramen ovale. (Reproduced with permission; see Figure Credits)

FIGURE 23.22 Aortic valve with associated vegetations. (Reproduced with permission; see Figure Credits)

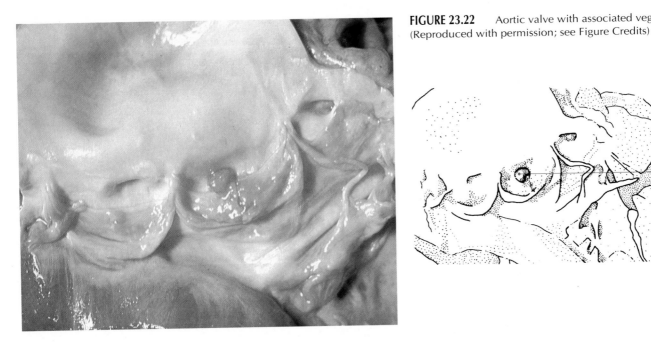

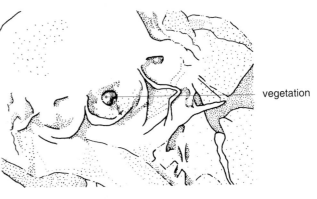

vegetation

THE HEART AND OTHER CONDITIONS

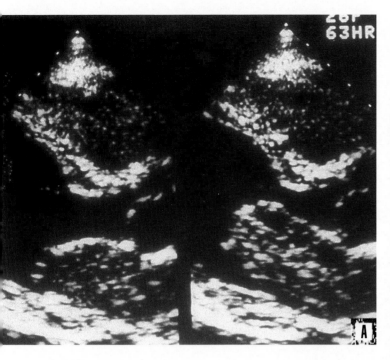

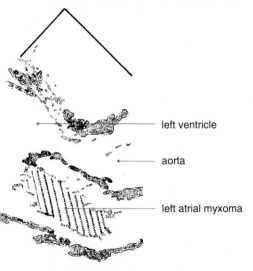

left ventricle

aorta

left atrial myxoma

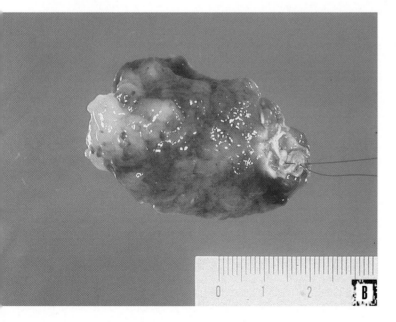

FIGURE 23.23 (A) Atrial myxoma well visualized by end-diastole (left) and late-diastole (right) echocardiograms. (B) Myxoma after surgical removal.

carotid arteries

vertebral arteries

aorta

heart

A = Mechanical injury to atheromatous plaque atheroma debris emboli

B = Intracatheter clot formation fresh clot emboli

catheter

FIGURE 23.24 Embolization during cardiac catheterization.

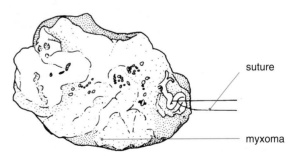

suture

myxoma

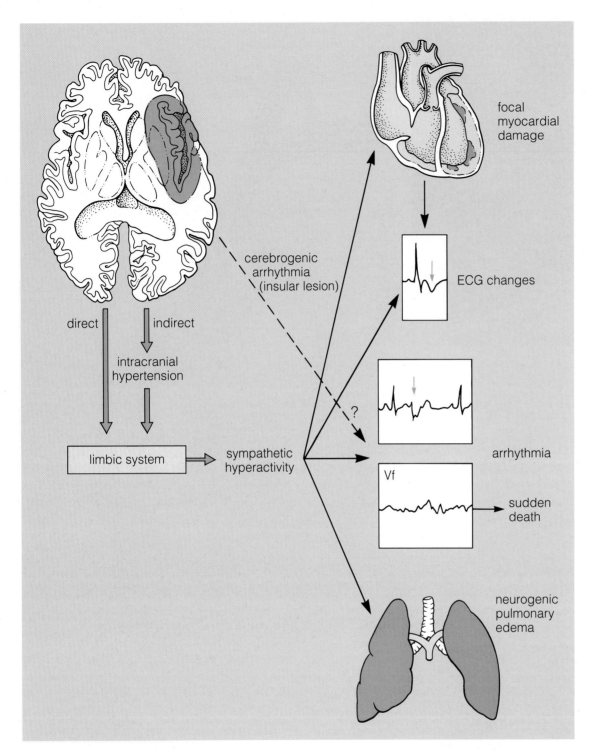

FIGURE 23.25   Cardiopulmonary effects of an intracranial lesion.

FIGURE CREDITS

Fig. 23.1 data compiled from Sacco RL: Current epidemiology of stroke. In Fisher M, Bogousslavsky J (eds): Current Review of Cerebral Vascular Disease. Current Medicine, Philadelphia, 1993.

Fig. 23.4 data compiled from Kase CS, Fisher M, Babikian VL, et al: Cerebrovascular Disease. In Rosenberg RN (ed): Comprehensive Neurology. Raven Press, New York, 1991.

Figs. 23.7A, 23.17B, 23.19, 23.20, 23.21B, 23.22 from Perkin Atlas of Clinical Neurology. Gower, New York, 1986.

Fig. 23.7B from Toole JF: Handbook of Clinical Neurology, Vol. 54: Vascular Disease, Part II. Elsevier, New York, 1989.

Fig. 23.14 from Tsuchiya T, Yasaka M, Yamaguchi T, et al: Imaging of the basal cerebral arteries and measurement of blood velocity in adults by using transcranial real-time color flow Doppler sonography. Am J Neurol Radiol 12:497–502, 1991.

Fig. 23.16 from Minematsu K, Yamaguchi T, Tagawa K, et al: A young man presenting sudden onset of left hemiplegia with a history of ischemia in the leg. Circ Sci (Tokyo) 2:484–494, 1982.

REFERENCES

1. Asinger RW, Oyken ML, Fisher M, et al. Cardiogenic brain embolism: The second report of the cerebral embolism task force. Arch Neurol 46:727, 1989.

2. Barnett HJM: Embolism in mitral valve prolapse. Ann Rev Med 33:489, 1982.

3. Bogousslavsky J, Van Melle G, Regli F: The Lausanne Stroke Registry: Analysis of 1000 consecutive patients with first stroke. Stroke 19:1083, 1988.

4. Broderick JP, Phillips SJ, Whisnant JP, et al: Incidence rates of stroke in the eightie The end of the decline. Stroke 20:577, 1989.

5. Kase CS, Fisher M, Babikian VL, et al: Cerebrovascular Disease. In Rosenberg R. (ed): Comprehensive Neurology. Raven Press, New York, 1991.

6. Kittner SJ, Sharkness CM, Price TR, et al: Infarcts with a cardiac source of embolis in the NINCDS Stroke Data Bank. Neurology 40:281, 1990.

7. Lechat P, Mas JL, Lascault G, et al: Prevalence of patent foramen ovale in patien with stroke. N Engl J Med 318:1148, 1988.

8. Okada Y, Yamaguchi T, Minimatsu K, et al: Hemorrhagic transformation in cerebr embolism. Stroke 20:598, 1989.

9. Ringelstein EB, Koschorke S, Holling A, et al: Computed tomographic patterns o proven embolic brain infarctions. Ann Neurol 20:759, 1989.

10. Talman WT: Cardiovascular regulation and lesions of the central nervo system. Ann Neurol 18:1, 1985.

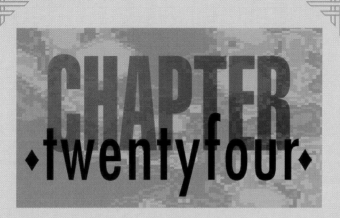

CHAPTER
◆twentyfour◆

ENDOCRINE
DISORDERS
AND THE HEART

STUART R. CHIPKIN, MD

Hormonal imbalances can lead to cardiovascular abnormalities involving rhythm, coronary vascular perfusion, or contractility. Some endocrine-related cardiac disorders are acute and reversible, whereas others, usually those occurring over longer periods of time, are permanent. Hormones can affect cardiovascular tissues either directly via hormone-receptor interactions or indirectly by altering electrolytes, fuels, lipoproteins, or coagulability. Because of the multiple levels at which hormones act, it is possible that treatment of a hormonal disorder may ameliorate one aspect of cardiac function only to adversely affect another. Similarly, correcting an endocrine disorder in a patient without cardiovascular symptoms may unmask or potentiate previously unrecognized cardiac disease. Thus, it is important to understand the ways in which endocrine disorders and their treatments affect cardiovascular tissues.

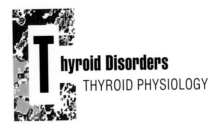

Thyroid Disorders
THYROID PHYSIOLOGY

Iodine is actively taken up by the thyroid gland and, after being oxidized by thyroid peroxidase, it is added to tyrosine residues carried by thyroglobulin to form monoiodotyrosine and diiodotyrosine. These iodinated tyrosines then combine

FIGURE 24.1 DIRECT EFFECT OF THYROID HORMONE ON THE HEART

A. Chronotropic—Heart rate
B. Inotropic—Contractility
  1. ↑ intracellular calcium via sarcoplasmic reticulum
  2. ↑ myosin ATPase activity
  3. Na⁺/K⁺ ATPase

FIGURE 24.2 CAUSES OF HYPOTHYROIDISM

	FTI*	TSH†
Primary	low	high
Hashimoto's disease		
Post-ablative (radioactive iodine, thyroidectomy, or external beam radiation)		
Impaired synthesis		
Iodine deficiency		
Amiodarone		
Lithium		
Secondary—hypopituitarism	low	low
Tertiary—hypothalamic defect	low	low
Resistance to thyroid hormone	high	high

*FTI = free thyroxine index: a calculated measure of the amount of free thyroxine (T_4) based on the total (bound and free) T_4 and the number of thyroid hormone–binding sites (derived from the T_3 resin uptake or T_3RU).
†TSH = thyroxine-stimulating hormone: synthesized and released from pituitary. This table assumes that a highly sensitive assay is used.

o form tetraiodothyronine (thyroxine or T_4) and triiodothyronine (T_3), which re released into the circulation in a ratio of 10:1. Thyroid hormone is carried by hyroid-binding globulin, albumin, and thyroid-binding pre-albumin. After being iffused across the cell membrane, T_4 (which contains four iodine molecules) is onverted to the more active T_3 by a deiodinase enzyme that removes an outer odine molecule. The intracellular thyroid hormone receptor, which binds T_3 nuch more avidly than T_4, then binds to a thyroid hormone response element hat activates a region of DNA containing nucleotide consensus sequences that esult in transcription. In the heart, the presence of thyroid hormone results in ecreased synthesis of myosin-heavy chain β and increased synthesis of myosin-eavy chain α, sarcoplasmic reticulum calcium ATPase, malic enzyme, Na^+/K^+ ATPase, atrial natriuretic factor, and β-adrenergic receptors.

Thyroid hormone has been shown to directly affect the heart (Fig. 24.1).[76] The ncrease in heart rate resulting from thyroxine administration is associated with n increase in the rate of diastolic depolarization and a decrease in the interval etween action potentials from the sinoatrial node. Thyroid hormone also ncreases intracellular Ca^{++} from the sarcoplasmic reticulum, thereby increasing nyosin-actin–generated force. Myosin ATPase activity, which is thought to regu-ate the turnover of myosin and the cross bridges between myosin and actin, is ncreased after thyroid hormone administration.[23,101] As opposed to contraction, elaxation is produced by reaccumulation of calcium by the sarcoplasmic reticu-um. Finally, thyroid hormone has been shown to increase Na^+/K^+ ATPase, lthough the effect of this ionic flux on heart muscle is not clear.[28]

HYPOTHYROIDISM

he major causes of hypothyroidism and the corresponding changes in thyroid unction tests are listed in Figure 24.2. Hashimoto's disease is the most common ause of hypothyroidism in the United States. Ablative therapy, depending on he amount of residual thyroid tissue, may take months to years before resulting n hypothyroidism.

Impaired thyroxine synthesis is usually related to abnormalities of iodine netabolism. Fifty percent of people with endemic goiter secondary to iodine defi-iency have elevated thyroxine-stimulating hormone (TSH) values consistent vith subclinical hypothyroidism.[51] Amiodarone can precipitate hypothyroidism luring the first year of use in nearly 20% of patients treated with this class III ntiarrhythmic drug. One mechanism appears to involve exacerbation of under-ying autoimmune disease; 60% of amiodarone-induced hypothyroid patients ave underlying antithyroid antibodies typically found in Hashimoto's disease. Amiodarone has also been postulated to cause hypothyroidism because of the arge amounts of iodine released into the circulation. Approximately 6 mg of odine (30 times the average U.S. daily dietary intake) are released from every 00-mg tablet of amiodarone. Amiodarone-induced hypothyroidism may be reated either by withdrawing the drug or by cautious addition of levothyroxine.

Iodine metabolism is also inhibited by lithium, which can inhibit iodide organifi-cation, thyroid hormone release, and peripheral metabolism. Secondary and ter-tiary hypothyroidism, as well as thyroid hormone resistance syndromes, are rare.

Clinical presentation of hypothyroidism frequently varies with age. Although younger patients manifest more classic symptoms, hypothyroidism may be diffi-cult to recognize in the elderly. The typical symptoms of hypothyroidism are also common complaints of elderly patients and include fatigue, weight gain, dry skin, cold intolerance, arthralgias, decreased hearing, constipation, depression, and memory loss. Conversely, patients with no detectable symptoms may be found to have elevated TSH levels (subclinical hypothyroidism). Finally, hypothyroidism in the elderly may present as toxicity to medications (e.g., digoxin or warfarin) because of changes in drug metabolism.

CARDIAC MANIFESTATIONS

Many of the cardiac abnormalities found in hypothyroidism are demonstrated in the case presented in Figure 24.3.[62] The patient's physical examination noted bradycardia and distant heart sounds secondary to a pericardial effusion. Diastolic hypertension is more common among hypothyroid patients.[96] Laboratory examination revealed hypothyroidism (elevated TSH with low T_4), most likely due to Hashimoto's disease (positive antithyroid antibodies). Hyperlipidemia is common in hypothyroidism; however, the elevated levels of low- and high-density lipoproteins are probably due to a decrease in clearance.[1]

The electrocardiogram shows low-voltage bradycardia and either flattened or inverted T waves throughout. QRS and Q–T intervals are often prolonged and may predispose to arrhythmias. Cardiomegaly is common in hypothyroidism.

Echocardiography can demonstrate a pericardial effusion in about one third of cases (readily seen on chest radiograph), which is due to increased capillary permeability, protein extravasation, and decreased lymphatic drainage. Pericardial effusions from hypothyroidism very rarely cause tamponade and will resolve with replacement therapy. The isovolumetric relaxation phase and the pre-ejection period are increased in hypothyroidism. Systolic time intervals are also increased while contractility, cardiac output, and stroke volume are de-creased (see Fig. 24.7).

The effect of hypothyroidism on coronary artery disease has been debated for many years. Studies have found hypothyroidism to be an independent risk fac-tor,[115] a risk factor in conjunction with hypertension,[108] or an insignificant risk factor for coronary atherosclerosis.[10] In animal models, hypothyroidism potenti-ates (and administration of thyroid hormone inhibits) atherosclerosis from cho-lesterol feeding. Interestingly, chest pain and myocardial infarction are less com-mon among patients with hypothyroidism, despite significant atherosclerotic disease.[58,115] Some explanations for this are the decreased platelet adhesiveness and the reduced levels of clotting factors VII, VIII, IX, and XI.[30]

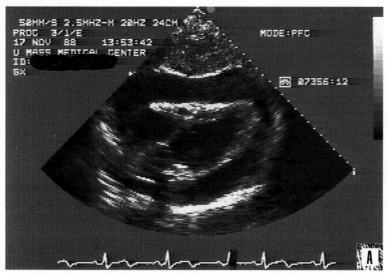

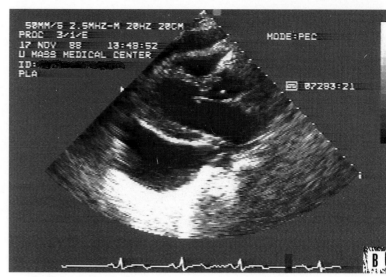

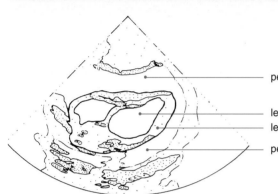

pericardial effusion

left ventricular cavity
left ventricular wall

pericardial effusion

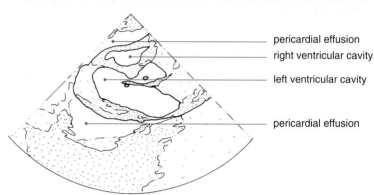

pericardial effusion
right ventricular cavity

left ventricular cavity

pericardial effusion

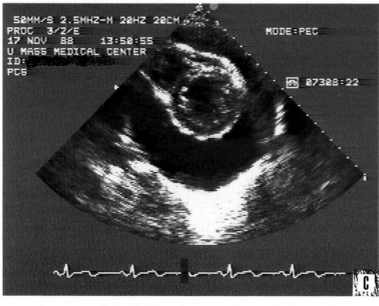

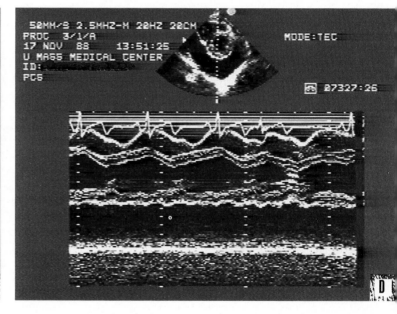

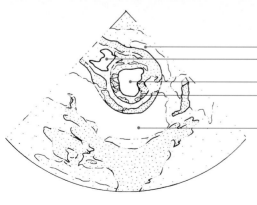

pericardial effusion
right ventricular cavity

left ventricular cavity
left ventricular wall

pericardial effusion

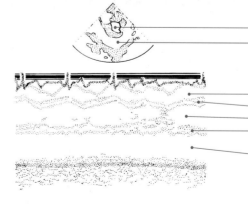

left ventricular cavity
pericardial effusion

pericardial effusion
septum
left ventricular cavity
posterior wall of left
  ventricle
pericardial effusion

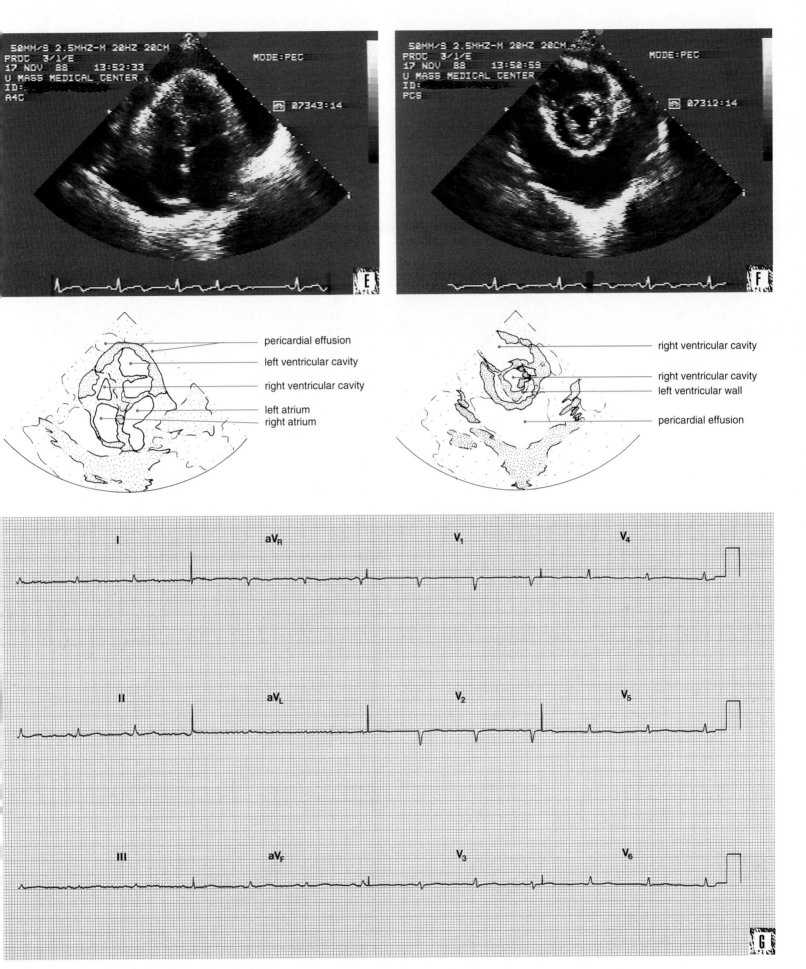

FIGURE 24.3 Echocardiography **(A–F)**, and ECG **(G)** studies of a 50-year-old woman who presented with complaints of fatigue and pedal edema. Physical examination revealed a pulse rate of 60 with distant heart sounds and a blood pressure of 140/95. Laboratory studies revealed the following: total T₄ was less than 1 ug/dL; TSH was greater than uU/mL; antithyroid antibodies were positive (1:3200); total cholesterol was 240 mg/dL; HDL-cholesterol was 60 mg/dL.

In the 1930's, the theoretical benefits of the hypometabolic state of hypothyroidism led to using radioactive iodine in patients with intractable angina or congestive heart failure. However, hypothyroidism was later shown to increase the risk for subendocardial ischemia and to complicate myocardial infarctions that did occur.

The coexistence of hypothyroidism and atherosclerosis raises two major concerns. The first is that thyroid replacement increases myocardial oxygen demand. Prior to 1980, under-replacement with thyroid hormone (especially with extracts of thyroid hormone) was frequently advocated because of the risk of myocardial infarction and precipitation of unstable angina. However, the development of specific antianginal medications (cardioselective beta blockers, calcium-channel blockers, etc.) and the improved ability to accurately prescribe doses of levothyroxine and evaluate replacement using highly sensitive TSH assays should reduce the risk for adverse events during treatment of hypothyroidism. In isolated cases, symptoms of chest pain have been reduced following replacement with thyroid hormone.[121]

The second concern for patients with hypothyroidism and atherosclerosis is the possible necessity of bypass graft surgery prior to initiating thyroid replacement (Fig. 24.4). The complications of surgery on hypothyroid patients and the utility of preoperative thyroid replacement have been reviewed.[9] In one case-control study, mild-to-moderate hypothyroidism did not affect the outcomes of the 59 hypothyroid patients undergoing coronary artery bypass grafting (CABG).[117] However, the hypothyroid patients tended to bleed more and to have longer times to extubation. A second case-control study documented higher risk among hypothyroid patients for perioperative congestive heart failure, prolonged anesthesia recovery, ileus, and central nervous system disturbances. In addition, despite comparable rates of infection, hypothyroid patients were less likely than non-hypothyroid patients to manifest a fever.[63]

In summary, hypothyroidism decreases inotropic and chronotropic actions of the heart but also reduces myocardial oxygen demand. While these abnormalities may impair cardiac function, they may also reduce symptoms of angina. The contribution of chronic hypothyroidism to atherosclerosis has not been well-defined.

Revascularization procedures can be performed safely in hypothyroid patients.

HYPERTHYROIDISM

Thyrotoxicosis is the general term describing an increase in plasma thyroid hormone concentration. *Hyperthyroidism* is a more specific term referring to disorders in which thyroid hormone production, as measured by increased iodine uptake, is increased (Fig. 24.5). There are four major causes of hyperthyroxinemia that do not involve increased hormone synthesis and therefore have decreased radioactive iodine uptake. Thyroiditis results in follicular cell disruption and release of preformed thyroid hormone. Because of the cellular damage, iodine is unable to be trapped or organified, resulting in a low radioactive iodine uptake. After an initial elevation in T_4, patients may have a transient hypothyroid phase prior to returning to an euthyroid state. Another cause of nonthyroidal thyrotoxicosis is iatrogenic hyperthyroidism, which can be prevented by periodic (every 6 to 12 months) thyroid function testing, especially if there is a change in the dose or preparation of thyroxine used. Iodine-induced thyrotoxicosis is more common in areas of iodine deficiency and in patients with underlying thyroid abnormalities.

CARDIAC MANIFESTATIONS

Increased activation of the sympathetic nervous system was previously proposed as the principal cause of many of the signs of thyrotoxicosis, including increased heart rate, increased cardiac output, increased cardiac contractility, increased hepatic glycogenolysis, increased gastrointestinal motility, muscle weakness, and emotional lability. Conversely, a lack of catecholamine action in hypothyroidism was thought to cause bradycardia, decreased cardiac contractility, decreased thermogenesis, narrow pulse pressure, and ptosis. However, increases in plasma or urinary measurements of norepinephrine and epinephrine have not been noted in hyperthyroidism;[7,24] paradoxically, catecholamines have been shown to be elevated in hypothyroidism.[25,109] Although some studies have documented an increased number of β-receptors in hyperthyroidism, changes in the

---

FIGURE 24.4 RISKS FOR HYPOTHYROID PATIENTS UNDERGOING CABG

Congestive heart failure
Prolonged anesthesia recovery
Prolonged constipation or ileus
CNS disturbances—confusion, coma, psychosis
Lack of fever with infection

FIGURE 24.5 CLASSIFICATION OF THYROTOXICOSIS

THYROTOXICOSIS WITH INCREASED RADIOACTIVE IODINE UPTAKE (HYPERTHYROIDISM)	THYROTOXICOSIS WITH DECREASED RADIOACTIVE IODINE UPTAKE
Graves' disease	Thyroiditis
Toxic multinodular goiter	Increased intake of thyroid hormone
Toxic adenoma	Iatrogenic
Hashitoxicosis	Factitious
TSH-producing tumors	Iodine-induced
Trophoblastic tumors	Struma ovarii

FIGURE 24.6 EFFECT OF THYROTOXICOSIS ON THE CARDIOVASCULAR SYSTEM

Bounding pulse and hyperdynamic precordium
Displaced PMI
Decreased systolic time intervals
Means-Lerman crunch
Widened pulse pressure
High-output congestive heart failure
Sinus tachycardia/atrial fibrillation

dose-response curve to epinephrine have not been demonstrated.[66] Possible explanations for an increase in adrenergic activity in states of excess circulating thyroid hormone include a novel neurotransmitter, a sympathomimetic action of iodotyrosines, or an alteration in post receptor signal transduction.[65]

A combination of increased adrenergic activity and direct effects of thyroxine on the cardiovascular system most likely explains the clinical abnormalities observed in thyrotoxicosis (Figs. 24.6, 24.7). The bounding pulse and hyperdynamic precordium are manifestations of increased contractility. The lateral displacement of the point of maximal impulse (PMI) in thyrotoxic patients is due to the increase in left ventricular mass. Shortening of the systolic time interval is among the earliest detectable abnormalities in thyrotoxicosis. The pulmonic component of S_2 is frequently forceful. The Means-Lerman scratch, or click, heard in systole is thought to reflect friction between the pleural and pericardial surfaces. In the subset of hyperthyroid patients with Graves' disease, mitral valve prolapse is more common than in euthyroid controls.[19] A widened pulse pressure is most likely produced by an increase in stroke volume and a 50% decrease in systemic vascular resistance. The large increase in flow to the skin helps dissipate excess heat generated by metabolically overactive tissue.[52] The reduction in vascular resistance could be a direct result of thyroid hormone on arteriolar smooth muscle tone or an indirect action mediated by local vasodilators.[60]

Despite increases in cardiac output, stroke volume, and coronary blood flow,

as well as a decrease in systemic resistance, hyperthyroid patients can present with congestive heart failure. Although thyrotoxic cardiac disease mostly occurs in a setting of heart disease, 43% of hyperthyroid patients with cardiac signs and symptoms have no evidence of underlying pathology.[97] The predisposition to thyrotoxic congestive heart failure may relate to abnormalities of either systemic vascular resistance or cardiac output. Whereas cardiac outputs have been found to be similar before and after thyrotoxicosis, systemic vascular resistance tends to be increased in thyrotoxic patients with congestive heart failure.[52] In addition, thyrotoxic patients do not display the normal increases in ejection fraction and cardiac output with exercise, causing some investigators to postulate a reversible cardiomyopathy in thyrotoxicosis.[36] Diastolic dysfunction has also been observed in thyrotoxic heart failure.[75] Thyrotoxic heart failure may ultimately be due to a combination of abnormal vascular responsiveness, increased blood volume, reversible muscle damage, and/or diastolic dysfunction.[60]

Although sinus tachycardia is the most common arrhythmia seen in hyperthyroidism, 10 to 22% of hyperthyroid patients exhibit atrial fibrillation.[2,6] Atrial fibrillation is more likely to occur in thyrotoxic patients who are male and greater than 60 years old and who have a history of hypertension or rheumatic heart disease.[6,35] Tachyarrhythmias appear to be caused by a shortening of the action potential duration;[38] however thyroxine levels do not consistently predict fibrillation.[50]

Hyperthyroidism is a common cause of atrial fibrillation accounting for 12% of

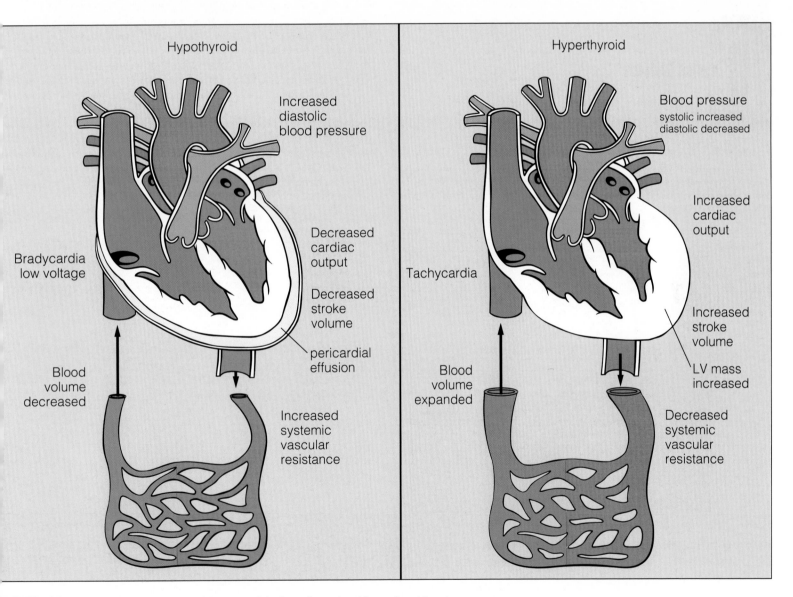

FIGURE 24.7   Cardiovascular hemodynamics of the hypothyroid and hyperthyroid patients.

patients with unexplained atrial fibrillation.[37] Conversion of atrial fibrillation often, but not always, occurs with return of the euthyroid state. Of 163 patients who were found to have thyrotoxic atrial fibrillation for up to 1 year, 62% reverted to normal sinus rhythm within 13 weeks of becoming euthyroid (Fig. 24.8).[80] Patients in whom atrial fibrillation persisted longer than 13 weeks did not spontaneously convert; these patients would be candidates for DC cardioversion. Evidence exists that disopyramide improves the likelihood of remaining in sinus rhythm.[79] Of the patients with thyroid-induced atrial fibrillation, arterial embolization has been observed in 10 to 40%.[6,105] Therefore, anticoagulation is indicated in thyrotoxic atrial fibrillation and should be continued until sinus rhythm has persisted for 3 months.[35] Doses of warfarin are typically lower in hyperthyroid patients because of enhanced degradation of vitamin K–dependent clotting factors.

In summary, excess thyroid hormone can produce increased cardiac output and decreased systemic vascular resistance. If compensation cannot be maintained for any reason, high output congestive heart failure can result. Atrial fibrillation can occur in hyperthyroidism, and hyperthyroidism can cause atrial fibrillation; anticoagulation is then indicated. Reversion to sinus rhythm usually occurs with normalization of thyroid function. Persistent atrial fibrillation with normal thyroid function will usually respond to cardioversion.

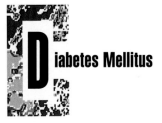

Diabetes Mellitus

Hyperglycemia is the common abnormality to both type I (insulin-dependent) and type II (noninsulin-dependent) diabetes mellitus. Although autoimmune destruction of pancreatic beta cells in type I diabetes creates an insulin-deficient state, these patients can develop some cellular resistance to insulin. In addition, subcutaneous administration of insulin results in increased peripheral concentrations relative to the normal secretion from the pancreas into the portal circulation. Type II diabetes is thought to be the result of resistance to some (e.g. glucose transport), but not all, of insulin's cellular effects.

Atherosclerotic cardiovascular disease is the leading cause of death among patients with diabetes mellitus.[61] Patients with diabetes manifest arteriosclerosis at an earlier age and are at increased risk for cardiogenic shock, congestive heart failure, and ventricular rupture. Female diabetic patients are at increased risk for coronary artery disease compared to nondiabetic females; the risk is similar to that of nondiabetic males.[5] Among minorities, Hispanic diabetic patients are at variable risk, depending on their particular ethnicity.[27,44] The increased risk among African-Americans for both diabetes and hypertension is thought to increase their risk for coronary disease.

Diabetes mellitus affects other vascular structures besides the heart. Patients with diabetes mellitus are at greater risk for stroke and have a higher mortality following stroke.[84] In addition, diabetic people are more likely to develop peripheral arterial disease.[85]

DIABETES AND ATHEROGENESIS

Diabetic vascular disease is usually classified as micro- or macrovascular, even though some affected end-organs (e.g., heart and kidney) possess both types of vessels. Microvascular abnormalities in diabetes are associated with endothelial damage, capillary basement membrane thickening, nonenzymatic glycosylation of proteins, increased free radical activity, and prostaglandin abnormalities. Some of these same mechanisms appear to be involved in diabetic macrovascular disease (e.g., nonenzymatic glycosylation of proteins, prostaglandin abnormalities). Microvascular disease may serve as a marker and may, in fact, be a risk factor for macrovascular disease; albuminuria has been shown to correlate with cardiovascular risk.[98] However, there also appear to be other distinct processes that participate in the formation of macrovascular lesions.

Some of the processes involving lipids, endothelial cells, platelets, monocytes/macrophages, and smooth muscle cells that predispose the patient with diabetes mellitus to atherosclerosis are depicted in Figure 24.9. Diabetic patients have abnormalities in cholesterol metabolism involving both the composition and the structure of lipoproteins. While the normal vasculature possesses the

FIGURE 24.8   Spontaneous conversion of atrial fibrillation with euthyroidism. (See Figure Credits)

bility to inhibit thrombus formation and to lyse existing clots, fibrinolysis in he diabetic patient is impaired. In addition, insulin resistance may play a role in nooth muscle proliferation and migration.

Diabetes is associated with abnormal amounts and composition of lipoproteins Fig. 24.10). Lipoprotein lipase (LPL) activity, which is responsible for releasing ee fatty acids from chylomicron-bound triglycerides, decreases with hyperlycemia and increases with improved glycemic control. Very low-density poproteins (VLDL), the most common lipid abnormality in diabetic patients, re elevated due to increased production and decreased clearance. Although DL levels vary in patients with type II diabetes, the amount of glycosylated LDL s increased and may bind abnormally to endothelial cells. Glycosylated LDL, because of its impaired catabolism, may be predisposed to become a more therogenic oxidized form. A peroxidized fraction of LDL, which may be a form f oxidized LDL, appears to be increased in diabetic patients.[68,82] Perhaps of reater significance, HDL-cholesterol is consistently decreased in patients with iabetes. Insulin therapy can increase the HDL$_2$ fraction by approximately 20%.

Because of the different patterns of hyperlipidemia in diabetes and the adverse effects of certain cholesterol-lowering agents on glycemia, the approach to treatment of lipid disorders may differ in the diabetic patient.

Endothelial damage is one of the initiating occurrences in atherogenesis. Hyperglycemia or increased free fatty acids can damage endothelial cells, thereby inhibiting normal fibrinolysis (plasminogen activator, prostacyclin) and promoting local thrombus formation (fibrinogen, von Willebrand factor [factor VIII], and glycosylated LDL-cholesterol). Diabetes can also increase platelet adhesiveness and aggregation via thromboxane and platelet-derived growth factor (PDGF).

As ambient glucose concentrations remain elevated, proteins become nonenzymatically glycosylated and create cross bridges that combine to form advanced glycosylation end products (AGEs). AGEs have been shown to facilitate migration of monocytes beneath the endothelial layer[59] and enhance binding of LDL to collagen within the arterial wall.[14] In addition, AGEs may inhibit the vasodilatory and antiproliferative effects of nitrous oxide.

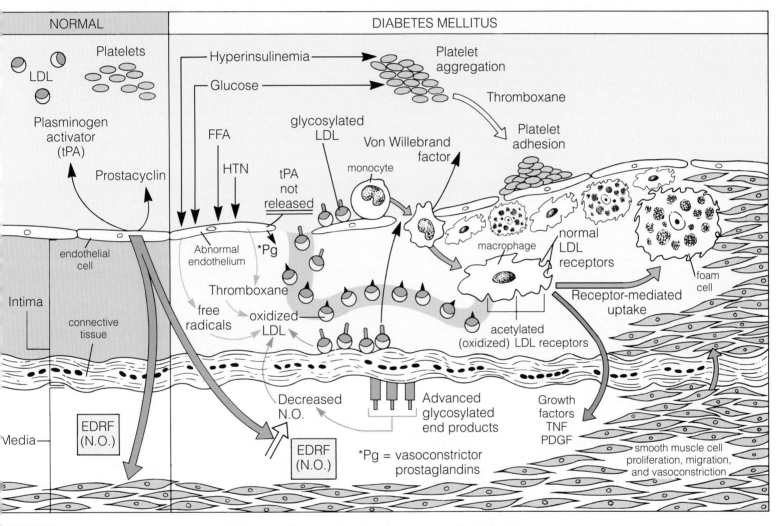

FIGURE 24.9   Hemodynamic processes of diabetes mellitus predisposing the patient to atherosclerosis.

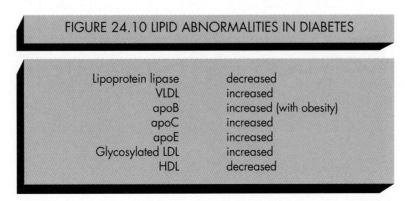

FIGURE 24.10 LIPID ABNORMALITIES IN DIABETES

Lipoprotein lipase	decreased
VLDL	increased
apoB	increased (with obesity)
apoC	increased
apoE	increased
Glycosylated LDL	increased
HDL	decreased

While elevated glucose levels are important in the genesis of diabetic cardiovascular disease, recent attention has focused on the role of insulin resistance and hyperinsulinemia in stimulating atherosclerosis.[110,111] Non-insulin–dependent diabetic patients as well as some obese nondiabetic patients and hypertensive patients will respond to a glucose challenge with exaggerated insulin secretion (Fig. 24.11). The maintenance of normal or near-normal glucose levels in the setting of hyperinsulinemia implies a partial resistance to the glucose-lowering actions of insulin. Increased insulin reponses to an oral glucose load have been demonstrated in patients who have, or who are at risk for, vascular disease.[29] Three prospective studies have consistently found hyperinsulinemia to be an independent risk factor for the development of coronary artery disease.[31,88,118]

The mechanisms by which insulin might stimulate atherosclerosis are not precisely known. In animals, chronic insulin therapy, despite lowering total cholesterol, produce early atherosclerotic lesions and also inhibits their regression.[72] In addition to stimulating intra-arterial lipid synthesis, insulin has been shown to stimulate proliferation[87] and enhance migration of vascular smooth muscle cells.[78] Insulin resistance and the resulting hyperinsulinemia might also increase the risk for atherosclerosis by adversely affecting blood pressure, lipid profiles, plasminogen activator, and smooth muscle activity.[29,110]

Along with endogenous insulin, proinsulin and partially degraded split products of insulin also circulate in patients with type II diabetes. A clinical trial using proinsulin for the treatment of type II diabetes was prematurely stopped after 2 years of investigation because of an increased number of myocardial infarctions.[39] Split products of insulin have been shown to have a better correlation with lipid profiles than intact insulin.[77]

Several types of abnormal cellular signal pathways have also been identified in insulin-resistant states associated with cardiovascular disease (Fig. 24.12).[92,104] Increases in intracellular calcium have correlated with hypertension and hyperinsulinemia. In hypertensive type II diabetic patients, decreased intracellular calcium flux due to decreased membrane Ca^{++} ATPase has been suggested to explain the observed increase in erythrocyte calcium levels.[120] An inverse relationship exists between intracellular magnesium and both insulin resistance and diastolic blood pressure. This intracellular defect may be of great importance in understanding the link between insulin and blood pressure; after correcting for intracellular magnesium concentrations, the usual relationship between insulin and blood pressure is no longer seen.

Intracellular pH also appears to be important in both hypertension and diabetes. Decreased intracellular pH varies inversely with fasting insulin concentrations, body mass index, and blood pressure. The role of cellular hydrogen ion balance may be particularly important in understanding hypertension in diabetic patients. Hypertensive diabetic patients have been shown to have a lower intra-

cellular pH than normotensive diabetic patients, despite similar calcium and magnesium concentrations.[93]

The role of intracellular sodium in hypertension has been investigated for many years.[49] Although little is known about intracellular sodium in type II diabetes, patients with type I diabetes do appear to have increased Na^+Li^+ transport, which is thought to reflect Na^+H^+ exchange. Increased Na^+Li^+ transport has been associated with family histories of hypertension and development of diabetic nephropathy.

PAINLESS ISCHEMIA AND INFARCTION IN DIABETES

The clinical presentation of atherosclerotic disease in diabetic patients often differs from that in nondiabetic people. While diabetic patients have been observed to have less pain[13] and more atypical presenting symptoms of myocardial infarction,[103] it may be that sudden deterioration in glycemic control prompts diabetic patients to seek medical care. The Framingham study was only able to detect a significant difference in frequency of painless infarction between diabetic and nondiabetic patients after 26 years of age.[56] Autopsy studies have also reported a greater frequency of diabetes in patients with unrecognized myocardial infarction.[17]

Myocardial ischemia can also occur without pain in patients with diabetes. Holter monitor studies have demonstrated that diabetic patients with coronary disease are more likely to have painless episodes of ST-segment depression and that they have these in greater number than nondiabetic patients with coronary disease.[20] When Bruce protocol testing is used, diabetic and nondiabetic patients appear to have equal frequency of painless ischemia.[21] However, when thallium scintigraphy is employed, diabetic patients, either with or without known coronary heart disease, are more likely to show evidence of ischemia without pain compared with controls.[22,81]

Since painless ischemia also occurs frequently in nondiabetic patients, autonomic neuropathy cannot entirely explain the absence of pain in diabetic patients. Although some studies have correlated autonomic neuropathy with a lack of pain in diabetic patients,[64] others have not.[21,48] Autonomic neuropathy has been identified as a strong predictor of mortality.[33] Although it is not specifically known if diabetic patients with autonomic neuropathy die more often from cardiovascular disease, a prolongation in the corrected Q–T interval has been observed[54] and raises the question of whether neuropathy may increase the risk for fatal arrhythmias.[32]

DIABETIC CARDIOMYOPATHY

An association between diabetes and cardiomyopathy was first reported in 1972[95] and has stimulated epidemiologic, basic, and clinical research. In the

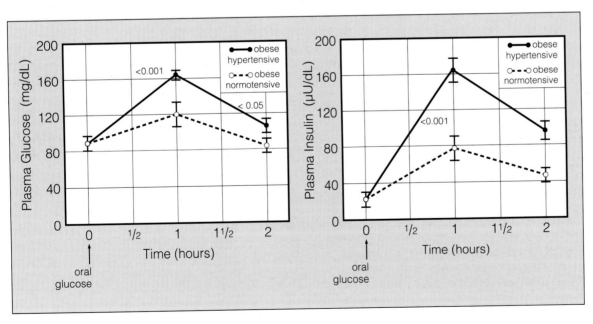

FIGURE 24.11 Plasma glucose and insulin concentrations during standard oral glucose tolerance tests performed in obese hypertensive (●) and obese normotensive (○) patients. (Redrawn with permission; see Figure Credits)

ramingham study, the risk of congestive heart disease among diabetic patients as found to be greater than expected from coronary disease alone (Fig. 24.13).[57] n addition, there is a higher prevalence of diabetes mellitus among patients with iopathic cardiomyopathies.[45] Among diabetic patients, noninvasive studies ave observed lower ejection fractions (either at rest or in response to exer-se)[74,91,116] and prolonged isovolumetric relaxation.[99] Improved diabetic control ems to ameliorate cardiac function.[18] While no single complication of diabetes as been predictive of impaired ventricular function, complications of diabetes nd to be associated with worse function.[100] Hypertension in combination with abetes confers a much worse prognosis.[43]

Histologic observations in the hearts of diabetic subjects include intimal prolif-ration and thickened walls, interstitial and perivascular fibrosis, glycoprotein eposition, thickened capillary basement membranes and microaneurysms; how-ver, these findings generally do not correlate with functional or clinical abnor-alities. It is unclear whether functional or histologic abnormalities are due to amaged ventricular myocytes, interstitial fibrosis, microvascular changes, or roximal coronary artery lesions.

Animal studies vary depending on the species used, but generally they have emonstrated decreased cardiac output and decreased ventricular compliance;[90] enetically diabetic mice are the only model that demonstrate abnormal ventricu-r myocytes.[41] Ten days of insulin therapy reversed the diabetes-induced decline the force-velocity curve for heart muscle.[34] At a cellular level, hearts from dia-etic animals have impaired calcium uptake by sarcoplasmic reticulum,[40] and ecreased myosin ATPase activity with an increase in the V_3 isoform of myosin.[69]

Thus, diabetes mellitus plays an important role in the pathology of cardiac vas-lar supply, neural innervation, and myocardial function. Much still needs to be arned about the impact of nutrition, ethnicity, gender, and socioeconomics on abetic cardiovascular disease. The contributions of glucose, AGEs, lipids, sulin resistance, and hyperinsulinemia are active areas of current research.

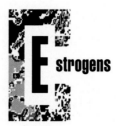

Estrogens

During the years between menarche and menopause in females, estrogen rises during the follicular phase while progesterone increases during the luteal phase. Estrogen therapy in premenopausal women is typically used in combination with progestin for contraception, and therefore sufficiently high doses are needed to prevent ovulation. While former use of oral contraceptives has not been associat-ed with a significant increase in coronary heart disease,[70,102,107] current users, especially older women who smoke,[26] consistently have an increased risk.[107] Because the estrogen content of newer oral contraceptives is less than that used in many of these studies, the risk for users of current oral contraceptives may be different than that previously reported. Taken together, oral contraceptives should be avoided in women who have hyperlipidemia, diabetes, hypertension, a family history of heart disease, or a history of cigarette smoking.

Following menopause, the decline in estrogen levels is associated with an increase in coronary heart disease. Although postmenopausal estrogen replacement therapy is frequently advocated for its role in decreasing cardiac risk, there has been no large-scale, randomized, double-blind, placebo-controlled study to evalu-ate the benefits and risks. Factors such as race, education, socioeconomic status, and body weight have not been fully investigated. The evidence in favor of estro-gen therapy is derived from controlled observational studies using either coronary heart disease risk[16,39,46,89,106] or angiographically documented coronary disease.[73,112]

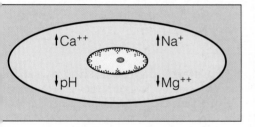

GURE 24.12   Cellular abnormalities associ-ed with insulin resistance.

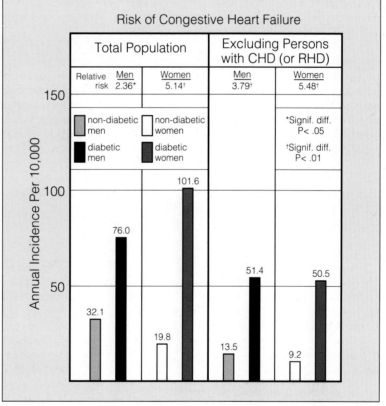

FIGURE 24.13
Risk of congestive heart failure accord-ing to diabetic status during biennial exami-nations. (Men and women between age 45 and 74; the Framingham study 18-year follow-up) (Redrawn with permis-sion; see Figure Credits)

These studies, evaluating primarily unopposed estrogen therapy (i.e., without progesterone), observed about a 50% lower cardiovascular risk in estrogen users. However, other studies have observed either no benefit[94,113] or an increase in risk.[53,114,119]

The beneficial effects of estrogen on cardiovascular disease are generally thought to be due to an improvement in lipid profile. HDL-cholesterol increases and LDL decreases in response to estrogen. Decreases in LDL-cholesterol have also been noted in women treated with tamoxifen.[67] However, using multivariate analysis, the changes in lipid levels do not fully explain all of the benefit derived from estrogen therapy. Other possible mechanisms involve the effect of estrogen on carbohydrate metabolism, coagulation, vascular action, or the secretion of steroids, prostacyclin, growth factors, or lipoproteins. When estrogen replacement therapy in postmenopausal women is being considered, other factors in the decision are the potential benefits to bone mineral density[47] and emotional well-being versus the potential risks for breast cancer and endometrial cancer (not a factor if progesterone is added).

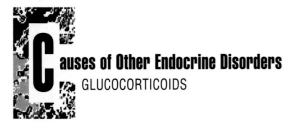

Causes of Other Endocrine Disorders
GLUCOCORTICOIDS

An excess in glucocorticoid can occur from pharmacologic administration or as a result of Cushing's syndrome. Pathologic overproduction of cortisol can be stimulated by a pituitary tumor (Cushing's disease), an adrenal adenoma, or an ectopic tumor producing either ACTH or corticotropin-releasing hormone (CRH). Cardiovascular disease is common in patients with untreated Cushing's syndrome, accounting for 40% of deaths.[15] Patients with hypercortisolemia are more likely to have hypertension, hyperlipidemia, hypokalemia, and a secondary form of diabetes mellitus. Possible mechanisms for corticosteroid-induced vascular disease include decreased insulin sensitivity and increased vascular responsiveness to catecholamines.[55] A rare inherited variant of Cushing's syndrome is associated with cardiac myxomas.

Hypoadrenalism, or Addison's disease, is most commonly caused by autoimmune destruction or granulomatous disease (most often tuberculosis). Cardiac contractility and blood volume are decreased in this syndrome, and hypotension with orthostasis is common. Bradycardia is typical and ECG tracings show flat P waves, first-degree block, prolonged Q–T intervals and T-wave abnormalities.

MINERALOCORTICOIDS
Hyperaldosteronism can occur from either an isolated adenoma (80%) or bilateral hyperplasia (20%). The salt-retaining properties of aldosterone lead to hypertension and can produce left ventricular hypertrophy and congestive heart failure.

Hypokalemia can present with abnormal T or U waves on the electrocardiogram. Surgical removal of an adenoma usually, but not always, results in resolution of the hypertension. However, bilateral hyperplasia does not respond to surgery; spironolactone can be an effective form of antihypertensive therapy.

CATECHOLAMINES
Pheochromocytomas are rare neuroendocrine tumors that typically (80% of the time) occur in the adrenals, but can occur anywhere in the sympathetic nervous system. The episodic secretion of epinephrine, norepinephrine, or dopamine precipitates spells of headache, sweating, palpitations, and severe anxiety. Physical examination usually notes baseline hypertension with orthostasis. The electrocardiogram reveals left ventricular hypertrophy and sinus tachycardia; abnormal ST–T segments and inverted T waves are also seen. Ventricular arrhythmias and conduction disturbances have been observed.[70] Pheochromocytomas can present with myocardial infarction, even in the absence of coronary artery disease.[89] Congestive heart failure has been reported in conjunction with myocarditis[4] and cardiomyopathy.[83] Beta blockers should not be started as sole therapy because the resulting unopposed α-receptor stimulation can precipitate a hypertensive crisis.

PARATHYROID HORMONE
Although much of the hypertension and rhythm disturbances observed with parathyroid disease are due to calcium, parathyroid hormone (PTH) also directly increases contractility and tachycardia.[12] Increased entry of calcium into cardiac myocytes decreases the action potential and shortens the Q–T interval. Hypertension occurs more frequently in hyperparathyroid patients; whether this is mediated by calcium or PTH is unclear. The hypertension often resolves after successful surgery. Hypoparathyroidism, with the resulting hypocalcemia, can prolong the Q–T interval and, if chronic, can result in congestive heart failure and a dilated cardiomyopathy.[42]

GROWTH HORMONE
Hypertension occurs in approximately 30% of acromegalic patients, and blood pressure correlates with age and duration of elevated plasma growth hormone levels. Cardiomegaly also is very common. Long-standing acromegaly may produce premature coronary artery disease and congestive heart failure. Histologic abnormalities include myocarditis, cellular hypertrophy, focal interstitial fibrosis, and myofibrillar degeneration. The presence of electrocardiographic, echocardiographic, and pathologic changes in acromegalic patients with or without hypertension has resulted in the postulation of an acromegalic cardiomyopathy. Many of these cardiac abnormalities revert to normal with therapy of the underlying acromegaly.

FIGURE CREDITS
Fig. 24.8 data from Nakazawa HK, et al: Management of atrial fibrillation in the post-thyrotoxic state. Am J Med 72:903. 1982.

Fig. 24.11 redrawn from Manicardi V, et al: Evidence for an association of high blood pressure and hyperinsulinemia in obese man. J Clin Endocrinol Metab 62:1302, 1986.

Fig. 24.13 redrawn from Kannel WB: Role of diabetes in cardiac disease: Conclusions from populations studies. In Zoneraich S (ed): Diabetes and the Heart. Charles C Thomas, Springfield, Ill, 1978.

REFERENCES
1. Abrams JJ, Grundy SM: Cholesterol metabolism in hypothyroidism and hyperthyroidism. J Lipid Research 22:323, 1981.

2. Agner T, Abundal T, Thorsteinzson B, et al: A re-evaluation of atrial fibrillation in thyrotoxicosis. Dan Med Bull 31:157, 1984.

3. Avila MH, Walker AM, Jick H: Use of replacement estrogens and the risk of myocardial infarction. Epidemiology 1:128, 1990.

4. Baker G, Zeller NY, Weitzner S, et al: Pheochromocytoma with hypertension presenting as cardiomyopathy. Am Heart J 83:688, 1972.

5. Barrett-Connor E, Wingard DL: Sex differential in ischemic heart disease mortality in diabetics: A prospective population-based study. Am J Epidemiol 118:489, 1983.

6. Bar-Sela S, Ehrenfeld M, Eliakim M: Arterial embolism in thyrotoxicosis with atrial fibrillation. Arch Intern Med 141:1191, 1981.

7. Bayliss RIS, Edwards OM: Urinary excretion of free catecholamines in Graves' disease. Endocrinology 49:167, 1971.

8. Beard CM, Kottke TE, Annegers JF, et al: The Rochester Coronary Heart Disease Project: Effect of cigarette smoking, hypertension, diabetes, and steroidal estrogen use on coronary heart disease among 40 to 59 year old women, 1960 through 1982. Mayo Clin Proc 64:1471, 1989.

9. Becker C: Hypothyroidism and atherosclerotic disease: Pathogenesis, medical management, and the role of coronary artery bypass surgery. Endo Rev 6:432, 1985.

10. Blumgart HL, et al: Hypercholesterolemia, myxedema and atherosclerosis. Am J Med 14:665, 1953.

1. Blumgart HL: Treatment of incapacitated euthyroid cardiac patients with radioactive iodine. Summary of results in treatment of 1070 patients with angina pectoris or congestive heart failure. JAMA 157:1, 1955.
2. Bogin E, Massry SG, Haray I: Effect of parathyroid hormone on rat heart cells. J Clin Invest 67: 1215, 1981.
3. Bradly RF, Schonfeld A: Diminished pain in diabetic patients with acute myocardial infarction. Geriatrics 17:322, 1962.
4. Brownlee M, Vlassara H, Cerami A: Nonenzymatic glycosylation products on collagen covalently trap low-density lipoprotein. Diabetes 34:938, 1985.
5. Burke CW, Beardwell CG: Cushing's syndrome. Q J Med 42:175, 1972.
6. Bush TL, Barrett-Connor E, Cowan LD, et al: Cardiovascular mortality and non-contraceptive estrogen use in women: Results from the Lipid Research Clinics' Program follow-up study. Circulation 75:1002, 1987.
7. Cabin HS, Roberts WC: Quantitative comparison of extent of coronary narrowing and size of healed myocardial infarct in 33 necropsy patients with clinically recognized and in 28 with clinically unrecognized ("silent") previous acute myocardial infarction. Am J Cardiol 50:677, 1982.
8. Carlstrom S, Karlefors T: Haemodynamic studies on newly diagnosed diabetics before and after adequate insulin treatment. Br Heart J 32:355, 1970.
9. Channick BJ, Adlin EV, Marks AD, et al: Hyperthyroidism and mitral-valve prolapse. N Engl J Med 305:497, 1981.
10. Chiarello MM, Indolfi C, Cotecchia MR, et al: Asymptomatic transient ST changes during ambulatory ECG monitoring in diabetic patients. Am Heart J 110:529, 1985.
11. Chipkin SR, Frid D, Alpert JS, et al: Frequency of painless myocardial ischemia during exercise tolerance testing in patients with and without diabetes mellitus. Am J Cardiol 59:61, 1987.
12. Chipkin SR, Gottlieb P, Lundstrom R, et al: Transient myocardial perfusion abnormalities in diabetic patients: A prospective study using thallium exercise tolerance testing. Cardiology, 79:172, 1991.
13. Conway G, Heazlitt RA, Fowler NO, et al: The effect of hyperthyroidism on the sarcoplasmic reticulum and myosin ATPase of dog heart. J Mol Cell Cardiol 8:39, 1976.
14. Coulombe P, Dussault JH, Letarte J, et al: Catecholamine metabolism in thyroid diseases. I. Epinephrine secretion rate in hyperthyroidism and hypothyroidism. J Clin Endocrinol Metab 42:125, 1976.
15. Coulombe P, Dussault JH, Walker P: Plasma catecholamine concentrations in hyperthyroidism and hypothyroidism. Metabolism 25:973, 1976.
16. Croft P, Hannaford PC: Risk factors for acute myocardial infarction in women: Evidence from the Royal College of General Practitioners' oral contraception study. Br Med J 298:165, 1989.
17. Cruz-Vidal M, Garcia-Palmieri MR, Costas R, et al: Abnormal blood glucose and coronary heart disease: The Puerto Rico heart health program. Diab Care 6:556, 1983.
18. Curfman GD, Crowley TJ, Smith TW: Thyroid-induced alterations in myocardial sodium and potassium-activated adenosine triphosphatase, monovalent cation active transport, and cardiac glycoside binding. J Clin Invest 59:586, 1977.
19. DeFronzo RA, Ferrannini E: Insulin resistance: A multifaceted syndrome responsible for NIDDM, obesity, hypertension, dyslipidemia, and atherosclerotic cardiovascular disease. Diab Care 14:173, 1991.
20. Edson JR et al: Low platelet adhesiveness and other hemostatic abnormalities in hypothyroidism. Ann Intern Med 82:342, 1975.
21. Eschwege E, Richard JL, Thibult N, et al: Coronary heart disease mortality in relation with diabetes, blood glucose and plasma insulin levels: The Paris prospective study, ten years later. Horm Metab Res 15(suppl):41, 1985.
22. Ewing DJ, Boland O, Neilson JMM, et al: Autonomic neuropathy, QT interval lengthening, and unexpected deaths in male diabetic patients. Diabetologia 34:182, 1991.
23. Ewing DJ, Campbell IW, Clarke BF: Mortality in diabetic autonomic neuropathy; Lancet I:7960, 1976.
24. Fein FS, Strobeck JE, Malhotra A, et al: Reversibility of diabetic cardiomyopathy with insulin in rats. Circ Res 49:1251, 1981.
25. Forfar JC, Caldwell GC: Hyperthyroid heart disease. Clin Endocrinol Metab 14:491, 1985.
26. Forfar JC, Juir AL, Sawers SA, et al: Abnormal left ventricular function in hyperthyroidism. N Engl J Med 307:1165, 1982.
27. Forfar JC, Miller HC, Toft AD: Occult thyrotoxicosis: A correctable cause of "idiopathic" atrial fibrillation. Am J Cardiol 44:9, 1979.
28. Freedberg AS, Papp JG, Williams EMV: The effect of altered thyroid stae on atrial intracellular potentials. J Physiol 207:357, 1970.
39. Galloway JA: Treatment of NIDDM with insulin agonists or substitutes. Diabetes Care 13:1209, 1990.
40. Ganguly PK, Pierce GN, Dhalla KS, et al: Defective cardiac sarcoplasmic reticular calcium transport in diabetic cardiomyopathy. Am J Physiol 244:E528, 1983.
41. Giacomelli F, Wiener J: Primary myocardial disease in the diabetic mouse: An ultrastructural study. Lab Invest 40:460, 1979.
42. Giles TD, Iteld BJ, Rires KL: The cardiomyopathy of hypoparathyroidism. Chest 79:225, 1981.
43. Giles TD, Sander GE; Myocardial disease in hypertensive-diabetic patients. Am J Med 87(suppl 6A):23S, 1989.
44. Haffner SM, Mitchell BD, Stern MP, et al: Macrovascular complications in Mexican Americans with type II diabetes. Diabetes Care 14(suppl 3):665, 1991.
45. Hamby RI, Zoneraich S, Sherman S: Diabetic cardiomyopathy. JAMA 229:1749, 1974.
46. Henderson BE, Paganini-Hill A, Ross RK: Estrogen replacement therapy and protection from acute myocardial infarction. Am J Obstet Gynecol 159:312, 1988.
47. Hillner BE, Hollenberg JP, Pauker SG: Postmenopausal estrogens in prevention of osteoporosis: Benefit virtually without risk if cardiovascular effects are considered. Am J Med 80:1115, 1986.
48. Hume L, Oakley GD, Boulton AJM, et al: Asymptomatic myocardial ischemia in diabetes and its relationship to diabetic neuropathy: An exercise electrocardiography study in middle-aged diabetic men. Diab Care 9:384, 1986.
49. Huot SJ, Aronson PS: Na+-H+ exchanger and its role in essential hypertension and diabetes mellitus. Diab Care 14:521, 1991.
50. Iasaki T, Naka M, Hiramatsu K, et al: Echocardiography studies on the relationship between atrial fibrillation and atrial enlargement in patients with hyperthyroidism of Graves' disease. Cardiology 76:10, 1989.
51. Ibbertson HK: Endemic goiter in cretinism. Clin Endocrinol Metab 8:97, 1979.
52. Ikram H: The nature and prognosis of thyrotoxic heart disease. Q J Med 54:19, 1985.
53. Jick H, Dinan B, Rothman KJ: Noncontraceptive estrogens and nonfatal myocardial infarction. JAMA 239:1407, 1978.
54. Kahn JK, Sisson JC, Vinik AI: QT interval prolongation and sudden cardiac death in diabetic autonomic neuropathy. J Clin Endocrinol Metab 64:751, 1987.
55. Kalsner S: Mechanism of hydrocortisone potentiation of response to epinephrine and norepinephrine in rabbit aorta. Circ Res 24:383, 1969.
56. Kannel WB: Detection and management of patients with silent myocardial ischemia. Am Heart J 117:221, 1989.
57. Kannel WB, Hjortland M, Castelli WP: Role of diabetes in congestive heart failure: The Framingham study. Am J Cardiol 34:29, 1974.
58. Keating FR Jr, Parkin TW, Selby JB, et al: Treatment of heart disease associated with myxedema. Prog Cardiovasc Dis 3:364, 1961.
59. Kirstein M, Brett J, Radoff S, et al: Advanced protein glycosylation induces transendothelial human monocyte chemotaxis and secretion of platelet derived growth factor: Role in vascular disease of diabetes and aging. Proc Nat Acad Sci 87:9010, 1990.
60. Klein I: Thyroid hormone and the cardiovascular system. Am J Med 88:631, 1990.
61. Kleinman JC, Donahue RP, Harris MI, et al: Mortality among diabetics in a national sample. Am J Epidemiol 128:389, 1988.
62. Ladenson PW: Recognition and management of cardiovascular disease related to thyroid dysfunction. Am J Med 88:638, 1990.
63. Ladenson PW, Levin AA, Ridgeway EC, et al: Complications of surgery in hypothyroid patients. Am J Med 77:264, 1984.
64. Langer A, Freeman MR, Josse RG, et al: Detection of silent myocardial ischemia in diabetes mellitus. Am J Cardiol 67:1073, 1991.
65. Levey GS, Klein I: Catecholamine-thyroid hormone interactions and the cardiovascular manifestations of hyperthyroidism. Am J Med 88:642, 1990.
66. Liggett SB, Shah SD, Cayer PE: Increased fat and skeletal muscle β-adrenergic receptors but unaltered metabolic and hemodynamic sensitivity to epinephrine in vivo in experimental human thyrotoxicosis. J Clin Invest 83:803, 1989.
67. Love RR, Wiebe DA, Newcomb PA, et al: Effects of tamoxifen on cardiovascular risk factors in postmenopausal women. Ann Intern Med 115:860, 1991.
68. Lyons TJ: Oxidized low density lipoproteins: A role in the pathogenesis of atherosclerosis in diabetes? Diab Med 8:411, 1991.
69. Malhotra A, Penpargkul S, Fein FS, et al: The effect of streptozotocin-induced diabetes in rats on cardiac contractile proteins. Circ Res 49:1243, 1981.
70. Manger WM, Gifford RW Jr: Pheochromocytoma. Springer Verlag, New York, 1977.

71. Mann JI, Inman WHW, Thorogood M: Oral contraceptive use in older women and fatal myocardial infarction. Br Med J 2:445, 1976.

72. Marquie G: Effect of insulin in the induction and regression of experimental cholesterol atherosclerosis in the rabbit. Postgrad Med J 54:80, 1978.

73. McFarland KF, Bonniface ME, Hormung CA, et al: Risk factors and noncontraceptive estrogen use in women with and without coronary disease. Am Heart J 117:1209, 1989.

74. Mildenberger RR, Bar-Shlomo B, Druck MN, et al: Clinically unrecognized ventricular dysfunction in young diabetic patients. J Am Coll Cardiol 4:234, 1984.

75. Mintz G, Pizzarello R, Goldman M, et al: Cardiac diastolic function in hyperthyroidism: Response to therapy. Clin Res 37:502A, 1989.

76. Morkin E, Flink IL, Goldman S: Biochemical and physiologic effects of thyroid hormone on cardiac performance. Prog Cardiovas Dis 25:435, 1983.

77. Nagi DK, Hendra TJ, Ryle AJ, et al: The relationships of concentrations of insulin, intact proinsulin and 32-33 split proinsulin with cardiovascular risk factors in type 2 (non-insulin-dependent) diabetic subjects. Diabetologia 33:532, 1990.

78. Nakao J, Ito H, Kanayasu T, et al: Stimulatory effect of insulin on aortic smooth muscle cell migration induced by 12-l-hydroxy 5,8,10, 14-eicosatetraenoic acid and its modulation by elevated extracellular glucose levels. Diabetes 34:185, 1985.

79. Nakazawa H, Ishikawa H, Noh J, et al: Efficacy of disopyramide in conversion and prophylaxis of post-thyrotoxic atrial fibrillation. Eur J Pharmacol 40:215, 1991.

80. Nakazawa HK, Sakurai K, Momotani N, et al: Management of atrial fibrillation in the post-thyrotoxic state. Am J Med. 72:903, 1982.

81. Nesto RW, Phillips RT, Kett KG, Hill T, Perper E, Young E, Leland OS; Angina and exertional myocardial ischemia in diabetic and nondiabetic patients: assessment by exercise thallium scintigraphy. Ann Intern Med 108:170-175, 1988.

82. Nishigaki I, Hagihara M, Tsunekawa H, et al: Lipid peroxide levels of serum lipoprotein fractions of diabetic patients. Biochem Med 25:373, 1981.

83. Northfield TL: Cardiac complications of pheochromocytoma. Br Heart J 29:588, 1967.

84. Olsson T, Viitanen M, Asplund K, et al: Prognosis after stroke in diabetic patients: A controlled prospective study. Diabetologia 33:244, 1990.

85. Osmundson PJ, O'Fallon WM, Simmerman BR, et al: Course of peripheral occlusive arterial disease in diabetes: Vascular laboratory assessment. Diab Care 13:143, 1990.

86. Petitti DB, Perlman JA, Sidney S: Noncontraceptive estrogens and mortality: Long-term follow-up of women in the Walnut Creek study. Obstet Gynecol 70:289, 1987.

87. Pfeifle B, Ditschuneit H: Effect of insulin on growth of cultured human arterial smooth muscle cells. Diabetologia 20:155, 1981.

88. Pyorala K: Relationship of glucose tolerance and plasma insulin to the incidence of coronary heart disease: Results from two population studies in Finland. Diab Care 2:131, 1979.

89. Radtke WE, Kazmier FJ, Rutherford BD, et al: Cardiovascular complications of pheochromocytoma crisis. Am J Cardiol 35:701, 1975.

90. Regan TJ, Ettinger PO, Kahn MI, et al: Altered myocardial function and metabolism in chronic diabetes mellitus without ischemia in dogs. Circ Res 35:222, 1974.

91. Regan TJ, Lyons MM, Ahmed SS, et al : Evidence for cardiomyopathy in familial diabetes mellitus. J Clin Invest 60:885-99, 1977.

92. Resnick LM: Calcium metabolism in hypertension and allied metabolic disorders. Diab Care 14:505, 1991.

93. Resnick LM: Gupta RK, Bhargava BK, et al: Cellular ions in hypertension, diabetes, and obesity: An NMR spectroscopic study. Hypertension, In press.

94. Rosenberg L, Slone D, Shapiro S, et al: Non-contraceptive estrogens and myocardial infarction in young women. JAMA. 244:339, 1980.

95. Rubler S, Dlugash J, Yuceoglu YZ, et al: New type of cardiomyopathy associated with diabetic glomerulosclerosis. Am J Cardiol 30:595, 1972.

96. Saito I, Ito K, Saruta T: Hypothyroidism as a cause of hypertension. Hypertension 5:112, 1983.

97. Sandler G, Wilson GM: The nature and prognosis of heart disease in thyrotoxicosis. Q J Med 28:247, 1959.

98. Schmitz A, Christensen T, Miller A, et al: Kidney function and cardiovascular risk factors in non-insulin-dependent diabetics (NIDDM) with microalbuminuria. J Intern Med 228:347, 1990.

99. Shapiro LM, Leatherdale BA, Coyne ME, et al: Prospective study of heart disease in untreated maturity onset diabetics. Br Heart J 44:342, 1980.

100. Shapiro LM, Leatherdale BA, MacKinnon J, Fletcher RF: Left ventricular function in diabetes mellitus. II. Relation between clinical features and left ventricular function. Br Heart J 45:129, 1981.

101. Skelton CL, Sonnenblick EH: The cardiovascular system in: Ingbar SH, Braverman LE (eds): Werner's The Thyroid, 5th ed. J B Lipincott, Philadephia, 1988.

102. Slone D, Shapiro S, Kaufman DW, et al: Risk of myocardial infarction in relation to current and discontinued use of oral contraceptives. N Engl J Med 305:420, 1981.

103. Soler NG, Bennett MA, Pentecost BL, et al: Myocardial infarction in diabetics. Q J Med 44:125, 1975.

104. Sowers JR, Standley PR, Ram JL, et al: Insulin resistance, carbohydrate metabolism, and hypertension. Am J Hypertens 4:466S, 1991.

105. Staffurth JS, Gibberd MC, Fui SNT: Arterial embolism in thyrotoxicosis with atrial fibrillation. Br Med J 3:688, 1977.

106. Stampfer MJ, Willet WC, Colditz GA, et al: A prospective study of postmenopausal estrogen therapy and coronary heart disease. N Engl J Med 313:1044, 1985.

107. Stampfer MJ, Willet WC, Colditz GA, Speizer FE, Hennekens CH: A prospective study of past use of oral contraceptive agents and risk of cardiovascular diseases. N Engl J Med 319:1313, 1988.

108. Steinberg AD: Myxedema and coronary artery disease: A comparative autopsy study. Ann Intern Med 68:338, 1968.

109. Stoffer SS, Jiang N, Gorman CA, et al: Plasma catecholamines in hypothyroidism and hyperthyrodism. J Clin Endocrinol Metab 36:587,1973.

110. Stolar MW: Atherosclerosis in diabetes: The role of hyperinsulinemia. Metabolism 37(suppl 1):1, 1988.

111. Stout RW: Insulin and atheroma: 20-year perspective. Diab Care 13:631, 1990.

112. Sullivan JM, Zwagg RV, Lemp GF, et al: Post-menopausal estrogen use and coronary atherosclerosis. Ann Intern Med 108:358, 1988.

113. Szklo M, Tonascia J, Gordis L, et al: Estrogen use and myocardial infarction risk: A case-control study. Prev Med 13:510, 1984.

114. Thompson SG, Meade TW, Greenberg G: The use of hormonal replacement therapy and the risk of stroke and myocardial infarction in women. J Epidemiol Comm Health 43:173, 1989.

115. Vanhaelst L, et al: Coronary artery disease in hypothyroidism: Observations in clinical myxedema. Lancet 1:800, 1967.

116. Vered A, Battler A, Segal P, et al: Exercise-induced left ventricular dysfunction in young men with asymptomatic diabetes mellitus (diabetic cardiomyopathy). Am J Cardiol 54:633, 1984.

117. Weinberg AD et al: Outcome of anesthesia and surgery in hypothyroid patients. Arch Intern Med 143:893, 1983.

118. Welborn TA, Wearne K: Coronary heart disease incidence and cardiovascular mortality in Busselton with reference to glucose and insulin concentrations. Diab Care 2:154, 1979.

119. Wilson PWF, Garrison RJ, Castelli WP: Post-menopausal estrogen use and heart disease. N Engl J Med 315:135, 1986.

120. Zemel MB, Beaford BA, Zemel PC, et al: Altered cation transport in non-insulin dependent diabetic hypertension. Effects of dietary calcium. J Hypertens 6:S228, 1988.

121. Zondek H: Association of myxedema heart and arteriosclerotic heart disease. JAMA 170:1920, 1959.

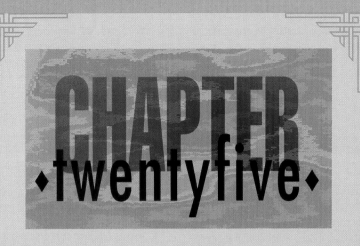

CHAPTER ·twentyfive·

DISEASES AFFECTING THE HEART AND KIDNEYS

DAVID M. CLIVE, MD

No medical disease is confined to one organ of the body. The human organism represents a network of interdependent physiologic systems; a malfunction in one area ultimately exerts an influence, even if trivial, upon another. Diseases of the heart and kidneys are illustrative of this principle; morbidity in either organ is likely to have quite serious consequences for the other. This is hardly surprising, considering the enormous role each organ plays in defining the internal milieu. This chapter explores the effects of primary renal disease on the heart, and the effects of heart disease on the kidneys. In addition, brief consideration is given to systemic disorders affecting both of these organs secondarily.

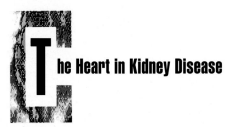

The Heart in Kidney Disease

The kidneys work to preserve homeostasis in four ways: maintenance of water and ion balance, maintenance of acid-base balance, regulation of systemic arterial blood pressure, and elimination of soluble metabolic wastes. Each kidney contains up to one million nephrons (Fig. 25.1). The microanatomy of the nephron is uniquely suited to its physiologic tasks (Fig. 25.2). A detailed description of nephron anatomy and physiology is outside the realm of this review, although it is worth mentioning that physiologic heterogeneity exists among nephrons depending on their location in the kidney.

The kidneys also serve a variety of metabolic and endocrine functions (e.g., synthesis of erythropoietin, renin, and 1,25-dihydroxycholecalciferol). However, it is chiefly through derangement of their homeostatic capacities that the heart may become a casualty of kidney disease.

ELECTROLYTE DISTURBANCES AND CARDIAC FUNCTION

The activity of the cardiac myosite, as is the case with all electrically excitable cells, is determined by ionic fluxes across its membrane. The most important ionic species in this regard is *potassium*. Either an excess or deficiency in potassium can alter the relative potassium concentrations on each side of the myosite membrane, resulting in abnormal membrane potentials. The earliest cardiac manifestations of potassium imbalance are revealed in the electrocardiogram (Fig. 25.3). The appearance of conduction abnormalities and arrhythmias should prompt emergent correction of the imbalance. Hyperkalemia predisposes to ventricular irritability, and represents potentially the most rapidly lethal electrolyte abnormality. Hypokalemia may pose a life-threatening problem as well, but generally only in the setting of underlying heart disease.

Divalent cation imbalances exert effects on the electrical and mechanical functions of the heart, albeit not as dramatic as those associated with potassium imbalance. Hypocalcemia, a reduced concentration of ionized calcium in the serum, impairs myocardial contractility. The contraction of cardiac muscle, like

that of other contractile tissues, is a calcium-dependent process. One of th salutary results of dialysis is improved myocardial performance felt, in part, to b due to replenishment of ionized calcium (see the discussion below on dialysis Hypomagnesemia is more apt to be associated with electrical dysfunction of th heart; magnesium deficiency can provoke ventricular irritability and tachycard (Fig. 25.4) and has been implicated as a cause of sudden death in geographi areas in which drinking water is poor in magnesium.

Although hypercalcemia is generally not a serious electrolyte disturbanc from the standpoint of cardiac function, several abnormalities have bee described, including prolongation of the A–V conduction, and shortening c the electrocardiographic Q–T interval. Because calcium predisposes to digitali toxicity, cardiac glycosides should be used with caution in hypercalcemi patients. Myocardial calcification may develop in patients with sustaine hypercalcemia or hyperphosphatemia (i.e., the "calcium × phosphorus prod uct"); these would appear similar to those shown in Figure 25.7. Hypertensio is common in hypercalcemia, but it probably arises through peripheral vasc constriction. Hypermagnesemia may induce subtle electrocardiographic find ings and changes in myocardial performance, but only when severe (serum magnesium ≥5 mEq/L).

Phosphorus depletion is less common than phosphorus overload in renal disease but it can occur in a variety of settings. Phosphorus is a critical factor in mos cellular aerobic and anaerobic metabolic pathways, as well as in transmembran transport processes. It is therefore not surprising that many significant patho physiologic phenomena have been reported in association with severe phos phate deficiency, including reversible myocardial dysfunction.[17]

METABOLIC ACIDOSIS AND THE HEART

It has been demonstrated, with the use of isolated heart muscle preparation that severe acidosis impairs myocardial contractility. In the intact organism, th effect is offset by the positive inotropic effects of beta-adrenergic hormones. A the degree of acidosis becomes increasingly profound (pH ≤ 7.0), cardiac an vascular smooth muscle become refractory to the stimulus of adrenergic hor mones, and hypotension may ensue.

EFFECTS ON THE HEART OF UREMIA AND DIALYSIS

Uremia is truly a multisystem disease; the ongoing retention of numerous meta bolic wastes and toxins, many of them incompletely identified, engenders mor bidity in virtually every organ system. There are two major cardiac morbiditie associated with uremia: (i) reversible cardiomyopathy and (ii) pericarditi *Uremic pericarditis* (see Fig. 9.12) is an inflammatory serositis, thought to aris from the direct actions of metabolic toxins on the pericardium. Fluid overloa may complicate this condition. Pericarditis was a common manifestation of ure mia in the pre-dialysis era. Today its prevalence in the dialysis population i probably under 10%. The occurrence of pericarditis in an established dialysi patient may be related to a comorbid state, such as a viral infection, but its pres ence usually bespeaks the need for more vigorous dialytic therapy.

The signs, symptoms, and pathophysiology of uremic pericarditis are similar t those of pericarditis of other etiologies (see Chapter 9). Fever, chest pain,

cardial effusion. Management consists of aggressive dialysis and optimal maintenance of body fluid balance. Pericardiocentesis or surgical pericardiectomy may be indicated in resistant or life-threatening effusions.

Congestive heart failure is a common problem in uremic patients. Most cases simply reflect fluid overload, a result of the kidneys' inability to excrete sodium and water normally. Nephrogenic fluid overload places a strain on the heart by increasing ventricular preload. Hypertension, arising for the same reason, further aggravates ventricular strain by raising the afterload. The most common cause of pulmonary edema in patients with renal failure is nephrogenic fluid overload and the attendant left ventricular strain. There have been rare reports, however, of pulmonary edema occurring in uremic patients without elevated filling pressures, raising speculation that uremic toxins may induce pulmonary capillary leakage. The term *uremic lung* should be reserved for patients of this sort.

The observation that congestive heart failure is occasionally alleviated by isovolemic dialysis led to the suggestion that there may be a dialyzable uremic toxin(s) that exerts a suppressive effect on myocardial performance and lent credence to the concept of a reversible *uremic cardiomyopathy*. Indeed, studies have shown that, following an acute hemodialysis or peritoneal dialysis treatment, echocardiographic indices of left ventricular contractility improve to an extent unattributable to altered Frank-Starling (preload) relationships alone. More recent investigations indicate that the salutary effect of dialysis on cardiac function is probably due less to waste removal than to the increase in serum ionized calcium that occurs during the procedure[12] (Fig. 25.5). Higher dialysate calcium concentration has been shown to reduce hemodialysis-associated hypotension, perhaps through the enhancement of cardiac output.

For many years, *acetate* was the most commonly used buffer base in commercial dialysate preparations. This substance is now known to impair myocardial performance. Replacement of acetate by bicarbonate has reduced the incidence of intradialytic hypotension. The relative hypoxemia commonly occurring during hemodialysis treatments may contribute to myocardial dysfunction on an ischemic basis. For this reason, patients with known organic heart disease should receive oxygen during dialysis, and their hemoglobin concentration should be maintained at a level sufficient to ensure adequate myocardial and peripheral oxygen delivery.

Nutritional cardiomyopathy is a rare cause of heart failure in the dialysis population, occurring on the basis of reduced vitamin intake and the loss of water-soluble vitamins into the dialysate. Two causes of high-output cardiac failure are anemia and arteriovenous dialysis fistulas. With the advent of recombinant human erythropoietin therapy, anemia can be controlled in most dialysis patients. Dialysis fistulas rarely cause heart failure, except in patients with substantial pre-existing cardiac disease or in those with multiple high-flow arteriovenous fistulas.

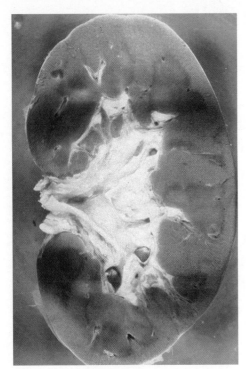

FIGURE 25.1 Gross specimen of a normal human kidney, cut longitudinally. (Reproduced with permission; see Figure Credits)

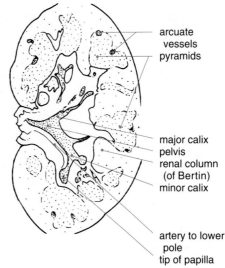

arcuate
vessels
pyramids

major calix
pelvis
renal column
(of Bertin)
minor calix

artery to lower
pole
tip of papilla

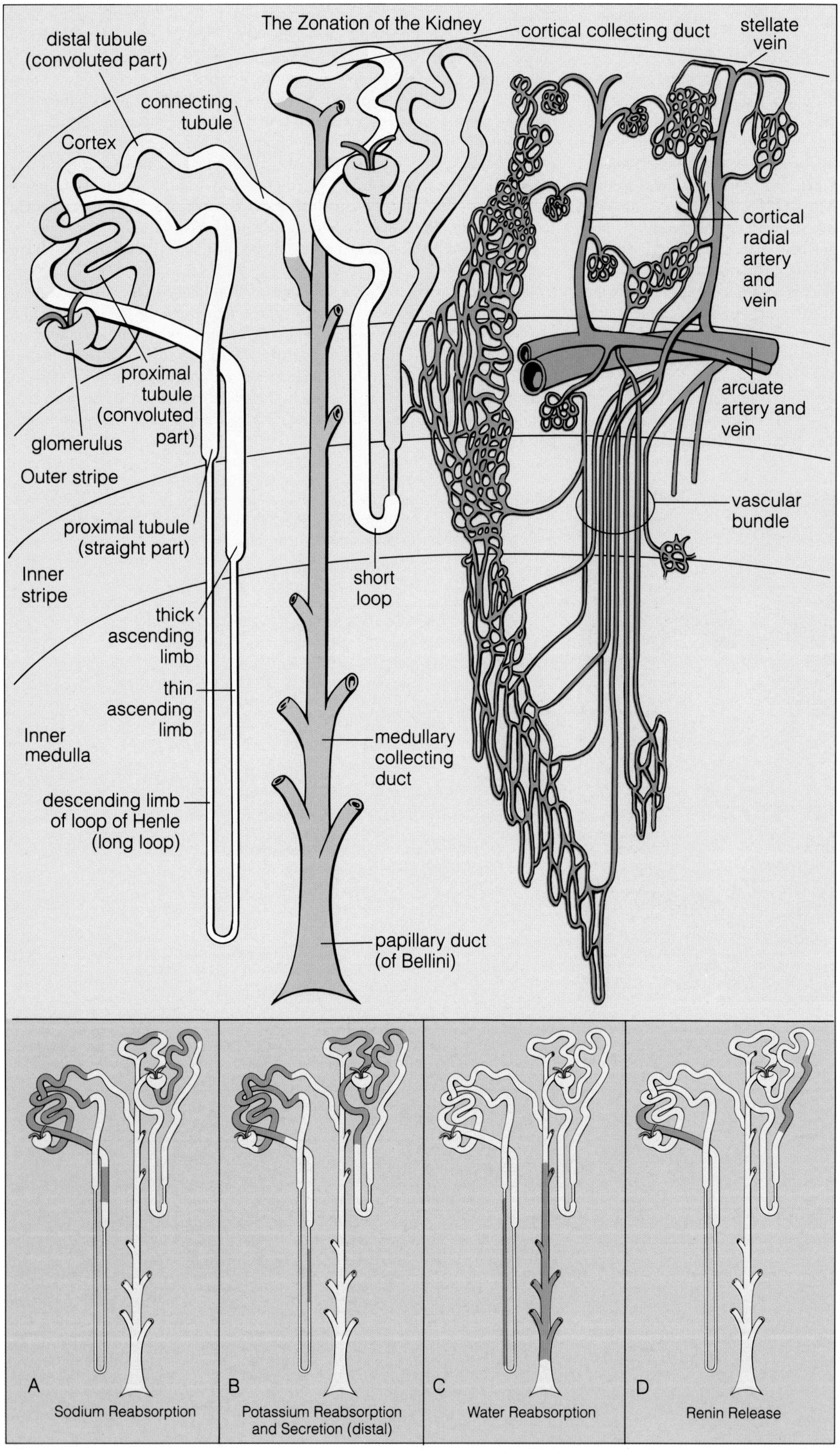

FIGURE 25.2   Anatomic relationship of vascular and tubular elements of a nephron. **(A–D)** The correlation between anatomic sites and specific physiologic functions. (Reproduced with permission; see Figure Credits)

The Zonation of the Kidney

distal tubule (convoluted part)

connecting tubule

Cortex

proximal tubule (convoluted part)

glomerulus

Outer stripe

proximal tubule (straight part)

Inner stripe

thick ascending limb

thin ascending limb

Inner medulla

descending limb of loop of Henle (long loop)

cortical collecting duct

short loop

medullary collecting duct

papillary duct (of Bellini)

stellate vein

cortical radial artery and vein

arcuate artery and vein

vascular bundle

A   Sodium Reabsorption

B   Potassium Reabsorption and Secretion (distal)

C   Water Reabsorption

D   Renin Release

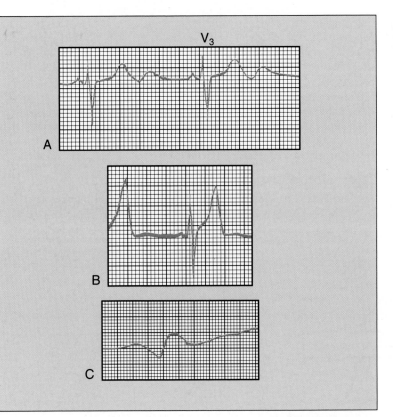

FIGURE 25.3   Electrocardiographic signs of potassium imbalance.
(A) Hypokalemia. Note presence of U waves. **(B)** Early hyperkalemia. The
T waves are peaked and the QRS complex has just begun to widen.**(C)** Late
hyperkalemia. Note gross distortion of QRS morphology.

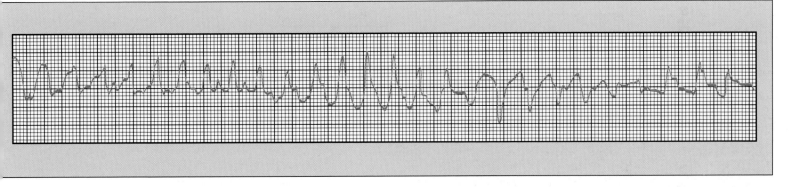

FIGURE 25.4   ECG showing a cyclical, polymorphic form of ventricular tachycardia referred to as "torsade de pointes."
This arrhythmia may be seen in hypomagnesemia.

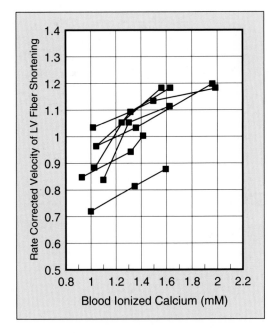

FIGURE 25.5   Effect on myocardial performance
of dialytically increasing the blood ionized calcium
level in a group of patients with chronic renal failure.
(Reproduced with permission; see Figure Credits)

Chronic renal failure may engender cardiac morbidity in several other fashions, even in patients who are not frankly uremic or on dialysis. *Phosphorus retention* initiates the vicious pathophysiologic cycle of secondary hyperparathyroidism (Fig. 25.6). It is likely that sustained, abnormally high levels of parathyroid hormone exert direct toxic effects on myocardial cells. Additionally, the deposition of calcium phosphate salts in myocardial tissue may lead to gross impairment of electrical and mechanical function (Fig. 25.7). With dietary phosphate restriction, use of phosphate-binding preparations, and satisfactory dialysis, myocardial calcification is relatively rare.

RENAL DISEASE, DIALYSIS, AND ATHEROSCLEROSIS

It is thought that atherosclerosis is more prevalent and progresses more rapidly in hemodialysis patients than in the normal population. When examined as an independent risk factor, i.e., with adjustment for other risk factors such as hypertension, diabetes mellitus, and advanced age, it is difficult to prove that hemodialysis alone accelerates atherosclerosis. However, it is well known that stroke and myocardial infarction are the leading causes of death in the dialysis population.

With or without renal failure, patients with the nephrotic syndrome are definitely predisposed to hyperlipidemia. The rate of hepatic lipoprotein synthesis in nephrotic patients has been shown to correlate with the rate of urinary albumin excretion[10] (Fig. 25.8). Patients with sustained nephrosis are felt to be at risk for accelerated atherogenesis on this basis.

HYPERTENSION AND CARDIAC DISEASE

Systemic arterial hypertension is one of the commonest diseases in our society.

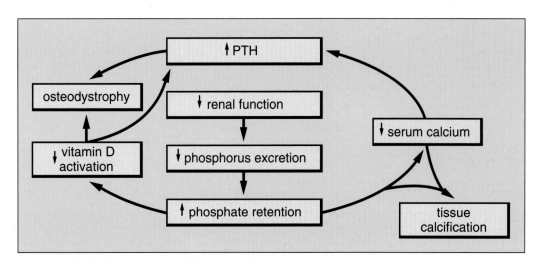

FIGURE 25.6   Pathogenesis of secondary hyperparathyroidism in chronic renal failure.

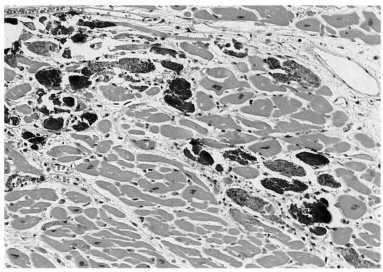

FIGURE 25.7   Myocardial calcifications in a uremic patient. (Reproduced with permission; see Figure Credits)

THE HEART AND OTHER CONDITIONS

ffecting perhaps 20% of the population of the United States. Hypertension ctually represents a spectrum of diseases; essential hypertension is by far the most common of these, accounting for up to 90% of hypertensive patients (Fig. 5.9). Hypertension resulting from endocrinopathies (such as primary hyperaldosteronism) and renal diseases (such as renovascular stenosis and renal arenchymal diseases) comprise the so-called secondary forms of hypertension. t is generally agreed that the kidney is the major organ of blood pressure regulaion, and plays a critical role in the pathophysiology of most forms of hypertenion. Hypertension is therefore included in this chapter, although it is discussed n greater detail in Chapter 15.

The relationship between hypertension and cardiac disease is intimate and has been the object of a great deal of study. The Framingham study has identified hypertension as an important predisposing factor for ischemic cardiac disease.[9] Hypertension is known to accelerate coronary atherogenesis. The enormous strain imposed on the left ventricle by severe systemic hypertension can lead to acute congestive heart failure in previously well-compensated patients presenting with malignant or accelerated-phase hypertension. Congestive heart failure may also occur at a more chronic pace; because arterial hypertension and coronary disease coexist so commonly, it may be difficult to attribute congestive failure to one or the other, particularly in a patient at midlife or beyond.

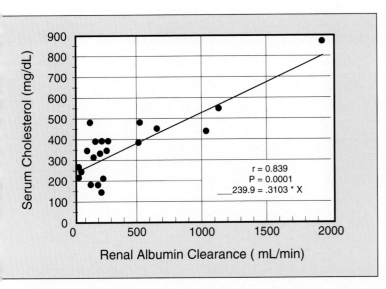

FIGURE 25.8 Effect of albumin excretion on serum cholesterol in patients with nephrotic syndrome. (Reproduced with permission; see Figure Credits)

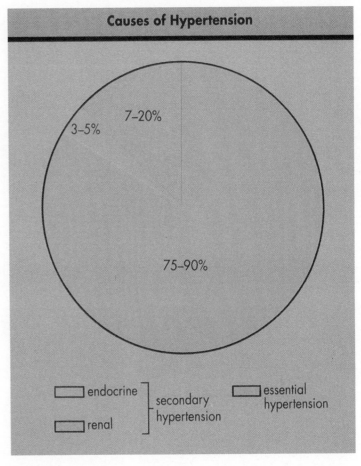

FIGURE 25.9 Causes of hypertension. (Reproduced with permission; see Figure Credits)

Chronic hypertension may lead to other forms of cardiac failure. The left ventricle, faced with a sustained elevation in afterload, undergoes hypertrophic changes (Fig. 25.10). These changes may be demonstrated early in the course of experimental hypertension. The term *hypertensive cardiomyopathy* has been used to designate the significant increase in ventricular mass that accompanies longstanding hypertension. Although the hypertrophic ventricle may have normal contractility, its reduced compliance impedes diastolic filling, and cardiac output may be reduced on this basis. Drug therapy, particularly with sym-

patholytic agents and calcium channel blockers, can reduce ventricular mass i patients undergoing hypertensive therapy, in addition to ameliorating the hypertension.

POLYCYSTIC KIDNEY DISEASE

The polycystic kidney diseases are a family of hereditary conditions marked b progressive cystic degeneration of the renal parenchyma (Fig. 25.11). Tw major disease types are recognized: an autosomal recessive form and an autoso

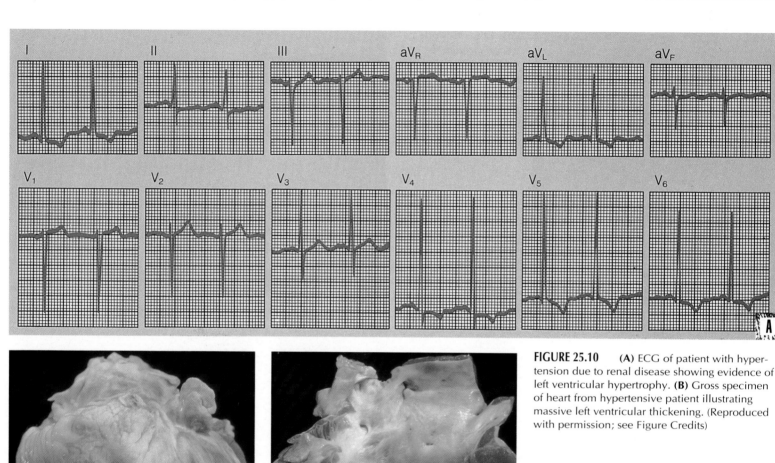

FIGURE 25.10 **(A)** ECG of patient with hypertension due to renal disease showing evidence of left ventricular hypertrophy. **(B)** Gross specimen of heart from hypertensive patient illustrating massive left ventricular thickening. (Reproduced with permission; see Figure Credits)

mal-dominant form (ADPKD). The latter is far more common, representing one of the most prevalent genetic disorders in the world.

Although considerable heterogeneity exists in the natural history of ADPKD, most patients develop hypertension and progressive renal failure in middle life as renal cysts expand. ADPKD is also associated with extrarenal complications. Liver cysts are present in 50% of patients, and cerebral berry aneurysms, and colonic diverticuli occur with increased frequency. Patients with ADPKD are at increased risk for valvular heart disease; prolapsed mitral valve and myxomatous degeneration of the mitral and aortic valves occur in as many as 18% of patients[13] (Fig. 25.12). It has been suggested that, in addition to the tendency for epithelial proliferation generating the cysts, ADPKD may manifest diffuse abnormalities in connective tissue formation leading to development of the extrarenal defects.

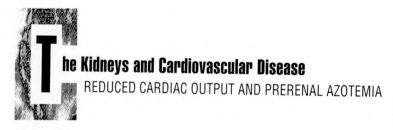

The Kidneys and Cardiovascular Disease
REDUCED CARDIAC OUTPUT AND PRERENAL AZOTEMIA

The renal circulation normally receives approximately 20% of the cardiac output, an appropriate amount for the kidneys' pivotal homeostatic function. Twenty percent of the plasma flow is made into filtrate during each pass through the glomerulus; this percentage is referred to as the *filtration fraction*.

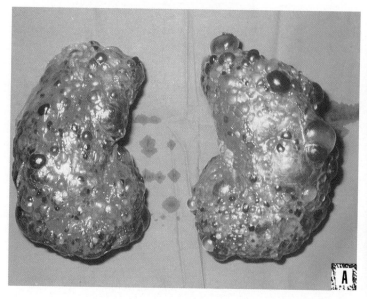

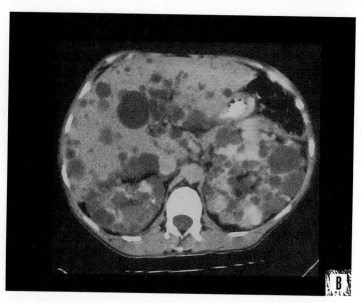

FIGURE 25.11 **(A)** Gross specimen of kidney in autosomal-dominant polycystic kidney disease. **(B)** Abdominal CT of patient with ADPKD showing numerous renal and hepatic cysts. (Reproduced with permission; see Figure Credits)

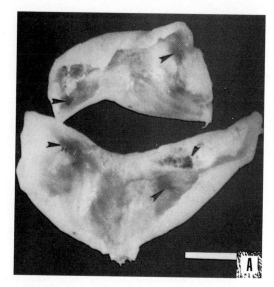

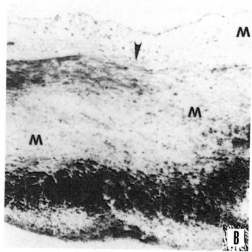

FIGURE 25.12 **(A)** Gross specimen of bicuspid aortic valve from patient with ADPKD. **(B)** Microscopic specimen of same valve showing myxomatous degeneration (M). (Reproduced with permission; see Figure Credits)

The hemodynamics of glomerular plasma flow and filtration are under tight autoregulatory control.

When renal perfusion is compromised by a reduction in cardiac output, compensatory mechanisms are activated. Dilatation of the afferent arteriole optimizes flow in the face of reduced perfusion pressure (Fig. 25.13). Constriction of efferent arterioles raises the hydrostatic pressure in each glomerular capillary. This increases their filtration fraction, maximizing the collective glomerular filtration rate despite the fall-off in renal perfusion. Although the renal autoregulatory mechanisms a

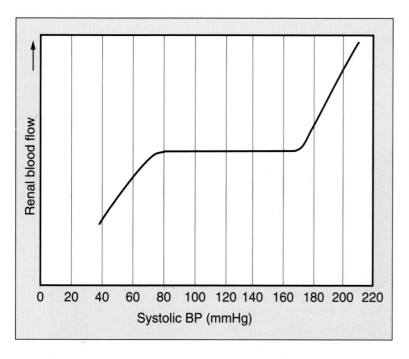

FIGURE 25.13 Autoregulation of renal blood flow maintains constancy of perfusion over a wide range of systolic blood pressure. (Reproduced with permission; see Figure Credits)

FIGURE 25.14 CAUSES OF PRERENAL AZOTEMIA

HYPOVOLEMIA
Gastrointestinal losses (vomiting, diarrhea)
Diuresis (diuretic therapy, osmotic diuresis, diabetes insipidus)
Excessive perspiration and other insensible losses
Mineralocorticoid deficiency

OTHER HEMODYNAMIC ABNORMALITIES
Hypotension (and overcontrol of hypertension)
Preglomerular renal vasoconstriction or occlusion (renal artery stenosis, scleroderma, vasculitis, hepatorenal syndrome)
Drugs (nonsteroidal anti-inflammatory drugs and other agents inducing preglomerular renal vaso-constriction)
"Edematous disorders" (low cardiac output, cirrhosis, nephrotic syndrome)

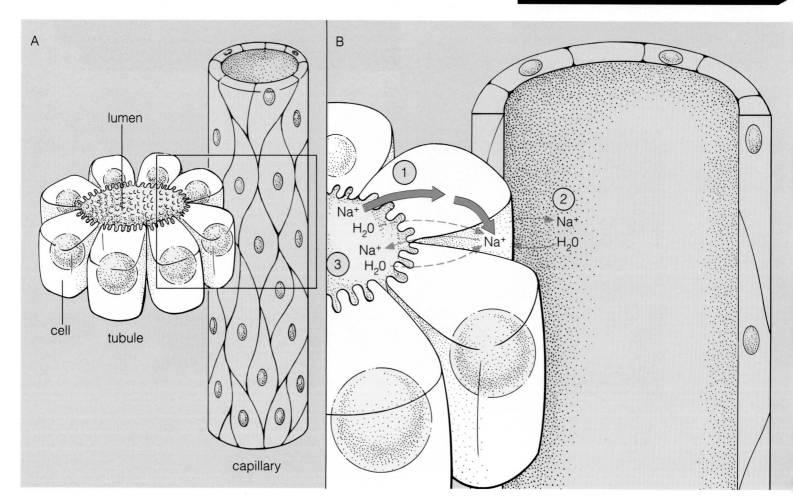

FIGURE 25.15 Mechanism of proximal tubular handling of sodium and water. **(A)** Anatomic relationship of proximal tubule and peritubular capillary. **(B)** Magnified view. (1) Sodium is actively transported by the tubular cell from lumen to paracellular space, (2) raising the concentration of sodium there. (3) Sodium backleaks from paracellular space to lumen (wavy arrow). The net proximal reabsorption of sodium, therefore, depends on balance between backleak and movement of sodium into capillary. Note that water moves passively, following sodium.

effective, the net glomerular filtration rate is not completely normalized, and nitrogenous wastes ultimately accumulate in the bloodstream. Azotemia resulting from reduced blood flow to an otherwise intact kidney is called *prerenal azotemia*. It can be caused by any of a number of pathophysiologic states (Fig. 25.14).

Autoregulation of glomerular filtration profoundly influences tubular reabsorption. Proximal reabsorption represents a balance between movement of sodium and water into the peritubular capillary versus backleak into the tubular lumen (Fig. 25.15). Normally, the net result of these two opposing processes is that about 80% of the filtrate is reabsorbed. When the efferent glomerular arteriole is constricted (Fig. 25.16), the resulting changes in the peritubular capillary Starling forces are more favorable to reabsorptive movement, and fractional proximal reabsorption may exceed 90%. Because less filtrate is delivered to the ascending limb of Henle's loop, where urinary dilution occurs, free water excretion is impaired. Other mechanisms promoting salt and water retention in the distal nephron, including antidiuretic hormone, aldosterone, and renal sympathetic neural activity, are activated in congestive heart failure as well. These mechanisms help preserve the integrity of the vascular compartment in hypovolemic patients. However, in patients with heart failure and various other edematous disorders, they contribute to a maladaptive expansion of the extracellular space, i.e., edema formation. Both hypovolemic and edematous patients with this "prerenal" pathophysiology are prone to hyponatremia because of their reduced ability to make and excrete free water.

REDUCED CARDIAC OUTPUT AND ACUTE TUBULAR NECROSIS

The high level of metabolic and transport activity in the renal parenchyma obligates a generous oxygen uptake. When a sustained reduction in blood flow to the kidneys exceeds their capacity to compensate by autoregulation, frank ischemic damage to the parenchyma is inevitable. Using isolated perfused kidney models, it has been elegantly demonstrated that the portions of the kidney most vulnerable to ischemic damage are the cells in the thick ascending limb of Henle's loop, particularly at the outer medullary zone.[4] These are cells normally engaged in a high rate of active transport. Ongoing ischemia gradually affects other portions of the nephron. Ischemic renal tubular damage is generally referred to as *acute tubular necrosis* (ATN), and is a clinically important disease.

One of the most mystifying aspects of ATN is that it is often associated with a degree of functional impairment totally disproportionate to the observed extent of the histopathologic abnormality. As a result of this discrepancy, the pathophysiology of renal failure in ATN remains a matter of debate. Vasomotor instability, intraluminal obstruction by sloughed cellular debris, and transepithelial backleak of filtered wastes into the circulation have all been espoused as explanations for this form of acute renal failure. Clinically, patients may or may not be oliguric; when present, oliguria bespeaks a longer course and a higher likelihood of needing interventional dialysis.

It is important to differentiate acute renal failure on a prerenal basis from that of ATN. The former requires treatment by volume resuscitation and/or hemodynamic interventions. Therapy of ATN is mainly supportive. The urine sediment and chemical composition often provide clues to aid in this differential process. Patients with ATN quite commonly have brown, granular casts (Fig. 25.17), thought to represent tubular cell debris, in the urinary sediment.

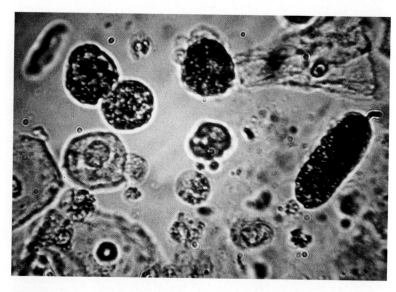

FIGURE 25.17   Urinary sediment from patient with acute tubular necrosis showing a brown granular cast and renal tubular epithelial cells.

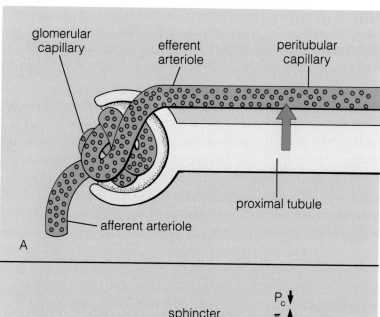

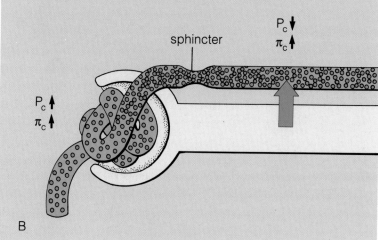

FIGURE 25.16   Effect of autoregulation of glomerular filtration on proximal reabsorption. **(A)** Normal balance of reabsorption and backleak. **(B)** In autoregulation, efferent arteriolar sphincter is constricted. This leads to alterations in the peritubular capillary Starling forces favoring reabsorption. (P_c = hydrostatic pressure; π_c = oncotic pressure)

These are generally not seen in uncomplicated prerenal azotemia. Patients with prerenal azotemia have a low urinary sodium concentration, reflecting the avid reabsorption of filtered sodium; the calculated fractional excretion of filtered sodium (FE_{Na}) is less than 1%. Patients with ATN, by virtue of the tubular injury, cannot avidly conserve sodium and will generally not show a low FE_{Na}.[16]

The cardiac patient is susceptible to ischemic ATN in the settings of cardiogenic shock, prolonged arrhythmia, and cardiac surgery. It has been observed anecdotally that ATN due to cardiogenic causes is rarer than that due to hypotension of other etiologies. This has prompted speculation on the existence of a protective "cardiorenal reflex" effected by atrial natriuretic peptide or other unknown humoral and neural factors. A more likely explanation is that survival associated with profound cardiogenic hypotension is too short to allow the full evolution of ATN.

Acute renal failure associated with nephrotoxins and radiocontrast agents is also included within the ATN classification, although these syndromes are probably distinct entities. The incidence of radiocontrast-induced acute renal failure following coronary angiography is low, but warrants vigilance.

EMBOLIC DISEASES AND THE KIDNEYS

Systemic thromboembolization from the heart occurs in several discrete clinical settings: following a transmural myocardial infarction; in infective endocarditis; in mitral stenosis; in dilated cardiomyopathy; and in paroxysmal atrial tachyarrhythmias. Infarction of renal parenchyma occurs when these emboli occlude the major renal arteries or their branches. Radiographically, vascular defects may be seen corresponding to the involved segments (Fig. 25.18). The most consistent laboratory finding is an elevation of the renal fraction of lactate dehydrogenase.[14] Azotemia is seen only if the embolic event causes massive bilateral loss of renal parenchyma.

Atheroembolic disease should be differentiated from major arterial thromboembolism. In this entity, showers of atheromatous microemboli from the aorta or its proximal branches lead to deposition of cholesterol crystals in small tissue vessels (Fig. 25.19). These showers occur in waves. Virtually any organ system may be involved, depending on the source of the atheroemboli. Atheroembolic disease of the kidneys usually produces a picture of subacute, progressive renal failure. Atheroemboli from the proximal aorta or coronaries may be deposited in the myocardial circulation. Cholesterol embolization usually arises following

surgical or angiographic manipulation of a plaque-ridden aorta, but may occasionally occur spontaneously. The prognosis depends on the duration of the atheroembolic process and the extent of target organ involvement.[20] There is no known treatment.

Systemic Diseases Affecting the Heart and Kidneys
DIABETES MELLITUS

Diabetes mellitus has become the leading cause of end-stage renal failure in the United States. Both the juvenile and adult-onset patterns are associated with nephropathy, the most characteristic of which is glomerulosclerosis. Virtually all patients with diabetic nephropathy have systemic hypertension and, in addition to microvascular disease, an enhanced tendency for atherosclerosis in larger vessels. Coronary artery disease and hypertensive heart disease are extremely common in patients with end-stage diabetic renal failure, contributing to their increased morbidity and reduced survival relative to other dialysis patients.

Diabetic atherosclerosis can effect the coronary circulation diffusely, and even involve small distal elements of the myocardial circulation, producing a congestive cardiomyopathy. The renal manifestations in such patients are similar to those of congestive heart failure occurring from other etiologies.

INFECTIVE ENDOCARDITIS

Glomerulonephritis is a well-known concomitant of bacterial endocarditis. The prevalence of glomerulonephritis among patients with endocarditis is not as high as it was in the earlier half of the century. The reasons for this decline in incidence are probably related to the changing nature of infective endocarditis. Since the development of glomerulonephritis is mediated by deposition of immune complexes, it is most likely to arise in the setting of prolonged antigenemia. A greater proportion of cases of infective endocarditis today represent the

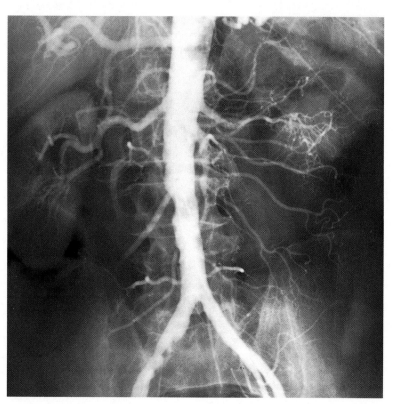

FIGURE 25.18 Angiogram of patient with left renal artery embolism. Note abrupt attenuation of contrast column (arrow) and absence of normal nephrogram on involved side.

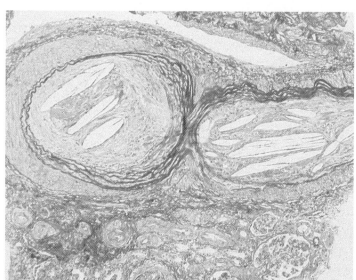

FIGURE 25.19 Cholesterol cleft in a renal arteriole from a patient with atheroembolic disease. (Reproduced with permission; see Figure Credits)

more virulent, or *acute*, form seen in parenteral drug abusers. The course of this illness often precludes the prolonged period of renal exposure to antigen-antibody complexes more typical of the indolent, or *subacute*, form. Furthermore, with more rapid recognition of the disease and the wide availability of antibiotic treatment, prolonged periods of immune complex exposure are less common. Immune complex glomerulonephritis of a diffuse or focal proliferative type may occur in patients with bacterial endocarditis. Additionally, endocarditis may cause septic embolization to the kidneys, with resultant infarction or cortical abscess formation.

AMYLOIDOSIS

Amyloidosis is a term applied to several disease states in which proteinaceous material is deposited in tissues throughout the body. The starchy-appearing material has a characteristic organized, fibrillar ultrastructure, although the constituent substances may vary among the amyloid types. Diffuse amyloid deposition is called *systemic amyloidosis*, and consists of two major types: (i) collections of immunoglobulin light chains (also called AL amyloid) in patients with plasma cell dyscrasias; and (ii) aggregated serum proteins or chronic phase reactants in patients with chronic inflammatory diseases. Other, rarer forms of amyloidosis are recognized, including some syndromes characterized by localized amyloid deposits.

The heart and kidneys may be affected by systemic amyloidosis. Cardiac deposition is most likely to occur in disorders marked by AL amyloid production, of which the two most important are primary amyloidosis and the amyloidosis associated with multiple myeloma.[7,8] Congestive cardiomyopathy results from myocardial infiltration with amyloid. In the kidneys, the disease is most likely to present with heavy proteinuria and progressive renal failure.

FABRY'S DISEASE

Few genetic or metabolic diseases cause significant morbidity of both the heart and kidneys. Fabry's disease, a hereditary cellular deficiency of the enzyme alpha-galactosidase A, is an exception. As a result of this deficiency, glycosphingolipids accumulate in numerous tissues. These are first manifest as cutaneous angiokeratomas; virtually all tissues of the body may become involved. Renal involvement begins with mild proteinuria and hematuria and may eventuate by midlife in renal failure. Renal histology reveals inclusions of lipid material in glomerular and tubular cells. The heart may also be involved in Fabry's disease; glycolipid deposition in the myocardium is not uncommon and an increased risk of coronary artery disease is observed.

Primary hyperoxaluria, or *oxalosis*, is a metabolic disorder characterized by overproduction of oxalic acid. Calcium oxalate deposits occur in many tissues; the kidney is particularly susceptible to this process, and renal failure early in life is common. Myocardial calcifications, occasionally severe enough to cause conduction abnormalities, are also reported.

AUTOIMMUNE AND VASCULITIC DISEASES

The systemic necrotizing vasculitides are a loosely related group of syndromes associated with widespread vascular inflammation. Those forms of vasculitis that mainly attack small vessels (e.g., Henoch-Schonlein purpura, hypersensitivity, cutaneous vasculitis) involve the kidneys much more often than the heart. Coronary and renal vasculitis may occur, however, in some of the other syndromes, albeit with differing frequencies.

The kidney is the most common site of involvement in *polyarteritis nodosa*. Hypertension is the predominant clinical manifestation of renal polyarteritis, presumably on a renovascular basis (Fig. 25.20). Coronary arteritis is seen in up to 70% of cases (Fig. 25.21), and may lead to myocardial infarction. Approximately 10% of patients have focal glomerulonephritis in association with polyarteritis. Glomerulonephritis is more common in the small vessel form of the disease, referred to as *microscopic polyarteritis*.

Renal lesions are frequent in *Wegener's granulomatosis* and include both classic necrotizing granulomatous arteritis, as well as aggressive glomerulitis. Pericarditis and arrhythmias have been reported with Wegener's granulomatosis, but are seen much less often than granulomatous manifestations in the renal and respiratory systems.

The recently described antineutrophil cytoplasmic antibodies (ANCA) are serologic markers frequently present in Wegener's granulomatosis, polyarteritis nodosa, and certain forms of idiopathic crescentic glomerulonephritis.[5] Their common expression in these disorders bespeaks an immunopathogenetic link. In addition, ANCA is of use in diagnosing and following the progress of these vasculitic syndromes, particularly Wegener's granulomatosis.

Takayasu's arteritis is a rare disease of the aorta and its major branches; the inflammatory process commonly involves all layers of the arterial wall. Loss of pulse transmission in these vessels may result, so the disease has acquired the sobriquet *pulseless disease*. Takayasu's disease can affect the heart in several ways; e.g., proximal aortitis may produce aortic insufficiency and thoracic aneurysms. Arteritis may also involve the major coronary arteries. Arteritis of the major renal vessels occurs less often, but, when present, may cause renovascular hypertension.

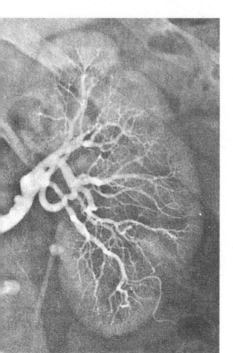

FIGURE 25.20
Angiogram of kidney of patient with polyarteritis nodosa. Note aneurysms of major and intrarenal renal arteries. (Reproduced with permission; see Figure Credits)

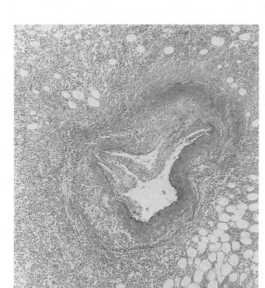

FIGURE 25.21
Polyarteritis involving a coronary artery. (Elastin stain). (Reproduced with permission; see Figure Credits)

Progressive systemic sclerosis (PSS) is a rheumatologic condition characterized by generalized vascular abnormalities and deposition of collagen in the skin and internal organs, including the viscera, lungs, heart, and kidneys. PSS is the most severe of a variety of related disorders sometimes referred to collectively as *scleroderma*; technically, this term should be reserved for the dermatologic changes seen with these syndromes. Although the histopathologic findings of PSS are less actively inflammatory than those of lupus erythematosus or the vasculitides, its distinctive immunoserologic abnormalities identify it as being autoimmune in nature.

The heart in PSS may become infiltrated with fibrotic tissue, leading, in advanced cases, to a restrictive cardiomyopathy (Fig. 25.22). Conduction abnormalities and arrhythmias commonly occur on a similar basis. Pulmonary hypertension results from fibrosis of the small pulmonary arteries, and may lead to right heart strain. The classic renal lesion in PSS is fibrosis and intimal hyperplasia of the distal intrarenal arteries (Fig. 25.23). The pathophysiology of scleroderma kidney disease is similar to that of renal artery stenosis. Patients may progress rapidly to malignant hypertension and renal failure, a situation often referred to as *scleroderma renal crisis*. Still a leading cause of death in PSS patients, renal crisis has been successfully reversed in reported cases with the aid of converting enzyme antagonists.[21]

Systemic lupus erythematosus (SLE) is the paradigm autoimmune disorder. With occasional exceptions, SLE is primarily a disease occurring in young women. The clinical observation that antibodies to native DNA are generally present in the serum of patients with active lupus, in levels correlating with disease activity, has provided the basis for a great deal of investigation and speculation regarding the pathogenesis of this disease. Nearly every organ system can be affected by SLE, including the heart and kidneys. In the days prior to steroid therapy, renal failure was the leading cause of death in patients with lupus. Most patients with SLE, with or without clinical evidence of renal disease, have demonstrable abnormalities of renal morphology at the electron microscopic level. Urinary abnormalities or frank renal dysfunction are present in at least 50% of adult patients.

Renal involvement in SLE is predominantly glomerular. Five basic histopathologic patterns are recognized by the World Health Organization, as listed in Figure 25.24.[1,2] The clinical manifestations of lupus may belie the degree of histopathologic abnormality. For example, diffuse proliferative glomerulonephritis has been reported in lupus patients with no clinical signs of renal disease. In general, however, the finding of a class IV lesion (Fig. 25.25) on renal biopsy identifies a patient at risk for chronic renal failure, and constitutes grounds for treatment. Pooled historical data indicate that steroids prolong survival in patients with lupus nephritis.[18] Since lupus nephritis is a disease marked by chronic flares and re-exacerbations, there is a rationale for combining steroids with cytotoxic agents, such as azathioprine or cyclophosphamide,[15] to minimize the long-term steroid exposure.

Three forms of cardiac disease have been described in association with SLE. Of these, sterile inflammatory pericarditis is the most familiar, occurring in up to 25% of patients. Lupoid serositis (i.e., pericarditis or pleuritis) constitutes one of the American Rheumatism Association's diagnostic criteria for SLE.

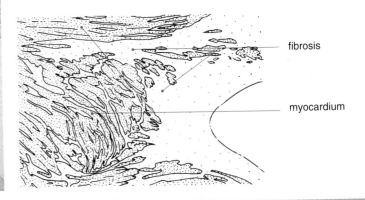

FIGURE 25.22   Histologic section of myocardial fibrosis in heart of a patient with progressive systemic sclerosis. (Reproduced with permission; see Figure Credits)

fibrosis

myocardium

FIGURE 25.24 WORLD HEALTH ORGANIZATION CLASSIFICATION OF LUPUS NEPHRITIS*

CLASS I:	Normal
CLASS II:	Mesangial lupus nephritis
CLASS III:	Focal proliferative nephritis
CLASS IV:	Diffuse proliferative nephritis
CLASS V:	Membranous lupus nephritis

***Classification system established by the World Health Organization.**

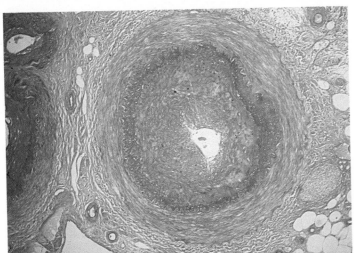

FIGURE 25.23   Histologic section of kidney from a patient with progressive systemic sclerosis showing marked intimal proliferation (PAS/Alcian blue stain). (Reproduced with permission; see Figure Credits)

Nonbacterial thrombotic endocarditis, or *Libman-Sacks endocarditis*, is quite common in patients with SLE[6] (Fig. 25.26), but is rarely of clinical significance. Myocarditis may also occur with active SLE,[3] but develops into cardiac failure in only the most aggressive cases. Lupus patients are at an increased risk for coronary artery disease, but this tendency is more likely to reflect the atherogenic effects of chronic steroid therapy and coexisting renal parenchymal hypertension, as opposed to direct involvement of the coronaries by lupus vasculitis; the latter, however, has been reported.[11]

HEMATOLOGIC DISORDERS

There are several common threads binding hematologic disease to the heart and kidneys. Anemia is the final common pathway of numerous hematologic diseases and can induce high-output cardiac failure (see Chapter 22). Hypercal-cemia associated with hematologic malignancies like lymphoma and myeloma may lead to polyuria and acute renal failure. Massive intravascular hemolysis, as occasionally seen in cold agglutinin disease, transfusion reaction, or severe microangiopathy, may produce hemoglobinuric acute renal failure.

The anemic disorder that affects the heart and kidneys in the most striking fashion is probably *sickle cell disease*. This is a common, hereditary disturbance of hemoglobin synthesis. The erythrocytes of patients homozygous for the sickle cell gene have a high content of hemoglobin S, which predisposes the erythrocytes to deform spontaneously in response to physical and chemical stimuli, notably hypoxemia. Hypertonic dehydration may also lower the threshold for this transformation. The deformed, or sickled, cells tend to become entrapped in small blood vessels, causing a variety of vaso-occlusive morbidities. The spleen, bone, and skin, among others, are sites of recurring focal infarcts and ischemic events.

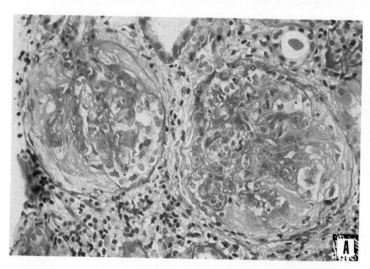

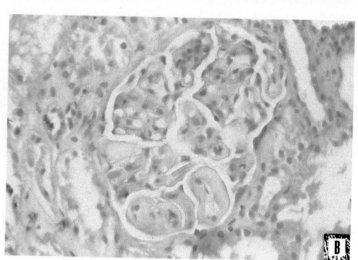

FIGURE 25.25   Diffuse proliferative lupus nephritis. **(A)** Glomeruli show early crescent formation and segmental areas of sclerosis. (PAS stain) **(B)** Note the thickened "wire loop" appearance of the capillary loops, corresponding to areas of the glomerular basement membrane heavily involved with immunodeposition (H&E stain). (Reproduced with permission; see Figure Credits)

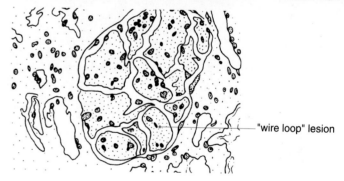

"wire loop" lesion

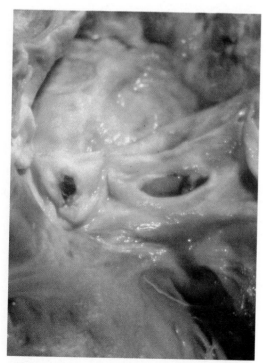

FIGURE 25.26   Libman-Sacks endocarditis. The holes in the cusps of this aortic valve represent areas of previous inflammation. (Reproduced with permission; see Figure Credits)

The kidneys are commonly affected by sickle cell disease. The low oxygen tension and high ambient tonicity of the renal medulla are conducive to sickling. The ongoing occlusion of the vasa recta leads to their rarefication (Fig. 25.27), and progressive fibrosis of the medulla. In advanced cases, papillary necrosis may result. The functional consequences of these changes typify those of a tubulointerstitial nephropathy; tubular functions, such as potassium secretion, urinary acidification, and urinary concentration, are impaired.

Sickling in the distal branches of the coronary arteries can cause repeated small myocardial infarctions. Other cardiac manifestations of the disease include flow murmurs and high-output failure.

THROMBOTIC THROMBOCYTOPENIC PURPURA

Thrombotic thrombocytopenic purpura (TTP) is a syndrome characterized by generalized thrombotic microangiopathy and platelet consumption. The classic triad of fever, neurologic abnormalities, and thrombocytopenic purpura characterize the presentation of most cases. Microangiopathic hemolytic anemia is invariably present. In some instances, acute renal failure may be seen; these cases are often referred to as the *hemolytic–uremic syndrome* (HUS).

Microthrombosis can be observed in virtually any organ that is affected by TTP/HUS, including the heart (Fig. 25.28).[19] Large infarctions of the myocardium are generally not seen, although focal areas of hemorrhage and necrosis, corresponding to microvascular thromboses, do occur. Involvement of the conduction system may produce arrhythmias and conduction disturbances.

The pathogenesis of TTP remains unclear. Evidence of several distinct abnormalities has been found in these patients, including a circulating plasma factor that causes platelet agglutination and aberrant endothelial production of Von Willebrand factor and prostacyclin. A number of therapeutic approaches have been employed, of which the most promising currently include infusion of fresh frozen plasma or exogenous prostacyclin.

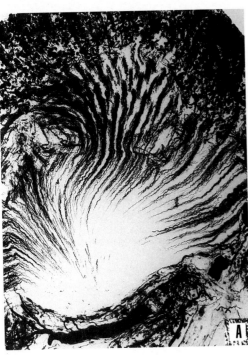
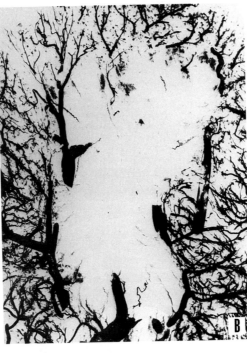

FIGURE 25.27 **(A)** Postmortem microangiogram of a normal kidney. The vasa recta are easily seen. **(B)** Microangiogram of kidney in patient with sickle cell disease. Note near absence of vasa recta vessels. (Reproduced with permission; see Figure Credits)

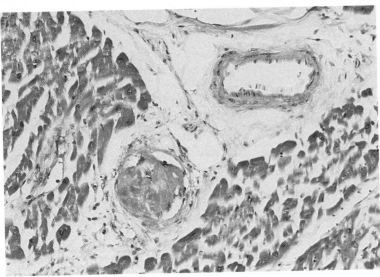

FIGURE 25.28 Heart from patient with thrombotic thrombocytopenic purpura. A thrombosed vessel is seen surrounded by a focus of necrotic myocardium. (Reproduced with permission; see Figure Credits)

FIGURE CREDITS

Figs. 25.1, 25.2, 25.9, 25.11, 25.13, 25.19, 25.20, 25.23, 25.25 from Williams JD, et al: Clinical Atlas of the Kidney. Gower, New York, 1991. Figure 25.2 has been redrawn.

Fig. 25.5 redrawn from Lang RM, et al: Left ventricular contractility varies directly with blood ionized calcium. Ann Intern Med 108:524, 1988.

Figs. 25.7, 25.28 courtesy of Henri Cuenoud, MD.

Fig. 25.8 Modified and redrawn from Kaysen GA, et al: Albumin synthesis, albuminuria and hyperlipidemia in nephrotic patients. Kid Int 31:1368, 1987.

Figs. 25.10A, B, 25.21, 25.22, 25.26 from Hurst JW (ed): Atlas of the Heart. Gower, New York, 1988. Fig. 25.10A redrawn from Hurst JW, Woodson GC: Atlas of Spatial Vector Electrocardiography. The Blakiston Company, New York, 1952.

Fig. 25.12 from Leier CV, et al: Cardiovascular abnormalities associated with adult polycystic kidney disease. Ann Intern Med 100:683, 1984.

Fig. 25.27 from Statius van Eps LWS, et al: Nature of concentrating defect in sickle-cell nephropathy. Lancet 1:450, 1970.

REFERENCES

1. Baldwin DS: Clinical usefulness of the morphological classification of lupus nephritis. In Hayslett JP, Hardin JA (eds): Advances in Systemic Lupus Erythematosus. Grune & Stratton, New York, 1983.
2. Balow JE, Austin HA, Tsokos GC, et al: Lupus nephritis. Ann Intern Med 106:79, 1987.
3. Borenstein DG, Fye WB, Arnett FC, et al: The myocarditis of systemic lupus erythematosus. Ann Intern Med 89:619, 1978.
4. Brezis M, Rosen S, Silva P, et al: Renal ischemia: A new perspective. Kid Int 26:375, 1984.
5. Falk RJ, Hogan S, Carey TS: Clinical course of anti-neutrophil cytoplasmic autoantibody-associated glomerulonephritis and systemic vasculitis. Ann Intern Med 113:656, 1990.
6. Galve E, Candell-Riera J, Pigrau C, et al: Prevalence, morphologic types, and evolution of cardiac valvular disease in systemic lupus erythematosus. N Engl J Med 319:817, 1988.
7. Glenner GG: Amyloid deposits and amyloidosis. The b-fibrilloses (Part I). N Engl J Med 302:1283, 1980.
8. Glenner GG: Amyloid deposits and amyloidosis. The b-fibrilloses (Part II). N Engl J Med 302:1333, 1980.
9. Kannel WB: Some lessons in cardiovascular epidemiology from Framingham. Am J Cardiol 37:269, 1976.
10. Kaysen GA, Gambertoglio J, Felts J, et al: Albumin synthesis, albuminuria and hyperlipidemia in nephrotic patients. Kid Int 31:1368, 1987.
11. Korbut SM, Schwartz MM, Lewis EJ: Immune complex deposition and coronary vasculitis in systemic lupus erythematosus. Am J Med 77:141, 1984.
12. Lang RM, Fellner SK, Neumann A, et al: Left ventricular contractility varies directly with blood ionized calcium. Ann Intern Med 108:524, 1988.
13. Leier CV, Baker PB, Kilman JW, et al: Cardiovascular abnormalities associated with adult polycystic kidney disease. Ann Intern Med 100:683, 1984.
14. Lessman RK, Johnson SF, Coburn JW, et al: Renal artery embolism. Clinical and long-term follow-up of 17 cases. Ann Intern Med 89:477, 1978.
15. McCune WJ, Golbus J, Zeldes W, et al: Clinical and immunologic effects of monthly administration of intravenous cyclophosphamide in severe systemic lupus erythematosus. N Engl J M.ed 318:1425, 1988.
16. Miller TR, Anderson RJ, Linas SL, et al: Urinary diagnostic indices in acute renal failure. Ann Intern Med 89:47, 1978.
17. O'Connor LR, Wheeler WS, Bethune JE: Effect of hypophosphatemia on myocardial performance in man. N Engl J Med 297:901, 1977.
18. Pollak VE, Dosekun AK: Evaluation of treatment in lupus nephritis: Effects of prednisone. In Hayslett JP, Hardin JA (eds): Advances in Systemic Lupus Erythematosus. Grune & Stratton, New York 1983.
19. Ridolfi RL, Hutchins GM, Bell WR: The heart and cardiac conduction system in thrombotic thrombocytopenic purpura. Ann Intern Med 91:357, 1979.
20. Smith MC, Ghose MK, Henry AR: The clinical spectrum of renal cholesterol embolization. Am J Med 71:174, 1981.
21. Steen VD, Costantino JP, Shapiro AP, et al: Outcome of renal crisis in systemic sclerosis: Relation to availability of angiotensin converting enzyme (ACE) inhibitors. Ann Intern Med 113:352, 1990.

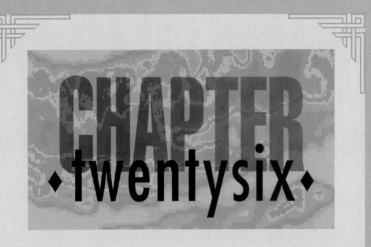

CHAPTER twentysix

PREGNANCY AND THE HEART

BRAD S. BURLEW, MD

HOWARD R. HORN, MD

JAY M. SULLIVAN, MD

Pregnancy, with its associated cardiovascular effects, places significant hemodynamic stresses on the woman with cardiac disease. The risk of cardiac complications from these stresses ranges from negligible (as in patients with mitral valve prolapse) to a prohibitively high likelihood of maternal death (as in patients with Eisenmenger's physiology). Successful management of the pregnant cardiac patient therefore depends on an understanding of the normal hemodynamic changes associated with the gravid state, on the recognition of cardiac disease in the pregnant woman, and on an understanding of the likely response of the patient's specific disorder to these hemodynamic changes.

Fortunately, the prevalence of heart disease is low in the reproductive female population, ranging between 0.4% and 4.1%.[2,3,17] Worldwide, rheumatic heart disease accounts for up to 90% of the cardiac disorders seen in pregnant women. Of these, mitral stenosis is the most common lesion, occurring in approximately 90% of women with rheumatic heart disease. In the United States, Canada, and western Europe, rheumatic heart disease now accounts for a diminishing portion (approximately 45% to 75%) of all heart disease.[2] Congenital heart disease accounts for much of the remainder, with surgically corrected congenital heart disease and patients with prosthetic valves forming a relatively new category of heart disorders among pregnant women.

After conception, a series of hematologic changes occur that are presumably hormonally mediated (Fig. 26.1). Within the first trimester of pregnancy, maternal total blood volume begins to increase, reaching maximal values of 50% above baseline (nongravid) values. The plasma volume increases relatively more than the red cell mass, which increases by only 10%. This results in a relative "hemodilution," accounting for the "physiologic anemia of pregnancy."[3]

Physiology of Pregnancy and Parturition

The resting cardiac output increases early in pregnancy as well (Fig. 26.2). The increased cardiac output is initially mediated through an increased stroke volume. As the pregnancy progresses, however, the stroke volume returns toward the normal range while the heart rate progressively rises. Early investigators demonstrated an apparent plateau in cardiac output during the final trimester, although it was eventually recognized that cardiac output is position dependent. The gravid uterus is currently believed to compress the inferior vena cava in the recumbent position, thereby reducing venous return and cardiac output (Fig. 26.3). With patients hemodynamically evaluated in the lateral decubitus position, which prevents caval obstruction, a continuing rise in the cardiac output is observed until term. In either event, the magnitude of this rise is on the order of 40% to 50% above the nongravid state.[15] Some contemporary studies suggest a slight decline in resting cardiac output just prior to term.[3,11,15]

The regional perfusion of various vascular beds within the body also changes during pregnancy (Fig. 26.4). An approximate tenfold increase of blood flow to the uterus is observed during the third trimester. The breasts often visibly

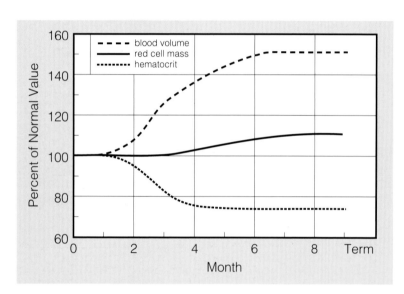

FIGURE 26.1   Hematologic effects of pregnancy.

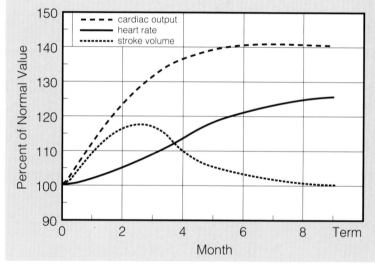

FIGURE 26.2   Hemodynamic effects of pregnancy.

FIGURE 26.3   Effect of gravid uterus on inferior vena cava pressure (uterus lifted between arrows). (Reproduced with permission; see Figure Credits)

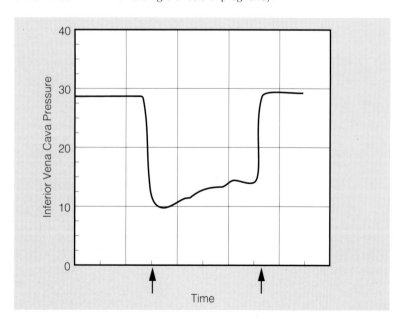

THE HEART AND OTHER CONDITIONS

enlarge with auscultatory souffles frequently heard, possibly secondary to increased blood flow. There are, however, no studies currently available documenting increased blood flow to the human breast at term. The perfusion of the kidneys is also increased by approximately 30%. Blood flow to the hands is also known to increase. The overall effect of these changes of regional perfusion is a reduction in the peripheral vascular resistance at term as compared to the nongravid state.[11] The arterial blood pressure is maintained without significant change throughout pregnancy. In view of the known elevations in cardiac output, this suggests that the degree of reduction of the systemic vascular resistance is significant.

With the onset of parturition, marked variations in hemodynamic function occur (Fig. 26.5). During the first stage of labor, the cardiac output increases an additional 25%; during the second stage, an additional 50%. At vaginal delivery with local anesthesia, cardiac output can increase as much as 80%.[19]

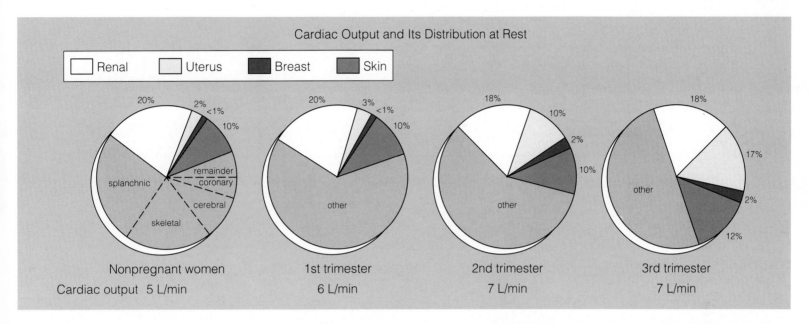

FIGURE 26.4   The increase in cardiac output during pregnancy is associated with a redistribution of blood flow. This results in an approximate ten-fold increase in uterine blood flow and a 1.5- to 2-fold increase in renal blood flow. There are few available data regarding the distribution of flow to the other systems of the body during pregnancy. (Reproduced with permission; see Figure Credits)

FIGURE 26.5   Effects of parturition (uterine contractions at arrows).

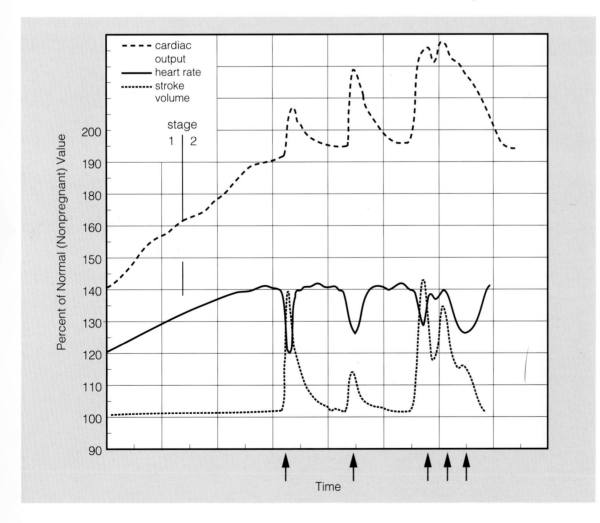

During each uterine contraction there is an expression of 300 to 500 mL of blood from the uterus to the central circulation. This is associated with an increase in both cardiac output (up to 24%) and stroke volume (up to 33%), in spite of frequently observed reflex bradycardia.[9,11] During uterine contraction there is often complete occlusion of the distal aorta as well, accounting for an increase in systemic vascular resistance.[20] Interestingly, cesarean section without labor is in itself associated with additional increases in cardiac output of up to 50% and increases in arterial blood pressure and central venous pressure.

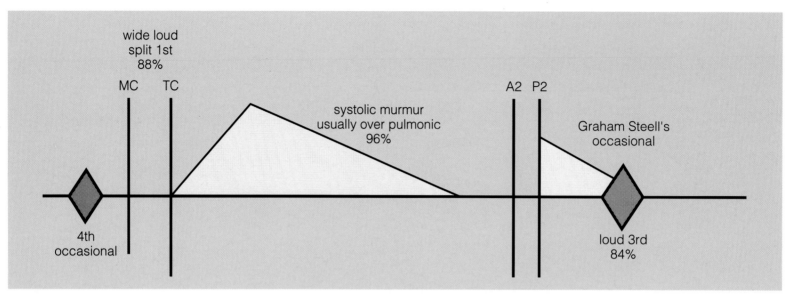

FIGURE 26.6   Auscultatory findings during pregnancy. (Reproduced with permission; see Figure Credits)

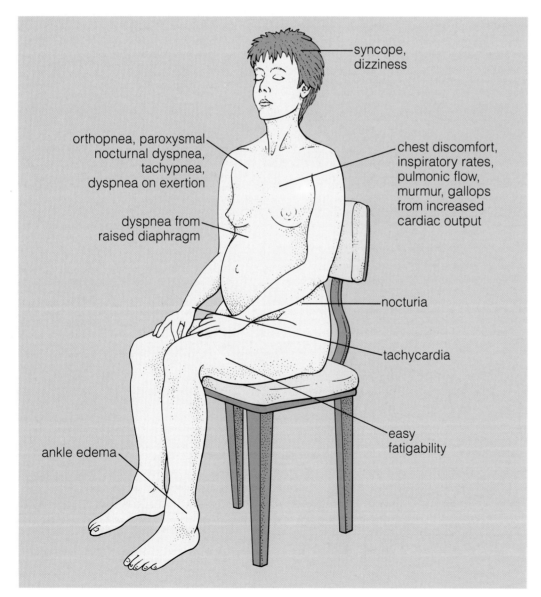

FIGURE 26.7   Signs and symptoms mimicking heart disease in pregnancy.

After parturition, the cardiac output often remains higher than values seen before parturition, presumably due to enhanced venous return, returning to pregravid values over the course of weeks. This is probably a reflection of the hormonal rather than mechanical nature of the hemodynamic changes of pregnancy.

Signs and Symptoms Associated with Pregnancy

The combined stresses of pregnancy and parturition can substantially challenge even a normal cardiovascular system. As mentioned, there are variations in cardiac output, stroke volume, regional perfusion patterns, and, as the uterus enlarges, venous return to the central circulation. These changes are associated with the development of symptoms and signs that may mimic heart disease. For example, exertional dyspnea occurs in over half of pregnant women. Orthopnea, paroxysmal nocturnal dyspnea, dizziness, and easy fatigability are quite common. Frank syncope may occur in the normal gravid woman. Patients may also experience chest discomfort mimicking angina pectoris.

On physical examination (Figs. 26.6, 26.7), normal patients may have prominent neck veins, inspiratory rales, S3 gallops, cardiomegaly, and peripheral edema. Murmurs, particularly systolic flow murmurs of up to 2 out of 6 intensity, are often heard. Although diastolic murmurs are unusual in pregnancy, a diastolic murmur over the pulmonic area similar to the Graham Steell's murmur is sometimes heard. This is felt to be related to a physiologic dilatation of the pulmonary artery and vanishes soon after delivery.[3] A diastolic flow murmur arising from the tricuspid valve is occasionally heard, likewise disappearing after delivery. Venous sounds such as venous hums and mammary souffles can also be heard.

Cardiac Conditions in Pregnancy
ACQUIRED VALVULAR HEART DISEASE

Worldwide, mitral stenosis probably represents the most frequently observed acquired valvular lesion in the reproductive female. It also poses one of the most substantial risks to the survival of the gravid female and the fetus. Depending on the degree of mitral valve stenosis, a pressure gradient will develop across the valve, resulting in elevated pressures in the left atrium and the pulmonary veins. Factors that will increase the left atrial pressure are those which will increase the diastolic mitral valvular flow rate through an increase in cardiac output or an increase in heart rate (which diminishes the duration of diastole, increasing the diastolic transvalvular gradient) (Fig. 26.8).

FIGURE 26.8   Pregnancy and mitral stenosis.

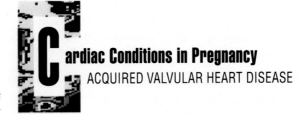

need for increased cardiac output to meet demands of growing fetus

increased atrial pressure and need for atrial contraction; vulnerabilities to atrial fibrillation

increased mitral valve pressure gradient

increased pressure

increased pressure with right ventricular lift

diminished diastolic filling

Recalling the normal physiologic increases in cardiac output and stroke volume during pregnancy and delivery, we can anticipate that the left atrial pressures will tend to be more severely elevated in the gravid state as the diastolic flow across the stenotic mitral valve increases. The elevation of left atrial pressure, if sufficient, can result in pulmonary interstitial edema and hypoxemia. Clinically, patients develop dyspnea, tachypnea, orthopnea, and paroxysmal nocturnal dyspnea, which can be difficult to differentiate from symptoms experienced by the normal gravid female. Frank pulmonary edema and hemoptysis can occur in patients in the third trimester and in the immediate postpartum period. Even patients who appear to be doing well can decompensate suddenly with the onset of atrial fibrillation or rapid atrial tachycardia. Symptomatic tachycardias must therefore be treated promptly, as pulmonary edema frequently ensues.

Infection and even mild hyperthyroidism also need to be treated promptly in this setting, as these disorders can similarly trigger tachycardia and subsequent pulmonary edema.

Aortic stenosis in pregnancy has not been as extensively studied as mitral stenosis. This is likely a reflection of the very low incidence of aortic stenosis in the reproductive female. Based on the data available, aortic stenosis appears to adversely affect pregnancy, with a 17% overall maternal mortality.[1] Patients with severe aortic stenosis are preload-dependent with a fixed stroke volume. Any increase in cardiac output is mediated through an increase in heart rate. Medications that decrease heart rate or preload should be avoided if possible. Vasodilators should also be avoided. If critical stenosis is diagnosed prior to pregnancy, surgical correction should be recommended.

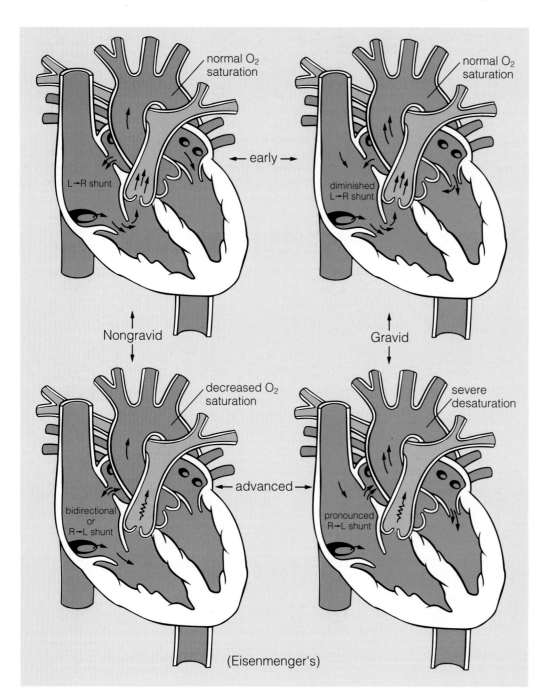

FIGURE 26.9   Early atrial septal defect and advanced (Eisenmenger's) atrial septal defect in the nongravid and gravid patient.

Mitral and aortic insufficiencies have diverse etiologies. Fortunately, valvular insufficiency is typically well tolerated in the gravid patient. The severity of valvular regurgitation may actually decrease during pregnancy because of the physiologic decrease in peripheral vascular resistance. Patients generally respond well to conservative therapy should they become symptomatic.

Mitral valve prolapse unassociated with other cardiovascular abnormalities does not increase maternal or fetal risk.[18] The use of prophylactic antibiotics in this setting remains controversial.

CONGENITAL HEART DISEASE

Atrial septal defect (ASD), particularly the secundum type, is the most common of congenital cardiac anomalies and is seen with relative frequency in the reproductive female population. Uncomplicated ASDs are almost predictably associated with uneventful pregnancies. Isolated ventricular septal defects (VSD) are also well-tolerated during pregnancy. However, when these lesions are associated with progressing pulmonary hypertension and intracardiac shunt reversal (Eisenmenger's syndrome), maternal and fetal mortality increase substantially. This is a consequence of the diminished systemic vascular resistance of pregnancy increasing the intracardiac right-to-left shunt (Figs. 26.9, 26.10). Eisenmenger's syndrome is associated with the highest maternal mortality rate, ranging from 36% to 56%, and a high infant mortality rate of up to about 40%. Maternal complications typically manifest as postpartum syncope and sudden death.[2] Therefore, pregnancy is strictly contraindicated in this setting, with sterilization being recommended by most authorities. When pregnancy occurs, therapeutic abortion is recommended.[10]

Unrepaired tetralogy of Fallot is also associated with increased mortality and morbidity of the mother. Again, the right-to-left shunt through the ventricular septal defect is exacerbated during pregnancy (Fig. 26.11). This relates to the increasing cardiac output and diminishing peripheral vascular resistance as pregnancy progresses. The increase in right-to-left shunt causes a fall in systemic

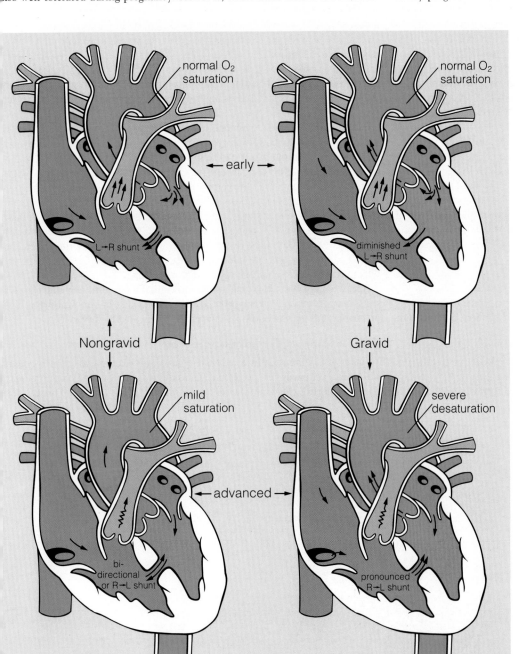

FIGURE 26.10 Early and advanced ventricular septal defect in the nongravid and gravid patient.

arterial oxygen saturation, with a subsequent rise in hematocrit and deepening cyanosis. This, in addition to increasing maternal morbidity, is associated with increased fetal wastage.[9]

There are suprisingly few available data on pulmonary valvular stenosis, a relatively common congenital defect. It appears to be well tolerated in pregnancy. Right ventricular failure is rare, particularly in previously asymptomatic individuals. No specific intervention is usually necessary.

Another congenital maternal anomaly, the patent arterial duct, is associated with aneurysmal dilatations of the circle of Willis. Complications arising from this association are uncommon, allowing for generally uneventful pregnancies.

Primary pulmonary hypertension is associated with high fetal and maternal mortalities. As a general rule, cardiac abnormalities associated with pulmonary hypertension, with or without right-to-left communication, are associated with a maternal mortality of approximately 50%.[18] Avoidance or interruption of pregnancy is indicated.

Other developmental abnormalities include Marfan's syndrome and hypertrophic cardiomyopathy. Marfan's syndrome, with its connective tissue abnormality, is associated with a high incidence of aneurysmal dilatation of the aortic root (Fig. 26.12). In this abnormality, dissection or rupture of the aortic root occurs in as many as 50% of affected pregnancies. Serial echocardiography has been recommended to monitor progression of dilatation or development of dissection of the aortic root. The risk of sudden death is felt to be proportional to the diameter of the aortic root.[14] Nonetheless, undetected dissections have occurred in spite of close echocardiographic monitoring.

Hypertrophic obstructive cardiomyopathy is usually associated with uneventful pregnancies. The outflow obstruction is dynamic and dependent on factors such as blood pressure and ventricular preload, both of which should be maintained if possible. During pregnancy, patients should be encouraged to preferably lie in the lateral decubitus position. This maneuver relieves inferior vena caval obstruction, thereby preserving ventricular preload. Because of the likelihood of marked worsening of the dynamic outflow obstruction, beta sympathomimetic tocolytic agents are strictly contraindicated in this disorder. Regional anesthesia with its risk of hypotension should also be avoided.[16]

PROSTHETIC CARDIAC VALVES

Hemodynamically, patients with prosthetic valves tend to fare quite well throughout pregnancy. However, the spontaneous abortion rate in patients with mechanical valve prostheses on anticoagulant therapy is approximately 50%. An additional concern in these patients relates to the teratogenesis associated with their warfarin therapy. Warfarin exposure at 6 to 9 weeks of gestation is reported to carry an 8% incidence of warfarin embryopathy[13] (Fig. 26.13). Although heparin does not cross the placenta, prolonged intravenous therapy is

associated with maternal complications—specifically, the development of heparin-induced osteopenia.

Bearing these issues in mind, widely followed recommendations for anticoagulation during pregnancy consist of the administration of intravenous heparin during the first trimester, followed by oral warfarin therapy during the second and third trimesters.[7] During the last weeks of pregnancy, intravenous heparin is again administered, as late exposure to warfarin is clearly associated with increased peripartum hemorrhage. Although this protocol was designed to minimize risk to the fetus and mother, the use of intravenous heparin does not appear to result in a significantly better outcome.[5] Because of this, pregnancy in patients requiring systemic anticoagulation is probably best avoided.

MYOCARDIAL INFARCTION

Ischemic heart disease due to coronary atherosclerosis in the face of pregnancy is fortunately quite uncommon. This low incidence is undoubtedly a reflection of the epidemiologic nature of ischemic heart disease in that reproductive females are at extremely low risk. Considering the current national trend toward bearing children later in life, myocardial infarction in the pregnant woman will likely be seen more frequently in the years to come. The present frequency of myocardial infarction in pregnancy is very low, with only 70 cases reported between 1922 and 1985.[6] The overall maternal mortality in this population was 35%. There does not appear to be any recent improvement in maternal mortality in this setting.

Current management recommendations include efforts to reduce cardiac workload, such as bedrest, parenteral nitrate therapy, and conduction anesthesia during delivery. In the past it had been recommended that oxytocin not be used in patients with ischemic heart disease. Currently, however, synthetic oxytocin that does not contain arginine vasopressin is available and, in appropriate doses, it is unlikely to increase coronary vasoconstriction. With intravenous bolus administration of 5 to 12 units, oxytocin does produce a 30% decrease in mean arterial pressure and a 50% increase in cardiac output in healthy patients undergoing tocolysis. These hemodynamic effects can be avoided by the administration of oxytocin as a dilute solution. Synthetic oxytocin has been used successfully in pregnant patients after myocardial infarction.

An extremely rare cause of maternal myocardial infarction is spontaneous dissection of a coronary artery (Fig. 26.14). This occurs in the ninth month of pregnancy and the early post partum period. There are few survivors.

PERIPARTUM CARDIOMYOPATHY

Peripartum cardiomyopathy is a disease of unknown etiology, which is associated with the development of congestive heart failure during the final month of pregnancy or during the 5 months following delivery (Fig. 26.15). This disorder

FIGURE 26.11   Unrepaired tetralogy of Fallot in the nongravid and gravid patient.

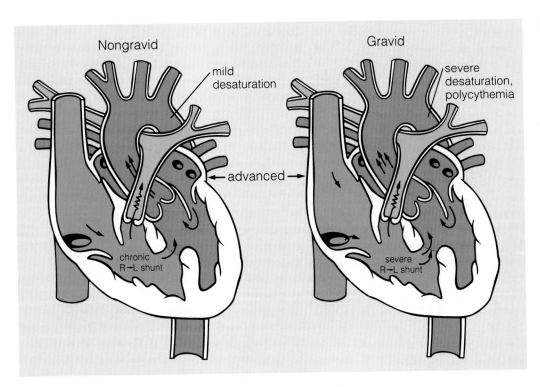

Nongravid

Gravid

mild desaturation

severe desaturation, polycythemia

←advanced→

chronic R→L shunt

severe R→L shunt

occurs initially in women who have not previously had heart disease and in whom other explanations for their congestive failure are not apparent. It occurs more commonly in the black population. Peripartum cardiomyopathy is more likely to occur in a woman who is (1) 30 years old or older, (2) pregnant with twins, (3) toxemic; also, it is more likely to occur in a third or subsequent pregnancy. If the patient has acquired peripartum cardiomyopathy during a previous pregnancy, it is likely to return in subsequent pregnancies, particularly if the patient had persistent postpartum cardiomegaly. It has been suggested that hypertension, myocarditis, and dietary factors may play etiologic roles in the development of peripartum cardiomyopathy.[8,12]

With careful medical care and appropriate hemodynamic monitoring, most patients with cardiac disease can be safely carried through pregnancy and delivery.[21] On occasion, unfortunately, termination of the pregnancy is still indicated. Patients in whom termination should be considered include those with severe congestive failure in early pregnancy, as continuation of the pregnancy is likely to result in an unacceptable outcome for both the mother and the fetus. Similarly, patients with Eisenmenger's syndrome, primary or secondary pulmonary hypertension, and cyanotic congenital heart disease should also be considered for therapeutic abortion. As discussed, these clinical conditions can be associated with maternal mortalities in excess of 50%. Termination of the pregnancy in the first or second trimester presents a more favorable outcome for the survival of the patient.[4]

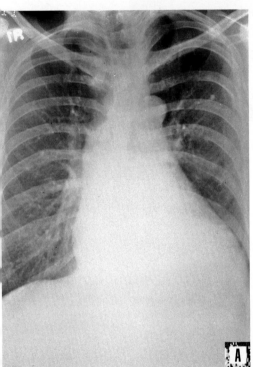

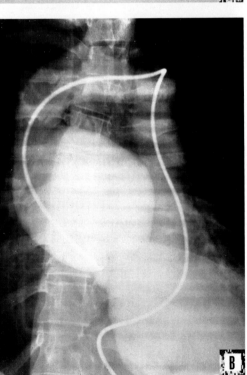

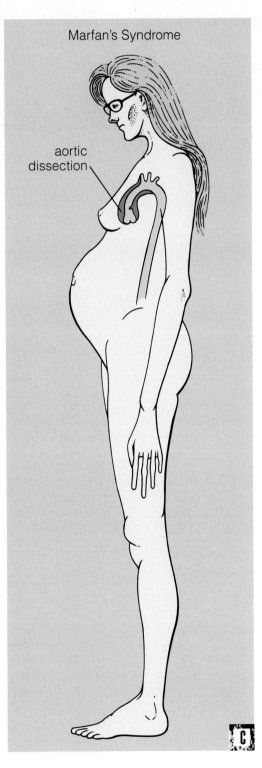

FIGURE 26.12   Pregnancy and Marfan's syndrome.

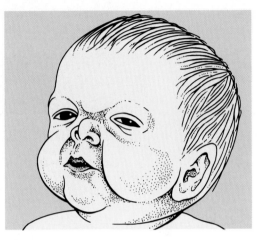

FIGURE 26.13   Effects of warfarin intake on the fetus as seen in the newborn. Note the hypoplastic nose with low nasal bridge and broad, flat face. (Reproduced with permission; see Figure Credits)

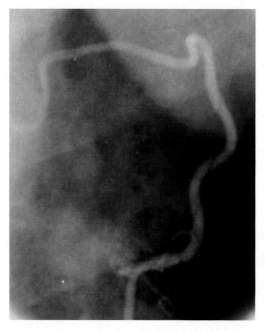

FIGURE 26.14   Spontaneous dissection of the right coronary artery in a 38 year old female. Extensive intimal flap is seen in vessel from proximal portion to just before the origin of the posterior descending artery. (Reproduced with permission; see Figure Credits)

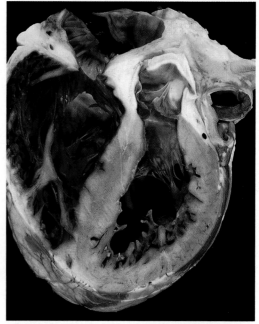

FIGURE 26.15   Biventricular chamber dilation with wall hypertrophy in dilated congestive cardiomyopathy. (Reproduced with permission; see Figure Credits)

FIGURE CREDITS

Fig. 26.3 from Kerr MG: The mechanical effects of the gravid uterus in late pregnancy. J Obstet Gynaecol Br Comm 72:513, 1986.

Fig. 26.4 from McAnulty JH, Metcalfe J, Ueland K: Pregnancy in the cardiac patient. In Chatterjee K, et al (eds): Cardiology: An Illustrated Text–Reference. Gower, New York, 1992.

Fig. 26.6 modified from Cutforth R, MacDonald CB: Heart sounds and murmurs during pregnancy. Am Heart J 71:742–747, 1966.

Fig. 26.13 redrawn from Shaul WL, Emery H, Hall JG: Am J Dis Child 129:360, 1975.

Fig. 26.14 courtesy of Paul Gerlach, MD, Memphis, TN.

Fig. 26.15 from Hurst JW: Atlas of the Heart. Gower, New York 1988.

REFERENCES

1. Arias F, Pineda J: Aortic stenosis and pregnancy. J Reproduct Med 20:229, 1978.

2. Burlew BS: Managing the pregnant patient with heart disease. Clin Cardiol 13:757, 1990.

3. Conradsson T, Werkö L: Management of heart disease in pregnancy. Prog Cardiovasc Dis 16:407, 1974.

4. Elkayam U, Gleicher N: Cardiac problems in pregnancy. JAMA 251: 2838, 1984.

5. Hall JG, Pauli RM, Wilson KM: Maternal and fetal sequelae of anticoagulation during pregnancy. Am J Med 68:122, 1980.

6. Hankins GDV, Wendel GD, Leveno KJ, et al: Myocardial infarction during pregnancy: A review. Obstet Gynecol 65:139, 1985.

7. Hirsch J, Cade JF, O'Sullivan EF: Clinical experience with anticoagulation therapy during pregnancy. Br Med J 1:270, 1970.

8. Homans D: Peripartum cardiomyopathy. N Engl J Med 312:1432, 1985.

9. Lang RM, Borow KM: Pregnancy and heart disease. Clin Perinatol 12:551, 1985.

10. Lieber S, Dewilde Ph, Huyghens L, et al: Eisenmenger's syndrome and pregnancy. Acta Cardiol 40:421, 1985.

11. Metcalf J, Ueland K: Maternal cardiovascular adjustment to pregnancy. Prog Cardiovasc Dis 16:363, 1974.

12. O'Connell JB, Costanzo-Nordin MR, Subramanian R, et al: Peripartum cardiomyopathy: Clinical, hemodynamic, histologic and prognostic characteristics. J Am Coll Cardiol 8:52, 1986.

13. Pauli RM, Hall JG, Wilson KM: Risks of anticoagulation during pregnancy. Am Heart J 100:761, 1980.

14. Pyeritz RE: Maternal and fetal complications of pregnancy in the Marfan syndrome. Am J Med 71:784, 1981.

15. Robson SC, Hunter S, Boys RJ, et al: Serial study of factors influencing changes in cardiac output during pregnancy. Am J Physiol 256:H1060, 1989.

16. Shah DM, Sunderji SG: Hypertrophic cardiomyopathy and pregnancy: Report of a maternal mortality and review of literature. Obstet Gynecol Surv 40:444, 1985.

17. Sullivan JM, Ramanathan KB: Management of medical problems in pregnancy—Severe cardiac disease. N Engl J Med 313:304, 1985.

18. Tang LCH, Chan SYW, Wong VCW, et al: Pregnancy in patients with mitral valve prolapse. Int J Gynaecol Obstet 23:217, 1985.

19. Ueland K, Hansen JM: Maternal cardiovascular dynamics III. Labor and delivery under local and caudal analgesia. Am J Obstet Gynecol 103:8, 1969.

20. Ueland K, Hansen JM: Maternal cardiovascular dynamics II. Posture and uterine contractions. Am J Obstet Gynecol 103:1, 1969.

21. Whittemore R, Hobbins JC, Engle MA: Pregnancy and its outcome on women with and without surgical treatment of congenital heart disease. Am J Cardiol 50:641, 1982.

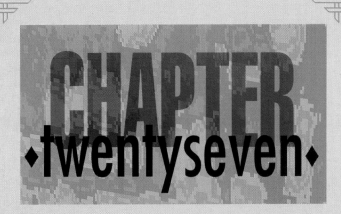

CHAPTER
◆twentyseven◆

COLLAGEN VASCULAR DISEASE AND THE HEART

J. WILLIS HURST, MD

BERNADINE P. HEALY, MD

J. O'NEAL HUMPHRIES, MD

ANTON E. BECKER, MD

JOSEPH S. ALPERT, MD

Collagen vascular diseases may affect the heart; the primary cardiac manifestations are listed in Figure 27.1. Also called connective tissue disorders, they include systemic lupus erythematosus, progressive systemic sclerosis (scleroderma), polyarteritis nodosa, ankylosing spondylitis, and rheumatoid arthritis. Although the etiology of these conditions is not known, most seem to be the result of an immunologic disorder.

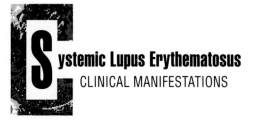

ystemic Lupus Erythematosus
CLINICAL MANIFESTATIONS

Systemic lupus erythematosus (SLE) occurs most often in women between the ages of 20 to 40 years. The symptoms and signs depend on the organ that is initially or predominately involved. Accordingly, the patient may have epilepsy, fever, arthritis, a characteristic skin rash (Fig. 27.2), pleurisy, pericarditis (frequently asymptomatic), myocarditis, or cardiac valve disease.

Pericarditis is a common manifestation of SLE, often being the presenting clinical problem. Cardiac tamponade and constrictive pericarditis occur rarely. Immunosuppressed patients are at greater risk for purulent pericarditis.

Endocarditis associated with SLE was described by Libman and Sacks before its relationship to lupus was appreciated. These sterile vegetations may be located on both sides of any of the four valve leaflets, but they are more commonly located on the undersurface of the mitral valve. While these sterile lesions are similar to marantic endocarditis, focal necrosis of the valve leaflets and mononuclear infiltrates may occur (Fig. 27.3). This type of endocarditis is more commonly observed at autopsy than during clinical examination. Healed stages of the lesions may lead to aortic or mitral regurgitation. The sterile lesions are subject to infection in the immunosuppressed patient.[5]

Myocarditis may occur rarely in patients with SLE. Heart failure, ventricular arrhythmias, and atrioventricular block also occur rarely.

The small coronary arteries may be involved in SLE. Fibrinoid necrosis with thromboembolism may occur, but myocardial necrosis and fibrosis are uncommon

FIGURE 27.1 PRIMARY CARDIAC MANIFESTATIONS OF COLLAGEN VASCULAR DISEASES*

DISEASE	PERICARDIUM	MYOCARDIUM	ENDOCARDIUM (VALVES)	CORONARY ARTERIES
Systemic lupus erythematosus	++	+	++	+/−
Progressive systemic sclerosis	+	++	o	++
Polyarteritis nodosa	+/−	+	o	++
Ankylosing spondylitis	o	+/−	++	o
Rheumatoid arthritis	++	+	+	o

*++, major site of involvement; +, may be involved, but less frequently; +/−, rarely involved; o, not involved. (Reproduced with permission; see Figure Credits)

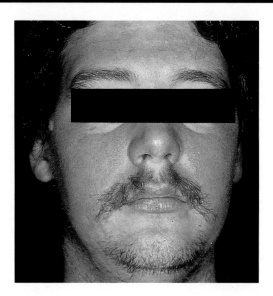

FIGURE 27.2   Face of a young man with SLE. The intense erythema of the cheeks and the forehead following exposure to the sun is evident. This type of rash is often seen with the subacute variant of lupus erythematosus but was part of the clinical picture of this patient who had SLE. (Reproduced with permission; see Figure Credits)

mon. James and colleagues[2] reported arteritis of the sinus node artery with scarring of the sinus and the atrioventricular nodes. These abnormalities may be responsible for the arrhythmias and the conduction disturbances that are seen on rare occasion in patients with SLE.

Hypertension is a common occurrence in patients with renal lupus; it may cause left ventricular hypertrophy and heart failure. Pericarditis related to uremia may develop.

LABORATORY ABNORMALITIES

Patients with lupus erythematosus exhibit LE cells, antinuclear antibodies, anticytoplasmic antibodies, and rheumatoid factor in their blood. Serum complement is decreased. Biopsy of the kidney may reveal the different stages of a membranoproliferative (mesangiocapillary) glomerulonephritis (Fig. 27.4); a skin biopsy may show a dense linear deposition of immunoglobulins along the epidermal–dermal junction (Fig. 27.5).

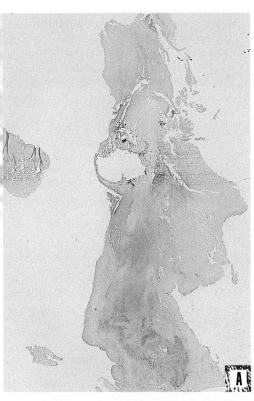
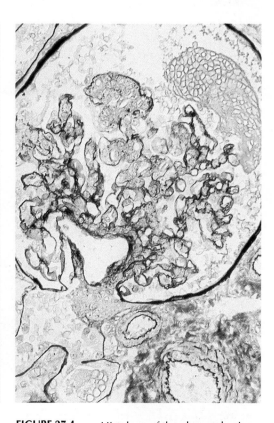

FIGURE 27.3 Histologic sections of an aortic valve resected from a patient with SLE (**A**, elastic tissue stain; **B**, H&E stain). There is evidence of necrosis of the valve tissue with a cellular infiltrate. Infective endocarditis is not present. (Reproduced with permission; see Figure Credits)

FIGURE 27.5 Histologic section of a skin biopsy revealing a dense line of immunoglobulin deposits along the epidermal junction with an immunoperoxidase technique (C1q). The so-called lupus line suggests the diagnosis of SLE. (Reproduced with permission; see Figure Credits)

FIGURE 27.4 Histology of the glomerulus in the acute stage of SLE. Extravasation of erythrocytes and early signs of a membranoproliferative (mesangiocapillary) glomerulonephritis are present (trichrome stain). (Reproduced with permission; see Figure Credits)

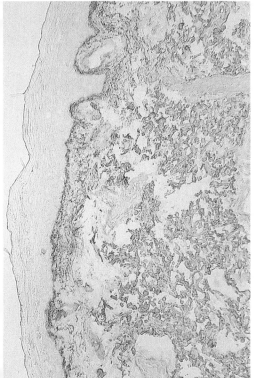

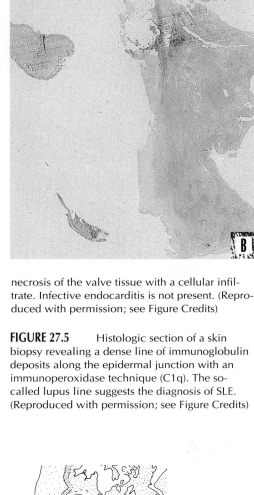

lupus band at dermal-epidermal junction

epidermis

dermis

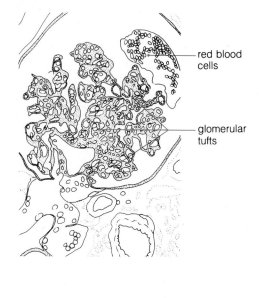

red blood cells

glomerular tufts

Progressive Systemic Sclerosis (Scleroderma)
CLINICAL MANIFESTATIONS

The vascular lesions of progressive systemic sclerosis produce fibrotic thickening of the skin, lesions of the fingertips and the fingers (Fig. 27.6), lesions of the esophagus, small bowel, large bowel, kidney, lung, and heart, and, usually, Raynaud's phenomenon. The CREST variant of scleroderma consists of calcinosis, Raynaud's phenomenon, esophageal abnormality, sclerodactyly, and telangiectasia.

Scleroderma can produce a multifaceted cardiac and cardiovascular picture (Fig. 27.7). Progressive systemic sclerosis is characterized by Raynaud's phenomena, fibroblast stimulation, small vessel disease, and extensive visceral involvement of the lungs, kidney, and heart. Cardiac involvement affects all layers of the heart. Pericarditis is seen in as many as 50% of patients with scleroderma. Usually only small pericardial effusions are present, but occasionally individuals develop tamponade. The effusion is nonspecific and does not contain mediators of immune response. A rare individual develops constrictive pericarditis. Myocardial fibrosis is common and occurs in a patchy distribution throughout both right and left ventricles. Myocardial fibrosis leads to heart failure, arrhythmias, and conduction defects. It has been suggested that myocardial fibrosis is the result of episodic epicardial coronary arterial vasospasm and/or small arterial obstruction.

Capillary devascularization has also been observed. Cold stimulation leads to reversible thallium-scan defects and regional wall motion abnormalities. Treatment with Nifedipine prevents these reversible abnormalities following cold stimulation. Hence, these changes are likely to be the result of cold-induced vasospasm.

Disease of small pulmonary arteries and aterioles leads to pulmonary hypertension, which can be severe. Pulmonary hypertension is only seen in the CREST variant of scleroderma. Individuals with marked pulmonary hypertension develop cor pulmonale, although this syndrome of scleroderma heart disease is uncommon. Involvement of renal vessels leads to renovascular hypertension, which can be severe and even malignant. Marked left ventricular dysfunction can result from the combination of myocardial fibrosis and severe systemic hypertension. Scleroderma is not associated with valvular abnormalities.

The smaller arteries and arterioles throughout the body appear to undergo spasm for unknown reasons; this may be responsible for target organ damage in the heart as well as in other tissues. Patients with myocardial involvement may develop congestive heart failure and dilated cardiomyopathy. Patients may have angina pectoris, myocardial infarction, and sudden death; they are often misdiagnosed as having coronary atherosclerosis. Patients may have cardiac arrhythmias and conduction disturbances.

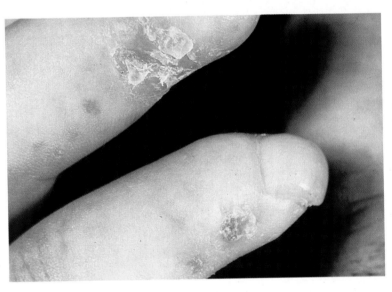

FIGURE 27.6   Fingers of a patient with the CREST variant of progressive systemic sclerosis (scleroderma). Note the sclerodactyly and distal digital scars. (Reproduced with permission; see Figure Credits)

FIGURE 27.7 CARDIAC MANIFESTATIONS OF PROGRESSIVE SYSTEMIC SCLEROSIS (PSS)—SCLERODERMA

Pericarditis/effusion

Abnormal vascular reactivity

Arteriolar and capillary abnormalities

Myocardial fibrosis

Arrhythmias and conduction disturbances

Pulmonary hypertension and cor pulmonale

Systemic hypertension and sequelae

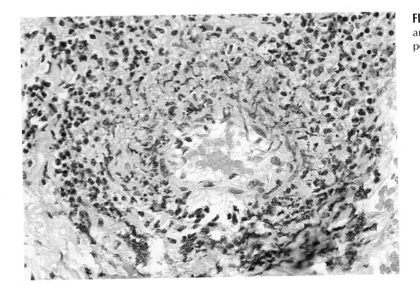

FIGURE 27.8   Histologic section of a skin biopsy from a patient with polyarteritis nodosa. There is a necrotizing arteritis (H&E stain). (Reproduced with permission; see Figure Credits)

Patients with renal disease due to progressive systemic sclerosis develop hypertension, left ventricular hypertrophy, and heart failure.

Pericarditis may be due to uremia. Patients with pulmonary disease due to progressive systemic sclerosis may develop cor pulmonale, right ventricular hypertrophy, and heart failure. Pulmonary arteriolar lesions may occur in the absence of pulmonary parenchymal disease. Lesions in the pulmonary arterioles may lead to a clinical syndrome that is similar to primary pulmonary hypertension. This is a serious form of the disease, and sudden death may occur.

Exercise tests disclose arrhythmias in approximately one third of patients; Holter monitoring discloses arrhythmias in approximately two thirds of patients compared with case controls. Conduction defects occur in approximately 15% to 20% of patients; first-degree atrioventricular block, left anterior hemiblock, and intraventricular conduction defect are the most common defects noted.

Approximately 50% of patients have normal ECGs; left ventricular hypertrophy is seen in 7% and right ventricular hypertrophy is noted in 7%.

LABORATORY ABNORMALITIES

Although the results of radiographic studies of the esophagus and the bowel may show abnormalities, biopsy of the skin and the kidney provides the most precise diagnosis.

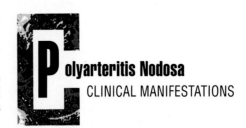

Polyarteritis Nodosa
CLINICAL MANIFESTATIONS

Polyarteritis nodosa is a necrotizing arteritis of the small and the medium-sized arteries that leads to occlusion of vessels and, hence, may produce infarcts in multiple organs. Accordingly the skin (Fig. 27.8), gastrointestinal tract, kidneys (Figs. 27.9, 27.10), brain, spleen, lymph nodes, musculoskeletal system, and heart may be involved.

The epicardial and the subepicardial coronary arteries may also be involved in polyarteritis nodosa. The inflammatory process extends through all arterial layers, leading to necrosis; inflammation is accompanied by thrombosis in the acute stage of the disease. Aneurysms of the coronary artery with thrombosis may appear in the healed stage. Myocardial infarction may occur. Since the disease has a tendency to affect multiple, smaller-sized coronary arteries, the ischemic myocardial changes may be focal in nature.[1]

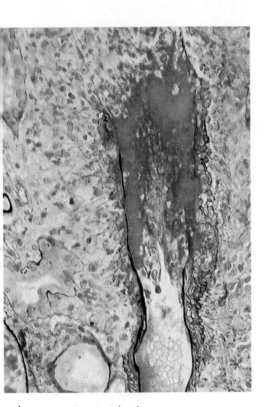

FIGURE 27.9
Histologic section showing fibrinoid necrosis of a small artery in the kidney in a patient with polyarteritis nodosa (trichrome stain). (Reproduced with permission; see Figure Credits)

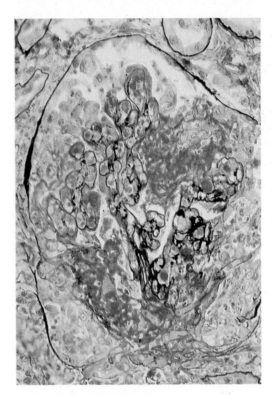

FIGURE 27.10
Extensive glomerular changes seen in histologic section of polyarteritis nodosa. These changes are characterized by an extracapillary proliferation with vasculitis of the tufts (trichrome stain). (Reproduced with permission; see Figure Credits)

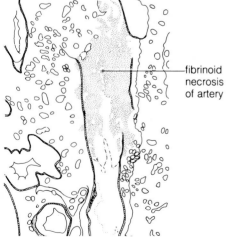

fibrinoid necrosis of artery

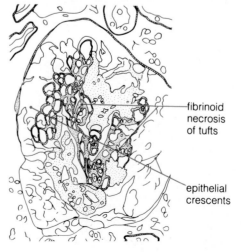

fibrinoid necrosis of tufts

epithelial crescents

Atrial arrhythmias and atrioventricular conduction defects occur when the arteries to the sinoatrial node and the atrioventricular node are involved.

Renal involvement with polyarteritis nodosa may result in hypertension, left ventricular hypertrophy, and heart failure. Kidney failure may produce uremia and pericarditis.

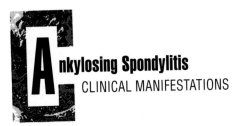

LABORATORY ABNORMALITIES

The sedimentation rate and the serum gamma globulin may be increased. Antinuclear antibodies and rheumatoid factor may be detected. The diagnosis is usually based on the clinical picture and biopsy.

Ankylosing Spondylitis
CLINICAL MANIFESTATIONS

Ankylosing spondylitis is due to inflammatory lesions of the spine, leading to chronic back pain, dorsal kyphosis, and fusion of the costovertebral and sacroili-ac joints. An inflammatory lesion may involve the aortic root, extending into the region below the aortic valve and the basal portion of the mitral valve. This process may cause aortic or mitral regurgitation and atrioventricular block (Fig. 27.11). The longer the duration of ankylosing spondylitis, the more likely that aortic regurgitation will develop.

Almost all patients with ankylosing spondylitis have HLA-B27 histocompatibility antigen. This suggests a genetic linkage; it also indicates a relationship to Reiter's syndrome and juvenile arthritis.

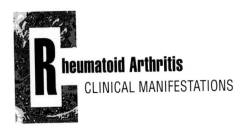

Rheumatoid Arthritis
CLINICAL MANIFESTATIONS

This common collagen vascular disease, characterized by synovial inflammation that destroys the joints, is more common in women; it may be familial. The patient has pain and deformity of the joints of the hands, wrists, and upper and lower extremities (Fig. 27.12). The temporomandibular and the sternoclavicular

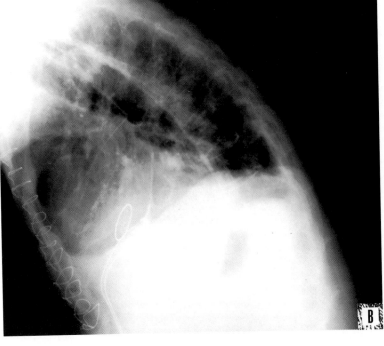

FIGURE 27.11 **(A)** Posteroanterior chest film of 70-year-old man with severe ankylosing spondylitis, aortic regurgitation, and complete heart block. The projection shows cardiac enlargement, the annular ring of the Hancock valve inserted in the aortic valve, and the electrodes of a cardiac pacemaker.

The large dense area at the upper portion of the film is the patient's head. **(B)** Left lateral view shows cardiac enlargement, the annular ring in the aortic valve position, and the electrodes of a cardiac pacemaker. (Reproduced with permission; see Figure Credits)

FIGURE 27.12 Hand of a patient with advanced rheumatoid arthritis. This appearance is typical of the deformity associated with this condition. (Reproduced with permission; see Figure Credits)

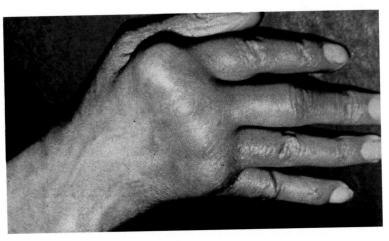

oints may also be involved. Patients may have fever, weight loss, rheumatoid nodules, iritis, rheumatoid lung disease, lymphadenopathy, pericarditis, pleurisy, heart disease, and arteritis.

Pericarditis and pericardial effusion may occur; cardiac tamponade and constrictive pericarditis are infrequent complications. Rheumatoid lung disease may occur, and rheumatic arteritis may produce disease of the gastrointestinal tract.

On rare occasion rheumatoid nodules may occur within the myocardium and heart valves (Figs. 27.13, 27.14). These lesions may produce sufficient myocardial damage and valvular insufficiency to produce heart failure, cardiac arrhythmias, and conduction defects. Amyloid involvement of the heart may also occur. In patients with rheumatoid myocardial involvement, elevated levels of rheumatoid factor are usually present in the blood.[4]

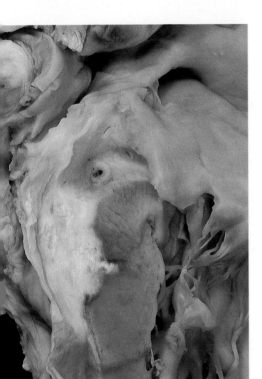

FIGURE 27.13
Rheumatoid nodule located in the back of the heart, partially within the epicardium and partially within the mural myocardial wall. (Reproduced with permission; see Figure Credits)

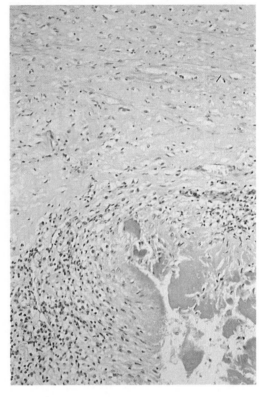

FIGURE 27.14
Histologic section of a rheumatoid nodule in the heart. There is fibrinoid necrosis with a histiocytoid cellular reaction and peripheral fibrosis (H&E stain). (Reproduced with permission; see Figure Credits)

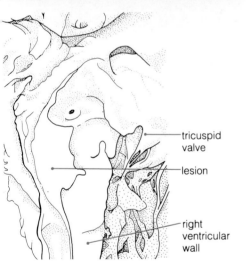

tricuspid valve

lesion

right ventricular wall

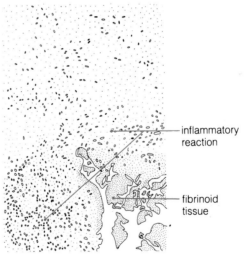

inflammatory reaction

fibrinoid tissue

ACKNOWLEDGMENT

This chapter is based in part on Bulkley BH, Humphries JO: The heart and collagen vascular disease. In Hurst JW (ed): The Heart, 6th ed. McGraw-Hill, New York, 1986.

FIGURE CREDITS

Fig. 27.1 from Hurst JW: The Heart, 6th ed. McGraw-Hill, New York, 1986.
Figs. 27.2, 27.6, 27.3–27.5, 27.8–27.14 from Hurst JW (ed): Atlas of the Heart. Gower, New York, 1988.
Figs. 27.2, 27.6 courtesy of Mark Holzberg, MD, Atlanta, GA.
Fig. 27.11 courtesy of William J. Casarella, MD, Atlanta, GA.
Fig.27.12 courtesy of William P. Maier, MD, Atlanta, GA.

REFERENCES

1. James TN, Birk RE: Pathology of the cardiac conduction system in polyarteritis nodosa. Arch Intern Med 117:561, 1966.
2. James TN, Rupe CE, Monto RW: Pathology of the cardiac conduction system in systemic lupus erythematosus. Ann Intern Med 63:402, 1965.
3. Libman E, Sacks B: A hitherto undescribed form of valvular and mural endocarditis. Arch Intern Med 33:701, 1924.
4. Liss JP, Bachmann WT: Rheumatoid constrictive pericarditis treated by pericardiectomy: Report of a case and review of the literature. Arthritis Rheumatism 13:869, 1970.
5. Paget SA, Bulkley BH, Grauer LE, et al: Mitral valve disease of systemic lupus erythematosus: A cause of severe congestive heart failure reversed by valve replacement. Am J Med 59:134, 1975.

INDEX*

---

* Page numbers in boldface refer to those pages on which a figure appears.